Textbook of Pediatric Allergy

Carlo Caffarelli • Gian Luigi Marseglia
Editors

Textbook of Pediatric Allergy

Springer

Editors
Carlo Caffarelli
Pediatric Clinic, Department of Medicine and Surgery
University of Parma
Parma, Italy

Gian Luigi Marseglia
Department of Pediatric, Clinical and Surgical. Science
Policlinico San Matteo Fondazione
Pavia, Italy

This work contains media enhancements, which are displayed with a "play" icon. Material in the print book can be viewed on a mobile device by downloading the Springer Nature "More Media" app available in the major app stores. The media enhancements in the online version of the work can be accessed directly by authorized users.

ISBN 978-3-031-71285-2 ISBN 978-3-031-71283-8 (eBook)
https://doi.org/10.1007/978-3-031-71283-8

This Springer imprint is published by the registered company Springer Nature Switzerland AG
The registered company address is: Gewerbestrasse 11, 6330 Cham, Switzerland

Preface

As editors, we are pleased to introduce the *Textbook of Pediatric Allergy*.

It is a valuable resource for healthcare professionals involved in the diagnosis, treatment, and management of allergic diseases in children and for researchers in the field. Although the knowledge in Pediatric Allergy is continually evolving, it remains relatively unfamiliar to many pediatric specialists today. Despite this, it is a specialty that significantly impacts the lives of millions of children globally. As a result, understanding the immunological, clinical, and therapeutic foundations of the allergic diseases in children is now a fundamental requirement for pediatricians. This comprehensive overview of Pediatric Allergy covers a wide range of topics from the epidemiology of allergic diseases to the mechanisms of allergy development and the fundamental principles guiding diagnostic processes. Specific conditions such as asthma, dermatitis, allergic conjunctivitis, rhinitis, and food allergy are explored in-depth. The text also discusses urticaria, angioedema, and less frequent conditions in the pediatric population, such as hymenoptera venom allergy and drug hypersensitivity. Emerging diseases that are of great clinical and scientific interest, such as eosinophilic esophagitis, and inborn errors of immunity with atopic manifestations are also comprehensively outlined. Furthermore, advanced diagnostic tools for all allergic diseases in the pediatric age are extensively discussed.

This textbook highlights the increasing significance of Pediatric Allergy in recent years. Scientific advancements have led to a "multiomic approach" that integrates and analyzes various biological datasets like genomics, transcriptomics, proteomics, and metabolomics. This has provided new insights into the mechanisms behind allergic diseases, leading to targeted therapies aligned with the Precision Medicine approach. This textbook covers the transformative impact of biological therapies and allergen immunotherapy on medical practices in Pediatric Allergy, as well as daily challenges faced by allergic children and strategies for allergy prevention.

What sets this textbook apart is its ability to present complex medical information in a clear and accessible format without sacrificing depth. Renowned authors have collaborated to offer a harmonious blend of theoretical and practical insights. The goal is to empower healthcare professionals with the latest evidence-based information and practical insights in the field of pediatric allergy. This textbook serves as an invaluable companion for students, residents, and expert practitioners navigating the dynamic landscape of pediatric allergy care.

In conclusion, we trust that our collective effort will not only enhance the knowledge base of medical professionals but, more importantly, contribute to the overarching goal of continually improving the care of our children.

Parma, Italy Carlo Caffarelli
Pavia, Italy Gian Luigi Marseglia

Introduction

Pediatric allergy is a rapidly changing field. Historically, mainstream pediatric literature and training had little focus on allergic diseases. There were fallacies based on myths, traditions, prejudices, and lack of reliable information regarding the pathology, physiology, and reactivity. Luckily, by the end of the twentieth century, new awareness and consideration had turned to the growing field of allergy. Efforts by national and international scientific societies have also helped in advancing knowledge on allergies. This textbook serves to create a foundation upon which an understanding of allergic diseases should be built. It is a comprehensive textbook written by dozens of nationally and internationally recognized experts in the field. This is most relevant as pointed out in Chap. 1 since the incidence of allergic diseases is increasing especially in Western countries from the 60s onwards. It contains chapters on biology, clinical features, and treatment of a myriad of diseases. An up-to-date reference on basic mechanisms of allergy is reported in Chap. 2. A comprehensive report on diagnostic pathways is offered in Chap. 3. A concise, well-written, recommendation on managing asthma that is consistent with the latest guidelines is reported in Chaps. 4 and 5. The differences between asthma and wheezing in pediatric patients as well as the clinical approach are discussed in Chap. 6. In Chap. 7, an unprecedented view of atopic dermatitis mechanisms in children illustrates novel treatments that have the highest efficacy. Allergic rhino conjunctivitis represents the most common allergic disease in childhood. In Chaps. 8 and 9, new advances for both patient and specialist are presented, but not so much as to lose the whole representation in the particulars. The conundrum of immunotherapy for hymenoptera venom allergy in children is solved in Chap. 10. In Chap. 11, the historical milestone on anaphylaxis reminds us from where we have come from, and how we have been able to make it this far, thanks to researcher's hard work. Chapter 12 contributes to resolve controversies in drug allergy and provides guidance for making clinical decisions. A comprehensive, yet extremely digestible update in both IgE-mediated and non-IgE-mediated food allergy is timely provided in Chaps. 13 and 14. In Chap. 15, all features of eosinophilic esophagitis in children including the relationship with food allergy and novel treatments are given. The role of allergy in urticaria and angioedema is presented in Chaps. 16 and 17. There is also Chap. 18 on structure, function, biology of eosinophils and Chap. 19 on mastocytosis. As our population is increasingly multiracial, the task of recognizing contact dermatitis in children with different skin colors is faced in Chap. 20. In Chap. 21, the benefit of understanding the allergic manifestations of inborn immunity errors is distinctly described. Specific guides to understanding allergy tests including new diagnostic technologies such as molecular diagnosis, and novel inflammatory markers, offer us an unprecedented view of the function of the immune system in allergic reactions and an unparalleled diagnostic mean for identifying allergic diseases (see Chaps. 22 and 23). Chapter 24 represents an invaluable tool to help the use of corticosteroids in the allergic child. There have been exciting changes in the treatment of pediatric allergies. Among them, detailed explanations of what monoclonal antibodies are and how they should be used in the treatment of allergies in children are reported in Chap. 25. Furthermore, the advantages of allergen-specific immunotherapy that is the only causative therapy for allergic diseases are clearly showed in Chap. 26. The part of the role of environmental changes and pollution on the development of allergies has not been left out (Chap. 27). A rich understanding of the influence of cultural habits, practices, beliefs of patients and parents on daily life of allergic children is presented in Chap. 28. Finally, the book closes with a hopeful note on progresses in allergy prevention. Together, these chapters concur in turning this work into a valued companion and handy tool for pediatricians and subspecialists assisting them in meeting the challenges of treating children with allergies.

Contents

Epidemiology of Allergic Diseases

1

Salvatore Tripodi, Alessandro Maria Marra, and Giuseppe Pingitore

Abstract

Allergy is not a disease itself, but a mechanism leading to disease. In clinical practice, allergy manifests in form of various different conditions such as anaphylaxis, urticaria, angioedema, allergic rhinoconjunctivitis, asthma, atopic dermatitis, as well as the colorful spectrum of food- or drug-induced hypersensitivity reactions. Since the discovery of immunoglobulin E (IgE) as a mediator of allergic diseases in 1967, our knowledge about the immunological mechanisms of IgE-mediated allergies has remarkably increased. Novel allergens are constantly being described and new allergen sources. In recent decades, the incidence of allergic diseases has continued to increase, affecting 20% of the worldwide population, especially children. Atopic diseases are becoming an epidemic and pandemic issue. Projections suggest that the global population is likely to reach 9–10 billion people by 2050, with 2–4 billion suffering from them. Studies have suggested that allergic diseases occur following a time-based order: from atopic dermatitis (AD) and food allergy in infancy to gradual development into allergic asthma (AA) and allergic rhinitis (AR) in childhood, even if some epidemiologic evidence outlines the existence of different allergic march trajectories. In recent decades, climate change has affected key aspects of human health, including allergic and respiratory diseases. The research programs contributed to the important concept of personalized medicine in many allergic diseases, and specific therapies were chosen based on specific clinical characteristics. We are witnessing important revolutions both in the diagnosis of allergic pathologies (component-resolved diagnosis, telemedicine, use of devices such as smartphones and tablet computers to support and improve health-related services) and in therapy, such as the use of biologics for many allergic pathologies, evolving toward personalized medicine.

Keywords

Hypersensitivity · Allergy · Asthma · Atopic march · Food allergies · Climate change · Environment · Exposome · Pollution · Hygiene hypothesis · Component-resolved diagnosis · Allergen immunotherapy · Biologic therapies · Mobile health technology Telemedicine

S. Tripodi (✉)
Policlinico Casilino Hospital, Allergology Service, Rome, Italy

A. M. Marra
Pneumology Unit, ASST Rhodense Garbagnate Milanese Hospital, Milan, Italy

G. Pingitore
Allergist, Professional, Rome, Italy

C. Caffarelli, G. L. Marseglia (eds.), *Textbook of Pediatric Allergy*,
https://doi.org/10.1007/978-3-031-71283-8_1

Test your learning and check your understanding of this book's contents: use the "Springer Nature Flashcards" app to access questions.
To use the app, please follow the instructions below:

1. Go to https://flashcards.springernature.com/login.
2. Create a user account by entering your e-mail address and assigning a password.
3. Use the following link to access your SN Flashcards set: ▶ https://sn.pub/nspbjm.

If the link is missing or does not work, please send an e-mail with the subject "SN Flashcards" and the book title to customerservice@springernature.com.

1.1 Historical Features: From the Atopic March to the Climate Change

The term "Allergy" was born on July 24, 1906, in the Münchener Medizinische Wochenschrift as "specifically altered reactivity of the organism." Today, we define allergy as immunological hypersensitivity that can lead to a variety of different diseases via different pathomechanisms, and thus, different approaches in diagnosis, therapy, and prevention can be taken [1]. Allergy is not a disease itself but a mechanism leading to disease. In clinical practice, allergy manifests in form of various different conditions such as anaphylaxis, urticaria, angioedema, allergic rhinoconjunctivitis, allergic asthma, serum sickness, allergic vasculitis, hypersensitivity pneumonitis, atopic dermatitis (eczema), contact dermatitis and granulomatous reactions, as well as the colorful spectrum of food- or drug-induced hypersensitivity reactions. Allergies can be seen in almost every organ. Most commonly, however, it is the skin and the mucous membranes that are involved since they represent the frontier between the individual organism and its environment. Allergy often starts in the first 3 months of life but very rarely at birth, although there is a strong genetic background [2]. Allergy in some cases does not persist over lifetime; it starts and some patients may outgrow their allergic disease spontaneously. Many allergic diseases have a chronic course, but there are ways to cure. Allergic diseases can be influenced by psychological processes in a positive or in a negative way [3]. Since the discovery of immunoglobulin E (IgE) as a mediator of allergic diseases in 1967, our knowledge about the immunological mechanisms of IgE-mediated allergies has remarkably increased. In addition to understanding the immune response and clinical symptoms, allergy diagnosis and management depend strongly on the precise identification of the elicitors of the IgE-mediated allergic reaction [4]. In the past four decades, innovations in bioscience and technology have facilitated the identification and production of well-defined, highly pure molecules for component-resolved diagnosis (CRD), allowing a personalized diagnosis and management of the allergic disease for individual patients [5]. In recent decades, the incidence of allergic diseases has continued to increase, affecting 20% of the worldwide population, especially children. Cross-sectional and longitudinal studies have suggested that allergic diseases occur following a time-based order: from atopic dermatitis (AD) and food allergy in infancy to gradual development into allergic asthma (AA) and allergic rhinitis (AR) in childhood [6]. In terms of anatomic structure, it follows the spatial evolution of skin–gastrointestinal tract–respiratory tract, and this phenomenon is defined as the "atopic march" (Fig. 1.1). Among the allergic diseases mentioned above, some resolve gradually to disappear with age, whereas others continue for many years [7]. Some studies have shown that the atopic march does not progress completely in a temporal pattern with genes and the environment. Nevertheless, the concept of the atopic march provides a new perspective for the mechanistic research, prediction, prevention, and treatment of allergic diseases [8]. AD is the first manifestation

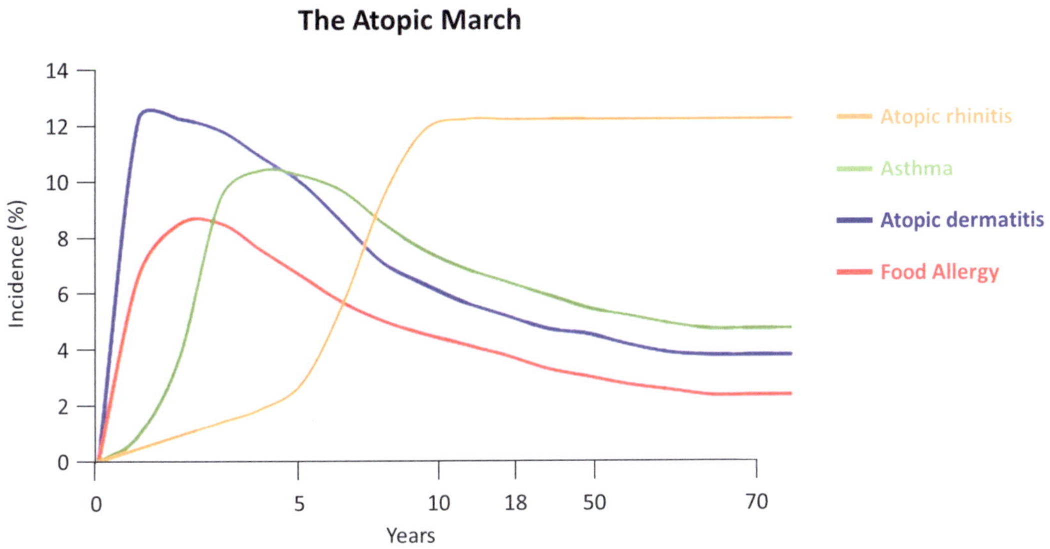

Fig. 1.1 Several studies have suggested that allergic diseases occur following a time-based order: from atopic dermatitis and food allergy in infancy to gradual development into allergic asthma and allergic rhinitis in childhood. In terms of anatomic structure, it follows the spatial evolution of skin—gastrointestinal tract–respiratory tract, and this phenomenon is defined as the "atopic march." Among the allergic diseases mentioned above, some resolve gradually to disappear with age, whereas others continue for many years

of the atopic march and is a chronic, recurrent skin disease. Its clinical manifestations are chronic inflammation of the skin, itching, and an impaired skin barrier. AD can affect 3% of adults and near 30% of children, and its prevalence tends to increase with age. Some epidemiology studies have shown that 45% of affected children had the condition before 6 months of age, 60% before 1 year of age, and up to 85% before 5 years of age [9]. AD patients can be classified into two types based on whether the IgE level is increased: intrinsic (normal IgE and non-allergic) and extrinsic (high IgE level associated with increased disease severity). Studies have shown that extrinsic AD increases the risk of developing the atopic march [10]. Dharmage et al. found, in infants who have AD within 2 years of age, that the incidence of AA and AR increased significantly during age 6–7 years. In particular, early-onset, persistent, and IgE-positive AD led to a higher risk of developing AA and AR [11]. AA is a common chronic airway disease characterized by the inflammation, hyperresponsiveness, and remodeling of airways. With modernization and industrialization, AA incidence has increased year by year [12]. Epidemiologic evidence has revealed a link between AA and AR. AR may lead to changes in the function of the lower airways through three main mechanisms. Firstly, stimulation of the nasal mucosa contracts bronchial smooth muscle through the nasal–tracheal reflex. Secondly, various chemical mediators and cytokines released by antigenic stimulation causing nasal mucosa allergy are absorbed into blood, are transported to the lung through circulation, and then act on the trachea and bronchi, causing smooth muscle spasm. Thirdly, nasal inflammatory mediators and secretions are discharged through the nasal passage to the lower airways, resulting in a reduced b-adrenergic receptor functional response. Many studies suggest that early-onset, persistent, and IgE-positive AD led to a higher risk of developing AA and AR [13]. A longitudinal study on a Canadian birth cohort (2311 children) has shown that AD with sensitization at 1 year of age increased the prevalence of AA and AR at 3 years of age more than 11- and 7-fold, respectively [14]. A prospective cohort study (3124 children aged 1–2 years) reported that, compared with children with no history of AD, those once having AD, particularly moderate-to-severe, early, and persistent AD, were more inclined to develop AA and AR [15]. The discoveries mentioned above strongly support the natural process of the atopic march. IgE-positive food allergy commonly coexists with AD in early childhood as the earliest manifestation of the atopic march. In 2011, Japanese scholars conducted a retrospective questionnaire survey on freshmen, and they found that AD occurred earlier in those with accompanying food allergy. Also, having food allergy was regarded as the biggest risk factor for the atopic march [16]. A family-based cohort study from Chicago revealed that symptomatic food allergy, especially severe or multiple food allergies, was closely related to AA in children aged ≥6 years. Children with food allergy developed AA earlier than those without food allergy [17]. A survey of 2222 infants with AD aged 11.5–25.5 months showed that 64% of children diagnosed with AD within 3 months of birth exhibited an IgE-mediated sensitivity to milk, peanuts, or eggs. Also, in infants <12 months of age, the proportion of infants with sensitivity to eggs, milk, or peanuts increased with AD severity, but this phenomenon was not manifested in children with AD after 1 year of age [18]. In addition, studies have shown that children sensitive to milk in infancy subsequently exhibited aggravated airway inflammation and increased airway responsiveness to histamine. Remarkably, food allergy commonly exists together with AD in infants. Therefore, it is worth exploring whether the link between food allergy and AA or AR is related to AD or is a direct consequence of the food allergy itself [19]. The prevalence of food allergies is increasing around the globe posing a significant public health issue [20]. In industrialized countries, food allergy is the leading cause of anaphylaxis seen in emergency departments. In developing countries, however, concerns are rising about managing and preventing complications [21].While the prevalence of food allergies in children born in the United Kingdom between 2005 and 2007 was about 3.5%, the prevalence in infants born between 2009 and 2012 was already twice as high (7.1–7.3%) [22]. Data from Asian countries show a similar development. In China, the prevalence of food allergies proved by an oral food challenge among 0–24 months old infants increased from 3.5% to 7.7% between 1990 and 2009 [23].The global increase in food allergy prevalence can be attributed in particular to a few specific allergies such as egg allergy and milk allergy. Atopic diseases are becoming an epidemic and pandemic issue. Projections suggest that the global population is likely to reach 9–10 billion people by 2050, with 2–4 billion of them suffering from allergic diseases, such as asthma, allergic rhinitis, and atopic dermatitis [24]. Therefore, it is important to find new and effective ways to prevent asthma and other atopic diseases. This is only possible if we understand the connection between the development of atopic diseases, the host, and the environmental factors involved. Environmental factors have a huge impact on the development of food allergies. At the population level, these factors play a major role in the development of all noncommunicable diseases. They are summarized under the term exposome, which is defined as "the totality of specific and nonspecific external environmental exposures to which a subject is exposed from preconception onward and their consequences at the organ and cell levels." [25] The increase in atopic diseases reflects the changed social and environmental conditions in which the world population lives [26]. There are different hypotheses that seek to explain the increase in atopic diseases. Many data suggest that genetic factors are important on allergy development, but their expression is filtered through environmental factors [27]. Looking at the world allergy map, the most affected regions with high incidence rates are Europe, North America, South America, and Australia. Hence, countries with a high gross net income per capita have the highest allergy rates. A study using the GINI index (an economic index indicating the equality of income distribution in a country) suggests a correlation between economic inequality and asthma prevalence [28].This means that allergies seem to be diseases of developed countries. The Hygiene Hypothesis fits into this picture. Postulated by Strachan more than 30 years ago, the Hygiene Hypothesis has undergone many revisions and adaptations. From an epidemiological perspective, it advanced to a comprehensive concept expanding beyond the initial focus on allergies. The Hygiene Hypothesis comprises immunological, microbiological and evolutionary aspects. Thus, the original postulate developed into a holistic model that explains the impact of post-modern lifestyle on humans, who initially evolved in close proximity to a more natural environment. Microbiology added fundamental knowledge about the micro-ecosystem that is established throughout the human body as a unique symbiosis between humans and microbes [29]. Urban environment is another factor that increases the risk of allergies. Living in a smaller city or village, on the other hand, seems to protect against allergies [30]. Living in neighborhoods with little green space, or to soil/soil bacteria can contribute to the development of food allergies. Further possible contributors to a higher allergy risk in urban areas could be air pollution (diesel fuel, ozone) as well as chemical contaminants in water, soil, or packaged foods. The exposure to these pollutants is associated with allergy development [31]. Contact with farm animals in early life seems to protect against allergy development. This farm effect was first observed in the allergy and endotoxin (ALEX) cohort. This cross-sectional study included more than 900 school-aged farm and non-farm children from Switzerland, Germany, and Austria and it showed a reduction in prevalence of hay fever, asthma, and atopy of approximately 50% in children with farm exposure [32]. Based on these data, the hypothesis of a farm effect as protection against allergy was postulated and described in different epidemiologic and prospective studies [33]. In the recent decades, climate change explicitly or implicitly affects key aspects of human health, including allergic and respiratory diseases. Increasing CO_2 and global temperatures have been linked to longer duration of pollen season, pollen concentration, and geographical distribution of pollens, leading to increased duration and severity of seasonal allergic rhinitis and allergic asthma [34]. Higher CO_2 levels increase photosynthesis in plants, leading to increased production of pollen [35]. An association between thunderstorms and asthma, termed thunderstorm asthma, has been observed. During thunderstorms, pollen and/or mold spores are swept up into the clouds, where they are fractured (either by electric charge or by absorption of moisture) into smaller more allergenic fragments. In addition, thunderstorms also alter the distribution of these pollen-derived particles making them more concentrated at the ground level. Thunderstorms during the pollen season are linked to increased asthma exacerbations and emergency room visits [36]. In November 2016, a catastrophic and deadly thunderstorm asthma epidemic struck Melbourne, Australia, and overwhelmed health services, leading to loss of many lives [37]. Wildfires and dust storms increase air pollution and indirectly enhance health risks. Wildfire smoke contains gases, particulate matter, complex hydrocarbons, trace minerals, and several other toxic and carcinogenic compounds. In a study investigating health effects of a 2013 wildfire season in Oregon, USA, a 10 $\mu g/m^3$ increase in wildfire smoke increased risk of asthma diagnosis [38]. A 5-year study in Kuwait found that dust storm events (defined as events with PM10 > 200 $\mu g/m^3$) were associated with respiratory disease in children [39]. In the aftermath of Hurricane Katrina in New Orleans, USA, higher fungal counts were recorded indoors and outdoors [40]. Higher temperatures and increased CO_2 also promote fungal growth. Increased exposure to mold and fungi has been associated with allergic exacerbations. Climate change is a key environmental factor for allergic respiratory diseases, especially in childhood. Recent findings on the direct effects of temperature and weather changes, as well as the influences of climate change on air pollution, allergens, biocontaminants and their interplays, are discussed in several papers that also focus on the impact of climate change on biodiversity loss and on migration status as a model to study environmental effects on childhood asthma onset and progression (Fig. 1.2). Adaptation and mitigation strategies are urgently needed to prevent further respiratory diseases and human health damage in general, especially in younger and future generations [41]. Although there is still no consensus on the role of individual countries and their respon-

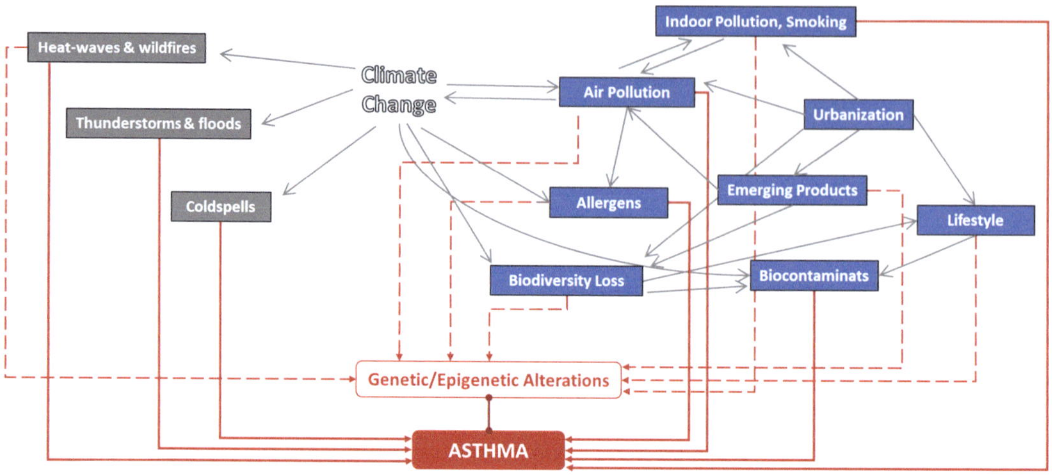

Fig. 1.2 The multiple roles of Climate Change on allergic respiratory diseases and in particular on childhood asthma

sibility for climate change, some progress has been achieved. Every country that signed up to the Paris Agreement has put forth a nationally determined contribution (NDC) for reducing greenhouse gas emissions by around 2030. These pledges, which are renewed every 5 years, are formulated by the countries based on their own priorities and needs and are non-binding. Currently, 192 parties have submitted their first NDCs. The evidence of current climate change caused by increased industrialization and human activity is irrefutable and this strongly suggest that we join and act now to build a healthier planet for the future [42].

1.2 Advances in Diagnosis and Treatment of Allergic Diseases and Future Perspectives

The identification of IgE antibodies to specific molecules can not only improve diagnosis but also have additional applications, such as the risk assessment of sensitized individuals, monitoring of environmental exposure, and detection of specific allergens in foods. Novel allergens are constantly being described and new allergen sources, such as edible insects, for example. The role of immunoactive substances, such as ligands, can contribute to an accurate diagnosis [5]. For example, component-resolved diagnosis (CRD) contributes to optimize the diagnosis in patients with allergic rhinitis, asthma, foods allergy and can be useful to treat the patients with the right immunotherapy. In clinical practice, although there are no "official" estimates, at least 11% of adults in Europe have grass pollen allergy [43] in the form of allergic rhinitis (hay fever), allergic asthma, or both. The burden associated with this allergenic source is therefore enormous [44]. Avoidance of grass pollen allergens is difficult, and therefore treatment is based mostly on drugs [45]. Pharmacotherapy has no direct effect on the immunologic mechanisms sustaining IgE sensitization, and the efficacy of drugs is dependent on their administration [46]. By contrast, allergen-specific immunotherapy (AIT) is the only treatment with long-lasting effects that continue after treatment discontinuation [47] and can contribute to prevention of disease progression [48]. AIT has been traditionally based on the administration of extracts of allergenic sources, which are supposed to contain all the major allergenic proteins. The exact composition of subcutaneous immunotherapy and sublingual immunotherapy preparations, however, it is often not precisely defined. Moreover, grass pollen extract preparations from different companies can change in their molecular composition, and this might reduce their efficacy [49, 50]. To optimize AIT efficacy, Valenta et al. proposed the concept of

Fig. 1.3 Profiles of IgE sensitization to 8 *P. pratense* molecules in 176 children with an IgE reaction to *P. pratense*. The figure shows the heterogeneity of IgE sensitization profiles. Reproduced with permission from Ref. [52]

Profile APCS code	profile's binary code (8 molecules): cut-off 0.35 kU/L	rPhl p 1	rPhl p 2	rPhl p 4	rPhl p 5	rPhl p 6	rPhl p 7	rPhl p 11	rPhl p 12	n pos. mol.	n	%	cum. %
128	10000000	●								1	36	20,8	21
248	11111000	●	●	●	●	●				5	21	12,1	33
160	10100000	●		●						2	10	5,8	39
184	10111000	●		●	●	●				4	8	4,6	43
186	10111010	●		●	●	●		●		5	8	4,6	48
251	11111011	●	●	●	●	●		●	●	7	8	4,6	53
192	11000000	●	●							2	7	4,0	57
216	11011000	●	●		●	●				4	7	4,0	61
249	11111001	●	●	●	●	●			●	6	7	4,0	65
250	11111010	●	●	●	●	●		●		6	7	4,0	69
32	100000			●						1	5	2,9	72
224	11100000	●	●	●						3	5	2,9	75
152	10011000	●			●	●				3	4	2,3	77
185	10111001	●		●	●	●			●	5	4	2,3	79
208	11010000	●	●		●					3	3	1,7	81
218	11011010	●	●		●	●		●		5	3	1,7	83
48	110000			●	●					2	2	1,2	84
64	1000000		●							1	2	1,2	85
144	10010000	●			●					2	2	1,2	86
162	10100010	●		●				●		3	2	1,2	87
187	10111011	●		●	●	●		●	●	6	2	1,2	88
193	11000001	●	●						●	3	2	1,2	90
217	11011001	●	●		●	●			●	5	2	1,2	91
225	11100001	●	●	●					●	4	2	1,2	92
16	10000				●					1	1	0,6	92
34	100010			●				●		2	1	0,6	93
58	111010			●	●	●		●		4	1	0,6	94
96	1100000		●	●						2	1	0,6	94
129	10000001	●							●	2	1	0,6	95
130	10000010	●						●		2	1	0,6	95
132	10000100	●					●			2	1	0,6	96
156	10011100	●			●	●	●			4	1	0,6	97
188	10111100	●		●	●	●	●			5	1	0,6	97
194	11000010	●	●					●		3	1	0,6	98
232	11101000	●	●	●		●				4	1	0,6	98
240	11110000	●	●	●	●					4	1	0,6	99
254	11111110	●	●	●	●	●	●	●		7	1	0,6	99
255	11111111	●	●	●	●	●	●	●	●	8	1	0,6	100
0	0									0	3	1,7	

component-resolved therapy (CRT) [51]. Accordingly, an AIT preparation should be characterized and standardized at a molecular level, and its composition should match the patient's molecular profile of IgE sensitization. To tailor a patient's CRT to grass species (e.g., *Phleum pratense*) is rather complex. In 2012 Tripodi et al. demonstrated a large number of different IgE sensitization profiles to *P. pratense* among a children population and that molecularly designed AIT preparations tailored to patients' needs should consider this high heterogeneity [52] (Fig. 1.3). CRD evaluating different allergen molecules can by very useful to find the right patient sensitization and choose the most suitable therapy. Molecules are also very important in diagnosis of food allergy and venom allergy. IgE-mediated sensitization to pollen allergens can be associated with a food allergy due to the co-recognition (cross-reactivity) of structurally homologous proteins present in plant-derived foods. Molecular IgE test methods have substantially advanced allergy diagnostics. Evaluation of patients' sensitization profiles contributes to our mechanistic understanding of allergies and the characterization of major allergens. Molecular IgE tests are an essential support for decision making. In food allergy, identification of specific IgE (sIgE)-sensitization patterns combined with the interpretation of the patients' history is essential for the management and guidance of patients. This information allows tailored recommendations regarding symptom severity based on the recognized allergen molecule. In allergology, a cross-reaction is the consequence of the binding of IgE to homologous, linear or conformational, allergen structures conserved among proteins that are characterized by a similar function. It has been estimated that up to 60% of food allergies in older children, adolescents, and adults are linked with an inhalant allergy [53]. Singleplex and Multiplex tests are now available to help clinicians to arrive to most possible patient's tailored diagnosis and this is an example of precision medicine [54]. From 2016 EAACI Molecular Allergology User's guide from the European Academy of Allergy and Clinical Immunology (EAACI), reviews current knowledge and aims to provide clinical guidance to healthcare professionals taking care of children and adults with respiratory, food and hymenoptera venom allergy [55] and it has been further improved in 2022 with the version 2.0 [5]. The research programs that led to their development have likewise contributed to the important concept of personalized medicine in many allergic diseases in which specific therapies are chosen based on specific clinical characteristics like asthma, atopic dermatitis, chronic spontaneous urticaria and most recently chronic rinosinusitis with nasal polyps (CRSwNP) and eosinophil-driven diseases [56]. Biologic therapies represent a major advance in the treatment of difficult-to-treat for example severe asthma, providing a therapeutic option that is highly effective in reducing severe exacerbation risk in selected patients with specific phenotypes. Omalizumab, benralizumab, mepolizumab, dupilumab, and tezepelumab have been approved. They also provide an opportunity to reduce patient dependence on high-dose oral corticosteroid (OCS) and inhaled corticosteroid (ICS) therapy and the associated risks of systemic adverse effects [57]. In children the potential use of other biologics in the management of food allergy is subject of speculation. Systematic reviews and meta-analysis demonstrated safety and effectiveness of omalizumab in the treatment of food allergy [58]. Another important revolution in allergology is the use of devices such as smartphones and tablet computers to support and improve health-related services. Allergology, as any other area of medicine, will be deeply influenced by mobile health technology. Allergists and their patients have a new way of communication, through the phone camera, sound recording system, motion sensors, texting, and ultimately by using diagnostic devices and diagnostic algorithms incorporated within the mobile phone itself. The revolution that these possibilities are bringing in epidemiology, care, and research has already arrived. The role of doctors, and in particular allergists, will be progressively altered. To contribute to this trend, the "EAACI Task Force for mobile health and allergy" has designed a two-year-long action plan that will be implemented [59]. In Italy, for example, the mobile application and back-office of AllergyMonitor (TPS software production, Rome, Italy) enable patients to record their daily allergy symptoms as well as drug and immunotherapy intake plus possible side effects in a customizable way. The results can be accessed by the patient and attending physician as concise reports via a smartphone or computer. This technology has been used in several clinical studies and routine practice since 2009 have proven the reliability and positive impact of a digital platform including an electronic diary on the diagnostic precision of allergic rhinitis in poly-sensitized patients as well as patient adherence to both, drug therapy and allergen immunotherapy [60] (Fig. 1.4). Since 2020, the coronavirus disease 2019 (COVID-19) has evolved into a pandemic infectious disease transmitted by the severe acute respiratory syndrome coronavirus (SARS-CoV-2). Allergists and other healthcare providers (HCPs) in the field of allergies and associated airway diseases are on the front line, taking care of patients potentially infected with SARS-CoV-2. Hence, strategies and practices to minimize risks of infection for

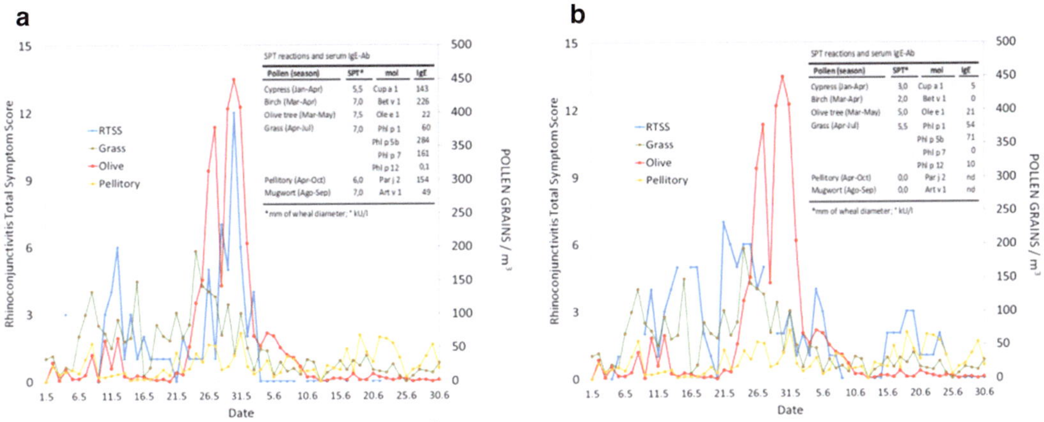

Fig. 1.4 Trajectories of symptom severity vs pollen counts in two pediatric patients (**a**: patient 1; **b**: patient 2) with allergic rhinitis, and similar allergic profile, according to SPT and CRD. Data on severity of symptoms—collected with AllergyMonitor—have been reported as Rhinoconjunctivitis Total Symptom Score (RTSS). Pollen counts (grains/m^3) were obtained from the local pollen trap. Reproduced with permission from Ref. [60]

both HCPs and treated patients must be developed and followed by allergy clinics [61]. HCPs providing care to allergic patients were affected during the pandemic in diagnostic, management, and therapeutic approaches, including AIT for respiratory, insect-venom, and food allergies. Most HCPs maintained controller treatments for both asthma, and allergic rhinitis consistent with international recommendations, as well as biological agents in asthma. Remote tools are valuable in delivering allergy care [62]. Various surveys have indicated a high degree of satisfaction in the use of telemedicine during the COVID-19 pandemic, both by doctors and patients. Digital health can have a very positive impact on the management of allergic patients, especially in epidemic situations [63].

References

1. Johansson SGO, Bieber C, Dahl R, Friedmann PS, Lanier BQ, Lockey RF, et al. Revised nomenclature for allergy for global use: report of the nomenclature committee of the World Allergy Organization. J Allergy Clin Immunol. 2004;113:832–6.
2. Ring J. Allergy in practice. Berlin: Springer; 2005.
3. Adkinson NF, Bochner BS, Burks AW, Busse WW, Holgate ST, Lemanske LF, O'Hehir RE. Middleton's allergy principles and practice. 8th ed. Philadelphia: Elsevier; 2014.
4. Ring J, Akdis C, Behrendt H, Lauener RP, Schäppi G, Akdis M, et al. Davos declaration: allergy as a global problem. Allergy. 2012;67:141–3.
5. Dramburg S, Hilger C, Santos AF, de Las Vecillas L, Aalberse RC, Acevedo N, et al. EAACI molecular allergology user's guide 2.0. Pediatr Allergy Immunol. 2023;34(Suppl 28):e13854.
6. Bantz SK, Zhu Z, Zheng T. The atopic march: progression from atopic dermatitis to allergic rhinitis and asthma. J Clin Cell Immunol. 2014;5:202.
7. Spergel JM, Paller AS. Atopic dermatitis and the atopic march. J Allergy Clin Immunol. 2003;112(6 Suppl):S118–27.
8. Gabryszewski SJ, Hill DA. One march, many paths: insights into allergic march trajectories. Ann Allergy Asthma Immunol. 2021;127:293–300.
9. Bieber T. Atopic dermatitis. N Engl J Med. 2008;358:1483–94.
10. Novembre E, Cianferoni A, Lombardi E, Bernardini R, Pucci N, Vierucci A. Natural history of "intrinsic" atopic dermatitis. Allergy. 2001;56:452–3.
11. Dharmage SC, Lowe AJ, Matheson MC, Burgess JA, Allen KJ, Abramson MJ. Atopic dermatitis and the atopic march revisited. Allergy. 2014;69:17–27.
12. James A. Airway remodeling in asthma. Curr Opin Pulm Med. 2005;11:1–6.
13. Yang L, Fu J, Zhou Y. Research Progress in atopic march. Front Immunol. 2020;11:1907.
14. Tran MM, Lefebvre DL, Dharma C, Dai DW, Lou YWY, Subbarao P, et al. Predicting the atopic march: results from the Canadian healthy infant longitudinal development study. J Allergy Clin Immunol. 2018;141:601–607.
15. von Kobyletzki LB, Bornehag CG, Hasselgren M, Larsson M, Lindstrom CB, Svensson A. Eczema in early childhood is strongly associated with the devel-

opment of asthma and rhinitis in a prospective cohort. BMC Dermatol. 2012;12:11.
16. Kijima A, Murota H, Takahashi A, Arase N, Yang L, Nishioka M, et al. Prevalence and impact of past history of food allergy in atopic dermatitis. Allergol Int. 2013;62:105–12.
17. Schroeder A, Kumar R, Pongracic JA, Sullivan CL, Caruso DM, Costello J, et al. Food allergy is associated with an increased risk of asthma. Clin Exp Allergy. 2009;39:261–70.
18. Hill DJ, Hosking CS, de Benedictis FM, Oranje AP, Diepgen TL, Bauchau V, et al. Confirmation of the association between high levels of immunoglobulin E food sensitization and eczema in infancy: an international study. Clin Exp Allergy. 2008;38:61–8.
19. Bousquet J, Khaltaev N, Cruz AA, Denburg J, Fokkens WJ, Togias A, et al. Allergic Rhinitis and its Impact on Asthma (ARIA) 2008 update (in collaboration with the World Health Organization, GA(2)LEN and AllerGen). Allergy. 2008;63(Suppl. 86):8–160.
20. Tang ML, Mullins RJ. Food allergy: is prevalence increasing? Intern Med J. 2017;47:256–61.
21. Hossny E, Ebisawa M, El-Gamal Y, Arasi S, Dahdah L, El-Owaidy R,et al. Challenges of managing food allergy in the developing world. World Allergy Organ J. 2019;12:100089.
22. Perkin MR, Logan K, Tseng A, Raji B, Ayis S, Peacock J, et al. Randomized trial of introduction of allergenic foods in breast-fed infants. N Engl J Med. 2016;374:1733–43.
23. Chen J, Hu Y, Allen KJ, Ho MH, Li H. The prevalence of food allergy in infants in Chongqing, China. Pediatr Allergy Immunol. 2011;22:356–60.
24. van de Veen, W. Mechanisms of immune regulation in allergy. Zurich Open Repository and Archive, 2014.
25. Cecchi L, D'Amato G, Annesi-Maesano I. External exposome and allergic respiratory and skin diseases. J Allergy Clin Immunol. 2018;141:846–57.
26. Fiocchi A, Dahdah L, Fierro V, Artesani MC, Valluzzi R. Food allergy trends at the crossing among socio-economics, history and geography. Curr Opin Allergy Clin Immunol. 2018;18:271–6.
27. Suaini NHA, Wang Y, Soriano VX, Martino DJ, Allen KJ, Ellis JA, et al. Genetic determinants of pediatric food allergy: a systematic review. Allergy. 2019;74:1631–48.
28. Uphoff EP, Cabieses B, Wright J, Pickett KE. International prevalence rates of asthma and allergy are associated with income inequality. J Allergy Clin Immunol. 2015;136:189–190.e2.
29. Pfefferle PI, Keber CU, Cohen RM, Garn H. The hygiene hypothesis – learning from but not living in the past. Front Immunol. 2021;16:635935.
30. Sbihi H, Boutin RC, Cutler C, Suen M, Finlay BB, Turvey SE. Thinking bigger: how early-life environmental exposures shape the gut microbiome and influence the development of asthma and allergic disease. Allergy. 2019;74:2103–15.
31. D'Amato G, Chong-Neto HJ, Monge Ortega OP, Vitale C, Ansotegui I, Rosario N,et al. The effects of climate change on respiratory allergy and asthma induced by pollen and mold allergens. Allergy. 2020;75:2219–28.
32. Riedler J, Braun-Fahrlander C, Eder W, Schreuer M, Waser M, Maisch S, et al. Exposure to farming in early life and development of asthma and allergy: across-sectional survey. Lancet. 2001;358:1129–33.
33. von Mutius E, Vercelli D. Farm living: effects on childhood asthma and allergy. Nat Rev Immunol. 2010;10:861–8.
34. Lind T, Ekebom A, Alm Kubler K, Ostensson P, Bellander T, Lohmus M. Pollen season trends (1973–2013) in Stockholm Area, Sweden. PLoS One. 2016;11:e0166887.
35. Kevat A. Thunderstorm asthma: looking back and looking forward. J Asthma Allergy. 2020;13:293–9.
36. D'Amato G, Annesi-Maesano I, Cecchi L, D'Amato M. Latest news on relationship between thunderstorms and respiratory allergy, severe asthma, and deaths for asthma. Allergy. 2019;74:9–11.
37. Campbell SL, Fox-Hughes PD, Jones PJ, Remenyi TA, Chappell K, White CJ, et al. Evaluating the risk of epidemic thunderstorm asthma: lessons from Australia. Int J Environ Res Public Health. 2019;16:837.
38. Gan RW, Liu J, Ford B, O'Dell K, Vaidyanathan A, Wilson A, et al. The association between wildfire smoke exposure and asthma-specific medical care utilization in Oregon during the 2013 wildfire season. J Expo Sci Environ Epidemiol. 2020;30:618–28.
39. Thalib L, Al-Taiar A. Dust storms and the risk of asthma admissions to hospitals in Kuwait. Sci Total Environ. 2012;433:347–51.
40. Barbeau DN, Grimsley LF, White LE, El-Dahr JM, Lichtveld M. Mold exposure and health effects following hurricanes Katrina and Rita. Annu Rev Public Health. 2010;31:165–78.
41. Biagioni B, Cecchi L, D'Amato G, Annesi-Maesano I. Environmental influences on childhood asthma: climate change. Pediatr Allergy Immunol. 2023;34:e13961.
42. Nadeau KC, Agache I, Jutel M, Annesi Maesano I, Akdis M, Sampath V, et al. Climate change: a call to action for the United Nations. Allergy. 2022;77:1087–90.
43. Bauchau V, Durham SR. Prevalence and rate of diagnosis of allergic rhinitis in Europe. Eur Respir J. 2004;24:758–64.
44. Natan R. The burden of allergic rhinitis. Allergy Asthma Proc. 2007;28:3–9.
45. Bousquet J, Schünemann HJ, Zuberbier T, Bachert C, Baena-Cagnani CE, Bousquet PJ, et al. Development and implementation of guidelines in allergic rhinitis: an ARIA-GA2LEN paper. Allergy. 2010;65:1212–21.
46. Durham SR, Walker SM, Varga EM, Jacobson MR, O'Brien F, Noble W, et al. Long-term clinical efficacy of grass-pollen immunotherapy. N Engl J Med. 1999;341:468–75.
47. Moller C, Dreborg S, Ferdousi HA, Halken S, Høst A, Jacobsen L, et al. Pollen immunotherapy reduces the development of asthma in children with seasonal

rhinoconjunctivitis (the PAT-study). J Allergy Clin Immunol. 2002;109:251–6.
48. Vogelberg C, Klimek L, Brüggenjürgen B, Jutel M. Real-world evidence for the long-term effect of allergen immunotherapy: current status on database-derived European studies. Allergy. 2022;77:3584–92.
49. Rossi R, Monasterolo G, Passalacqua G. The biological potency of different extracts for sublingual immunotherapy assessed by skin prick tests. Eur Ann Allergy Clin Immunol. 2010;42:112–4.
50. Schmidt H, Gelhaus C, Nebendahl M, Janssen O, Petersen A. Characterization of Phleum pratense pollen extracts by 2-D DIGE and allergen immunoreactivity. Proteomics. 2010;10:4352–62.
51. Valenta R, Lidholm J, Niederberger V, Hayek B, Kraft D, Gronlund H. The recombinant allergen-based concept of component-resolved diagnostics and immunotherapy (CRD and CRIT). Clin Exp Allergy. 1999;29:896–904.
52. Tripodi S, Frediani T, Lucarelli S, Macrì F, Pingitore G, Di Rienzo BA, et al. Molecular profiles of IgE to Phleum pratense in children with grass pollen allergy: implications for specific immunotherapy. J Allergy Clin Immunol. 2012;129:834–839.e8.
53. Asero R, Ariano R, Aruanno A, Barzaghi C, Borrelli P, Busa M, et al. Systemic allergic reactions induced by labile plant-food allergens: seeking potential cofactors. A multicenter study. Allergy. 2021;76:1473–9.
54. Diem L, Neuherz B, Rohrhofer J, Koidl L, Asero R, Brockow K, et al. Real-life evaluation of molecular multiplex IgE test methods in the diagnosis of pollen associated food allergy. Allergy. 2022;77:3028–40.
55. Alvaro-Lozano M, Akdis CA, Akdis M, Alviani C, Angier E, Arasi S, et al. EAACI allergen immunotherapy User's guide. Pediatr Allergy Immunol. 2020;31(Suppl 25):1–101.
56. Ramírez-Jiménez F, Pavón-Romero GF, Velásquez-Rodríguez JM, López-Garza MI, Lazarini-Ruiz JF, Gutiérrez-Quiroz KV, et al. Biologic therapies for asthma and allergic disease: past, present, and future. Pharmaceuticals (Basel). 2023;16:270.
57. Beasley R, Hatter L. Biologics and personalized medicine in severe asthma: one step at a time. J Allergy Clin Immunol Pract. 2023;11:1771–2.
58. Mutarelli A, Giavina-Bianchi B, Arasi S, Cafarotti A, Fiocchi A. Biologicals in IgE-mediated food allergy. Curr Opin Allergy Clin Immunol. 2023;23:205–9.
59. Matricardi PM, Dramburg S, Alvarez-Perea A, Antolín-Amérigo D, Apfelbacher C, Atanaskovic-Markovic M, et al. The role of mobile health technologies in allergy care: an EAACI position paper. Allergy. 2020;75:259–72.
60. Tripodi S, Giannone A, Sfika I, Pelosi S, Dramburg S, Bianchi A, et al. Digital technologies for an improved management of respiratory allergic diseases: 10 years of clinical studies using an online platform for patients and physicians. Ital J Pediatr. 2020;46:105.
61. Alvaro-Lozano M, Sandoval-Ruballos M, Giovannini M, Jensen-Jarolim E, Sahiner U, Tomic Spiric V, et al. Allergic patients during the COVID-19 pandemic-clinical practical considerations: an European academy of allergy and clinical immunology survey. Clin Transl Allergy. 2022;12:e12097.
62. Pfaar O, Klimek L, Jutel M, Akdis CA, Bousquet J, Breiteneder H, et al. COVID-19 pandemic: practical considerations on the organization of an allergy clinic-an EAACI/ARIA position paper. Allergy. 2021;76:648–76.
63. Pattini S, Pingitore G, Cardinale F, Licari A, Miraglia Del Giudice M, Calvani M, et al. Digital health in the management of allergic diseases. Acta Biomed. 2021;92(S7):e2021529.

Basic Mechanisms of Allergy

2

Riccardo Castagnoli, Antonio Andrea Senatore, Martina Solfa, Gian Luigi Marseglia, and Raffaele Badolato

Abstract

Allergy is a complex condition characterized by immune responses triggered by allergens, involving both the innate and adaptive immune systems. Macrophages and mast cells are key players in initiating allergic reactions, while T cells, B cells, and regulatory T cells have crucial roles in adaptive immunity. Allergic inflammation is mediated by various cytokines, including IL-4, IL-5, IL-9, and IL-13, which contribute to mast cell degranulation, cellular infiltration, and tissue remodeling. Mast cells, eosinophils, and basophil release mediators play significant roles in allergic responses. In addition to immune cells, structural epithelial cells and the neurological system contribute to allergic inflammation. Therapeutically, proinflammatory cytokines and upstream regulatory cytokines represent potential targets for precision medicine. By understanding the underlying mechanisms of allergic inflammation, targeted therapies can be developed to alleviate symptoms and improve patient outcomes.

Keywords

Allergy · Th2 response · Cytokines · Inflammation · Targeted therapies

Test your learning and check your understanding of this book's contents: use the "Springer Nature Flashcards" app to access questions using ▶ https://sn.pub/nsphjm. To use the app, please follow the instructions in Chap. 1.

R. Castagnoli · A. A. Senatore · M. Solfa
G. L. Marseglia
Pediatric Unit, Department of Clinical, Surgical, Diagnostic and Pediatric Sciences, University of Pavia, Pavia, Italy

Pediatric Clinic, Fondazione IRCCS Policlinico San Matteo, Pavia, Italy

R. Badolato (✉)
Department of Clinical and Experimental Sciences, University of Brescia, Brescia, Italy

Pediatric Clinic, ASST Spedali Civili, Brescia, Italy
e-mail: raffaele.badolato@unibs.it

2.1 Allergy

The term "Allergy" encompasses multiple pathogenetic mechanisms in which several actors are involved.

From an immunological point of view, allergy is primarily based on the IgE-mediated response induced by allergens, which, in predisposed individuals, cause an altered immune response. This

C. Caffarelli, G. L. Marseglia (eds.), *Textbook of Pediatric Allergy*,
https://doi.org/10.1007/978-3-031-71283-8_2

complex pathogenesis involves both innate and adaptive immune responses.

2.2 Allergens

Allergens are proteins capable of inducing a type 1 hypersensitivity immune response, resulting in the production of IgE. Not all proteins are allergens; to be defined as such, they must have unique characteristics. Most allergens have a molecular weight between 10 and 70 kDa, a size suitable for interaction with APRs (antigen-presenting cells). Allergens often contain proteases, which have the ability to disrupt the skin and mucosal barrier, thus promoting the entry of other allergens into tissues. Some allergens, such as drugs, have a low molecular weight but can bind to serum or membrane proteins, acting as full-fledged allergens.

2.3 Introduction to the Immune System

The immune system is divided into two broad categories: innate immunity and adaptive immunity.

Innate immunity is already effective at birth and is based on the ability to readily recognize microbe-specific "highly conserved molecular features," defined as PAMPs (pathogen-associated molecular patterns) via PRRs (pattern recognition receptors). PRRs are divided into AMPs (antimicrobial peptides), which are released proteins that provide a microbicidal barrier against microbial adhesion and invasion when produced on skin and mucous membranes, and TLRs (toll-like Receptors), transmembrane molecules expressed by many cell types of innate immunity. Once PRRs are activated, the first responders of the innate immune system, such as tissue macrophages, fibrocytes, epithelial cells, and mast cells, are in frontline positions for detection. Innate immune cells process allergens and can trigger pathologic allergic/inflammatory immune reactions. Although it is unclear what causes allergy immunity in humans, the innate immune system might play an important role in allergic susceptibilities.

The innate immune system activates and directs the response of the adaptive immune system, which is characterized by increased antigen specificity and immunological memory.

Adaptive immunity is characterized by the development of antigen-specific immunological memory. Once established, adaptive immunity is characterized by a specific, rapid, and robust response to a previously recognized antigen. In particular, T- and B cell clonal growth in response to antigens (including allergens) results in the development of immunological memory. The development of clonal populations of antigen-specific lymphocytes, which includes both T- and B-cell immune responses, accounts for antibody diversity.

The immunological response begins when the antigen comes into contact with APCs (antigen-presenting cells), such as dendritic cells, monocytes, and macrophages. It is subsequently captured and internalized by endocytosis by APCs which associates with class II MHC (major histocompatibility complex) molecules and re-exposed on the cell surface. Certain cytokines, including IL-1 (Interleukin-1) and IL-2 (which is an autocrine stimulator), activate CD4+ T cells which detect antigenic peptides when they are associated with a class II MHC molecule and to the appropriate costimulatory signals.

Upon activation, CD4 T-lymphocytes undergo immunological differentiation into three pathways: Th1, Th2, or Th17. Th1 response is mediated by IL-12 and interferon-alpha (IFN-alpha) and induces T-cell-mediated cytotoxicity; it is involved in the eradication of intracellular organisms, such as mycobacteria and viruses. Th2 response is mediated by IL-4, IL-5, and IL-13; it is responsible for the production of IgE (immunoglobulin E) and eosinophilia-mediated allergic illness. Th17 response depends on the cytokines transforming growth factor beta (TGF), IL-23, and IL-6; it is involved in the immune defense against extracellular bacteria and fungi, and results in a distinctive neutrophilic inflammatory response [1].

2.4 T-lymphocytes

Adaptive immune responses involve two types of T cells expressing CD4 or CD8 co-receptors. CD4+ T cells, known as helper T (Th) cells, activate and orchestrate immune response by cell surface interaction with other immune cells and release of cytokines. They include CD4+ regulatory T (Treg) cells which regulate immune responses in an inhibitory fashion. CD4+ T cells can specifically recognize antigen-derived peptides presented by MHC class II molecules on APCs, such as dendritic cells, B cells, and macrophages. Conversely, CD8+ cytotoxic T-lymphocytes (CTLs) are specifically activated by microbial antigen-derived peptides presented on MHC class I molecules by any nucleated cell type. Upon antigen recognition, activated CTLs release cytolytic effector molecules which result in the targeted killing of infected cells.

Activated CD4+ T cells differentiate into effector cells that release specific cytokines, defining their functional capabilities (Fig. 2.1). Th1 cells secrete IFN-gamma, while Th2 cells release IL-4, IL-5, IL-9, IL-10, and IL-13. Th17 cells generate IL-17A, IL-17F, and IL-22. Treg cells can produce IL-10 and transform TGF-1, acting as inhibitory regulators rather than effector cells of other immune cells. CD4+ T cells polarization into Th1, Th2, or Th17 cell type is mediated by specific cytokines secreted by other immune cells. IFN-gamma and IL-12 promote Th1 cell development, while IL-4 supports Th2 cell differentiation. IL-13 contributes to Th2 cell induction through an unknown mechanism, not directly impacting CD4+ T cells. Th17 cell growth is induced by IL-6, IL-1, TGF-beta, and in specific circumstances, by IL-23.

2.5 B-lymphocytes

B cells play a crucial role in the development of humoral immune response. They express immunoglobulin on their cell surface, which constitutes the antigen-specific B-cell receptor (BCR).

Naive B-lymphocytes re-circulate among secondary lymphoid organs until they encounter a specific antigen that can bind and cross-link the surface-expressed BCR, thereby leading to becoming activated (which provides signal 1). Most antibody responses, including those to protein antigens, require a second signaling event, which is provided by antigen-specific T cells.

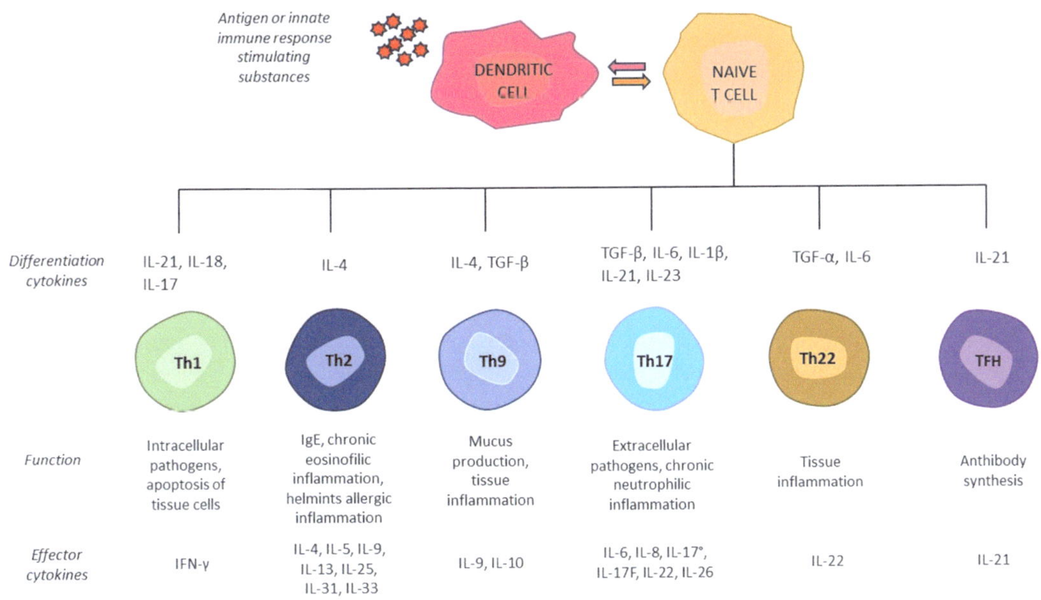

Fig. 2.1 Effector T-cell subsets

The antigen bound to BCR is internalized, digested, and presented on the cell surface in the context of MHC class II molecules. The second activation signal is provided by primed CD4+ T cells that recognize the peptide-MHC class II complex on the B-cell. Cytokines produced by CD4+ helper T cells during B-cell activation control the selection of immunoglobulin heavy-chain constant regions during class-switch recombination, thereby supporting the specific immune response's requirements. In the case of allergens, Th2 cells induce activate B-cell class switch recombination, resulting in elevated levels of allergen-specific IgE.

2.6 Immunoglobulin Structure and Function

B-lymphocyte activation occurs through complex intracellular molecular cascades involving signaling molecules such as the tyrosine kinases LYN, spleen tyrosine kinase (SYK), Bruton tyrosine kinase (BTK), and the mitogen-activated protein (MAP) kinase pathway. This activation pathway is regulated by a co-receptor complex that enhances the BCR's signals and also helps activate B cells. This complex is composed of CD19, complement receptor type 2 (CR2, also known as CD21), and CD81. These signaling steps result in the activation of several transcription factors including the nuclear factor of activated T cells (nfAT), nuclear factor B (nf-B), and activator protein 1 (AP-1). BCR cross-linking of naive and memory B cells results in the activation of their transcription programs and circulation between draining lymph nodes and target organs.

Each type of immunoglobulins is constituted by two identical heavy chains and two identical light chains. Light chains are connected to heavy chains by disulfide bonds but lack transmembrane domains. A unique set of disulfide bonds binds the two heavy chains together. Both heavy and light chains include a constant region (C) and a variable region (V). Through DNA recombination in the bone marrow, B cells generate a diverse repertoire of immunoglobulins by combining variability (V), diversity (D), and joining (J) regions of both heavy and light chains. Immunoglobulin diversity is what characterizes the fine response to pathogens. It is due to four mechanisms: multiple V(D)J genes in the germline, a random distribution of heavy chains and light chains, junctional nucleotide variability introduced during pre-B-cell immunoglobulin gene rearrangement, and somatic hypermutation of immunoglobulin variable regions following encounters with antigens. The five primary constant-region variants are specific of IgM, IgD, IgG, IgE, and IgA [2].

2.7 Immune Tolerance

To counteract inflammation, a counter-regulatory system is required. It acts by downregulating the immune response once the threat has been removed, preventing tissue damage, and blocking the inflammatory response activated against host tissues or harmless substances. All of these mechanisms contribute to immunological tolerance, which is organized into peripheral and central tolerance.

Central Tolerance It affects primary lymphoid organs like the thymus. In the thymus, mature thymocytes interact with cortical epithelial cells, enabling the presentation of self-antigens through major histocompatibility complex (MHC) molecules to T-cell receptors (TCRs) on thymocytes. This interaction leads to the removal of self-reactive T cells through negative selection. At the corticomedullary junction, various cells present autoantigens to further negatively select autoreactive T cells. Those CD4+ T cells that evade negative selection differentiate into central regulatory T (Treg) cells. These Treg cells play a crucial role in controlling immune reactions to self-antigens in the periphery, ensuring immune tolerance.

Peripheral Tolerance It affects peripheral lymph nodes, Peyer's patches, and tonsils. Various mechanisms, such as apoptosis induced by neighboring cells, suppressive cytokines, and regulatory T cells, contribute to the tolerance of effector T cells and to the maintenance of low tissue inflammation. Tissue cells in immunologically privileged organs employ strategies to inhibit or eliminate highly activated effector cells that could harm the tissues. The activation of CD4+ T cells occurs through the interaction of the TCR with antigens presented on APCs by MHC class II molecules. Costimulatory receptors, such as CD28 and ICOS, play a role in T-cell activation, while the absence of costimulatory signals can lead to T-cell anergy to activatory stimuli.

T-regulatory (or regulatory T) **cells (Tregs)** suppress the immune response, express CD4 + CD25+ surface molecules the transcription factor FOXP3, and produce immunosuppressive cytokines such as IL-10 and transforming growth factor-beta (TGF-beta1), playing an important role in suppressing allergic reaction in healthy subjects [3].

2.8 Allergy Immunology

2.8.1 Type-2 Innate Lymphoid Cells (ILC2)

Innate lymphoid cells (ILC) have been identified as populations of lymphoid cells that partially lack rearranged antigen receptors, differently from B- and T-lymphocytes, but they share phenotypic and functional features with these cells. ILLC populations can be divided into three groups, mirroring the adaptive immunity. Type 1 ILC (ILC1) expresses the transcription factor T-bet by default and secretes IFN-gamma when activated. Type 2 ILC (ILC2) expresses the transcription factor GATA 3 constitutively and produces IL-5 and IL-13 in response to IL-25, IL-33, and TSLP stimulation. Type 3 ILC (ILC3) expresses the transcription factor ROR-gamma and produces IL-17, IL-22, and IFN-gamma in response to IL-1beta and IL-23. ILC2 is involved in the development of allergy and regulates the mucosal environment.

2.8.2 Antigen-Presenting Dendritic Cells

Dendritic cells (DCs) and Langerhans cells are the most significant antigen-presenting cells for their ability to elicit a primary immune response and allergen sensitization. Immature DCs are located in the context of tissues where they can encounter and capture antigens such as the skin, the intestinal lamina propria, and the lungs. After capturing antigens, these cell types migrate to the lymph nodes, where they become mature and capable of inducing differentiation of T-cells. Mature DCs are divided into myeloid and plasmacytoid based on inducing Th1 or Th2 differentiation. In allergy, plasmacytoid DCs induce the T-cell polarization to Th2 response. These cells are also known for creating continuous effector responses, critical in maintaining allergic inflammation. Monocytes and macrophages are involved in the elicitation phase of allergy, activating memory T-cells through a re-exposure to a specific allergen.

2.8.3 IgE and IgE Receptor

IgE is the immunoglobulin type which is involved in the allergic response. Their synthesis requires two steps: the first is mediated by IL-4 and IL-13 and results in isotype-specific transcription, and the second involves the interaction on B- and T-lymphocytes, mediated by CD40 and CD40Ligand, respectively, and induces the class recombination mechanism.

The linkage between IgE and their receptor is important for inducing the allergic response. There are different types of receptors for IgE, but the most important ones are the high-affinity IgE receptor (FcεRI) and the low-affinity IgE receptor FcεRII (CD23). Once they meet the antigen, they trigger an intracellular signaling cascade that results in allergic inflammation, which involves mast cells, eosinophils, and basophils. The presence of a high-affinity IgE receptor (FcεRI) associated with an allergen-specific IgE also on APCs' cell surface is an important step for the allergic response because this complex promotes the initial antigen uptake and presentation.

2.8.4 Development of the Allergic Response

Central to the development of the allergic response is the Th2 response, which is mainly activated in subjects with atopy. It is the pivotal point for the mechanisms that lead to the activation of allergy effectors.

Once the allergen is encountered, Th2 lymphocytes expand rapidly. This is also due to the secretion by the epithelial cells of cytokines such as IL-25, IL-33, and TSLP (thymic stromal lymphopoietin). Once the Th2 response is activated, lymphocytes release cytokines such as IL-4, IL-5, and IL-13, which induce IgE formation and eosinophilia (Fig. 2.2). In particular, IL-4 and IL-13 enable the isotype switching to IgE in antigen-specific B cells; IL-5 and IL-9 enable eosinophil activation; IL-3, IL-4, and IL-9 contribute to mast cell activation; IL-9 is responsible for mucus secretions.

To a lesser extent, Th1 and Th17 responses also participate in the development of allergy. The Th1 response is important for the development in the "effector phase." Eczematous lesions in atopic dermatitis and bronchial cell detachment in asthma are mediated by the secretion of IFN-gamma, TNF-alpha, and Fas-ligand. The Th1 response and the Th17 response contribute to the activation of eosinophils, thus contributing to determining the severity of the allergy [4].

2.9 Cytokines and Chemokines in Allergic Inflammation (Table 2.1)

2.9.1 IL-4

Its main role of IL-4 is to induce the isotypic class switch of B cells from IgM to IgE-expressing cells. It also regulates the lymphocyte differentiation response to become Th2. Finally, it induces the endothelial expression of VCAM-1 (vascular cell adhesion molecule-1), which promotes the migration of T-lymphocytes, eosinophils, basophils, and monocytes, but not of neutrophils, as a hallmark of the allergic reaction. The receptor for IL-4 is present on the surface of mast cells, where it stimulates the expression of the receptor for IgE and the synthesis of leukotriene C4 (LTC4). The receptor for IL-4 includes

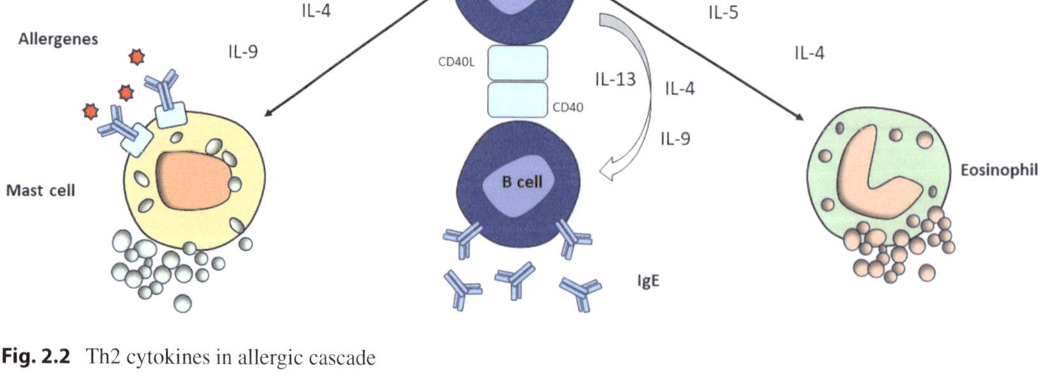

Fig. 2.2 Th2 cytokines in allergic cascade

Table 2.1 Cytokines in allergy

IL-4	Istotipic class switch of IgM to IgE Differentiates lymphocyte response in Th2 direction Induces endothelial expression of VCAM1 with migration of T lymphocytes, eosinophils, monocytes, and basophils
IL-5	Stimulates differentiations of basophils Promotes eosinophils formation Attracts and activates mature eosinophils inducing their secretion and toxicity and increasing their survival
IL-9	Induces synthesis of mast-cells proteases, inflammatory cytokines, and chemokines Stimulates T-cell and eosinophil chemotactic factors in airway epithelial cells
IL-13	Istotipic class switch of IgM to IgE Induces endothelial expression of VCAM1 Induces mucus secretion, bronchial hyper-reactivity, and metaplasia in asthma
IL-25	Drives Th2 immune deviation in adaptive immune response Promotes release of adattive IL-4, IL-5, and IL-13 from Th2 lymphocytes Stimulates release of IL-5 and IL-13 from ILC2 (innate lymphoid cells 2)
IL-33	Increases cytokines secretions by Th2 cells Stimulates ILC2 secretion of IL-5 and IL-13
IL-10	Inhibits production of pro-inflammatory cytokines Induces activation of Th1 and Th2 cells Produces T-ref and B-reg cells crucial for allergy tolerance

the IL4R-alpha chain and the IL-13 receptor; its signaling is mediated by activation of STAT6.

2.9.2 Interleukin-5 (IL-5)

The most important growth factor for eosinophils is IL-5, which can also stimulate the differentiation of basophils. In addition to promoting eosinophil formation, IL-5 attracts and activates mature eosinophils, inducing their secretion and increasing cytotoxicity. IL-5 enhances eosinophil accumulation by regulating chemokine responses and d2 integrin on eosinophils, allowing them to adhere to endothelial cells expressing VCAM-1. By inhibiting apoptosis, IL-5 increases eosinophil survival.

2.9.3 Interleukin-9 (IL-9)

Through its ability to induce the synthesis of mast cell proteases, inflammatory cytokines, and chemokines, IL-9, which is produced primarily by the Th2 lymphocytes, contributes to mast cell-mediated allergic reactions. It also acts synergically with IL-4 and IL-5. IL-9 stimulates T-cell and eosinophil chemotactic factors, such as CCL11 (eotaxin), CCL2 (MCP-1), CCL3 (MIP-1alpha), and CCL7 (MCP-3), in airway epithelial cells.

2.9.4 Interleukin-13 (IL-13)

IL-13 shares many functional activities with IL-4, such as induction of class isotype switching and VCAM-1 expression, due in part to the shared receptor chain of the two cytokines. IL-13 is particularly important for mucus secretion and for induction of nonspecific airway hyperreactivity (AHR). It is also the cause of the characteristic metaplasia present in asthma and the replacement of epithelial cells by Goblet cells.

2.9.5 Interleukin-25 (IL-25)

Injured epithelial cells produce IL-25, a key innate immunological signal that drives Th2 immune polarization in the ensuing adaptive immune response. IL-25 promotes the release of IL-4, IL-5, and IL-13 by Th2 lymphocytes, but it also stimulates the release of IL-5 and IL-13 from type 2 innate lymphoid cells (ILC2).

2.9.6 Interleukin-33 (IL-33)

IL-33 increases cytokine secretion by Th2 cells and, like IL-25, increases ILC2 secretion of IL-5 and IL-13. It is largely expressed by bronchial epithelial cells, but it is also expressed by fibroblasts and smooth muscle cells, and it is inducible in lung and dermal fibroblasts, keratinocytes, activated DCs, and macrophages. Th2-like cells, macrophages, hematopoietic stem cells, eosinophils, basophils, mast cells, ILC2, and fibroblasts share the expression of the IL-33 receptor.

2.9.7 Thymic Stromal Lymphopoietin (TSLP)

TSLP is expressed by skin, gut, and lung epithelial cells and primes local DC, resulting in Th2 immune deviation. TSLP levels are elevated in the keratinocytes of atopic dermatitis patients and in the lungs of asthmatic patients.

Through its ability to produce IL-25, IL-33, and TSLP, injured epithelium plays a critical role in promoting allergic inflammation. TSLP predominantly acts on DCs to elicit a Th2-like response. Furthermore, both IL-25 and IL-33 operate directly on mast cells to stimulate their production of Th2-associated cytokines. More importantly, IL-25, TSLP, and IL-33 stimulate ILC2 to produce more selectively the cytokines IL-5 and IL-13. These cytokine activities on ILC2 and mast cells can occur in the absence of continued allergen exposure, implying an allergen-independent mechanism for the persistence of allergic inflammation.

2.9.8 TGF-Beta

TGF-beta function has been related to immune response inhibition and the formation of Treg cell populations. TGF-beta, on the other hand, has a complex impact on allergic illness, including evidence of disease promotion and disease inhibition. TGF-beta may play a role in a negative feedback mechanism that regulates asthmatic airway repair and inflammation, inducing remodeling and fibrosis and so exacerbating disease progression in people.

2.9.9 IL-10

IL-10 inhibits the production of proinflammatory cytokines and the activation of Th1 and Th2 cells, which is primarily due to IL-10's mediated effects on APCs and direct effects on T-cell activity. The activity of IL-10 and IL-10-producing Treg and Breg cells is crucial for allergy tolerance. IL-10 helps to regulate allergy and asthma symptoms [5].

2.9.10 Mast Cells

Mast cells originate from CD34 hematopoietic progenitor cells in the bone marrow and undergo maturation in specific tissues. Their development and survival depend on interactions between the c-kit receptor and the stem cell factor derived from fibroblasts. Unlike mature basophils, mast cells are not commonly found in the bloodstream. Instead, they are widely distributed in connective tissues, positioned near blood vessels, and epithelial surfaces. Mast cells maintain tissue homeostasis by participating in wound repair, vascularization, and protection against bacterial infection and envenomation. Activation of mast cells by allergens contributes to the development of allergic symptoms.

The primary pathway for mast cell activation in allergies involves the FcεRI receptor, which has a high affinity for IgE. When a multivalent allergen attaches to allergen-specific IgE on FcεRI, it triggers mast cell activation. This activation leads to granule enlargement, crystal breakdown, fusion, and the subsequent release of mediators through anaphylactic degranulation. Additionally, mast cells produce arachidonic acid metabolites upon IgE-dependent activation. Human mast cells can be categorized into two subpopulations: those with tryptase and those with both tryptase and chymase.

Mast cells contain a diverse range of mediators that have various effects on allergic inflammation and organ function. These include preformed granule-associated mediators like histamine, serine proteases, and proteoglycans, as well as lipid, cytokine, and chemokine mediators synthesized and released upon appropriate stimulation. Notably, mast cell-derived lipid mediators, such as prostaglandin D2 and leukotrienes (LTC4, LTD4, and LTE4), exhibit potent pro-inflammatory activities. Mast cells also produce cytokines that promote Th2-type responses, inflammation, and regulate tissue remodeling. Immunologic activation of mast cells begins with the cross-linkage between IgE bound to FcεRI and a multivalent allergen. The levels of FcεRI on mast cell surfaces can be influenced by IL-4, IgE, and therapeutic agents targeting serum IgE levels.

2.9.11 Eosinophils

Eosinophils, derived from bone marrow, play a crucial role in the pathogenesis of various disorders, including asthma, allergies, and parasitic infections. Unlike other white blood cells, eosinophils produce a diverse range of mediators, such as proteins, cytokines, lipids, and enzymes. They express receptors that recognize different immunoglobulin components. Although eosinophils degranulate when exposed to certain types of immunoglobulins, the extent of degranulation is not significant. IL-5 stimulates various activities of eosinophils, including the production of certain compounds, phagocytosis, and degranulation. Other cytokines like TSLP and IL-33 also stimulate eosinophil functions such as adhering to matrix proteins, producing cytokines, and degranulation.

Allergic diseases are characterized by an increase in eosinophil count in the blood and by eosinophil tissue infiltration. Eosinophils contribute to both innate and adaptive immune responses. Similarly to mast cells, they contain granules that release inflammatory proteins. These proteins, including major basic proteins, eosinophil-derived neurotoxin, peroxidase, and cationic protein, damage epithelial cells, induce airway hyperresponsiveness, and trigger degranulation of basophils and mast cells. Major basic proteins released from eosinophils can interfere with the function of the M2 muscarinic receptor, leading to increased levels of acetylcholine and enhanced airway hyperreactivity. Eosinophils are also a significant source of prostaglandins, leukotrienes, cytokines (such as IL-4, IL-5, and TNF-α), proteolytic enzymes, and reactive oxygen intermediates, all of which contribute to allergic tissue inflammation.

The function of eosinophils in allergic disease is regulated by several cytokines. Eosinophils develop and mature in the bone marrow under the influence of IL-3, IL-5, and GM-CSF. Allergen exposure activates hematopoietic CD34 cells, leading to the expression of the IL-5 receptor and subsequent eosinophil maturation, synthesis of granule proteins, prolonged survival, enhanced degranulation, and release from the bone marrow. GM-CSF also promotes eosinophil proliferation, survival, cytokine production, and degranulation. Chemokines like CCL11, CCL5, and CCL3 play a crucial role in recruiting eosinophils to sites of allergic tissue inflammation. Eotaxin mobilizes eosinophil colony-forming progenitor cells from the bone marrow, which are quickly cleared from the blood and either return to the bone marrow or migrate to inflamed tissues [6].

2.9.12 Basophils

Basophils, which account for less than 1% of blood leukocytes, are mature cells that originate in the bone marrow. They contribute to the development of allergic reactions by infiltrating sites of allergic inflammation and releasing mediators and cytokines that promote type I immediate hypersensitivity reactions. Degranulation, triggered by the interaction between allergens and specific IgE molecules attached to high-affinity IgE receptors on basophils, leads to the release of these mediators. This IgE-dependent activation also results in the production of immunomodulatory cytokines. Moreover, basophils are particularly significant as a major source of IL-4 and IL-13.

2.10 Mechanism of Allergic Inflammation

IgE-mediated immune responses can be categorized into three distinct reaction patterns based on the timeline (Table 2.2). The **early-phase response** occurs immediately after allergen exposure and involves mast cell degranulation and release of preformed mediators within 1–30 min, resolving within 1–3 h. Acute reactions result in increased vascular permeability, leading to plasma protein leakage, tissue swelling, and symptoms like itching, sneezing, wheezing, or abdominal cramps, depending on the affected organ.

A second reaction pattern, known as the **late-phase response**, occurs within hours of allergen exposure, peaking at 6–12 h and resolving within 24 h. Neutrophils, eosinophils, basophils, monocytes, macrophages, and Th2-type cells infiltrate the affected tissue, facilitated by adhesion molecules and cytokine control. Chemokines, such as CCL5, CCL3, CCL7, and CCL13, attract eosinophils and mononuclear cells, while eotaxins selectively attract eosinophils to the site of late-phase responses and allergic inflammation. Blocking these chemokines reduces the migration of allergic effector cells to the affected tissue. This response is characterized by edema, redness, induration, nasal blockage, airway obstruction, and persistent wheezing.

In the third reaction pattern, **chronic allergic disease**, tissue inflammation can persist for extended periods. Factors like recurrent allergen and microbial exposure contribute to ongoing inflammation. Stimulated allergic effector cells, along with Th2-type cytokines, prolong the survival of these cells and induce local differentiation of eosinophils, exacerbating tissue damage. Chronic allergic disease involves tissue remodeling, leading to irreversible changes in organs, such as thickening of airway walls, smooth muscle hypertrophy, and hyperplasia. Generally, asthma, atopic dermatitis, chronic rhinosinusitis, and allergic rhinitis are characterized by a type 2 immune response. Th2 cells, type 2 B cells, ILC2, IL-4-secreting NK, T cells, basophils, eosinophils, and mast cells, along with their major cytokines, play significant roles in this response. Epithelial cells secrete IL-25, IL-31, IL-33, and TSLP, which further contribute to eosinophilic asthma-like airway inflammation through the activation of lung ILC2s.

By activating resident cells in target organs, Th2 cytokines not only support allergic inflam-

Table 2.2 Allergic inflammation patterns

Early-phase response	Immediately after allergen exposure
	Involves mast cell degranulation and release of preformed mediators
	Peak in 1–30 min resolving within 1–3 h
	Symptoms like itching, sneezing, wheezing, or abdominal cramps
	Reactions: acute rhinoconjunctivitis, acute asthma attack, urticaria, gastrointestinal reactions in food allergy, anaphylaxis
Late-phase response	Within hours of allergen exposure
	Local recruitment of neutrophils, eosinophils, basophils, monocytes, macrophages, and Th2 cells
	Peak at 6–12 h resolving within 24 h
	Symptoms like edema, redness, induration, nasal blockage, airway obstruction, and persistent wheezing
Chronic allergic disease	Can persist for extended periods
	Repeated stimulation of mast cells, basophils, eosinophils, and Th2 cells exacerbates tissue damage
	Tissue remodeling
	Reactions: Asthma, atopic dermatitis, chronic rhinosinusitis, allergic rhinitis

mation but also have an impact on tissue remodeling. They induce mucus hypersecretion, fibroblast growth, synthesis of extracellular matrix proteins, and fibrosis. TGF-β produced by eosinophils and fibroblasts enhances subepithelial fibrosis. IL-11 expressed by eosinophils and epithelial cells contributes to subepithelial fibrosis and collagen deposition. These tissue injury steps amplify proinflammatory cytokine release, extracellular matrix deposition, and angiogenesis.

Genetic predisposition and subsequent infiltration of Th1 and Th17 cells enhance the inflammatory potential of allergic effector cells, leading to chronic tissue inflammatory responses. Autoimmune responses involving IgE and IgG autoantibodies, as well as autoreactivity of Th1 and Th17 cells, may also contribute to allergic inflammation in genetically predisposed individuals.

2.11 Genetic Bases of Atopy

Allergic diseases result from a complex interplay of genetic factors and environmental triggers. Multiple genes are implicated in allergic diseases, including those involved in regulating systemic atopy expression, controlling barrier function in specific organs, and encoding pattern-recognition receptors of the innate immune system. Genetic predisposition contributes to prolonged inflammation and aberrant tissue remodeling once an allergic response has started.

Atopic diseases show a strong familial predisposition, as suggested by twin studies which have revealed approximately 60% heritability for asthma and atopic dermatitis in twins. Genes on 5q23-35 region, such as Th2 type cytokine related genes (IL-3, IL-4, IL-5, IL-9, IL-13, GM-CSF), contribute to genetic predisposition. Notably, IL-4 and IL-13 variants are associated with asthma and atopic dermatitis. Chromosome 16 also contributes to atopy, with a gain-of-function polymorphism in the IL-4R alpha subunit gene. Genome-wide searches have linked atopy to the 11q13 region, proposing the beta subunit of FcεRI (FcεRI-β) gene as a candidate gene. Additionally, chromosome 6 harbors genes encoding human leukocyte antigen (HLA) class I and class II molecules, influencing the immune responses to specific allergens. TNF-alpha and genetic polymorphisms in IL-33 and its receptor IL-1RL1 (ST2) are also strongly associated with asthma.

Barrier dysfunction plays a crucial role in the pathogenesis of allergic diseases. Genetic studies highlight the importance of chromosome 1q21 region, which contains genes involved in epidermal differentiation. In particular, filaggrin, essential for stratum corneum formation, and SPINK5, a serine protease inhibitor gene, which are associated with atopic dermatitis. Mutations in SPINK5 increase the risk of developing atopic dermatitis and asthma. Candidate genes for asthma susceptibility, including GPRA, ADAM-33, and DPP10, have been identified through positional cloning. Pattern-recognition receptors, such as CD14 and Toll-like receptor 2, also influence disease susceptibility by recognizing microbial components. Overall, dysregulation of genetic factors involved in atopy, barrier function, immune response, and pattern recognition contributes to the development of allergic diseases.

2.12 Asthma

Asthma is a chronic lung disease characterized by inflammation of the airways, excessive mucus production, and heightened bronchial sensitivity. The inflammatory cells involved in asthma include eosinophils, lymphocytes, mast cells, basophils, and neutrophils to varying degrees.

Exposure of the airways to proteases from common allergens, like mites and molds, disrupts the integrity of the airway epithelium and triggers the production of TSLP by the epithelial cells. TSLP promotes the expansion of basophils, prolongs the survival of eosinophils, and increases the production of inflammatory chemokines CCL2, CXCL1, and CXCL8 by eosinophils. In addition to TSLP, also IL-25 and IL-33 are produced by the epithelial cells, induced by allergen exposure or epithelial damage. IL-25 and IL-33 enhance the production of TSLP by epithelial cells and mast cells, stimulate mast cells to release IL-4, IL-5, IL-13, CCL1, and CXCL8, promote eosinophil survival, and increase eosinophil production of CCL2 and CCL3. Basophils, when activated, release IL-4, IL-13, granulocyte-macrophage colony-stimulating factor (GM-CSF), CCL3, histamine, and LTC4, leading to vasodilation and increased vascular permeability.

The activation and differentiation of naïve T cells into Th2 cells involve the downregulation of L-selectin and CCR7 and the appearance of CCR4, CCR8, CRTh2 (chemoattractant receptor-homologous molecule expressed on Th2 cells), and the BLT1 receptor for leukotriene B4 (LTB4). These receptors enable Th2 cells to migrate toward higher concentrations of CCL17, CCL22, CCL1, prostaglandin D2 (PGD2), and LTB4, which are released by dendritic cells (DCs) and activated mast cells.

The asthma reaction involves many distinct events, including the contraction of airway smooth muscle (ASM) in response to a variety of stimuli, but also the production of extracellular matrix (ECM) proteins, and proteases that control these proteins, and the production of a plethora of growth hormones and cytokines. These factors combine together to cause airway remodeling, which includes thickening of the airway wall, enhanced angiogenesis, mucous cell hyperplasia, basement membrane thickening, and muscle mass increase. It is now clear that inflammation and remodeling occur along different paths. This is consistent with the discovery that bronchoconstriction can cause airway remodeling in the absence of an inflammatory or allergic trigger. ASM expresses TLR1–TLR10 messenger RNAs (mRNAs) as well as functional TLR2 and TLR3, showing that these cells can respond to bacterial and viral infections. By activating cell adhesion molecules and secreting chemokines and cytokines, ASM affects leukocyte trafficking and function in asthma [7].

2.13 Atopic Dermatitis

Atopic dermatitis is a chronic inflammatory skin condition characterized by persistent itching and by the presence of immune cells such as CD4+ memory T-lymphocytes, dendritic cell subsets, eosinophils, and mast cells in the subepidermal, intraepidermal, and perivascular regions. The pathogenesis of atopic dermatitis begins with intense itching and subsequent mechanical damage caused by chronic scratching. This mechanical trauma triggers the release of histamine, neuropeptides, proteases, kinins, and cytokines by mast cells, which contribute to subsequent worsening the itching. Additionally, mechanical assault leads to increased levels of TSLP in the skin, which stimulates dendritic cell activation and the synthesis of CCL17 and CCL22 by dendritic cells. The leukocyte infiltration is primarily due to the excessive production of various chemokines, including CCL13, CCL11, and CCL26, which bind CCR2 and CCR3 ligands and recruit eosinophils and mast cells, CCL22 and CCL1, which bind CCR4 and CCR8 and recruit Th2 cells, and CCL27, which binds CCR10 and facilitates T-cell migration into the epidermis.

The interaction between cutaneous lymphocyte antigen (CLA) and E-selectin, produced on inflamed endothelium cells, is essential for the trafficking of memory T-lymphocytes into the skin. CLA, together with CCR4, and CCR6 are the trafficking molecules that T cells express most abundantly in healthy skin, followed by CCR8. CCL27, the only known CCR10 ligand, and skin endothelial cells and keratinocytes express CCL17, one of the CCR4 ligands, which is elevated during inflammation.

Keratinocyte apoptosis, which is linked to multiple elements including the cytokines IFN-gamma, TNF-alpha, TNF-related weak inducer of apoptosis (TWEAK), and IL-32, and the Fas-Fas-ligand interaction is a feature of both allergic contact dermatitis and atopic dermatitis.

2.14 Structural Cells' Contribution to Allergic Inflammation

Despite carrying out their specific tasks, structural cells like epithelium, bone, smooth muscle cells, and fibroblast also produce cytokines, chemokines, lipid mediators, and growth factors that control immune cell mobility and the environment's inflammatory state. Allergy airway sickness symptoms are "neuronally" mediated in response to inflammation. As a result, these structural cells play important roles in the genesis and symptoms of allergic disease and asthma, working in tandem with immune cells.

The epithelium plays a crucial role as a protective barrier between the lung's interior environment and the external surroundings. It encounters inhaled particles, contaminants, respiratory viruses, and allergens present in the air, making it an important physical and immunological barrier. The epithelium detects PAMPs on inhaled foreign substances through PRRs and regulates airway homeostasis by producing various mediators such as GM-CSF, TSLP, IL-25, and IL-33. These mediators induce a Th2 bias in dendritic cell precursors, bridging the gap between innate and adaptive immune responses and converting environmental exposures into disease phenotypes.

The structure and function of the airway epithelium are altered in people with asthma. Asthmatic epithelium differs significantly from that of nonasthmatic individuals. Goblet cell hyperplasia and excessive mucus production are commonly detected in asthma and contribute significantly to the disease's morbidity and mortality. Additionally, epithelial cells from asthma patients exhibit a weakened innate immune response to type I antiviral interferons.

Tight junctions (TJs) play a central role in sealing the epithelial layers and forming a barrier between the external environment and the underlying tissues. They regulate the flow of substances through the spaces between cells and control epithelial permeability, preventing the entry of foreign particles like allergens and toxins into subepithelial tissues. Abnormalities in TJ function and integrity have been observed in allergic and inflammatory conditions such as atopic dermatitis, asthma, and chronic rhinosinusitis. Additionally, TJ dysfunction in smooth muscle cells has been implicated in the development of asthma.

The neurological system also plays an important role in host defense within the airways. In reaction to inflammation, the neurological system protects the airways by orchestrating reflexes such as sneezing, coughing, mucus secretion, and bronchospasm. As a result, the nervous system serves as the primary link between the immunologic components of allergic inflammation and the symptoms of acute hypersensitivity. As with allergy, nerve-immune interactions can be inappropriate and harmful; allergen exposure can activate an immune response that involves the recruitment of the nervous system, which can have detrimental effects on the host and contribute to the development or worsening of allergic disease symptoms. These symptoms include irritation, itching, sneezing, coughing, excessive mucus production, reversible bronchospasm, and difficulty breathing (dyspnea). Allergic reactions in the respiratory tract are also linked to overt activation, increases in electrical excitability, and phenotypic alterations in sensory, central, and autonomic neurons [8].

2.15 Cytokine Networks in Allergic Inflammation

Allergic diseases have been associated with several proinflammatory cytokines, including IL-4, IL-5, IL-9, IL-13, IL-1beta, IL-6, TNF-alpha, and GM-CSF. They are released by various cell types, such as macrophages and epithelial cells, and they play a role in amplifying the allergic inflammatory response. These cytokines are selectively targeted and neutralized by biological immune response modifiers, which give new details on each of their unique activities. For example, IL-4 and IL-13 are involved in IgE synthesis through B-cell isotype switching and have been found to be critical in animal models of asthma.

However, blocking IL-4, IL-13, or their common receptor IL-4Ralpha has not yet shown significant clinical benefits in asthma, although numerous clinical trials are currently underway. IL-5 plays a vital role in the differentiation, survival, and activation of eosinophils. Mepolizumab is a humanized monoclonal antibody that neutralizes IL-5 and has demonstrated a substantial reduction in eosinophil counts in the blood and induced sputum of patients with mild asthma. However, it had no effect on the response to inhaled allergens. In carefully selected patients with severe asthma and eosinophilic sputum, despite high doses of corticosteroids, mepolizumab reduced the frequency of exacerbations and decreased the need for oral corticosteroids, although it did not alleviate symptoms or improve airway hyperresponsiveness (AHR). This suggests that targeting individual cytokines may only provide clinical benefits in specific patient populations.

Current research has shifted focus to upstream regulatory cytokines in asthma pathogenesis, as they are believed to hold greater therapeutic potential. One such cytokine is TSLP, which acts similarly to IL-7 and is involved in initiating and sustaining allergic immune responses. TSLP is predominantly produced by airway and nasal epithelial cells and stimulates immature myeloid dendritic cells, which express the TSLP receptor, leading to their differentiation into mature dendritic cells. TSLP-activated dendritic cells promote the differentiation of naïve CD4+ T cells into a Th2 phenotype, enhancing the expansion of Th2 memory cells and suppressing the IL-12 p40 receptor in dendritic cells. TSLP also contributes to allergic inflammation by activating IL-4 gene transcription in Th2 cells, promoting IL-13 production from mast cells, recruiting eosinophils, and amplifying basophil responses.

TSLP may consequently be crucial in the development of allergic rhinitis, atopic dermatitis, and asthma. It is highly expressed in asthmatic patients' airways, and it is also found in epithelial cells of individuals with allergic rhinitis and atopic dermatitis. Overexpression of TSLP in skin keratinocytes is also thought to be one of the mechanisms of the "allergic march," in which the onset of atopic dermatitis frequently predicts the onset of asthma in children.

IL-25 (also known as IL-17e) promotes allergic inflammation by increasing the production of Th2 cytokines. It is released by various cell types, including mast cells, basophils, eosinophils, macrophages, and epithelial cells. IL-25 blocking has demonstrated efficacy in animal models of allergy illness, leading to the development of IL-25-neutralizing antibodies that are currently undergoing clinical investigation.

IL-33 is instead a member of the IL-1 family. It is constitutively expressed at mucosal surfaces like the airways, located within the nucleus, where it potentially regulates chromatin structure and gene expression. It is released upon damage to epithelial or endothelial cells. In allergic inflammation, it acts as a potential link between innate and adaptive immunity, enhancing ILC2 and Th2 cell function and leading to eosinophilia, mast cell activation, and mucus overproduction. IL-33 also directly activates eosinophils, mast cells, epithelial cells, and dendritic cells and appears to induce the alternative activation of alveolar macrophages (M2 phenotype) observed in animal models of asthma, where its expression is elevated in the airway epithelium, and its levels are correlated with disease severity. IL-33 is also expressed in activated mast cells through IgE receptors and further contributes to mast cell activation. Antibodies that inhibit IL-33 are currently being developed for clinical use [9, 10].

References

1. Akdis M, Akdis CA. Mechanisms of allergen-specific immunotherapy: multiple suppressor factors at work in immune tolerance to allergens. J Allergy Clin Immunol. 2014;133:621–31.
2. Sonnenberg GF, Mjösberg J, Spits H, Artis D. SnapShot: innate lymphoid cells. Immunity. 2013;39:622–622.e1.
3. Dullaers M, De Bruyne R, Ramadani F, Gould HJ, Gevaert P, Lambrecht BN. The who, where, and when of IgE in allergic airway disease. J Allergy Clin Immunol. 2012;129:635–45.
4. Pierce SK, Liu W. The tipping points in the initiation of B cell signalling: how small changes make big differences. Nat Rev Immunol. 2010;10:767–77.
5. Schmitz J, Owyang A, Oldham E, Song Y, Murphy E, McClanahan TK, et al. IL-33, an interleukin-1-like cytokine that signals via the IL-1 receptor-related protein ST2 and induces T helper type 2-associated cytokines. Immunity. 2005;23:479–90.
6. Holgate ST. Epithelium dysfunction in asthma. J Allergy Clin Immunol. 2007;120:1233–44.; quiz 1245-6.
7. Esnault S, Kelly EA. Essential mechanisms of differential activation of eosinophils by IL-3 compared to GM-CSF and IL-5. Crit Rev Immunol. 2016;36:429–44.
8. Kubo T, Morita H, Sugita K, Akdis CA. Introduction to mechanisms of allergic diseases. Robyn E. O'Hehir

Stephen T. Holgate Aziz Sheikh Middleton's allergy essentials 2022; 31: 1–27. Elsevier.
9. Barnes PJ. The cytokine network in asthma and chronic obstructive pulmonary disease. J Clin Invest. 2008;118:3546–56.
10. Fort MM, Cheung J, Yen D, Li J, Zurawski SM, Lo S, et al. IL-25 induces IL-4, IL-5, and IL-13 and Th2-associated pathologies in vivo. Immunity. 2001;15:985–95.

Principles of Allergy Diagnostics

3

Maria Angela Tosca, Matteo Naso, and Giorgio Ciprandi

Abstract

Adequately mastering the principal diagnostic tests available in pediatric allergy is fundamental for correctly managing the patient. This chapter introduces the main tools available to physicians for the diagnosis of allergic diseases, in particular, in vivo and in vitro tests will be discussed, such as skin tests, intradermal tests, serum total immunoglobulin E (IgE) dosage, serum allergen-specific immunoglobulin E (sIgE) for allergens and allergen components dosage, basophil activation test (BAT), fraction exhaled nitric oxide (FeNO), blood count with eosinophil count, eosinophil count in induced sputum, and allergen provocation test. Furthermore, each method's relative indications, advantages, and disadvantages are analyzed. Currently, the skin prick test (SPT) remains the first level of investigation in most cases; the serum dosage of IgE against allergenic extracts or components allows us to define more precise diagnoses through molecular allergy diagnostics. The BAT is a relatively new method that has to be validated internationally. In some cases, such as for food and drug allergies, challenge tests still represent the gold standard for diagnosis; in others, they play an almost marginal role and are relegated to particular situations.

Keywords

Skin prick test · Prick by prick test
Intradermal test · Total immunoglobulin E
Specific immunoglobulin E · Basophil
activation test · Eosinophil · Provocation test
Oral food challenge · Molecular diagnostic
Fraction exhaled of nitric oxide · Eosinophil
count in induced sputum

Test your learning and check your understanding of this book's contents: use the "Springer Nature Flashcards" app to access questions using ▶ https://sn.pub/nspbjm. To use the app, please follow the instructions in Chap. 1.

M. A. Tosca (✉) · M. Naso
Allergy Unit, IRCCS Istituto Giannina Gaslini (IGG), Genoa, Italy
e-mail: mariangelatosca@gaslini.org

G. Ciprandi
Allergy Center, Casa di Cura Villa Montallegro, Genoa, Italy

C. Caffarelli, G. L. Marseglia (eds.), *Textbook of Pediatric Allergy*,
https://doi.org/10.1007/978-3-031-71283-8_3

3.1 Introduction

The diagnosis of allergic diseases represents the initial step in managing allergic patients. The diagnostic work-up is paramount because identifying the causative allergen could correspond to the treatment of the allergic disease. Avoiding the causative allergen may be the only solution to the problem.

Classically, the diagnostic procedure consists of several steps. The first step is the subject's medical history, which aims at defining the type of symptoms, their severity, chronology, and especially the correlation with exposure to the suspected allergen. In principle, the diagnosis of allergic disease is based on two basic requirements: documentation of the production of specific IgE (sensitization) and the demonstration of a causal link, that is, the appearance of symptoms immediately after exposure to the sensitizing allergen (true allergy). This process is fundamental, and only with this reasoning can a true allergy be diagnosed. The most common mistake is to confuse a simple sensitization with a confirmed allergy.

Sensitization can be documented with allergy testing, which is divided into three levels. The first-level test is the skin prick test. The second-level examination is the serum allergen-specific IgE assay. This examination can be conducted using raw extracts or allergic molecules. Finally, the third level is organ-specific provocation tests. In addition, other additional tests may be performed as detailed further.

Physical examination plays a pivotal role in allergy diagnostics by providing valuable insights into a patient's clinical presentation and aiding in the identification of potential allergens. While laboratory tests and medical histories are essential to the diagnostic process, physical examination complements them by offering direct observations and tangible evidence. Physical findings help guide further investigations and allow for more accurate diagnoses. Additionally, physical examination enables the identification of potential triggers in the environment, such as pollen or animal dander, by evaluating the patient's responses to specific stimuli. A thorough physical examination is crucial in the allergy diagnostic process, facilitating personalized treatment plans and improved patient outcomes (Fig. 3.1).

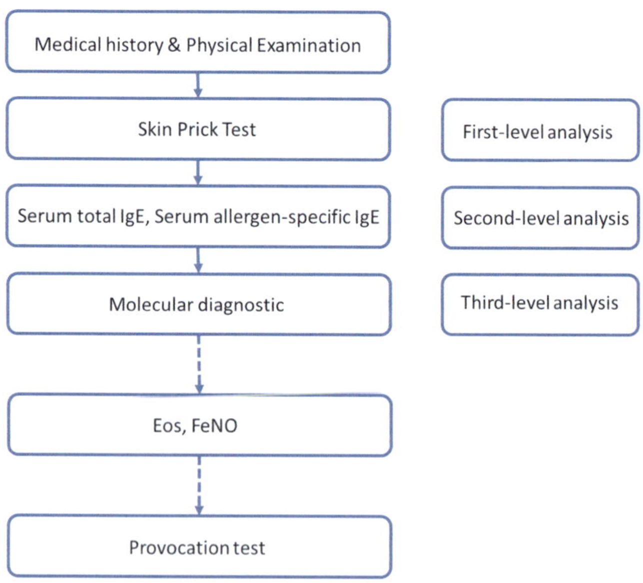

Fig. 3.1 Allergy diagnostic flowchart. *IgE* immunoglobulin E, *Eos* eosinophils, *FeNO* fraction exhaled nitric oxide

3.2 Skin Prick Test

Skin prick test (SPT) is the first level assay to document sensitization, such as the production of allergen-specific IgE. Namely, SPT is the simplest in vivo method to assess the presence of specific **Immunoglobulin E** (IgE) in a patient in whom a sensitization to inhalant, food, drug, or occupational allergen is suspected. SPT can be performed at any age, has high sensibility and specificity, is easy to perform, reliable, moderately cheap, and safe with rare anaphylaxis and no fatalities reported [1].

SPT provides objective confirmation of an IgE-mediated process that expresses sensitivity to allergens and should be evaluated in light of the patient's clinical history. SPT is performed with lancets generally designed to penetrate the skin for 1 mm [2]. A droplet of the allergen can be applied on the skin, and a prick through the drop can be made. When an antigen is applied to the skin of a sensitized patient, the antigen crosslinks IgE antibodies on the surface of cutaneous mast cells. This event results in the degranulation of mast cells and releasing mediators such as histamine, leading to a wheal and flare reaction that occurs in 15–20 min [3].

In children, the site of choice for the procedure is the volar surface of the forearms. Suppose the overall surface of the forearms is too small or there are active lesions on the skin. In that case, it is at the doctor's discretion to perform the test at a different site, bearing in mind that the reactivity to skin prick tests varies in different body districts. For example, the back is much more reactive than the volar surface of the forearms [4].

The location of every allergen can be marked with a pen or by using a test grid. Every prick should be performed at a minimum distance of 2 cm to avoid false-positive reactions due to direct contamination of a nearby test or secondary to an axon reflex [5].

As mentioned above, lancets are generally designed to limit skin penetration depth to 1 mm. Different degrees of pressure exerted through the lancets can result in different depth penetrations. A more profound or superficial prick can alter the test leading to a false positive or negative result. Induced bleeding raises the probability of a false positive [6].

Skin prick tests can be performed only on healthy skin. Patients affected by urticaria, **atopic dermatitis**, allergic contact dermatitis, or other inflammatory skin conditions cannot be tested with SPT in the active area of the disease. Up to 2–5% of the population may have **dermographism** and, as a consequence, an exaggerated response to minor skin trauma such as a skin prick test that may alter the result [7] (Table 3.1). Consequently, sensitization should be evaluated through in vitro tests such as dosing allergen-specific immunoglobulin E (sIgE).

Several medications can influence skin prick tests. It is always necessary to ask the patient about his recent drug history. Medications that inhibit mast cell degranulation or block histamine H1 receptors may suppress skin response to the test [8]. **Antihistamines** are the drugs that most frequently can alter the test result. The suppressive effect of antihistamines varies with the tissue concentration and half-life [9, 10]. Oral antihistamines typically suppress the cutaneous response to skin prick tests for 2–11 days after the last intake (Table 3.2).

Other drugs interfere with SPT: **Omalizumab**, a monoclonal anti-IgE antibody, may alter the result for 8–16 weeks after the last administration [11]; topical steroids inhibit the wheal and flare reaction in treated skin areas [12]; short-term systemic corticosteroid therapy seems not to affect the result of SPT, while long-term systemic corticosteroids might suppress skin reaction [13, 14]. **Leukotriene** receptor antagonists do not appear to interact with SPT results [15]. Furthermore, antidepressant with antihistaminic properties, such as tricyclic antidepressants, alters the wheal and flare [16], and even H2 receptor antagonists like ranitidine might reduce the wheal dimension [17, 18] (Table 3.3).

Table 3.1 Most common errors in skin tests

Most common errors in skin test
Do not investigate patient's drug history
Perform prick test on skin with active lesions
Inadequate distance between allergens
Do not mark allergen locations properly
Induction of bleeding during the procedure
Insufficient penetration of allergen (especially with plastic devices)
Spreading of allergen solution during the procedure
Too short or too long interval between application and reading

Table 3.2 Suppressant effects of H1-antihistamines on immediate skin testing

H1-antihistamine	Days suppressed
First generation	
Chlorphenamine	2–6
Clemastine	5–10
Cyproheptadine	9–11
Hydroxyzine	5–8
Second generation	
Bilastine	4–5
Cetirizine	3–10
Ebastina	3–10
Fexofenadine	2
Loratadine	7–10
Rupatadine	3–7
Topical H1-antihistamine	
Nasal levocabastine	Do not suppress skin test
Nasal azelastine	Do not suppress skin test
Nasal olopatadine	Do not suppress skin test

Modified from Ref. [7]

Table 3.3 Suppressant effects of other medication on immediate skin testing

Drugs	Days suppressed
Anti-IgE monoclonal antibody	
Omalizumab	At least 6 weeks. False negatives can occur for up to 1 year
Leukotriene receptor antagonist	
Montelukast	Does not suppress skin test
H2-antagonists	
Ranitidine	1
Tricyclic antidepressants and tranquilizers	
Desipramine	2
Imipramine	>10
Doxepin	6–11
Corticosteroids	
Oral short term	Does not suppress skin test
Oral long term	May suppress skin test
Topical long term	Suppress skin test in the area where has been applied
Local anesthetic	
EMLA (eutectic mixture of local anesthetic) cream	1 h—Only suppress erythema in the area where has been applied

IgE immunoglobulin E; Modified from Ref. [7]

The doctor should evaluate the choice and number of allergens to be tested based on the patient's clinical history [4, 19, 20]. It is recommended to set up an allergen panel that represents an appropriate geographical profile of allergens to which the patient may have been routinely exposed [21, 22].

The panel should always include a positive control (histamine) and a negative control (e.g., saline). Allergen extracts can consist of a mix of allergens belonging to the same taxonomic family, purified single allergens, or, thanks to new advances in technology in molecular biology, recombinant allergens [22, 23]. It should be noted that there is wide variability in quality and potency among the products available on the market. As a consequence, it is always recommended to use standardized allergens. When assuming the loss of relevant allergens due to extract preparation and storage, it is possible to perform SPT with fresh foods, i.e., **prick by prick** (PbP) [24], where a fresh allergen is pricked by a lancet and then immediately pricked into the skin [25].

The reading of the tests should be done at the peak of the reaction and in standardized mode. SPT induces a response between 8–10 min for histamine and 15–20 min for allergens. The least variable, most reproducible, and objective measurement method is using a ruler to measure the wheal size in millimeters (mm) [4].

The measurement of the reaction should be performed by adding the major diameter (D) with the minor diameter (d) of the wheal and dividing the sum by two [(D+d)/2]. Pseudopods should not be included in the measurement but may be marked separately. Wheal diameters >3 mm are considered positive compared to the negative control [7].

SPT may be associated with some discomfort during testing. However, PbP may be associated with a rare risk of anaphylaxis. Foods were identified as the most relevant trigger (75%), with nuts having the highest risk. A history of severe allergic symptoms and large skin test reactions were considered predictors of possible severe adverse reactions to allergy skin testing. The use of SPT is recommended in situations where the confirmation of sensitization is needed and may be performed at any age, recognizing that positive reactions tend to be smaller in infants and younger children (<2 years) and older people [7].

SPT has some contraindications (uncontrolled and severe asthma, severe and unstable cardiovascular disease, and pregnancy) and relative contraindications, such as Beta-blocker therapy and recent anaphylaxis, but overall is a safe and moderately cheap procedure [6].

3.3 Intradermal Test

Introduced by Cooke in 1911, the **Intradermal Test** (IDT) is one of the oldest techniques for allergy testing [26]. This method can be considered in patients with high clinical suspicion and negative SPT or those with lower skin reactivity, but it is fundamentally used in drug and venom allergy. This technique injects 0.02–0.05 ml of diluted antigen (100–1000 fold or more) into the dermis with a small needle to produce a bleb. Then the response is measured after 10–15 min from the injection [1]. A significant wheal and flare is the expression of preformed IgE bound to the surface of mast cells. IDT should always be preceded by SPT, including negative and positive controls.

Skin endpoint titration can be defined as the intradermal injection of allergens at increasing concentrations to measure their allergic response. The endpoint, typically, is the concentration of antigen that causes an increase in the size of the wheal. This method allows us to quantify the individual's skin response grossly and their degree of allergic sensitivity. Skin endpoint titration is used for drugs or **Hymenoptera** venom allergy, while IDTs for foods are potentially dangerous and overly sensitive [27].

IDT has several disadvantages compared to SPT. It is more invasive and, therefore, less tolerated by children due to the discomfort of the procedure. It has a lower safety profile with an increased risk of severe and anaphylactic reactions [28, 29]. Moreover, IDT is not an easy procedure and requires experience.

Diffuse eczema, urticaria, and dermographism are contraindications for IDT, such as poor subject cooperation and inability to stop antihistamines or other interfering drug treatments listed above [7].

3.4 Immunoglobulin E

In 1967, Kimishige Ishikaka and his wife, Teruko Ishizaka, isolated the fifth immunoglobulin class from the serum of a person highly sensitive to ragweed pollen. They called it erythema (E)-induced gamma globulin (immunoglobulin E, IgE). The two scientists described the binding of IgE to mast cells and basophils, demonstrated that antigen bridging of cell-bound IgE is required for histamine release, and studied the regulatory mechanisms of IgE production. Concurrently with Ishizaka's, two Swedish researchers at Uppsala University, Hans Bennich, and S.G.O. Johansson isolated IgE from a patient with multiple myeloma. In 1968, during the WHO International Reference Center for Immunoglobulins conference in Lausanne, these researchers agreed to call IgE this fifth class of serum immunoglobulin [30].

Like other immunoglobulins, IgE is a tetramer comprised of two identical pairs of heavy and light chains with a total molecular weight of 188 kDa. Variable regions at the N-termini of the heavy and light chains create unique binding pockets that determine the antigen specificity of the antibody. The C-terminal regions of the heavy chains contain a constant region comprised of four Cε repeats that confers the isotype-specific functions of IgE, including interaction with its cellular and soluble receptors. The incorporation of hydrophobic sequences encoded by M1 and M2 exons in transmembrane splice variants gives rise to membrane-bound IgE in B cells [31].

Mature B cells leave the bone marrow producing immunoglobulin D (IgD) and immunoglobulin M (IgM) of defined antigen specificity. The presence of IL-4 and IL-13 induces immunoglobulin class switching to IgE. These two cytokines interact with receptors on the surface of B-cells to initiate a signaling cascade mediated by Janus kinase 3 (JAK3) and signal transducer and activator of transcription 6 (STAT6). CD 40 on the B cell interacts with CD40-ligand on the T cell, offering the required second signal for IgE switching. Once allergen-specific B-cells produce IgE, it is released into the circulation [32, 33].

There are two receptors for IgE: **FcεRI** and **CD23 (FcεRII)**. FcεRI has a high affinity for IgE and has a tetrameric form on basophil and mast cells, while a trimeric form on other cells, such as monocytes, dendritic cells, eosinophils, smooth-muscle cells, and platelets. The tetrameric form is responsible for immediate hypersensitivity reactions.

CD23 is a low-affinity receptor for IgE and can both stimulate and inhibit the production of IgE. Interestingly, it can facilitate antigen processing and help transport the IgE-antigen complex across the intestinal epithelium [32]. Beyond these two principal receptors, a protein known as galectin-3 can bind both IgE and FcεRI and activate mast cells or basophils by crosslinking receptor-bound IgE, FcεRI, or both [34]. IgE is the immunoglobulin isotype with the lowest concentration in the circulation and a short half-life (2 days), which is unable to fix complement and has little ability to cross the placenta, nevertheless is quite an active molecule. Antigen-specific IgE antibodies are markers of T-helper 2 response and, together with mastocytes, are the key effector cells in the development of the acute manifestation of allergies [35].

Since their discovery, measuring the total amount of IgE was thought to be the simplest method to identify allergic subjects. But, it soon became evident that total IgE was not a reliable marker of atopy [7].

Very high IgE levels are also observed in parasitic infestations, rarely in multiple myeloma patients producing IgE, and in some primary immunodeficiencies (e.g., Immune dysregulation polyendocrinopathy enteropathy X-linked syndrome [IPEX], Omenn syndrome, Wiskott–Aldrich syndrome, Comel-Netherton syndrome, hyper-IgE syndrome, and atypical complete Di George syndrome). Total serum IgE is also elevated in allergic broncho-pulmonary aspergillosis (ABPA), the only condition where high levels of IgE are surely related to disease severity.

Table 3.4 Modified from Ref. [37]

Age	Range (kUI/L)
0	0,1-1,5
6 weeks	0,1-2,8
3 months	0,3-3,1
6 months	0,9-28,0
9 months	0,7-8,1
1 year	1,1–10,2
2 years	1,1-49,0
3 years	0,5-7,7
4 years	2,4-34,8
7 years	1,6-60,0
10 years	0,3-215,0
14 years	1,9–159

Table 3.5 Modified from Ref. [36]

Age (year)	Range (kUI/L)
<1	0,0-6,6
1	0,0-20,0
2	0,1–15,8
3	0,0-29,2
4	0,3-25,0
5	0,2-17,6
6	0,2-13,1
7	0,3-46,1
8	1,8-60,1
9	3,6-81,0
10	8,0-95,0
11	1,5-99,7
12	3,9-83,5
13 to 16	3,3-188,0

Total IgE values are currently reported in International Units of IgE per volume (IU/mL); a conversion factor (1 IU = 2.42 ng) is sometimes applied. Nowadays, it is prevalent to be reported in its equivalence of kU/L [7].

Normal total serum IgE levels are age-dependent and range widely both in children and in adults from <2 to 200 kU/L [36, 37] (Tables 3.4 and 3.5), but atopic infants have earlier and steeper increases in their levels than nonatopic infants [38].

3.5 Serum Allergen-Specific IgE

IgE is the least abundant of all immunoglobulins; nevertheless, high specific serum IgE levels against otherwise harmless environmental antigens are the hallmarks of IgE-mediated atopic diseases.

There is, therefore, the need to determine and measure the serum levels of allergen-specific immunoglobulins E with precision and accuracy to diagnose suspected allergic conditions. The measurement of IgE against specific allergenic epitopes can be achieved through serological immunoassays. The assay of allergen-specific IgE represents a second-level step in the allergy diagnostic.

The first laboratory test for allergy diagnosis was introduced in 1967 and was called the Radio Allergo Sorbent Test (**RAST**). In this technique, an antigen coupled to an insoluble polymeric support is added to the patient's serum. Then, I^{125} labeled IgE antibodies are added. The antibody uptake is then measured in terms of radioactivity, which is proportional to the amount of IgE directed against the allergen [39]. Classically, the diagnosis of allergic diseases was based exclusively on the search for sIgE class antibodies for different allergenic extracts. Allergen extracts are made up of mixtures of allergens [40].

The reaction may be triggered by another allergen contaminating the extract, or there may be an error in the interpretation of the diagnostic test when an allergen is not present in the extract used because it was degraded during the extraction procedures. Moreover, many allergic subjects present reactions on contact with apparently unrelated allergic sources, as happens in patients allergic to birch pollen, who frequently present reactions on the oral mucosa after contact with some types of fruit. This phenomenon is explained by cross-reactive allergens or pan-allergens in various allergenic sources [41].

In clinical practice, using an allergen extract may be sufficient to diagnose allergy to one or more allergenic sources. Still, it cannot provide information on the molecular components responsible for the symptomatology.

Innovations and advances in molecular biology have revolutionized the assay methods that can measure the levels of sIgE. Nowadays, it is possible to use serum sIgE immunoassays with recombinant or highly purified allergens, which considerably increase the sensitivity and specificity of the tests and, as a consequence, the diagnostic capacity and accuracy [42].

RAST test wrote the history of allergy diagnosis but is now surpassed in terms of accuracy by new immunoassay methods like **enzyme-linked immunosorbent assay** (ELISA), **fluorescent enzyme immunoassays,** and/or **chemiluminescent assays**.

New methods are quite similar to RAST and automated. The allergen, in a fluid or solid phase, depending on the assay, binds to serum-specific IgE. A second IgE recognizes the specific IgE conjugated to an enzyme that catalyzes the transformation of a specific substrate with quantifiable properties such as color or fluorescence. Hence, the levels for specific IgE are extrapolated from a dose-response curve of total IgE according to a reference IgE standard [43].

The dosage of specific IgE for allergens can be performed in **singleplex**, i.e., testing one allergen per sample, or in **multiplex**, i.e., testing a large panel of allergens on a single sample. The former allows the clinician to decide which allergen test is based on clinical history; the latter plays an important role in diagnosing polysensitized patients.

Three types of immunoassays are available: qualitative, semi-quantitative, and quantitative.

- A **qualitative assay** only generates positive or negative results and demonstrates the presence of sIgE above a specific threshold value. Still, it does not provide the concentration of sIgE. If the measured level is close to the cut-off point, then the results might be borderline.
- A **semi-quantitative assay** produces a response by reporting a series of increasing classes based on the concentration of specific IgE (e.g., from I to VI).
- A **quantitative assay** reports sIgE concentration.

In the last two decades, a new tool in molecular allergy diagnostics has emerged, a multiplex technology for determining specific IgE [44]. Thanks to advances in biochip technology, protein **microarrays** were developed, allowing small amounts of homogeneous components to be added to a glass slide. Microarray proved effective because many components were on a small surface with only a few drops of serum to be tested.

The most important advantage of this tool lies in the potential to investigate a large number of allergens in parallel, offering higher diagnostic accuracy in polysensitized patients and providing information in the interpretation of cross-reactivity phenomena, prediction of severe reaction, and tolerance of some food allergens [45].

It should be noted that the results obtained from these allergen chips cannot be compared with IgE measurements obtained with other analysis systems, even if the same company manufactures them and uses the same allergen source [46]. Microarray is a semi-quantitative method, meaning, as mentioned above, that variations in the positive signal are expressed as an increasing series and in arbitrary units relative to the dose-response curve [43]. Moreover, microarrays can produce false negative results, mainly in patients with a very low concentration of IgE antibodies. For this reason, microarrays should represent a second-third line of investigation in allergic diagnostics [47].

3.6 Molecular Diagnostics

The ability to identify, clone, and reproduce recombinant allergens has introduced precision molecular diagnostics into clinical practice. This diagnostic strategy has been termed component-resolved diagnostics (**CRD**), molecular-based allergy diagnostics (**MBAD**), or molecular allergy diagnostics (**MAD**), and now is termed precision allergy molecular diagnostic applications (**PAMD@**) [46, 48]. Molecular diagnostics constitute the third-level step in allergy diagnosis.

The number of identified and cloned antigens is increasing every day, hence the need to use an international nomenclature to identify each allergen. The World Health Organization and the International Union of Immunological Species (WHO/IUIS) developed a systematic nomenclature for allergenic molecules, accessed at http://www.allergen.org [49].

Allergenic molecules are named using their Latin binomial name comprehensive of genus and species (Betulla verucosa→Bet v) and a number added to the name in order of identification to distinguish the various allergens from the same species (Bet v1, Bet v2). Moreover, allergenic molecules are classified into protein families according to their structure and biological function.

One of the cornerstones of molecular diagnostics is that many molecules share common epitopes (binding site IgE) and that, consequently, a sIgE can bind to different allergenic molecules with similar structures from different allergenic sources and generate an immune response. These allergenic molecules are called cross-reactive allergens. In contrast, some molecules are unique markers for specific allergen sources, allowing for the identification of the primary sensitizer.

Molecular diagnostics also help the clinician to determine the likelihood of local versus systemic reactions and to predict the persistence of clinical symptoms, identify allergens stable to heat and digestion, and then predict the severity of the reaction.

PAMD@ supports the clinician in identifying whether the sensitization is primary and likely to be clinically relevant or due to clinically irrelevant cross-sensitization, and it helps evaluate the likelihood of reaction upon exposure to different allergen sources [42] (Table 3.6).

Above all, molecular diagnostics makes it possible, in the context of personalized medicine, to obtain clinically relevant information. In respiratory allergy, it allows a precise diagnosis and, thus, the correct choice of allergen extract for allergen-specific immunotherapy [50]. Also, molecular diagnostics makes it possible to identify a risk profile of severe allergic reactions concerning food allergy according to the family of sensitizing molecules (Fig. 3.2) [51].Clinical decisions, even important ones from a psychological point of view (prescription of self-injected adrenaline), must always underlie a true allergy diagnosis and not be based on mere sensitization [52].

Table 3.6 Principal allergen families

Plant origin molecules	Prolamins	Cereal prolamins
		A-amylase inhibitors
		2S albumins
		Non-specific lipid transfer proteins (nsLTP)
	Globulins	7S globulins
		11S globulins
	Pathogenesis-related proteins	PR-10
		PR-3
	Snakin/gibberellin protein (GRP)	
Animal origin molecules	Mammals allergens	Caseine
		Serum albumin
		Lipocalin
	Avian allergens	Ovomucoid
		Ovalbumin
		Ovotransferrin
		Lysozyme
	Fish allergens	Tropomyosin
		ß-Enolase
		ß-Parvalbumin

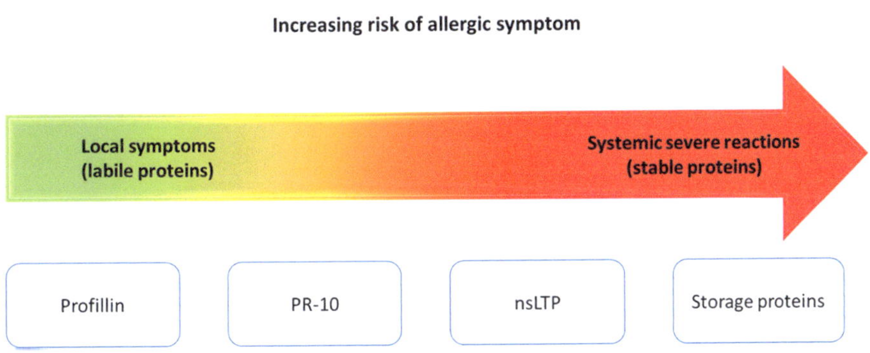

Fig. 3.2 Risk profile of allergic reaction

3.7 Basophil Activation Test

Basophils and mast cells are key effector cells in IgE-mediated allergy. Blood basophil granulocytes contain and release histamine on stimulation with an allergen they are sensitized to.

In 1991, Knol and colleagues [53] discovered **CD63** as a basophil activation marker. Upregulation of CD63 correlates with the release of histamine in IgE and non-IgE mediated basophil activation, as CD63 is a membrane protein localized to the same secretory lysosomal granule containing histamine [54]. **CD203c** is another activation marker with different kinetic, is already expressed on resting cells, and is upregulated slightly earlier than CD63 [55].

The **Basophil Activation Test** (BAT) uses flow cytometry to measure the translocation of CD63 on the surface membrane during the degranulation of secretory lysosomal granules contained into the basophil following the cross-linking of IgE antibodies bound to FcεRI in response to an allergen or anti-IgE stimulation.

BAT is often performed in food, medication, and venom allergies, as it avoids bothersome or high-risk provocations. The sensibility and specificity vary according to the tested allergen.

BAT can be performed using whole or isolated peripheral blood mononuclear cells (PBMC). Manipulation of PBMC may increase the risk of test alteration [56]. Moreover, using whole blood may recreate the physiologic situation that closely resembles the in vivo environment.

Whole blood BAT should be performed within 4 h of blood collection, as basophil activity decreases considerably over time [57]. Moreover, whole blood should be collected in heparin or another anticoagulant like ethylenediaminetetraacetic acid (EDTA) or acid citrate dextrose (ACD) to prevent basophil degranulation [54].

Antigens should be tested within 6 months/1 year from the most recent exposure to an allergen [58, 59]. Antihistamines should not affect BAT; systemic steroids and cyclosporine A may affect the result.

Although commercial basophil activation assays are available, these are rarely validated, and their interpretation must be made in the patient's clinical context. Further studies are needed to integrate this method into mainstream clinical practice. International agreement and standardization are still lacking, so each laboratory should establish its cut-off values. Threshold values also differ based on the allergen analyzed; for proteinaceous allergens, a reliable basophil activation test cut-off is at least 15%, possibly associated with a stimulation index of at least 2, compared to the negative control. For drugs considered substances with lower stimulating potency, a lower cut-off, for example, of 5%, can be considered reliable. However, it is advisable not to rely on arbitrary cut-offs blindly but constantly to evaluate the results in the clinical context [7].

One of the biggest pitfalls of BAT is the presence within the general population of a significant percentage, around 10%, of subjects with basophil anergy, defined as nonresponders to the BAT [60].

BAT could play a decisive role in diagnosing food allergy, especially in doubtful cases. Many studies have demonstrated high sensitivity and specificity for certain food species such as milk, eggs, and nuts. While it seems to be unreliable in plant-derived food allergy [61–64].

One primary application of BAT is immediate **drug hypersensitivity**, as other in vitro tests are frequently lacking, and skin test is still associated with considerable uncertainty. Unfortunately, sensitivity ranges between 50 and 60%, and specificity is around 80% [65, 66].

In venom allergy, BAT can be performed using native extracts but also with recombinant venom proteins. This assay has demonstrated remarkable utility in the diagnostic work-up of complex cases, for instance, patients demonstrating double positive sIgE and at risk for inappropriate venom immunotherapy or patients with a clinical history of allergy but with negative sIgE. Moreover, another application is the monitoring of treatment in venom immunotherapy [67, 68].

3.8 Peripheral Eosinophils

Eosinophils are multifunctional leukocytes implicated in the pathogenesis of numerous inflammatory processes, including parasitic helminth infections and allergic diseases. Eosinophil precursors differentiate in the bone marrow (BM) mediated by specific transcription factors, and eosinophil maturation occurs in response to eosinophilopoietic cytokines (interleukin (IL)-3, granulocyte-macrophage colony-stimulating factor, and most importantly, IL-5 [69].

In the peripheral blood, eosinophilia can be characterized as mild (500–1500 eosinophils per microliter), moderate (1500–5000 eosinophils per microliter), or severe (greater than 5000 eosinophils per microliter). **Hypereosinophilia** refers to blood eosinophils levels exceeding 1500 eosinophils per microliter [70].

In most cases, eosinophilia and hypereosinophilia occur in response to the overproduction of IL-5, which is reactive. The sources of IL-5 capable of stimulating eosinophilopoiesis are relatively limited and include activated T-cells with a "type-2" cytokine profile (Th2 cells), which differentiate in response to helminth infection or allergen; other causes are lymphomas, malignant cells in the setting of solid tumors, hyper-IgE syndrome, and Omenn's syndrome. Organ-specific eosinophilic disorders may also be associated with blood eosinophilia [69].

3.9 Fraction Exhaled of Nitric Oxide

In the respiratory tract, nitric oxide is produced by a variety of structural and inflammatory cells, including eosinophils, macrophages, epithelial cells, and smooth muscle cells. Exhaled nitric oxide fraction (FeNO) is a noninvasive method to assess allergic airway inflammation. It might be useful to evaluate potential response or failure to inhaled corticosteroids, to guide changes in therapy, to evaluate adherence to therapy, and can aid in the diagnosis of allergic asthma. FeNO levels are considered as low, less than 20 ppb; intermediate, 20–35 ppb; or high, greater than 35 ppb [71, 72].

3.10 Eosinophil Count in Induced Sputum

Induced sputum is a semi-invasive method of assessing airway inflammation. The identification of sputum eosinophilia currently has great clinical value as it predicts a favorable response to corticosteroids and can therefore guide treatment. The use of fluorocytometric analysis of induced sputum cells might shorten the process and provide complementary information on activated cells in the bronchial mucosa. Unfortunately, this technique requires a substantial amount of time to perform and process and also technical support and expertise to process, stain, and interpret the samples. As a consequence, this procedure is only of value in specialized centers [73].

3.11 Allergen Provocation Test

In addition to skin tests, allergens can be applied to the conjunctival, oral, nasal, and bronchial mucosa to elicit symptoms and demonstrate the presence of specific IgE if the history is suspicious. Still, if skin and in vitro tests are inconclusive, these methods are subject to a risk of a systemic reaction, especially in inhalation challenges.

The **oral food challenge test** (OFC) is the most reliable clinical procedure for diagnosing food allergies. The general methodology for the OFC is to administer the suspected food in gradually increasing doses in a medical setting and must be performed by well-trained clinicians.

Take-Home Messages

1. The diagnostic work-up is crucial in managing allergic diseases, as it helps identify the causative allergen, essential for effective treatment. The choice and interpretation of allergy tests should be based on the patient's clinical history, and tests should be performed and evaluated by experienced healthcare professionals.
2. The diagnostic procedure involves a combination of medical history, physical examination, and allergy testing to confirm specific IgE sensitization and establish a causal link between symptoms and allergen exposure (true allergy).
3. Skin prick test (SPT) is a reliable, safe, and moderately cheap method to assess IgE sensitization to allergens. It should be evaluated with the patient's clinical history and performed using standardized allergen extracts with proper controls.
4. SPT involves pricking the skin with allergens and observing the wheal and flare reaction, which indicates an IgE-mediated response. It can be performed at any age, but the choice of testing site and interpretation of results may vary.
5. Intradermal test (IDT) is an alternative to SPT, in drug allergy and may be considered in patients with high clinical suspicion and negative SPT or lower skin reactivity. IDT carries a higher risk

(continued)

of severe and anaphylactic reactions and is less tolerated, particularly by children, due to its invasive nature.
6. Using different immunoassay methods, serum-specific IgE assays help measure allergen-specific IgE levels. These tests have evolved with advances in molecular biology, allowing for more accurate and precise results. Molecular diagnostics are vital in identifying primary sensitizers, predicting reactions, assessing cross-reactivity, and defining allergy severity.
7. Basophil activation test (BAT) is a flow cytometry-based assay that measures the activation of basophils in response to allergen stimulation. BAT can help diagnose food allergies and immediate drug hypersensitivity, but further standardization and validation are needed.
8. Peripheral eosinophils are involved in allergic inflammation and can indicate eosinophilic disorders when elevated in the blood. Eosinophil levels may suggest type 2 inflammation intensity. Eosinophilia is often associated with IL-5 overproduction and can be seen in response to allergic and nonallergic causes.

References

1. Bernstein IL, Li JT, Bernstein DI, Spector SL, Tan R, Sicherer S, et al. Allergy diagnostic testing: an updated practice parameter. Ann Allergy Asthma Immunol. 2008;100(Suppl 3):S1-148.
2. Brown HM, Su S, Thantrey N. Prick testing for allergens standardized by using a precision needle. Clin Exp Allergy. 1981;11:95–8.
3. Kim BJ, Mun SK. Objective measurements using the skin prick test in allergic rhinitis. Arch Otolaryngol Head Neck Surg. 2010;136:1104–6.
4. Bousquet J, Heinzerling L, Bachert C, Papadopoulos NG, Bousquet PJ, Burney PG, et al. Practical guide to skin prick tests in allergy to aeroallergens. Allergy. 2012;67:18–24.
5. Nelson HS, Knoetzer J, Bucher B. Effect of distance between sites and region of the body on results of skin prick tests. J Allergy Clin Immunol. 1996;97:596–601.
6. Wise SK, Damask C, Roland LT, Ebert C, Levy JM, Lin S, Luong A, et al. International consensus statement on allergy and rhinology: allergic rhinitis—2023. Int Forum Allergy Rhinol. 2023;13:293–859.
7. Ansotegui IJ, Melioli G, Canonica GW, Caraballo L, Villa E, Ebisawa M, et al. IgE allergy diagnostics and other relevant tests in allergy, a world allergy organization position paper. World Allergy Organ J. 2020;13;100080.
8. Shah KM, Rank MA, Davé SA, Oslie CL, Butterfield JH. Predicting which medication classes interfere with allergy skin testing. Allergy Asthma Proc. 2010;31:477–82.
9. Almind M, Dirksen A, Nielsen NH, Svendsen UG. Duration of the inhibitory activity on histamine-induced skin weals of sedative and non-sedative antihistamines. Allergy. 1988;43:593–6.
10. Cook TJ, MacQueen DM, Wittig HJ, Thornby JI, Lantos RL, Virtue CM. Degree and duration of skin test suppression and side effects with antihistamines: a double blind controlled study with five antihistamines. J Allergy Clin Immunol. 1973;51:71–7.
11. Noga O, Hanf G, Kunkel G. Immunological and clinical changes in allergic asthmatics following treatment with Omalizumab. Int Arch Allergy Immunol. 2003;131:46–52.
12. Narasimha SK, Srinivas CR, Mathew AC. Effect of topical corticosteroid application frequency on histamine-induced wheals. Int J Dermatol. 2005;44:425–7.
13. Slott RI, Zweiman B. A controlled study of the effect of corticosteroids on immediate skin test reactivity. J Allergy Clin Immunol. 1974;54:229–34.
14. Des RA, Paradis L, Bougeard YH, Godard P, Bousquet J, Chanez P. Long-term oral corticosteroid therapy does not alter the results of immediate-type allergy skin prick tests. J Allergy Clin Immunol. 1996;98:522–7.
15. Simons FE, Johnston L, Gu X, Simons KJ. Suppression of the early and late cutaneous allergic responses using fexofenadine and montelukast. Ann Allergy Asthma Immunol. 2001;86:44–50.
16. Rao KS, Menon PK, Hilman BC, Sebastian CS, Bairnsfather L. Duration of the suppressive effect of tricyclic antidepressants on histamine-induced wheal-and-flare reactions in human skin. J Allergy Clin Immunol. 1988;82:752–7.
17. Kupczyk M, Kupryś I, Bocheńska-Marciniak M, Górski P, Kuna P. Ranitidine (150 mg daily) inhibits wheal, flare, and itching reactions in skin-prick tests. Allergy Asthma Proc. 2007;28:711–5.
18. Miller J, Nelson HS. Suppression of immediate skin tests by ranitidine. J Allergy Clin Immunol. 1989;84:895–9.
19. Bousquet PJ, Burbach G, Heinzerling LM, Edenharter G, Bachert C, Bindslev-Jensen C, et al. GA2LEN skin test study III: minimum battery of test inhalent aller-

gens needed in epidemiological studies in patients. Allergy. 2009;64:1656–62.
20. Burbach GJ, Heinzerling LM, Edenharter G, et al. GA(2)LEN skin test study II: clinical relevance of inhalant allergen sensitizations in Europe. Allergy. 2009;64:1507–15.
21. Sander I, Fleischer C, Meurer U, Brüning T, Raulf-Heimsoth M. Allergen content of grass pollen preparations for skin prick testing and sublingual immunotherapy. Allergy. 2009;64:1486–92.
22. Curin M, Reininger R, Swoboda I, Focke M, Valenta R, Spitzauer S. Skin prick test extracts for dog allergy diagnosis show considerable variations regarding the content of major and minor dog allergens. Int Arch Allergy Immunol. 2011;154:258–63.
23. Van Ree R, Chapman MD, Ferreira F, Vieths S, Bryan D, Cromwell O, et al. The CREATE project: development of certified reference materials for allergenic products and validation of methods for their quantification. Allergy. 2008;63:310–26.
24. Patti ML, De Rose C, Brancato F, Gambacorta A, Sopo SM. Sensitivity of prick test with walnut commercial extracts and of prick by prick with raw walnut compared with open food challenge in walnut allergy. Acta Biomed 2021;92(S1):e201067.
25. Dreborg S, Foucard T. Allergy to apple, carrot and potato in children with birch pollen allergy. Allergy. 1983;38:167–72.
26. Calabria CW, Hagan L. The role of intradermal skin testing in inhalant allergy. Ann Allergy Asthma Immunol. 2008;101:337–47.
27. Sampson HA. Food allergy. Part 2: diagnosis and management. J Allergy Clin Immunol. 1999;103:981–9.
28. Bernstein DI, Wanner M, Borish L, Liss GM. Twelve-year survey of fatal reactions to allergen injections and skin testing: 1990–2001. J Allergy Clin Immunol. 2004;113:1129–36.
29. Amin HS, Liss GM, Bernstein DI. Evaluation of near-fatal reactions to allergen immunotherapy injections. J Allergy Clin Immunol. 2006;117:169–75.
30. Bennich H, Ishizaka K, Johansson SG, Rowe DS, Stanworth DR, Terry WD. Immunoglobulin E, a new class of human immunoglobulin. Bull World Health Organ. 1968;38:151–2.
31. Gould HJ, Sutton BJ, Beavil AJ, Beavil RL, McCloskey N, Coker HA, et al. The biology of IGE and the basis of allergic disease. Annu Rev Immunol. 2003;21:579–628.
32. Kelly BT, Grayson MH. Immunoglobulin E, what is it good for? Ann Allergy Asthma Immunol. 2016;116:183–7.
33. Burton OT, Oettgen HC. Beyond immediate hypersensitivity: evolving roles for IgE antibodies in immune homeostasis and allergic diseases. Immunol Rev. 2011;242:128–43.
34. Gould HJ, Sutton BJ. IgE in allergy and asthma today. Nat Rev Immunol. 2008;8:205–17.
35. Galli SJ, Tsai M. IgE and mast cells in allergic disease. Nat Med. 2012;18:693–704.
36. Lindberg RE, Arroyave C. Levels of IgE in serum from normal children and allergic children as measured by an enzyme immunoassay. J Allergy Clin Immunol. 1986;78:614–8.
37. Kjellman NM, Johansson SGO, Roth A. Serum IgE levels in healthy children quantified by a sandwich technique (PRIST). Clin Exp Allergy. 1976;6:51–9.
38. Ozcan E, Notarangelo LD, Geha RS. Primary immune deficiencies with aberrant IgE production. J Allergy Clin Immunol. 2008;122:1054–62.
39. Wide L, Bennich H, Johansson SG. Diagnosis of allergy by an in-vitro test for allergen antibodies. Lancet. 1967;2:1105–7.
40. Barber D, Diaz-Perales A, Escribese MM, Kleine-Tebbe J, Matricardi PM, Ollert M, et al. Molecular allergology and its impact in specific allergy diagnosis and therapy. Allergy. 2021;76:3642–58.
41. Ebner C, Hirschwehr R, Bauer L, Breiteneder H, Valenta R, Ebner H, et al. Identification of allergens in fruits and vegetables: IgE cross-reactivities with the important birch pollen allergens Bet v 1 and Bet v 2 (birch profilin). J Allergy Clin Immunol. 1995;95:962–9.
42. Steering Committee Authors; Review Panel Members. A WAO – ARIA – GA2LEN consensus document on molecular-based allergy diagnosis (PAMD@): update 2020. World Allergy Organ J. 2020;13:10001.
43. Goikoetxea MJ, Sanz ML, García BE, Mayorga C, Longo N, Gamboa PM, et al. Recommendations for the use of in vitro methods to detect specific immunoglobulin E: are they comparable? J Investig Allergol Clin Immunol. 2013;23:448–54.
44. Hiller R, Laffer S, Harwanegg C, Huber M, Schmidt WM, Twardosz A, et al. Microarrayed allergen molecules: diagnostic gatekeepers for allergy treatment. FASEB J. 2002;16:414–6.
45. Melioli G, Compalati E, Bonini S, Canonica GW. The added value of allergen microarray technique to the management of poly-sensitized allergic patients. Curr Opin Allergy Clin Immunol. 2012;12:434–9.
46. Jahn-Schmid B, Harwanegg C, Hiller R, Bohle B, Ebner C, Scheiner O, et al. Allergen microarray: comparison of microarray using recombinant allergens with conventional diagnostic methods to detect allergen-specific serum immunoglobulin E. Clin Exp Allergy. 2003;33:1443–9.
47. Melioli G, Bonifazi F, Bonini S, Maggi E, Mussap M, Passalacqua G, et al. The ImmunoCAP ISAC molecular allergology approach in adult multi-sensitized Italian patients with respiratory symptoms. Clin Biochem. 2011;44:1005–11.
48. De Knop KJ, Bridts CH, Verweij MM, Hagendorens MM, De Clerck LS, Stevens WJ, et al. Component-resolved allergy diagnosis by microarray: potential, pitfalls, and prospects. Adv Clin Chem. 2010;50:87–101.
49. Davies JM, Gadermaier G, Hilger C, et al. WHO/IUIS allergen nomenclature: providing a common language. Mol Immunol. 2018;100:3–13.

50. Alvaro-Lozano M, Akdis CA, Akdis M, Alviani C, Angier E, Arasi S, et al. EAACI allergen immunotherapy user's guide. Pediatr Allergy Immunol. 2020;31:1.
51. Mastrorilli C, Tripodi S, Caffarelli C, Perna S, Di Rienzo-Businco A, Sfika I, et al. Endotypes of pollen-food syndrome in children with seasonal allergic rhinoconjunctivitis: a molecular classification. Allergy. 2016;71:1181–91.
52. Ciprandi G, Tosca MA. LTP allergy: a pragmatic and reasonable approach in clinical practice. Eur Ann Allergy Clin Immunol. 2019;51:84–5.
53. Knol EF, Mul FPJ, Jansen H, Calafat J, Roos D. Monitoring human basophil activation via CD63 monoclonal antibody 435. J Allergy Clin Immunol. 1991;88:328–38.
54. Hoffmann HJ, Santos AF, Mayorga C, Nopp A, Eberlein B, Ferrer M, et al. The clinical utility of basophil activation testing in diagnosis and monitoring of allergic disease. Allergy. 2015;70:1393–405.
55. Keswani T, Patil SU. Basophil activation test in food allergy: is it ready for real-time? Curr Opin Allergy Clin Immunol. 2021;21:442–7.
56. Ebo DG, Bridts CH, Hagendorens MM, Aerts NE, De Clerck LS, Stevens WJ. Basophil activation test by flow cytometry: present and future applications in allergology. Cytometry B Clin Cytom. 2008;74:201–10.
57. Hemmings O, Kwok M, McKendry R, Santos AF. Basophil activation test: old and new applications in allergy. Curr Allergy Asthma Rep. 2018;18:77.
58. Kvedariene V, Kamey S, Ryckwaert Y, Rongier M, Bousquet J, Demoly P, et al. Diagnosis of neuromuscular blocking agent hypersensitivity reactions using cytofluorimetric analysis of basophils. Allergy. 2006;61:311–5.
59. Fernández TD, Torres MJ, Blanca-López N, Rodríguez-Bada JL, Gomez E, Canto G, et al. Negativization rates of IgE radioimmunoassay and basophil activation test in immediate reactions to penicillins. Allergy. 2009;64:242–8.
60. Puan KJ, Andiappan AK, Lee B, Kumar D, Lai TS, Yeo G, et al. Systematic characterization of basophil anergy. Allergy. 2017;72:373–84.
61. Rubio A, Vivinus-Nébot M, Bourrier T, Saggio B, Albertini M, Bernard A. Benefit of the basophil activation test in deciding when to reintroduce cow's milk in allergic children. Allergy. 2011;66:92–100.
62. Carroccio A, Brusca I, Mansueto P, Pirrone G, Barrale M, Di Prima L, et al. A cytologic assay for diagnosis of food hypersensitivity in patients with irritable bowel syndrome. Clin Gastroenterol Hepatol. 2010;8:254–60.
63. Sato S, Tachimoto H, Shukuya A, Ogata M, Komata T, Imai T, et al. Utility of the peripheral blood basophil histamine release test in the diagnosis of hen's egg, cow's milk, and wheat allergy in children. Int Arch Allergy Immunol. 2011;155(Suppl 1):96–103.
64. Ford LS, Bloom KA, Nowak-Węgrzyn AH, Shreffler WG, Masilamani M, Sampson HA. Basophil reactivity, wheal size, and immunoglobulin levels distinguish degrees of cow's milk tolerance. J Allergy Clin Immunol. 2013;131:180–6.
65. Mangodt EA, Van Gasse AL, Decuyper I, Uyttebroek A, Faber MA, Sabato V, et al. In vitro diagnosis of immediate drug hypersensitivity: should we go with the flow. Int Arch Allergy Immunol. 2015;168:3–12.
66. Ebo DG, Faber M, Elst J, Van Gasse AL, Bridts CH, Mertens C, et al. In vitro diagnosis of immediate drug hypersensitivity during anesthesia: a review of the literature. J Allergy Clin Immunol Pract. 2018;6:1176–84.
67. Ebo DG, Van Vaerenbergh M, De Graaf DC, Bridts CH, De Clerck LS, Sabato V. In vitro diagnosis of hymenoptera venom allergy and further development of component resolved diagnostics. Expert Rev Clin Immunol. 2014;10:375–84.
68. Blank S, Bilò MB, Ollert M. Component-resolved diagnostics to direct in venom immunotherapy: important steps towards precision medicine. Clin Exp Allergy. 2018;48:354–64.
69. Roufosse F, Weller PF. Practical approach to the patient with hypereosinophilia. J Allergy Clin Immunol. 2010;126:39–44.
70. Rothenberg ME, Hogan SP. The eosinophil. Annu Rev Immunol. 2006;24:147–74.
71. Dweik RA, Boggs PB, Erzurum SC, Irvin CG, Leigh MW, Lundberg JO, et al. An official ATS clinical practice guideline: interpretation of exhaled nitric oxide levels (FENO) for clinical applications. Am J Respir Crit Care Med. 2011;184:602–15.
72. Morphew T, Shin HW, Marchese S, Pires-Barracosa N, Galant SP. Phenotypes favoring fractional exhaled nitric oxide discordance vs guideline-based uncontrolled asthma. Ann Allergy Asthma Immunol. 2019;123:193–200.
73. Araújo L, Moreira A, Palmares C, Beltrão M, Fonseca J, Delgado L. Induced sputum in children: success determinants, safety, and cell profiles. J Investig Allergol Clin Immunol. 2011;21:216–21.

4 Asthma in the Pediatric Patient

Sara Manti, Federico Motta, Davide Fabio, Lucia Caminiti, Grigorios Chatziparasidis, and Ahmad Kantar

Abstract

Asthma is a chronic and heterogeneous respiratory disease characterized by chronic airway inflammation, resulting in reversible respiratory symptoms, such as wheezing, shortness of breath, chest tightness, cough, and variable expiratory airflow limitation. Asthma affects 1–18% of the global population. Despite the recent advances in diagnostic and therapeutic strategies, asthma still poses a substantial health and socioeconomic burden, in particular in its uncontrolled and severe forms. To improve outcomes, accurate management and diagnosis are crucial, as well as follow-up, monitoring of lung function and inflammation, education, and supported self-management advice.

Keywords

Asthma · Children · Diagnosis · Guidelines Management · Treatment

Test your learning and check your understanding of this book's contents: use the "Springer Nature Flashcards" app to access questions using ▶ https://sn.pub/nspbjm. To use the app, please follow the instructions in Chap. 1.

4.1 Asthma: From Definition to Diagnosis

4.1.1 Definition

Asthma is a chronic and heterogeneous respiratory disease that affects 1–18% of the global population. It is characterized by chronic airway inflammation, resulting in reversible respiratory symptoms, such as wheezing, shortness of breath, chest tightness, cough, and variable expiratory

Authors Federico Motta and Davide Fabio contributed equally.

S. Manti (✉) · F. Motta · D. Fabio · L. Caminiti
Pediatric Unit, Department of Human Pathology of Adult and Evolutive Age "Gaetano Barresi", University of Messina, Messina, Italy
e-mail: smanti@unime.it

G. Chatziparasidis
Paediatric Respiratory Unit, IASO Hospital, Larissa, Thessaly, Greece and Faculty of Nursing, Thessaly University, Larissa, Greece

A. Kantar
Pediatric Asthma and Cough Centre, Istituti Ospedalieri Bergamaschi, University and Research Hospitals, Bergamo, Italy

C. Caffarelli, G. L. Marseglia (eds.), *Textbook of Pediatric Allergy*,
https://doi.org/10.1007/978-3-031-71283-8_4

airflow limitation. However, not all of these characteristics are present in each patient at all times. In fact, while most asthmatic children experience intermittent and mild symptoms, a minority exhibit persistent symptoms or even life-threatening exacerbations, which are linked to the underlying pathophysiology [1].

The multifaceted presentation of childhood asthma supports the argument that "asthma" is an umbrella term encompassing a constellation of symptoms (referred to as "phenotypes") that are observable in each child. It should be noted that the underlying pathophysiology (also known as "endotype") leading to these symptoms may vary among children who present with identical phenotypic features. Various asthma patterns with different responses to treatment have been identified [2].

The most common symptom patterns in childhood asthma include atopic asthma with airway eosinophilia, nonatopic asthma with airway eosinophilia, neutrophilic asthma, asthma with persistent airflow limitation, and asthma associated with obesity (Table 4.1) [3, 4]. It is important to note that these patterns should not be regarded as constant, as they may evolve throughout the course of the disease. Regular follow-ups and adjustments to the treatment plan are necessary [5].

4.2 Diagnosis

The diagnosis of asthma relies on identifying characteristic symptom patterns, documenting variable expiratory airflow limitation, assessing the response to anti-asthma medications, and ruling out alternative diagnoses. In children who are capable of performing pulmonary function tests (typically over 5 years of age), these tests can provide additional support for the diagnosis.

A family history of atopy and allergic diseases and a personal history of allergic rhinitis or atopic dermatitis during childhood can increase the likelihood that respiratory symptoms are related to asthma. However, these factors are not specific indicators. Nevertheless, it is important to inquire specifically about respiratory symptoms in children with allergic diseases [3].

Typical respiratory symptoms associated with asthma include wheezing, coughing, shortness of breath, chest tightness, and cough. These symptoms can coexist and occur intermittently, varying in intensity. They often manifest or worsen during viral infections and are typically more pronounced at night or upon waking. Additionally, they can be triggered by factors such as cold air, physical activity, allergens, household pollutants (such as molds and dust mites), exposure to pets

Table 4.1 Clinical phenotype and corresponding endotype

Atopic asthma with airway eosinophilia (Type 2-high airway inflammation endotype)	Generally associated with a personal or familial history of allergic disease (atopic dermatitis, allergic rhinitis, food or drug allergy). It is characterized by raised immunoglobulin (Ig)E and Fractional Exhaled Nitric Oxide (FeNO) levels and the predominance of eosinophils in the airways. This asthma phenotype is usually well controlled by inhaled corticosteroid (ICS) treatment
Nonatopic asthma with airway eosinophilia	Primed by I innate lymphoid cells (ILC)2 that produce small amounts of interleukin (IL)4, there is no associated IgE response from B cells. This endotype may or may not respond to ICS and responds well to biologics
Asthma with persistent airflow limitation	Uncommon in childhood, characterized by a persistent or incompletely reversible airflow limitation possibly due to long-lasting asthma and airway wall remodeling or antenatal /genetic factors
Asthma with obesity	Some obese children have eosinophilic airway inflammation, others neutrophilic airway inflammation or dysanaptic airway growth (normal forced expiratory volume in the first second—FEV1—with greater than normal forced vital capacity (FVC) and thus a reduced FEV1/FVC ratio)
Neutrophilic asthma (Type 2-low airway inflammation endotype)	Seen in preschool wheezers and some obese asthmatics, IL17, IL8, and pro-inflammatory cytokines may play a central role in this endotype

and animals, laughter, changes in weather, and environmental pollutants or irritants (such as car exhaust fumes, tobacco smoke, and strong odors) [6–10].

Due to the variability of symptoms, the physical examination of children with asthma may appear normal. However, any signs of allergic rhinitis or nasal polyposis are worth noting. The primary characteristic of asthma is expiratory wheezing, which can be auscultated, although it may be absent or only heard during forced expiration. Wheezing is a high-pitched, expiratory whistling sound that arises from inflammation, narrowing, and bronchospasm in the small airways of asthmatic children. This constriction of the airway diameter causes vibrations in the airway walls, resulting in the production of wheezing sounds. It should be noted that wheezing requires a certain airflow velocity, so children experiencing severe asthma exacerbation, where the airways are significantly constricted, may exhibit a "silent chest." Crackles (crepitations) and wheezing limited to inspiration are not indicative of asthma, and if wheezing is consistently absent during repeated examinations when the child is acutely ill, the diagnosis of asthma becomes less likely [11].

4.2.1 Lung Function and Other Tests

Lung function should be assessed using spirometry in school-age children. The Global Initiative for Asthma (GINA) recommends the use of either peak expiratory flow (PEF) or spirometry for diagnosing asthma in children over 5 years of age [12]. Performing lung function tests in preschoolers outside of a research setting can be challenging. In this age group, the diagnosis of asthma should rely on accurate documentation of wheezing by a physician when the child is acutely ill. Additionally, the response of wheezing intensity (along with other acute asthma symptoms and signs such as tachypnea, chest wall retractions, and oxygen saturation) to inhaled β-2 agonists should be investigated. It is essential to exclude other serious underlying diseases that may present with wheezing as part of the diagnostic procedure [13]. Research on oscillometry is increasing, and there is growing interest in and feasibility of its clinical application. In asthma, the impulse oscillometry system has already been utilized to assess the bronchodilator response and the therapeutic effects of different medications. It is a sensitive technique for evaluating disease control [14].

In older children, baseline spirometry provides several important parameters, including forced vital capacity (FVC), first-second forced expiratory volume (FEV_1), and PEF. A reduction in FEV_1 below 1.69 z-scores or an FEV_1 to FVC ratio less than 80% ($FEV_1/FVC < 80\%$) indicates airway obstruction, and bronchodilator reversibility (BDR) should be assessed. An increase of 12% or more in FEV_1 after bronchodilation confirms the diagnosis of asthma. In children with normal FEV_1 but a strong suspicion of asthma, fractional exhaled nitric oxide (FeNO) testing should be considered. If FeNO levels are elevated (>25 ppb), the physician should suggest either a 2-week trial of twice-daily PEF measurement at home or an on-site challenge test with methacholine or exercise. If both FEV1 and FeNO are normal, the diagnosis of asthma is called into question, and alternative pathologies should be considered as potential causes of the child's symptoms. Table 4.2 summarizes the data supporting the diagnosis of asthma with the use of spirometry of PEF devices.

The European Respiratory Society (ERS) clinical practice guidelines for diagnosing asthma in children aged 5 years recommend against using skin prick tests (SPTs) for aeroallergens or serum total and specific IgE (sIgE) tests as diagnostic tools for asthma in this age group. However, an exception to this rule is made for children with problematic severe asthma. In such cases, negative SPTs should prompt a comprehensive diagnostic review because although non-atopic pediatric severe asthma does exist, it is rare [15].

For preschoolers exhibiting asthmatic symptoms, the combination of peripheral blood eosinophil counts greater than 300/μl and aeroallergen sensitization strongly predicts response to ICS

Table 4.2 Data supporting the diagnosis of asthma

Positive bronchodilator responsiveness test	It is significant when there is an improvement in FEV1 > than 12% from baseline. The test consists of administering 400 mcg of salbutamol (albuterol) or equivalent and noting FEV1 variation after 15 min, comparing the value with pre-bronchodilator readings
Excessive variability in twice-daily PEF over 2 weeks	Average daily diurnal PEF variability >12%
Positive exercise challenge test	Fall in FEV1 of ≥15% from baseline, or PEF >15%
Positive methacholine challenge test	A provocative concentration of methacholine that results in a 20% drop in FEV1 (PC20) value equal to or less than 8 mg/ml should be considered a positive test

[16]. Furthermore, peripheral blood eosinophilia is an excellent biomarker as it reflects airway eosinophilia, aiding in diagnosing asthma in this age group [17].

In preschoolers, neutrophilic asthma is relatively common, and if there are suspicions of airway infection and primary bronchiolitis obliterans (PBO), it is advisable to document the infection through a cough swab or induced sputum, particularly if the child has undergone numerous or prolonged courses of antibiotics [18].

4.3 Differential Diagnosis

Underdiagnosis and overdiagnosis of asthma remain significant problems with high rates of occurrence. Overdiagnosis poses a problem as it subjects children to unnecessary medication and its adverse effects while also delaying the diagnosis of potentially serious underlying respiratory conditions. On the other hand, underdiagnosis deprives children of appropriate treatment, negatively impacting the quality of life for both the child and their family. It also exposes children to the risk of repeated courses of oral steroids and/or antibiotics, emergency department visits, and hospital admissions. For individuals with severe asthma, underdiagnosis of their condition can even pose a risk to their lives.

Several conditions associated with chronic cough, wheezing, and/or shortness of breath in children can mimic asthma (Table 4.3) [19, 20]. Due to the challenges in diagnosing these conditions, especially in young children where objective testing may not be feasible, it is crucial to reassess the diagnosis of asthma during each clinical presentation.

4.4 Management of Pediatric Asthma

The goals of asthma management include:

- Achieving good optimal disease control with least or absent asthma symptoms and minimal use of rescue medications.
- Preventing the future risk of exacerbations, medication side effects, and death.
- Acquiring normal or near-normal lung function.
- Achieving an age-appropriate level of physical activity and minimizing the number of off-school days due to asthma.
- Improving the quality of life of children and families.

Treatment of asthma is multipronged and involves nonpharmacological and pharmacological approaches.

4.4.1 Nonpharmacological Management

Educating caregivers and patients about modifiable risk factors and comorbidities and conducting annual asthma evaluations to evaluate current disease control and assess future risks are essential components of nonpharmacological asthma management.

Table 4.3 Differential diagnosis of asthma

Condition	Clues to differentiate
Chronic lung disease of prematurity	History of prematurity, home oxygen
Cystic fibrosis	Delayed passage of meconium Failure to thrive and malabsorption since birth Chronic wet cough Fingernail clubbing
Primary ciliary dyskinesia	Unexplained respiratory distress in a full-term neonate Daily, year-round, wet cough starting in the first year of life (usually first months of life) that does not go away with the change of seasons. It may improve with antibiotic treatment, but never fully resolves Daily, year-round nasal congestion starting in the first year of life (usually first months of life) that does not go away with a change of seasons Any laterality/situs (organ placement) anomaly and/or organ development issue
Immunodeficiency	Chronic diarrhea with failure to thrive Wheeze with infections that are severe, persistent, unusual or recurrent
Foreign body aspiration	History of chocking Sudden onset of respiratory symptoms Unilateral chest findings
Bronchiectasis	Recurrent (>3/year) episodes of protracted bacterial bronchitis Chronic wet cough that fails to resolve after 4 weeks of appropriate antibiotic treatment Persistent unilateral chest findings Persistent chest X-ray findings
Gastro-oesophageal reflux or primary aspiration	Vomiting Feeding difficulties Sandifer syndrome Hoarse voice Postprandial cough Recurrent chest infections Neurodevelopmental abnormality
Structural airway or lung abnormality, e.g., trachea-bronchomalacia, bronchogenic cyst	Noisy breathing Stridor or wheezing not responding to conventional treatment Recurrent chest infections Chronic wet cough Brassy quality of cough Symptoms started early in life
Cardiac abnormality	Tachycardia Murmur Hepatomegaly Basal crackles

Family education is crucial in enhancing understanding of asthma and its management. This includes explaining the risks associated with smoking, exposure to household pollutants (and other triggers), and obesity. It also offers an opportunity to emphasize the importance of treatment adherence for achieving better symptom control and reducing asthma-related mortality [21]. Encouraging physical activity is another important aspect, as it is an integral part of normal child development and promotes overall health in patients. Furthermore, it may slightly benefit respiratory function and symptom control [22].

Asthmatic children and teenagers should undergo an annual review, during which personal asthma action plans should be discussed along with their current symptom control, history of attacks, potential triggers, and modifiable risk factors. These consultations provide an opportunity to assess the child's and caregiver's understanding of asthma and offer valuable education. Part of this assessment involves evaluating the inhaler technique (and use of a spacer, if appropriate for their age), allowing physicians to intervene and provide re-training on the correct use of asthma devices. It is also important to have a brief but comprehensive discussion on the importance of proper techniques for achieving optimal asthma control. By taking the time to understand the perspectives of both the young person and their caregivers regarding the diagnosis and management of the condition, the outcomes for young people with asthma can be improved [23–27].

4.4.2 Asthma Action Plan

Asthma action plans are written instructions provided to patients with asthma, serving as a "road map" for managing their asthma when symptoms are well controlled and providing guidance on what steps to take during an asthma exacerbation. These action plans should be shared with individuals involved in the child's asthma management, such as grandparents, school nurses, and teachers. Their effectiveness and applicability should be regularly reviewed, discussed with the child and their family, and amended as needed.

A 2018 survey in the UK involving asthmatic children revealed that approximately 50% of them had never received an asthma action plan from their treating physician, and 20% of caregivers did not seek medical advice during an asthma exacerbation. However, written action plans have been shown to reduce emergency hospital visits, decrease school absenteeism, and enhance caregivers' ability to handle asthma flare-ups [28, 29].

4.4.3 Pharmacological Management

4.4.3.1 Medications and Asthma Severity Classification

Two primary categories of medications are used for treating asthma: maintenance medications (e.g., ICS) and rescue drugs (e.g., short-acting beta 2-agonists, SABA). Before initiating any treatment for a child with asthma, it is important to classify the severity of asthma based on the child's daytime symptoms, nighttime awakenings, activity limitations, frequency of SABA use, and lung function (when age permits). This classification helps determine the appropriate course of action.

Asthma severity is currently assessed retrospectively based on the level of treatment required to manage daily symptoms and flare-ups. A child is considered to have mild asthma if their symptoms are controlled with the as-needed use of ICS-formoterol (formoterol being a long-acting β2 agonist that provides a relatively rapid onset of action within 2–3 min) or with a low dose of ICS. On the other hand, a child with asthma symptoms that remain uncontrolled despite optimized high-dose ICS-LABA (inhaled corticosteroids and long-acting β2 agonists) combined with another controller medication (e.g., leukotriene receptor antagonist, LTRA), or require this high-dose treatment to prevent symptoms from becoming uncontrolled, is classified as having a severe asthma phenotype. The frequency of asthma symptoms should also be considered, as it aids in assigning patients to an intermittent phenotype (asthma symptoms occurring less than twice a month) or a persistent phenotype. It is worth noting that the distinction between intermittent and persistent asthma is arbitrary and should not affect treatment decisions regarding the use of ICS in patients over the age of 6 years, even when SABA is used twice a week or less as a baseline. Data have shown that using ICS-formoterol on an as-needed basis instead of SABA significantly reduces the risk of severe exacerbations in this age group.

4.4.3.2 Concerns About SABA Use in Asthma

The primary emphasis in asthma care is on maintenance therapy, aiming to ultimately eliminate the reliance on SABA. When a patient frequently uses reliever therapy, it indicates poor asthma control. In such cases, the physician should investigate factors such as inhalation technique, treatment compliance, and the patient's exposure to tobacco smoke or other environmental triggers. If symptoms persist despite reliever therapy, the next action is to consider stepping up asthma treatment or referring the patient to a respiratory center for further evaluation and management.

Recently, the GINA recommended against using SABA (short-acting beta 2-agonists) alone for treating intermittent asthma symptoms in children over 6 years and adolescents. Instead, they advised combining SABA with ICS. This recommendation is based on strong evidence indicating that SABA-only treatment while providing short-term relief of asthma symptoms does not offer protection against severe exacerbations. Moreover, it is a risk factor for lower lung function and future asthma attacks. The regular use of SABA can also increase allergic responses and airway inflammation, reduce the bronchodilator response when it is needed, and, most importantly, overusing SABA (defined as three or more SABA canisters dispensed in a year) is associated with an increased risk of asthma-related death. Instead, GINA recommends using as-needed low-dose ICS-formoterol as the preferred treatment for asthmatic adolescents, and low-dose ICS is taken whenever SABA is used for patients aged 6–18 years. This recommendation is supported by data showing the presence of airway inflammation in most individuals with asthma, even those with intermittent symptoms, and the occurrence of severe exacerbations in children with a mild asthma phenotype [12].

4.4.3.3 Comorbidities Involved in Asthma Management

The clinical course of asthma in children may be accompanied by extra-pulmonary conditions that can contribute to respiratory symptoms, exacerbate asthma, and increase the overall burden of the disease. These conditions include allergic rhinitis, chronic rhinosinusitis, obesity, gastroesophageal reflux, obstructive sleep apnea, depression, and anxiety. It is important to address these comorbidities alongside managing asthma symptoms, as treating them can lead to improved asthma control and potentially reduce the use of ICS.

4.4.3.4 Other Factors Affecting Treatment Decisions

Current recommendations regarding the preferred treatment for asthma vary based on the specific characteristics of the target population. Age is a significant factor influencing treatment decisions, and separate guidelines exist for preschoolers, children aged 6–11 years, and adolescents. In the GINA document [12], patients at step 5 of asthma treatment may require different treatment approaches, including the use of biologics, based on their inflammatory phenotype categorized as type 2-high or type 2-low.

Certain factors contribute to a child's increased risk of experiencing poor asthma outcomes and should be assessed at the time of diagnosis and periodically afterward. These factors include the overuse of SABA, the underuse of ICS, poor adherence to treatment or incorrect inhalation technique, the presence of comorbidities, exposure to asthma triggers, low lung function (e.g., $FEV_1 < 60\%$), the evidence of excessive type 2 inflammation (elevated blood eosinophils, high FeNO despite ICS use), and history of intubation, intensive care unit (ICU) admission, or at least one severe exacerbation within the previous year. The presence of one or more of these factors in an individual child influences the type and level of treatment required [16, 30–32]. In preschoolers, an eosinophil count >300/μl and/or aeroallergen sensitization predicts a favorable response to ICS.

4.4.3.5 Stepwise Approach to Asthma Medications

Different guidelines are utilized worldwide for determining the escalation or de-escalation of treatment in children with asthma. These guidelines uniformly recommend adjusting therapy to a higher step to achieve asthma control and mitigate the risk of future severe attacks.

These guidelines recommend the use of various control agents to manage asthma, including ICS, long-acting bronchodilators, leukotriene modifiers, long-acting antimuscarinic agents (LAMA), and biologics such as anti-IgE antibodies (e.g., omalizumab), anti-IL5 monoclonal antibodies (e.g., mepolizumab), and anti-IL4 receptor α monoclonal antibody (e.g., dupilumab) [33, 34]. The core components of asthma guidelines are summarized in Fig. 4.1.

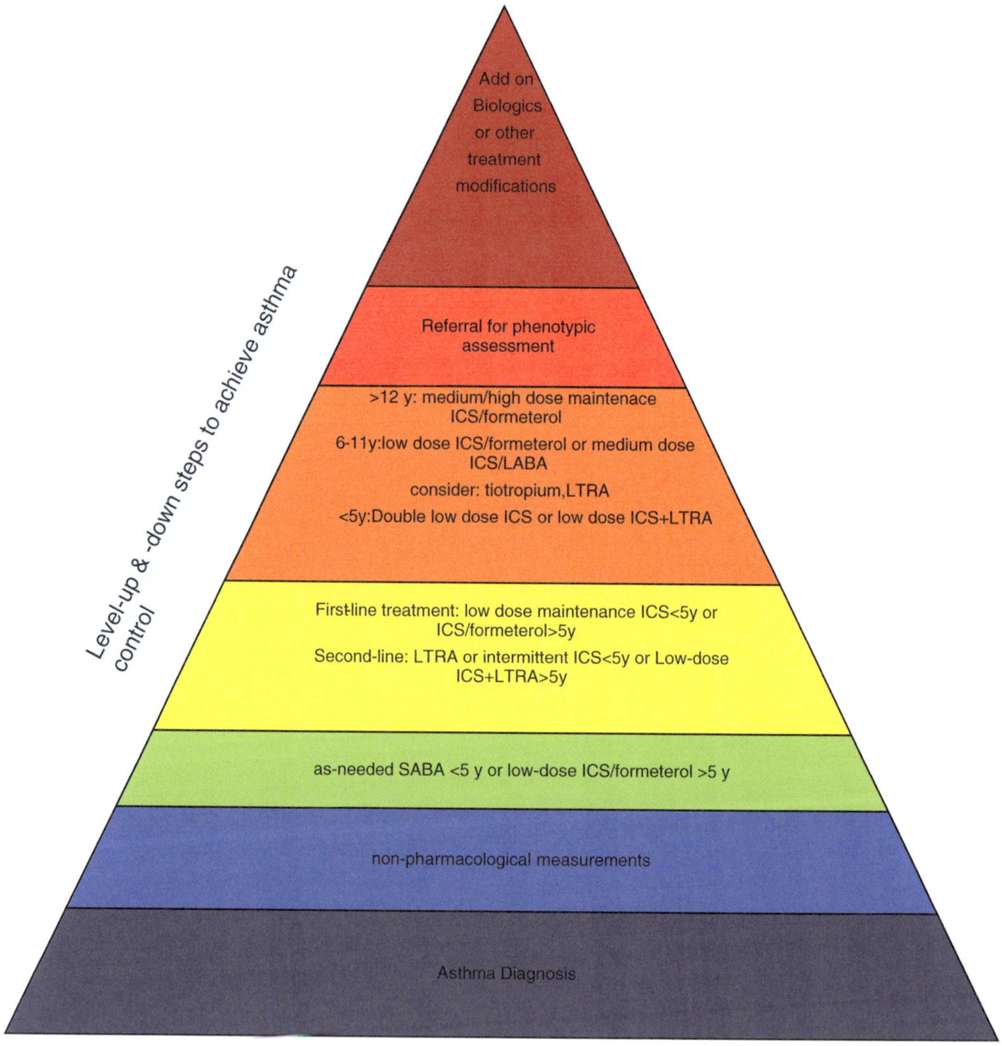

Fig. 4.1 A summary of different pediatric asthma guidelines. A confirmed asthma diagnosis is a pre-requisite before commencing asthma treatment of any level. If asthma is not adequately controlled on low daily doses of ICS with good adherence and inhalation technique, a step up of ICS dose or additional treatment is proposed. If asthma symptoms remain uncontrolled at a certain level of treatment (orange zone), a referral to a specialist for airway phenotypic assessment must be considered. Depending on the type of airway phenotype (type 2-high or type 2-low), further treatment steps are decided (e.g., the use of biologics, anti-fungal, high-dose ICS, antibiotics)

4.4.3.6 Treatment Peculiarities in Pre-School Asthma and Infantile Wheeze

There are still controversies regarding the treatment of these two forms of asthma. The rational approach is to identify the treatable traits exhibited by infants or preschoolers. For the latter, basic tests such as eosinophil count and aeroallergen sensitization tests should be performed to determine the presence of an eosinophilic phenotype in the child's airway [30]. If one or both tests suggest the presence of an eosinophilic phenotype, the child is highly likely to respond differentially to ICS. If primary bronchial ciliary dyskinesia or an airway infection is suspected, a cough swab or induced sputum should be conducted to detect the presence of bacteria. In such cases, a prolonged course of antibiotics may be used to manage symptoms.

Infantile wheezing remains a diagnostic challenge, with limited medical knowledge on this topic. Eosinophils do not appear to play a role in this type of asthma; therefore, prescribing ICS is not recommended. In this age group, symptoms may be caused by gastroesophageal reflux, primary aspiration, congenital airway anomalies (such as tracheobronchomalacia), inherited diseases that affect mucociliary clearance (such as cystic fibrosis and primary ciliary dyskinesia), prematurity, immunodeficiency, and rarely interstitial lung diseases. A thorough history and examination, along with basic tests such as a chest x-ray, a sweat test, and basic immunology studies, can aid in the diagnostic process. Treatment should be based on the underlying disorder, focusing on avoiding unnecessary or excessive therapies such as steroids or antibiotics [18].

4.4.3.7 When to Step Down the Asthma Treatment

According to the GINA 2021 report, when asthma symptoms have been well controlled for at least 3 months, it should be considered to stop or decrease the dose of medications to the lowest effective regimen [12]. A follow-up appointment is necessary to confirm the efficacy and safety of any treatment adjustments that are made.

4.4.3.8 When to Seek an Expert Opinion

Most pediatric asthma patients are diagnosed and treated in primary care without the involvement of general pediatricians or pediatric respiratory experts. However, certain children with asthma may require referral to an asthma specialist for consultation or co-management. There are several reasons for referral, including:

- Diagnostic ambiguity.
- Children who are not managed on moderate dose ICS despite proper inhalation technique and adequate medication adherence.
- Confirmed or suspected severe asthma.
- A history of an asthma-related ICU admission.
- Any hospitalization for asthma, or at least two emergency department visits or at least two courses of systemic steroids in the previous months.

4.4.4 Management of Worsening Asthma and Exacerbations

An asthma exacerbation is defined as an acute or subacute deterioration of symptom control that leads to respiratory distress or poses a health risk. It is characterized by a sudden or gradual worsening of symptoms such as difficulty breathing, coughing, wheezing, chest tightness, and decreased lung function. This deterioration necessitates a modification in treatment [34]. Asthma exacerbations can occur in patients already diagnosed with asthma, or they can be the first manifestation of asthma in a previously unaffected individual. Relapses often occur due to exposure to external triggers (such as allergens, pollutants, seasonal changes, or respiratory tract infections), persistent inflammation, or poor adherence to therapy [35] (Table 4.4).

Through history collection, objective examination, and vital parameters, the flare-up can be classified as mild, moderate, severe, or danger to life (Table 4.5).

Table 4.4 Assessing exacerbation severity

1. History.
   - Timing of onset and cause (if known) of the present exacerbation.
   - The severity of asthma symptoms, including any limiting exercise or disturbing sleep.
   - Any symptoms of anaphylaxis.
   - Any risk factors for asthma-related death.
   - All current reliever and controller medications, including doses and devices prescribed, adherence pattern, any recent dose changes, and response to current therapy.
2. Physical examination.
   - Signs of exacerbation severity.
   - Vital signs (e.g., level of consciousness, temperature, pulse rate, respiratory rate, blood pressure, ability to complete sentences, use of accessory muscles, wheeze).
   - Complicating factors (e.g., anaphylaxis, pneumonia, pneumothorax).
   - Signs of alternative conditions that could explain acute breathlessness (e.g., cardiac failure, inducible laryngeal obstruction, inhaled foreign body, or pulmonary embolism).
3. Objective measurements.
   - Pulse oximetry.
   - PEF.

PEF peak expiratory flow

Table 4.5 The severity of exacerbation

Mild or Moderate	Severe	Life -threatening
Talks in phrases The respiratory rate increased (but accessory muscles were not used) Pulse rate: 100–120bpm O_2 saturation: 90–95% PEF >50% predicted or best	Talks in words Agitated Respiratory rate >30/min Accessory muscles in use Pulse rate: > 120bpm O2 saturation: < 90% PEF <50% predicted or best	Drowsy Confused Silent chest

PEF peak expiratory flow

Table 4.6 Factors that increase the risk of asthma-related death. SABA: short-acting beta$_2$-agonist

Factors that increase the risk of asthma-related death
A history of near-fatal asthma requiring intubation and mechanical ventilation
Currently using or having recently stopped using oral corticosteroid
Several comorbidities, including pneumonia, diabetes and arrhythmias
A history of psychiatric disease or psychosocial problems
Food allergy
Overuse of SABAs, especially the use of more than one canister of salbutamol (or equivalent) monthly
Poor adherence to treatment
Hospitalization or emergency care visit for asthma in the past year

Severe asthma attacks can even lead to death. Factors associated with an increased risk of asthma-related death are reported in Table 4.6.

Initial treatment of acute asthma exacerbations, including beta-agonist therapy and oral glucocorticoids, is sometimes provided in the primary care setting or even at home. However, children with moderate-to-severe exacerbations require close observation for clinical deterioration, frequent treatments, and repeated evaluation. Therefore, most children with moderate or severe asthma exacerbations should be managed in an emergency department setting. The general approach to the treatment of an acute asthma exacerbation may involve the administration of inhaled bronchodilators (such as salbutamol), magnesium sulfate, systemic bronchodilators (such as salbutamol or theophylline), systemic glucocorticoids, and oxygen treatment. In severe cases, admission to the intensive care unit may be necessary. Following an asthma attack, reviews are crucial opportunities to assess maintenance medication and current symptom control.

4.5 Conclusion

Pediatric asthma outcomes currently remain poor, and many deaths are preventable. To improve outcomes, accurate diagnosis and management are crucial. Effective asthma care goes beyond providing medication and should encompass periodic follow-up, monitoring of lung function and inflammation, education, and supported self-management advice. Promoting lifestyle changes such as adopting a healthy diet, increasing physical activity, reducing sedentary activities, and minimizing children's exposure to environmental tobacco smoke is essential. Smoking and vaping cessation, as well as reducing barriers to vaccination, are recommended for asthmatic children. Encouraging regular exercise can enhance the quality of life (QoL) and lung function in patients with asthma [36]. Moreover, emerging evidence regarding the role of the microbiomes in asthma suggests that paying greater attention to dietary components and their impact on the gut microbiome may benefit obese individuals with asthma [37].

References

1. Manti S, Licari A, Leonardi S, Marseglia GL. Management of asthma exacerbations in the paediatric population: a systematic review. Eur Respir Rev. 2021;30:200367.
2. Bush A, Pavord ID. The lancet asthma commission: treating children in primary care. Prescriber. 2018;29:28–32.
3. Reddel HK, Bacharier LB, Bateman ED, Brightling CE, Brusselle GG, Buhl R, et al. Global initiative for asthma strategy 2021: executive summary and rationale for key changes. Am J Respir Crit Care Med. 2022;205:17–35.
4. Bel EH. Clinical phenotypes of asthma. Curr Opin Pulm Med. 2004;10:44–50.
5. Kuruvilla ME, Lee FE, Lee GB. Understanding asthma phenotypes, Endotypes, and mechanisms of disease. Clin Rev Allergy Immunol. 2019;56:219–33.
6. Levy ML. The national review of asthma deaths: what did we learn and what needs to change? Breathe (Sheff). 2015;11:14–24.
7. Gautier C, Charpin D. Environmental triggers and avoidance in the management of asthma. J Asthma Allergy. 2017;10:47–56.
8. Win PH, Hussain I. Asthma triggers: what really matters? Clin Asthma. 2008;22:149–56.
9. Manti S, Leonardi S, Rezaee F, Harford TJ, Perez MK, Piedimonte G. Effects of vertical transmission of respiratory viruses to the offspring. Front Immunol. 2022;14:853009. https://doi.org/10.3389/fimmu.2022.853009.
10. Manti S, Piedimonte G. An overview on the RSV-mediated mechanisms in the onset of non-allergic asthma. Front Pediatr. 2022;20.:998296.
11. Chatziparasidis G, Priftis KN, Bush A. Wheezing as a respiratory sound. In: Priftis K, Hadjileontiadis L, Everard M, editors. Breath sounds. Cham: Springer; 2018.
12. 2022 GINA Report, Global Strategy for Asthma Management and Prevention. https://ginasthma.org/gina-reports/.
13. Chatziparasidis G, Bush A. Enigma variations: the multi-faceted problems of pre-school wheeze. Pediatr Pulmonol. 2022;57:1990–7.
14. Grell AV, Vera RG, Yarur AM, Castro-Rodriguez JA, Montenegro MAP, Colodro OF, et al. Impulse oscillometry in pre-school children with persistent asthma can predict spirometry at school age. Pediatr Pulmonol. 2023;58:1411–6.
15. Gaillard EA, Kuehni CE, Turner S, Goutaki M, Holden KA, de Jong CCM,et al. European Respiratory Society clinical practice guidelines for the diagnosis of asthma in children aged 5–16 years. Eur Respir J. 2021;58:2004173.
16. Fitzpatrick AM, Jackson DJ, Mauger DT, Boehmer SJ, Phipatanakul W, Sheehan WJ, et al. Individualized therapy for persistent asthma in young children. J Allergy Clin Immunol. 2016,138.1608–1618.e12.
17. Jochmann A, Artusio L, Robson K, Nagakumar P, Collins N, Fleming L, et al. Infection and inflammation in induced sputum from pre-school children with chronic airways diseases. Pediatr Pulmonol. 2016;51:778–86.
18. Bush A. Pathophysiological mechanisms of asthma. Front Pediatr. 2019;7:68.
19. Marseglia GL, Manti S, Chiappini E, Brambilla I, Caffarelli C, Calvani M,et al. Chronic cough in childhood: a systematic review for practical guidance by the Italian Society of Pediatric Allergy and Immunology. Allergol Immunopathol (Madr). 2021;49:133–54.
20. Manti S, Parisi GF, Giacchi V, Sciacca P, Tardino L, Cuppari C,et l. Pilot study shows right ventricular diastolic function impairment in young children with obstructive respiratory disease. Acta Paediatr. 2019;108:740–4.
21. Wanrooij VH, Willeboordse M, Dompeling E, van de Kant KD. Exercise training in children with asthma: a systematic review. Br J Sports Med. 2014;48:1024–31.

22. Lu KD, Forno E. Exercise and lifestyle changes in pediatric asthma. Curr Opin Pulm Med. 2020;26:103–11.
23. Boutopoulou B, Koumpagioti D, Matziou V, Priftis KN, Douros K. Interventions on adherence to treatment in children with severe asthma: a systematic review. Front Pediatr. 2018;6:232.
24. Guevara JP, Wolf FM, Grum CM, Clark NM. Effects of educational interventions for self management of asthma in children and adolescents: systematic review and meta-analysis. BMJ. 2003;326:1308–9.
25. Gillette C, Rockich-Winston N, Kuhn JA, Flesher S, Shepherd M. Inhaler technique in children with asthma: a systematic review. Acad Pediatr. 2016;16:605–15.
26. Capanoglu M, Dibek Misirlioglu E, Toyran M, Civelek E, Kocabas CN. Evaluation of inhaler technique, adherence to therapy and their effect on disease control among children with asthma using metered dose or dry powder inhalers. J Asthma. 2015;52:838–45.
27. Searle A, Jago R, Henderson J, Turner KM. Children's, parents' and health professionals' views on the management of childhood asthma: a qualitative study. NPJ Prim Care Respir Med. 2017;27:53.
28. Lakupoch K, Manuyakorn W, Preutthipan A, Kamalaporn H. The effectiveness of newly developed written asthma action plan in improvement of asthma outcome in children. Asian Pac J Allergy Immunol. 2018;36:88–92.
29. Asthma care in a crisis. Annual asthma survey 2020. Available https://www.asthmaandlung.org.uk › sites › files.
30. Fitzpatrick AM, Bacharier LB, Guilbert TW, Jackson DJ, Szefler SJ, Beigelman A, et al. Phenotypes of recurrent wheezing in pre-school children: identification by latent class analysis and utility in prediction of future exacerbation. J Allergy Clin Immunol Pract. 2019;7:915–924.e7.
31. Licari A, Manti S, Castagnoli R, Marseglia A, Foiadelli T, Brambilla I, et al. Immunomodulation in pediatric asthma. Front Pediatr. 2019;12:289.
32. Licari A, Manti S, Castagnoli R, Leonardi S, Marseglia GL. Measuring inflammation in paediatric severe asthma: biomarkers in clinical practice. Breathe (Sheff). 2020;16:1903011.
33. Reddel HK, Taylor DR, Bateman ED, Boulet LP, Boushey HA, Busse WW, et al. An official American Thoracic Society/European Respiratory Society statement: asthma control and exacerbations: standardizing endpoints for clinical asthma trials and clinical practice. Am J Respir Crit Care Med. 2009;180:59–99.
34. Licari A, Manti S, Castagnoli R, Parisi GF, Salpietro C, Leonardi S, etal. Targeted therapy for severe asthma in children and adolescents: current and future perspectives. Paediatr Drugs. 2019;21:215–37.
35. Ramnath VR, Clark S, Camargo CA Jr. Multicenter study of clinical features of sudden-onset versus slower-onset asthma exacerbations requiring hospitalization. Respir Care. 2007;52:1013–20.
36. Jing Z, Wang X, Zhang P, Huang J, Jia Y, Zhang J, et l. Effects of physical activity on lung function and quality of life in asthmatic children: an updated systematic review and meta-analysis. Front Pediatr. 2023;11:1074429.
37. Tashiro H, Shore SA. Obesity and severe asthma. Allergol Int. 2019;68:135–42.

5 Severe Asthma in the Pediatric Patient

Giulia Roberto, Beatrice Andrenacci, Maria De Filippo, Martina Votto, Alessia Marseglia, Sara Manti, Gian Luigi Marseglia, and Amelia Licari

Abstract

Severe asthma is a rare, yet health-resource consuming and potentially lethal condition among children and adolescents. The severe asthma definition currently includes three different entities, according to the presence of concomitant addressable treatable traits (*difficult-to-treat-asthma*), not addressable or not identifiable complex treatable traits (*refractory difficult asthma*) or the absence of coexisting modifiable factors (the real *severe therapy-resistant asthma*, STRA). Compared to evidence among asthmatic adults, STRA has unique features in pediatrics. Therefore, this chapter will focus on severe asthma definition, classification, proper diagnosis, and management in pediatrics, with a brief overview of novel biomarkers and imaging techniques.

Keywords

Airflow obstruction · Airway inflammation Allergy · Alternative diagnosis · Biologic therapies · Biomarkers · Comorbidities Endotypes · Pediatrics · Severe asthma

Test your learning and check your understanding of this book's contents: use the "Springer Nature Flashcards" app to access questions using ▶ https://sn.pub/nspbjm. To use the app, please follow the instructions in Chap. 1.

Key Points

- Severe asthma is a rare yet resource-demanding and potentially fatal disease.
- Severe asthma has unique features in pediatrics. Such features must be considered in the attempt to provide target

(continued)

Giulia Roberto and Beatrice Andrenacci contributed equally to this work.

G. Roberto · B. Andrenacci · M. De Filippo · M. Votto A. Marseglia · G. L. Marseglia · A. Licari (✉)
Pediatric Unit, Department of Clinical, Surgical, Diagnostic and Pediatric Sciences, University of Pavia, Pavia, Italy

Pediatric Clinic, Fondazione IRCCS Policlinico San Matteo, Pavia, Italy
e-mail: amelia.licari@unipv.it

S. Manti
Pediatric Unit, Department of Human and Pediatric Pathology "Gaetano Barresi", AOUP G. Martino, University of Messina, Messina, Italy

C. Caffarelli, G. L. Marseglia (eds.), *Textbook of Pediatric Allergy*,
https://doi.org/10.1007/978-3-031-71283-8_5

anti-asthmatic treatments in children and adolescents.
- Since the management is different, real *severe therapy-resistant asthma* must be distinguished from *difficult-to-treat asthma* and *refractory difficult asthma.*
- Chest CT and novel, noninvasive urinary or exhaled biomarkers are promising tools to identify patients with poorer prognoses and response to therapies early.

5.1 Introduction

Most patients affected by asthma benefit from standard treatments to obtain symptom control and minimize acute attacks, but there is a subgroup of pediatric patients with persistent symptoms [1]. Severe asthma is a rare entity, affecting about 2–5% of asthmatic children, and because of its pleiomorphic aspects, a shared universal definition is still lacking. Many factors can influence asthma severity and symptom control. Severe asthma has been subclassified into three distinct entities: difficult-to-treat asthma; refractory difficult asthma; and severe therapy-resistant asthma (STRA) [2, 3]. More in detail, difficult-to-treat asthma is a form of severe asthma where clinical control can be reached after the identification and correction of all the modifiable cofactors ("treatable traits"), which include adherence to therapies, incorrect inhaler techniques, comorbidities, exposure to allergens, pollutants, and irritants, psychological issues, and the socioeconomic status of the family. Refractory difficult asthma is a more challenging form of severe asthma, complicated by the presence of "treatable traits" that, once identified, cannot be resolved—as complex psychological or sociocultural factors. Finally, STRA is severe asthma that remains uncontrolled despite good adherence to maximal anti-asthmatic therapies and proper management of all the concomitant "treatable traits." Such heterogeneity in the definition reflects that severe asthma is an "umbrella term," including many different clinical and molecular entities with unique characteristics. In this chapter, we have decided to adopt the general definition according to the ATS/ERS guideline reviewed in 2020 [4]: severe asthma is defined as asthma that requires high-dose inhaled corticosteroids (ICS) plus a second controller (and/or systemic corticosteroid) as a therapy to prevent it from becoming "uncontrolled" or remaining "uncontrolled" despite maximal therapy. The global prevalence of severe asthma in the pediatric population is not homogenously stratified; according to the International Study of Asthma and Allergies in Childhood (ISAAC), it has been calculated at 6.9%, ranging from 3.8% in Asia-Pacific and Northern and Eastern Europe to 11.3% in North America [1]. Hence, severe asthma represents a serious health problem responsible for about half of the global asthma burden worldwide (medication-related side effects, life-threatening exacerbations, and impaired quality of life). The progressive airflow limitation is also a feature of severe asthma, which can lead to airway remodeling and irreversible bronchial obstruction.

5.1.1 Severe-Therapy-Resistant Asthma Classification: From Phenotypes to Endotypes

Asthma is defined by the presence of bronchial inflammation resulting from a complex interplay among many different molecular and cellular actors, such as innate and adaptative immunity, microbiome, allergens, pollutants, and irritants. Increasing evidence has recently highlighted the relevant role of airway *redox imbalance* [5] and respiratory structural cells in asthma and severe asthma pathogenesis [6]. It is now known that the airway epithelial cells are much more than an inert physical barrier. Their involvement in airway remodeling may be a precocious step in asthma pathogenesis, which may even precede and promote bronchial inflammation in the pediatric age [6, 7].

Based on this evidence, asthma (and STRA in particular) is no longer considered a single disease but an umbrella term that covers many different entities with unique clinical and inflammatory features. Over the years, evidence led to the attempt to further classify asthma into discrete *phenotypes* (defined as "a set of observable characteristics resulting from the genotype-environment interaction") and *endotypes* (defined as "distinct molecular and functional pathways underlying different pathophysiologic processes"), to provide severe asthmatics with targeted therapies [8]. Studies like the longitudinal Severe Asthma Research Program (SARP), promoted by the National Heart, Lung and Blood Institute, or the Unbiased Biomarkers for the Prediction of Respiratory Disease Outcomes (U-BIOPRED) promoted by the European Innovative Medicines Initiative, helped in the initial definition of adult and pediatric severe asthma phenotypes and endotypes, combining unbiased hypothesis-free statistics and system biology [9]. Since clinical phenotypes showed poor consistency among different studies and a lack of correspondence to specific pathogenetic pathways, increasing efforts have been invested in defining STRA inflammatory endotypes. The gold standard for a proper definition of asthma STRA endotypes is using invasive techniques such as bronchoscopy or bronchoalveolar lavage (BAL), which are rarely performed in pediatrics. Therefore, most pediatric evidence is improperly extrapolated from adult studies or derived from a few monocentric, cross-sectional studies with small sample sizes. Despite these limitations, pediatric STRA is currently subclassified into five distinct endotypes according to BAL characteristics [10, 11].

- **Allergic eosinophilic asthma:** A form of "type 2 high" asthma (asthma whose bronchial inflammation is associated with a high level of T helper 2 cytokines such as interleukin 4, 5, and 13) triggered by allergens. This is the most common pediatric STRA endotype so far and can be favorably addressed using biological therapies such as anti-IgE (omalizumab), anti-interleukin 5 (mepolizumab), or anti-interleukin 4 receptor (dupilumab).
- **Nonallergic eosinophilic asthma**: A form of "type 2 high" asthma not triggered by allergens. In that case, the production of T helper 2 cytokines depends not on T helper (TH) cells but on type 2 innate lymphoid cells (ILC2). Those immune cells are activated in response to the release of molecular "danger signals" (the so-called "alarmins" IL-25 and IL-33) by damaged bronchial epithelium [7]. Anti-interleukin 5 (Mepolizumab) and anti-interleukin 4 receptor (Dupilumab) can be beneficial in addressing this specific kind of STRA.
- **Neutrophilic asthma**: A rare form of "type 2 low" asthma (which means: asthma whose bronchial inflammation is not associated with a high level of TH2 cytokines) with evidence of neutrophilic bronchial inflammation and high levels of IL-8. This STRA entity is quite rare and controversial in pediatrics. Some authors suggest that the neutrophilic inflammation in BAL can result from confounding factors, such as concomitant infections, microbiome alterations, or chronic, long-term treatments with ICS [10]. Currently, no biological therapies are available for that specific STRA endotype. Therapeutic options may include add-on tiotropium, long-term low-dose macrolide, and weight loss in the case of concomitant obesity [11].
- **Paucigranulocytic asthma**: A form of "type 2 low" asthma with few inflammatory cells and molecules detectable on BAL, in which the role of airway structural cells is predominant. Omalizumab is a promising therapy for addressing airway remodeling in paucigranulocytic asthma [12], thanks to its action against IgE-binding smooth muscle cells. Biologic treatments antagonizing alarmins, such as the anti-IL33 Tezepelumab, are another promising therapeutic option, currently approved by

the European Medicine Agency (EMA) from 12 years of age [13].
- **Mixed asthma**: A form of asthma with concomitant eosinophilic and neutrophilic bronchial inflammation. Since this form of asthma is often steroid-resistant, it is currently considered a form of "type 2 low" asthma.

Finally, although it is the most widespread and used, it is important to remember that this classification does not take into account three additional emerging features in severe asthma pathogenesis.

- The role of intraepithelial airway neutrophils seems to correlate with better lung function outcomes [14]. This has led to the hypothesis that inflammatory cells may have different roles according to their micro-compartmentalization in the bronchi.
- The emerging capability of different T cells to co-express mixed TH1/TH2/TH17 cytokines, escaping the current, binary classification of "type 2 high" and "type 2 low" inflammation [15].
- The documented presence, in some severe asthma mice models and pediatric STRA, of eosinophilic airway inflammation without the typical "type 2 high" cytokines [16], or the presence of "type 2 high" cytokines in the absence of detectable TH2 or ILC2 cells [17]. This contradictory evidence may be, respectively, the result of a long-term ICS therapy or of some innate cells capable of producing "type 2 high" cytokines, such as macrophages, but further studies are needed.

5.2 Evaluation of Pediatric Severe Asthma and Diagnostic Work-Up

The first step of the diagnostic work-up is the high degree of suspicion regarding the diagnosis of asthma (Fig. 5.1). Misdiagnosis of nonasthmatic conditions such as uncontrolled asthma has been reported up to 12–30%. A careful and detailed anamnesis history must focus on asthma symptoms, including dyspnea related to exercise, cough (dry/wet), wheezing, chest tightness, and nocturnal awakenings. In addition, the clinician should look for exacerbating triggers and environmental factors that may be contributing. Asthma masquerades must always be ruled out. It is important to confirm whether children with suspected asthma have variable airflow obstruction documented by spirometry. Post- bronchodilator response of 12% and/or 200 mL increase in Forced Expiratory Volume in the first second (FEV1) compared with baseline FEV1 suggest a "significant" bronchodilator response. In some cases, an 8% increase in FEV1 after bronchodilator may be more sensitive to evaluate response in children. Children with a normal FEV1 both before and after bronchodilatation may show a bronchodilator response in terms of forced expiratory flow at 25–75% of FVC (FEF25–75%), but the utility of FEF25–75% in the assessment or treatment of severe asthma is currently unknown. However, children with severe asthma often have normal lung function and no acute response to bronchodilators, and if there is no evidence of obstruction on spirometry, then bronchoprovocation testing with methacholine or exercise challenge needs to be performed. A chest radiograph is also necessary to rule out anatomic abnormalities of airways, lung parenchyma, and heart. Additional diagnostic procedures to rule out alternative diagnoses should be guided by clinical suspicion or atypical presentation: high-resolution computed tomography (HRCT), bronchoscopy with bronchoalveolar lavage (BAL), sweat chloride testing, nasal or airway ciliary biopsy, basic immune work-up including quantitative immunoglobulin levels with antibody responses, pH/impedance probe or videofluoroscopic swallow study needs to be considered in the assessment of differential diagnosis. Particularly, bronchoscopy is not considered in the current consensus statements regarding asthma management and has been relegated to ruling out asthma mimickers. More recently, however, there have been questions surrounding the clinical utility of bronchoscopy in severe childhood asthma. In practice, performing BAL will help to rule out protracted bacterial

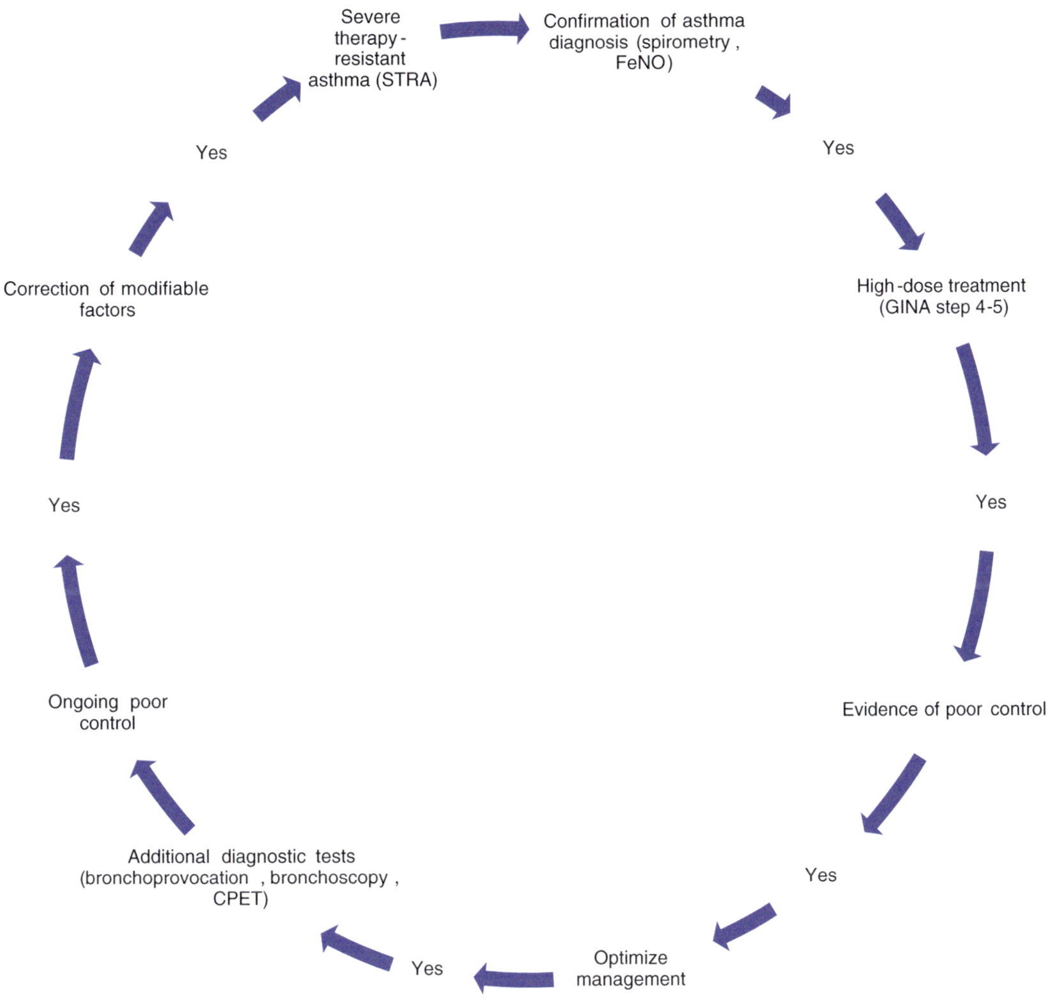

Fig. 5.1 summarizes the needed steps to confirm pediatric STRA diagnosis, according to European Respiratory Society (ERS) indications [3]

bronchitis, and it plays a key role in differentiating phenotypes of airway inflammation in severe asthma (eosinophilic inflammation, paucigranulocytic inflammation, and neutrophilic inflammation) [1]. Furthermore, ongoing studies are trying to understand if bronchoscopy could be part of treatment management (especially biological therapies), but results are now insufficient to come up with a confident answer. Ullman et al. were the first to analyze surrogate markers of airway inflammation prospectively and rigorously in children with severe asthma, concluding that "peripheral blood counts are not reliable in characterizing airway inflammation in severe asthmatic children exposed to high dose steroid therapy, therefore bronchoscopy with BAL should be considered." More recently, Ribeiro et al. demonstrated similar discordance between blood and BAL eosinophils, also highlighting the possibility that analysis of BAL eosinophils may help to identify patients who might be candidates for anti-IL-5 therapy despite blood values outside the recommended parameters for treatment [18]. The other diagnostic procedure with a controversial role is HRCT. The last ERS/ATS documents on pediatric severe asthma published in 2014 do not recommend routine chest HRCT scans and suggest it only when the presentation is atypical (such as excessive mucus production, rapid decline in lung function, reduced carbon monoxide transfer factor coefficient, absence of atopy in a child with difficult asthma) or in the assessment for complications in case of acute asthma exacerbation (i.e., pneumothorax, atelectasis). Conversely, a chest HRCT could identify alternative diagnoses and comorbidities essential in managing the patients. The main deterrents that limit chest CT execution today are the oncologic risk due to ionizing exposure and the cost. CT scanning may also be useful for diagnosing asthma-related diseases, such as allergic bronchopulmonary aspergillosis, eosinophilic pneumonia, and eosinophilic granulomatosis with polyangiitis. Subepithelial thickening of the bronchial reticular layer is an early feature of severe asthma in children and appears to be characteristic of the eosinophilic phenotype. Qualitative studies of CT scans performed on severe asthmatic adults have shown relatively high rates of bronchiectasis and bronchial wall thickening, associated with worse lung function and longer disease duration [19]. Quantitative analysis of CT images has shown that airway thickening and air trapping measures are associated with lung function impairments; however, most of the studies involved adults with severe asthma. Future improvements in HRCT may improve assessments of small airway damage and include it for determining optimal treatment. However, CT scans will continue to involve irradiation of the subject, justifying the development of other non-irradiating techniques. Lung imaging with hyperpolarized helium-3 magnetic resonance techniques seems to be a promising approach for monitoring changes in gas distribution in the lungs [20].

5.3 Differential Diagnosis of Severe Asthma in Pediatrics

Since clinical asthma symptoms are not specific, misdiagnosis due to nonasthmatic conditions is still frequent. Currently, it is thought that up to 30% of severe asthma diagnoses could instead underlie other alternative diagnoses [21], which need to be properly addressed and ruled out before starting anti-asthmatic treatments. Many conditions may mimic severe, uncontrolled pediatric asthma, the most common of which are summarized in Table 5.1. The presence of wheezing, cough, chest tightness, and shortness of breath of variable intensity, often worsening late at night or early in the morning, suggests asthma [22]. On the contrary, atypical signs and symptoms (such as failure to thrive, heart murmurs, wet cough, stridor, concomitant dizziness or paresthesia, or symptoms associated with meals) must be carefully evaluated, as they make asthma diagnosis less likely [22, 23]. In the suspicion of alternative diagnoses [23], additional tests can be performed according to clinical judgment, such as serum immunoglobulin dosage, flow cytometry, sweat chloride testing, nasal brushing, nasal nitric oxide, fungal precipitins, high-resolution computer tomography, laryngoscopy, bronchoscopy with bronchoalveolar lavage, pH-impedancemetry or video-fluoroscopy [22, 23].

5.4 Pediatric Severe Asthma Comorbidities

Asthma comorbidities frequently cause adverse outcomes, such as poor asthma control, frequent asthma attacks, reduced quality of life, and higher healthcare costs. Comorbidities are still a potential cause of misdiagnosis, and under or overtreatment and proper management can help to achieve optimal asthma control. Over the years, growing scientific evidence highlighted an epidemiological correlation between asthma and its comorbidities and possible common pathogenetic mechanisms. Therefore, during the first medical assessment for severe asthma, comorbidities should be identified to treat any of them if present and optimize asthma control [24].

Atopic conditions such as rhinosinusitis, dermatitis, or food allergies can all be associated with severe asthma and poor control, deserving appropriate treatments.

Allergic rhinitis is the most common comorbidity (70–80% of asthmatic patients) and shares

Table 5.1 Most frequent differential diagnoses of pediatric severe asthma

Upper airway diseases	Vocal cord dysfunction Tracheobronchomalacia
Chronic lung diseases	Bronchopulmonary dysplasia Cystic fibrosis Primary ciliary dyskinesia Alpha-1 antitrypsin deficiency Bronchiectasis Bronchiolitis obliterans Childhood diffuse interstitial lung diseases (chILD)
Infective diseases	Protracted bacterial bronchitis Tuberculosis Pertussis
Gastroenteric diseases	Dysphagia and swallow dysfunction Tracheoesophageal fistula
Extrinsic or intrinsic bronchial compression	Mediastinal masses Enlarged lymph nodes Endobronchial masses
Cardiovascular diseases	Vascular rings Congenital heart diseases
Immunorheumatological diseases	Congenital immune deficiency Acquired immune deficiency Connective diseases
Others	Dysfunctional breathing and hyperventilation Panic attacks Deconditioning Pulmonary embolism Foreign body aspiration

numerous pathogenetic and pathophysiological mechanisms with asthma. Based on the concept of "united airway disease," proper treatment of allergic rhinitis can reduce inflammation of the lower airways. When prescription criteria are fulfilled, allergen immunotherapy (AIT) can be considered the ideal therapy for simultaneous treatment of both upper and lower airways, and it is included in the latest GINA review among the additional treatment options for improving asthma control. Additionally, allergic rhinitis is considered a risk factor for asthma exacerbations [24].

The prevalence of food allergy is estimated to be around 10% in children with asthma. Regarding IgE-mediated forms, food allergy can lead to increased nocturnal symptoms, asthma flare-ups, and increased consumption of oral steroids and health care resources, as demonstrated in the National Cooperative Inner-City Asthma Study. The simultaneous presence of food allergies and asthma is an important risk factor for severe, though not fatal, allergic reactions.

Furthermore, asthma is present in approximately 15–50% of pediatric individuals with atopic dermatitis (AD), and the severity of dermatitis carries an increased risk of developing or presenting with concomitant asthma. For many years, the loss of skin integrity typical of AD (and the loss of function and structure of filaggrin, an integral epidermal barrier protein) has been considered the first step for the longitudinal development of other allergic diseases (the "atopic march"). However, it is known how the classic evolution of atopic march—from AD, to allergic rhinitis, to bronchial asthma—is often disregarded, as shown by recent studies, such as the Avon Longitudinal Study of Parents and Children, which found this time sequence in <4% of children. In adolescents with moderate-to-severe AD and children aged 6–11 years with severe AD, anti-IL4 and IL4a can finally be proposed, which are able not only to improve skin symptoms and quality of life but also to treat simultaneously other allergic comorbidities frequently present, such as asthma, allergic rhinitis, and chronic rhinosinusitis [11].

Finally, to 30–50% of individuals with eosinophil esophagitis (EoE) have concurrent asthma and severe asthma. Although the pathogenetic relationship between asthma and EoE has not been well defined yet, a recent retrospective single-center pediatric study of 24 patients aged 2–16 years who underwent combined esophagogastroduodenoscopy, bronchoscopy, and laryngoscopy detected the presence of elevated levels of eosinophils at both the esophageal and bronchial levels, suggesting the common trafficking of eosinophils in the airway and gastrointestinal systems. In addition, in subjects with both diseases, the extent of esophageal eosinophil infiltrate and allergic sensitizations, as well as fibroblast growth factor 2 (FGF2) and total serum IgE values, is higher than those found in subjects with EoE alone [11].

Chronic rhinosinusitis (CRS) can be distinguished into CRS without nasal polyposis (CRS-SNP) and with nasal polyposis (CRSWNP). While CRSsNP is more frequently associated with IL17-mediated neutrophilic inflammation, the pathogenesis of CRSwNP is more often eosinophilic, with elevated serum levels of IL5 and specific anti-enterotoxin IgE of *S. aureus*. Chronic rhinosinusitis afflicts up to 20–45% of pediatric (especially adolescent) subjects and, in the case of concomitant asthma, worsens its clinical control, increasing its severity and worsening the quality of life, in particular for CR-SwNP, which is more frequently associated with severe asthma. In a reciprocal relationship, bronchial asthma may worsen the outcomes of CRS and conversely, as evidenced by the increased levels of TNF-alpha, epithelial growth factor (EGF), fibroblast growth factor 2 (FGF2), and platelet-derived growth factor subunit A (PDGFA) in the mucosa of sinuses and adenoid tissue [24].

Obesity is a well-recognized risk factor for severe asthma, although a clear relationship is still lacking [25]. Several mechanisms can explain this correlation. First, obesity is a low-grade systemic proinflammatory condition, with leptin overexpression (an adipokine also produced by alveolar macrophages and type 2 pneumocytes) and an increase in the Th2-pathway [3]. On the other hand, asthma in obesity can be addressed by the "noneosinophilic" phenotype mediated by IL-6-driven inflammation, a systemic cytokine that results in the dysfunction of cytotoxic NK and T lymphocytes and increases the risk of asthma flare-ups secondary to viral infections [26]. In addition to inflammatory aspects, abdominal fat with diaphragm elevation may also mechanically interfere with respiratory activity, significantly limiting lung expansion.

Moreover, when obesity occurs in early life, it can lead to "dysanaptic growth," a disproportionate growth of lung parenchyma and airway caliber (longer and narrower than normal), which can contribute to steroid resistance. Conversely, asthma may itself predispose to the development of obesity because personal or parental fear of physical activity, seen as a potential asthma trigger, promotes sedentary behaviors. Furthermore, cardiopulmonary deconditioning is often associated with obesity and may contribute easily to mimicking asthma symptoms [27].

Breathing pattern disorders like vocal cord dysfunction, hyperventilation, and exercise-induced laryngeal obstruction (EILO) are often associated with asthma and anxiety and can significantly affect asthma control. Dysfunctional breathing has been found in up to 5% of children with severe asthma followed up in the outpatient clinic, and 23% of a cohort of children with problematic severe asthma admitted to the hospital [28]. Common symptoms include asthenia and malaise, dyspnea at rest, chest constriction sensation, and frequent yawning and sighing; association with obesity, anxiety, depression, and asthma is common. Asthmatics with dysfunctional breathing have a worse quality of life and severe limitations in daily activities. When assessing problematic severe asthma, a multidisciplinary team with a psychologist and a physiotherapist should always be present to teach breathing exercises and relaxation exercises (nose breathing, appropriate use of the diaphragm) and possibly cope with anxiety. Recall that dysfunctional breathing could be confused with asthma itself, leading to the prescription of unnecessary therapies.

Obstructive sleep apnea syndrome (OSAS) afflicts about 5% of pediatric subjects and up to 30% of children and adolescents with asthma, although its prevalence in severe asthma is thought to be even higher. Probably, the continuous alternation of hyper- and hypoxia typical of OSAS increases oxidative stress on the airways and vagus-mediated bronchial hyperreactivity, thus predisposing to the development of asthma and worsening in asthmatic subjects, the quality of life and symptom control, especially during sleep time [29]. Polysomnography in a clinical setting remains the gold standard for the diagnosis, and all asthmatic subjects with poor nocturnal symptom control should undergo it.

Frequently, gastroesophageal reflux (GER) is suspected in children with persistent dry cough, but until now, no evidence has been found between therapy with protonic pump inhibitors (PPI) and asthma control; hence GER should be treated only in the presence of gastroesophageal symptoms [30]. The prevalence of symptomatic reflux in the asthmatic population is about 5% in children and up to 15% among adolescents. This frequency may be secondary to inhaled relievers or oral steroids, which can induce lower esophageal sphincter relaxation, or by increased broncho-reactivity due to micro-aspirations of gastric material. The role of GER in asthma has been partially downplayed over the years; while it is true that symptomatic reflux is sometimes associated with poorly controlled asthma, it does not seem to correlate with the severity of asthma. Therefore, in GINA documents, GER is more considered as a mimicking condition of asthma than actual comorbidity, and its routine screening should be reserved mainly for subjects with uncontrolled asthma with a prevalence of nocturnal symptomatology [22]. In symptomatology suggestive of GER, an empiric trial with PPI for 3 months is indicated.

As the organic conditions described so far, psychological and emotional aspects can also strongly impact asthmatic subjects' quality of life and symptom control. Anxiety and depression are commonly found in asthmatic subjects and their caregivers, affecting up to ¼ of pediatric patients, especially adolescents [31, 32]. The relationship between asthma and emotional and psychological distress appears to be bidirectional and multifactorial: individuals with psychological comorbidities have a greater perception of their symptoms, but they often have markedly reduced adherence to therapy. Furthermore, stressful conditions can worsen eosinophilic inflammation, and hyperventilation associated with anxiety can induce bronchospasm. The pediatrician's task is to distinguish appropriately, in an emergency setting, acute asthma attacks from panic attacks, which can easily mimic asthma flare-ups, and to identify, in the outpatient setting, patients who need psychological support. Anxiety about asthma, family relationships, poor adherence, difficulty in understanding the disease, school problems, and refusal of symptoms are all issues that can be encountered when assessing problematic severe asthma.

5.5 Adherence to Anti-asthmatic Therapies

Adherence to anti-asthmatic therapies is a crucial topic in the management of difficult-to-treat asthma. According to the literature, <40% of asthmatic patients of all ages carry out their therapy regularly, at the proper dosage, and with good inhalation techniques [33]. The problem is even more widespread in pediatrics since poor adherence may involve up to 70% of asthmatic children and adolescents [34]. In turn, low adherence to ICS paves the way to higher short-acting beta2-agonist (SABA) abuse, which has been proven to be associated with an increased risk of asthma death [35]. Poor adherence may be due to unintentional obstacles (such as overestimation of asthma control, poor understanding of the therapeutic scheme or the proper inhaler technique, therapy forgetfulness, family logistic difficulties), intentional issues (such as economic difficulties, fear of side effects, rejection of the diagnosis, and unawareness of the potential danger of uncontrolled asthma), or both [11]. Adolescence is particularly critical regarding intentional poor adherence due to the many physiological and psychological changes related to puberty and the increasing independence from caregivers [36]. In that regard, it is vital for pediatricians always to check the proper understanding of asthma and asthma therapies by both the patients and their relatives and to promote increasing patient self-efficacy from childhood onward in a gradual, personalized, and developmentally-based way [36]. Many strategies could be used to improve adherence and self-efficacy among asthmatic children and adolescents. Among them, the use of written therapeutic action plans using plain, age-appropriated language, the choice of simplified therapeutic schemes, such as the maintenance-and-reliever-therapy (MART), the timely step-down of therapies in the case of a favorable response to biological drugs, the use of electronic inhaler monitors or the personal check of inhalers (in terms of expiring dates or residual doses at the time of the visit), and proper inhaler technique, may be extremely beneficial [11]. Regarding the pubertal age, the use of *transition readiness assessment tools* or the schedule of more frequent follow-up visits can be considered additional strategies to improve asthma management [36].

5.6 Pediatric Severe Asthma Biomarkers

Biomarkers identification is an emerging field in pediatric STRA, since it can provide noninvasive or minimally invasive, endotype-specific, low-priced tools to assess long-term response to anti-asthmatic treatments and the early identification of acute asthma attacks or subgroups of STRA patients with poorer prognosis, suggesting the need additional treatments [12, 37, 38].

Since the most common pediatric STRA endotype is the eosinophilic allergic one, the leading biomarkers to assess pediatric STRA are the same used in the evaluation of both mild and moderate "type 2 high" asthma—such as blood eosinophilia, total and specific serum immunoglobulin E (IgE), fractional exhaled nitric oxide (FeNO) and, eventually, sputum eosinophilia [22]. Elevated FeNO levels are evocative of persistent bronchial eosinophilic inflammation, which can depend on poor adherence to ICS therapies, protracted allergen exposure, or intrinsic asthma severity. It is important to remember that many conditions may lead to false positive and false negative results (Table 5.2) and that low FeNO levels do not completely exclude asthma diagnosis [39].

Alongside those classic biomarkers, novel promising, noninvasive biomarkers such as exhaled breath condensate (EBC), induced sputum biomarkers, urinary metabolites, or multi-sample-transcriptomics are currently emerging in the literature, although their use is currently still limited to research purposes [12].

EBC consists of a noninvasive sampling of volatile, semi-volatile, and nonvolatile compounds collected from respiratory droplets derived from the respiratory epithelial lining fluid, such as cytokines, leukotrienes, or oxidative metabolites like nitric oxide derivatives or peroxides [40, 41]. Its capability to reflect airway inflammation more faithfully than serum

Table 5.2 False positive and false negative in assessing fractional exhaled nitric oxide levels

False positive (Higher FeNO in nonasthmatic subjects)	False negative (Lower FeNO in asthmatic subjects)
Atopy	Active and passive smoking
Allergic rhinitis	Caffeine or alcohol intake
Atopic dermatitis	Cystic fibrosis
Chronic exposure to allergens	Early phase of allergic response
Chronic exposure to pollutants	Ongoing acute asthma attack
Eosinophilic bronchitis	PCD
Nitrates-rich diet	Physical exercise
Obesity	Prematurity
Viral infections	"Type 2 low" asthma endotypes
	Viral infections

PCD primary ciliary dyskinesia, *FeNO* fractional exhaled nitric oxide biomarkers makes EBC a promising STRA biomarker source in the imminent future [42].

Together with EBC, sputum biomarkers are more reliable than blood samples in assessing bronchial inflammation in asthmatic subjects. The sputum collection requires 20 minutes of nebulization of the airways with a 3% saline solution. The expectorate thus induced is centrifuged, stained, and possibly refrigerated. Finally, cells and molecules in it are analyzed. Among all sputum biomarkers, sputum eosinophilic cationic protein (derived from eosinophil degranulation) may be useful in detecting eosinophilic allergic asthma and ICS titration [42].

Urinary metabolites are another expanding field of research in pediatric STRA. Many different urinary compounds, such as eicosanoids, organic acids, or oxidative metabolism products, can be detected in the urine of the asthmatic subjects, suggesting eosinophilic inflammation (such as urinary leukotriene E4) or mast cell activity (such as urinary prostaglandin D2). Although they correlate with airway inflammation less well than EBC or induced sputum, urinary biomarkers seem particularly useful, especially in the early detection of asthma attacks [43]. Moreover, together with induced sputum and EBC, urine is the best sample to detect indirect derivatives of oxidative metabolism, which is supposed to play a relevant role in the pathogenesis of "type 2 low" asthma [44, 45]. As a matter of fact, reactive oxygen species (ROS) are too reactive and unstable to be directly measured.

Another promising source of STRA biomarkers is transcriptome analysis. This can regard both coding and noncoding RNAs and can be performed in many different biological samples to be collected minimally invasive (such as blood samples, induced sputum, or nasal brushing). Detecting specific sputum microRNA (miRNA) may help clinicians discriminate between eosinophilic and neutrophilic asthma [46]. Interestingly, it has been recently proved that a unique molecular signature of ten specific miRNA is higher among children with STRA than children with nonsevere asthma [47].

Noteworthy, although used among adults with uncontrolled severe eosinophilic asthma, serum and blood periostin are not desirable biomarkers in pediatrics since they are affected by the constitutional production of periostin by the children's growing bones [48].

Finally, since no single biomarker is currently enough to identify specific asthma endotypes and prognosis, a composite co-assessment of many different cells, molecules, and metabolites with multiple panels may be deeply beneficial in pediatric STRA to provide patients with tailored therapies.

Table 5.3 summarizes the currently validated and under-studying biomarkers for pediatric "type 2 high" or "type 2 low" STRA.

5.7 Severe Asthma Therapy

Treatment choices are guided first by the patient's inflammatory endotype (type 2 high or low). The cornerstone of asthma therapy (corticosteroid) may be insufficient in type 2 inflammation with relative refractoriness to high-dose ICS. It may be a positive response to oral corticosteroids (OCS), but potentially serious adverse effects limit their use in pediatrics. The possibility of refractory type 2 inflammation should be considered if any of the following are found while the patient is taking high-dose ICS or daily OCS: blood eosinophils ≥150/μl and/or FeNO ≥20 ppb, and/or sputum eosinophils ≥2%, and/or asthma is clinically allergen driven [22]. Patients requiring maintenance OCS may also have underlying type 2 inflammation, and they should be tested before starting OCS, at least 1-2 weeks after a course of OCS, or on the lowest possible OCS dose because OCS often suppresses biomarkers of type 2 inflammation. Biologic drugs represent a therapeutic innovation that has revolutionized the approach to severe asthma. They can be schematically classified, according to their therapeutic target, into drugs that target Th2-type mediators of inflammation [immunoglobulins (Ig)E and IL-5, -4 and -13] and drugs that target cytokines produced by innate lymphoid cells [i.e., the so-called "alarmins," such as IL-33 and thymic stromal lymphopoietin (TSLP)], which are characteristic of non-Th2 inflammation.

Table 5.3 Currently validated and under-studying biomarkers for pediatric "type 2 high" or "type 2 low" STRA

"Type 2 high" asthma	"Type 2 low" asthma
EBC – IL-5 – LTB4, LXA4 – 15-HETE	EBC – 8-isoprostane – Angiogenin, angiopoietin, DPP, TSP1, MMP-9, VEGF – IL-2, IL-10 – NOx
Serum – Eosinophils – Specific IgE – Total IgE – PGD2	Serum – Galectin-3 – IL-6, IL-8, IL-17 – MMP-9 – Progranulin – TNFa, TGFb – TSLP, IL-25, IL-33 – VOCs – YKL-40
Sputum – ECP – EDN, EPx, MBP, LTE4 – Eosinophils – Eosinophilic peroxidase – HMGB1 – IL-4, IL-5, IL-13 – ILC2 – miRNA	Sputum – Grx1 – IL-1, IL-6, IL-8 – IL-12, IL-17, IL-18, IL-21, IL-22 – ILC3 – Macrophages – MCP-1 – miRNA – Neutrophils – Neutrophil elastase – Neutrophilic myeloperoxidase – TNFa, TGFb – TSLP, IL-25, IL-33 – TWEAK
Urine – LTE4	Urine – Bromotyrosine – Isoprostane – Galectin-3

15-HETE 15-hydroxyeicosatetraenoic acid, *DPP* dipeptidyl peptidase IV, *EBC* exhaled breathe condensate, *ECP* eosinophilic cationic protein, *EDN* eosinophil derived neurotoxin, *EPX* eosinophil peroxidase, *HMGB1* high mobility group box-1, *IgE* immunoglobulin E, *IFN* interferon, *IL* interleukin, *ILC* innate lymphoid cells, *Grx1* glutaredoxin, *LTB4* leukotriene B4, *LTE4* leukotriene E4, *LXA4* lipoxin A4, *MBP* major basic protein, *miRNA* microRNA, *MMP-9* matrix metalloproteinase-9, *Nox* nitrite/nitrate, *STRA* severe-therapy resistant asthma, *PGD2* prostaglandin D2, *TGFb* transforming grow factor beta, *TNFa* tumor necrosis factor alpha, *TSLP* thymic stromal lymphopoietin, *TSP-1* thrombospondin-1, *TWEAK* tumor necrosis factor-like weak inducer of apoptosis, *VEGF* vascular endothelial growth factor, *VOCs* volatile organic compounds, *YKL-40* chitinase-3-like protein 1

Some of them are not approved yet for the pediatric population, and safety and effectiveness results from clinical trials are expected. Usually, response to the biological is evaluated after 4 months, and if favorable, it is continued with re-evaluation every 3–6 months [22]. GINA recommends switching to another biological if the patient fails to respond to the initial agent but is still eligible for T2 targeted treatment. Underlying the choice of biologicals is the fundamental difference between eosinophilic asthma and allergic asthma: the first one is characterized by a sputum eosinophil count >1%, peripheral blood eosinophil count ≥150 cells/μL, or FeNO ≥20 ppb; in the second one, there are asthma symptoms due to exposure to a perennial aeroallergen and serum total IgE levels should be 30–1300 IU/mL [22]. Generally, the criteria evaluated for a good response to biologics are exacerbation frequency, symptom control, lung function, medication side effects, treatment intensity, and patient/family satisfaction. Currently, five biologicals are approved for pediatric severe asthma (chronological order): omalizumab, mepolizumab, dupilumab, benralizumab, and tezepelumab [8].

Table 5.4 summarizes the molecular targets, mechanism of action, posology, and beneficial effects.

Table 5.4 Biologic therapies currently available in severe-therapy-resistant asthma

Drug name	Mechanism of action	Posology	Significant effects	Pediatric age approval
Omalizumab	IgG1 kappa humanized monoclonal antibody Binds to free lgE and inhibits the binding of IgE to both the high- and low-affinity IgE receptors (FeRl and CD23, respectively) It also enhances the production of IFN-a by pDCs, thus reducing viral-induced exacerbations	SC every 2–4 weeks based on total IgE level and body weight (30–1500 kU/L)	Reduced exacerbations, hospitalizations, oral CS, symptoms, increased asthma control, and quality of life	6–12 years old and >12 years old: add-on therapy to improve asthma control in patients with severe persistent allergic asthma who have a positive skin test or in vitro reactivity to a perennial aeroallergen and reduced lung function (FEV1<80%) as well as frequent daytime symptoms or night-time awakenings, and who have had multiple documented severe asthma exacerbations
Mepolizumab	IgG1 kappa humanized monoclonal antibody specific for IL-5 Inhibits the maturation, activation, proliferation, and recruitment of eosinophils	>12 years old: 100 mg SC (prefilled pen) once every 4 weeks 6–11 years old: 40 mg SC (powder for solution) once every 4 weeks	Reduced exacerbations, oral CS, symptoms	Severe refractory eosinophilic asthma in adults, adolescents, and children aged 6 years and older
Reslizumab	IgG4 kappa humanized monoclonal antibody. Binds to a specific epitope IL-5 and prevents it from binding to IL-5Ra Inhibits the maturation, activation, proliferation, and recruitment of eosinophils	IV every 4 weeks	Reduced exacerbations, serum eosinophils, increased FEV1, asthma control, and quality of life	Adult patients with severe eosinophilic asthma inadequately controlled despite high-dose ICS plus another maintenance treatment
Benralizumab	IgG1 kappa humanized monoclonal antibody Binds to a subunit of the IL-5 receptor (IL-5Ra) with inhibition of the hetero-oligomerization of a and B subunits and thus no signal transduction occurs Depletes the eosinophils and reduces basophil levels	30 mg SC every 4 weeks for the first three doses, and then every 8 weeks thereafter	Reduced exacerbations, oral CS, and symptoms	Add-on maintenance treatment in adult and adolescent patients with severe eosinophilic asthma

(continued)

Table 5.4 (continued)

Drug name	Mechanism of action	Posology	Significant effects	Pediatric age approval
Dupilumab	IgG4 human monoclonal antibody Binds to a subunit of the IL-4 receptor (IL-4Ra) shared by IL-4 and IL-13 receptor complexes, thus simultaneously inhibiting both IL-4- and IL-13-mediated signaling pathways. IL-4 and IL-13 are key cytokines for orchestration of type 2 immune responses	On OCS or with comorbid AD, initial dose of 600 mg followed by 300 mg every other week SC For all other patients, initial dose of 400 mg followed by 200 mg every other week SC	Reduced exacerbations, increased FEV1	Adults and adolescents 12 years and older as add-on maintenance treatment for severe asthma with type 2 inflammation characterized by raised blood eosinophils (>150) and/or raised FeNO (>20)

5.7.1 Omalizumab

The first and, to date, only available biologic drug that therapeutically targets serum IgE is the humanized monoclonal antibody omalizumab. Omalizumab is currently indicated for the treatment of moderate-to-severe persistent allergic asthma in patients older than 6 years since 2009 and for the treatment of chronic spontaneous urticaria in patients aged > 12 years whose symptoms are poorly controlled despite conventional antihistamine treatment (since 2014). It can be prescribed in children sensitized to aero-allergens and have a total IgE of 30 and >1500 IU/ml. However, approximately one-third of children with STRA have an IgE > 1500 IU/ml and are not eligible for omalizumab, and only approximately 50% respond to the treatment. Administered in a hospital setting subcutaneously every 2–4 weeks at a dosage that depends on the patient's weight and pretreatment total IgE value, omalizumab can bind circulating free IgE and prevent its binding to high- and low-affinity receptors present on the surface of mast cells, basophils, dendritic cells, and other cells of the immune system; such binding prevents their activation and subsequent release of cytokines and other mediators of allergic inflammation. In addition, the reduction of IgE results, through a down-regulation mechanism, in reduced expression of high-affinity receptors for IgE and, in general, can block the mechanisms that amplify the allergic-type immune response. Moreover, through the reduction of circulating free IgE, it would have the ability to restore innate antiviral defenses and reduce the number of seasonal flare-ups triggered predominantly by respiratory virus infections [49]. Overall, the therapeutic efficacy of omalizumab coexists with an excellent safety and tolerability profile, and its use is associated with a high degree of adherence to therapy. Some critical issues, however, are the definition of the optimal duration of therapy and the lack of predictive biomarkers of drug response that are useful for monitoring therapy. The registrational clinical trials seem to agree that a minimum period of 16 weeks represents an adequate treatment time to see drug efficacy, while the presence of comorbidities (atopic dermatitis, food allergy) with serum eosinophils above 300/μL and elevated exhaled nitric oxide (FeNO > 20 ppb) levels have emerged as descriptive parameters of pediatric patients' responder to omalizumab [8].

5.7.2 Mepolizumab, Benralizumab, and Reslizumab

IL-5 is a cytokine that plays a key role in the recruitment of eosinophilic granulocytes from the bone marrow and stimulates their survival, proliferation, and activation at the peripheral tissue level. It has now been shown that, in patients with severe asthma, the degree of bronchial infiltration of eosinophils correlates with the severity of the disease itself, and a direct relationship between peripheral blood eosinophil count and clinical exacerbations of asthma has also been described. Bone marrow recruitment and eosinophil activation occur through the binding between IL-5 and its receptor complex (IL-5R) on the surface of eosinophilic granulocytes. Therefore, IL-5R represents a significant therapeutic target in eosinophilic asthma. The three approved biologic drugs targeting IL5 are mepolizumab, reslizumab, and benralizumab [8]. In current guidelines, anti-IL-5 drugs are indicated as a possible adjunctive treatment in all those patients with uncontrolled severe asthma characterized by eosinophilic inflammation. These three biological drugs intervene in the IL-5 immune pathway by binding to the interleukin itself (mepolizumab and reslizumab) or its receptor (benralizumab). Mepolizumab and reslizumab are fully humanized antibodies, while benralizumab is a recombinant antibody. Of these three biological drugs, only mepolizumab is indicated in maintenance therapy in patients with severe eosinophilic asthma (>150 cells/μL) in pediatric patients aged 6 years or older through a subcutaneous administration. Benefits of mepolizumab use, initially demonstrated in adult population studies, include a reduction in asthma exacerbations and symptoms, a modest effect on FEV1, reduction or discontinuation of oral glucocorticoids, and significant improvement in quality of life [50]. Although more limited, available data on the pediatric population demonstrated a positive pharmacokinetic, pharmacodynamic, and safety profile for mepolizumab, as well as marked reductions in blood eosinophil counts and a 40% reduction in clinically significant flare-ups. Recently, the European Commission approved the marketing authorization of the monoclonal antibody benralizumab in patients aged 12 years and older with uncontrolled severe eosinophilic asthma despite prolonged inhaled corticosteroids and long-acting beta-agonists. The established dosing regimen is in fixed doses to be administered as a subcutaneous injection with prefilled syringes once every 4 weeks for the first 3 doses and once every 8 weeks thereafter. The potential advantage of benralizumab, compared with other monoclonal antibodies that target IL-5, lies in the peculiar ability to induce significant depletion of circulating eosinophils and those in the bone marrow and target tissues [50]. The consequence of this different mechanism of action is reflected in the absence of overexpression of IL-5 and IL-5R, reduced activation of eosinophils, and reduced risk of flare-ups of asthmatic events after drug withdrawal. Lastly, it is not possible to draw conclusions about the efficacy in the pediatric population for reslizumab, so further clinical trials are needed.

5.7.3 Dupilumab

Dupilumab is a fully humanized monoclonal antibody directed against IL-4 and IL-13 receptors, and it is administered subcutaneously. Its main target is the alpha subunit of the receptor for IL-4 (anti-IL-4Ralpha), which can block signal transduction mediated by both IL-4 and IL-13. These two interleukins are key factors in type 2 inflammation: while IL-4 is responsible for the regulation of IgE production by B cells and stimulates the differentiation of Th0- to Th2-naïve T helper (Th) cells, IL-13 stimulates mucus production by bronchial calyciform cells, subepithelial fibrosis, and is involved in the recruitment of eosinophils. Hence, supported by a strategic mechanism of action inhibiting T2-mediated inflammation, the efficacy of dupilumab has been evaluated in a variety of other atopic diseases, such as atopic dermatitis and chronic rhinosinusitis with nasal polyps (CRSwNP), which often present together as comorbidities [51]. Dupilumab may be prescribed in children older than 6 years of age as an adjunctive maintenance treatment for severe asthma with type 2 inflammation characterized by increased blood eosinophils and/or increased FeNO fraction, which is inadequately controlled with mid- to high-dose ICS plus another drug for maintenance treatment [22].

5.7.4 Tezepelumab

Tezepelumab blocks TSLP and prevents the initiation of inflammation caused by allergic and nonallergic disease triggers. This antibody is indicated in adults and adolescents 12 years of age and older with severe asthma that is not adequately controlled despite taking high doses of ICS and another medication for maintenance treatment. The PATHWAY and NAVIGATOR efficacy studies demonstrated a reduction in severe asthma flare-ups requiring emergency room intervention or hospitalization by 85% and 79%, respectively, in a patient population 12 years of age and older [8].

In conclusion, biological drugs for asthma are an innovative technology that targets key effectors of the pathologic inflammatory response underlying poor asthma symptom control. These new therapeutic options allow for a pharmacological "tailor-made" approach. Biologic drugs are helping patients with severe eosinophilic asthma, both allergic and nonallergic, to significantly improve symptom control, frequency of flare-ups, lung function, and overall health status. The significant positive impact on the quality of life of patients and their caregivers should also be considered. The ultimate goal of the research is to improve existing and emerging treatments and advance personalized medicine for severe asthma. For this reason, further research efforts must be made in the coming years to identify new therapeutic targets and improve knowledge of the drugs already in use.

5.8 Conclusion

Severe asthma (and STRA in particular) is a rare disease in pediatrics, yet it is responsible for more than 50% of asthma healthcare costs. Moreover, it is still a potentially lethal condition, so early diagnosis and proper management are mandatory. Severe asthma is considered an umbrella term, including different clinical entities and endotypes whose proper characterization is needed to provide tailored therapies. Differential diagnosis, comorbidities, and adherence to inhaled treatments are key features in the initial assessment of suspected severe asthma. Proper diagnosis requires a combination of clinical signs and symptoms, lung function tests, and imaging. Although biomarkers are not part of the diagnostic algorithm in everyday clinical practice, they could be promising tools to evaluate prognosis and therapy effectiveness in the next few years. According to age and inflammatory characteristics, many different biologic therapies are available in pediatric STRA. Since their introductions, significant improvements have been recorded in STRA children regarding symptom control, prevention of asthma attacks, and improvement of patients' and caregivers' quality of life. New targeted treatments will follow in the early future, together with a better understanding of the multiple facets of pediatric STRA.

References

1. Haktanir Abul M, Phipatanakul W. Severe asthma in children: evaluation and management. Allergol Int. 2019;68:150–7.
2. Licari A, Brambilla I, Marseglia A, De Filippo M, Paganelli V, Marseglia GL. Difficult vs. severe asthma: definition and limits of asthma control in the pediatric population. Front Pediatr. 2018;6:170.
3. Pijnenburg MW, Fleming L. Advances in understanding and reducing the burden of severe asthma in children. Lancet Respir Med. 2020;8:1032–44.
4. Holguin F, Cardet JC, Chung KF, Diver S, Ferreira DS, Fitzpatrick A, et al. Management of severe asthma: a European Respiratory Society/American Thoracic Society guideline. Eur Respir J. 2020;55:1900588.
5. Fitzpatrick AM, Jones DP, Brown LA. Glutathione redox control of asthma: from molecular mechanisms to therapeutic opportunities. Antioxid Redox Signal. 2012;17:375–408.
6. Elliot JG, Noble PB, Mauad T, Bai TR, Abramson MJ, McKay KO, et al. Inflammation-dependent and independent airway remodelling in asthma. Respirology. 2018;23:1138–45.
7. Gon Y, Hashimoto S. Role of airway epithelial barrier dysfunction in pathogenesis of asthma. Allergol Int. 2018;67:12–7.
8. Licari A, Manti S, Castagnoli R, Parisi GF, Salpietro C, Leonardi S, et al. Targeted therapy for severe asthma in children and adolescents: current and future perspectives. Paediatr Drugs. 2019;21:215–37.
9. Fitzpatrick AM. Severe asthma in children: lessons learned and future directions. J Allergy Clin Immunol Pract. 2016;4:11–9; quiz 20-1.
10. Fainardi V, Esposito S, Chetta A, Pisi G. Asthma phenotypes and endotypes in childhood. Minerva Med. 2022;113:94–105.
11. Andrenacci B, Ferrante G, Roberto G, Piacentini G, La Grutta S, Marseglia GL, et al. Challenges in

uncontrolled asthma in pediatrics: important considerations for the clinician. Expert Rev Clin Immunol. 2022;18:807–21.
12. Diamant Z, Vijverberg S, Alving K, Bakirtas A, Bjermer L, Custovic A, et al. Toward clinically applicable biomarkers for asthma: an EAACI position paper. Allergy. 2019;74:1835–51.
13. Menzies-Gow A, Corren J, Bourdin A, Chupp G, Israel E, Wechsler ME, et al. Tezepelumab in adults and adolescents with severe, uncontrolled asthma. N Engl J Med. 2021;384:1800–9.
14. Andersson CK, Adams A, Nagakumar P, Bossley C, Gupta A, De Vries D, et al. Intraepithelial neutrophils in pediatric severe asthma are associated with better lung function. J Allergy Clin Immunol. 2017;139:1819–29.e11.
15. Lloyd CM, Hessel EM. Functions of T cells in asthma: more than just T(H)2 cells. Nat Rev Immunol. 2010;10:838–48.
16. Liou CJ, Huang WC. Dehydroepiandrosterone suppresses eosinophil infiltration and airway hyperresponsiveness via modulation of chemokines and Th2 cytokines in ovalbumin-sensitized mice. J Clin Immunol. 2011;31:656–65.
17. Steinke JW, Lawrence MG, Teague WG, Braciale TJ, Patrie JT, Borish L. Bronchoalveolar lavage cytokine patterns in children with severe neutrophilic and paucigranulocytic asthma. J Allergy Clin Immunol. 2021;147(2):686–93.
18. Januska MN, Goldman DL, Webley W, Teague WG, Cohen RT, Bunyavanich S, et al. Bronchoscopy in severe childhood asthma: irresponsible or irreplaceable? Pediatr Pulmonol. 2020;55:795–802.
19. Ash SY, Diaz AA. The role of imaging in the assessment of severe asthma. Curr Opin Pulm Med. 2017;23:97–102.
20. de Blic J, Scheinmann P. The use of imaging techniques for assessing severe childhood asthma. J Allergy Clin Immunol. 2007;119:808–10.
21. Chung KF, Wenzel SE, Brozek JL, Bush A, Castro M, Sterk PJ, et al. International ERS/ATS guidelines on definition, evaluation and treatment of severe asthma. Eur Respir J. 2014;43:343–73.
22. Global Initiative for Asthma. Global strategy for asthma management and prevention, 2022. Available from: https://ginasthma.org.
23. Barsky EE, Giancola LM, Baxi SN, Gaffin JM. A practical approach to severe asthma in children. Ann Am Thorac Soc. 2018;15:399–408.
24. Licari A, Andrenacci B, Di Cicco ME, Leone M, Marseglia GL, Tosca M. Respiratory comorbidities in severe asthma: focus on the pediatric age. Expert Rev Respir Med. 2023;17:1–13.
25. Lang JE. Obesity and childhood asthma. Curr Opin Pulm Med. 2019;25:34–43.
26. Peters MC, McGrath KW, Hawkins GA, Hastie AT, Levy BD, Israel E, et al. Plasma interleukin-6 concentrations, metabolic dysfunction, and asthma severity: a cross-sectional analysis of two cohorts. Lancet Respir Med. 2016;4:574–84.
27. Di Cicco M, Ghezzi M, Kantar A, Song WJ, Bush A, Peroni D, et al. Pediatric obesity and severe asthma: targeting pathways driving inflammation. Pharmacol Res. 2023;188:106658.
28. de Groot EP, Duiverman EJ, Brand PL. Dysfunctional breathing in children with asthma: a rare but relevant comorbidity. Eur Respir J. 2013;41:1068–73.
29. Portel L, Parrat E, Nocent-Ejnaini C, Mangiapan G, Prud'homme A, et al. Phenotyping to target Obstructive Sleep Apnoea Syndrom (OSAS) in adults patients with severe asthma. Respir Med Res. 2022;82:100888.
30. Writing Committee for the American Lung Association Asthma Clinical Research Centers; Holbrook JT, Wise RA, Gold BD, Blake K, Brown ED, et al. Lansoprazole for children with poorly controlled asthma: a randomized controlled trial. JAMA 2012;307:373–381.
31. Licari A, Ciprandi R, Marseglia G, Ciprandi G. Anxiety and depression in adolescents with severe asthma and in their parents: preliminary results after 1 year of treatment. Behav Sci (Basel). 2019;9:78.
32. Licari A, Ciprandi R, Marseglia G, Ciprandi G. Anxiety in adolescents with severe asthma and response to treatment. Acta Biomed. 2020;91:e2020186.
33. Klok T, Kaptein AA, Duiverman EJ, Brand PL. Long-term adherence to inhaled corticosteroids in children with asthma: observational study. Respir Med. 2015;109:1114–9.
34. Desager K, Vermeulen F, Bodart E. Adherence to asthma treatment in childhood and adolescence—a narrative literature review. Acta Clin Belg. 2018;73:348–55.
35. Nwaru BI, Ekström M, Hasvold P, Wiklund F, Telg G, Janson C. Overuse of short-acting β2-agonists in asthma is associated with increased risk of exacerbation and mortality: a nationwide cohort study of the global SABINA programme. Eur Respir J. 2020;55:1901872.
36. Roberts G, Vazquez-Ortiz M, Knibb R, Khaleva E, Alviani C, Angier E, et al. EAACI Guidelines on the effective transition of adolescents and young adults with allergy and asthma. Allergy. 2020;75:2734–52.
37. Licari A, Castagnoli R, Brambilla I, Marseglia A, Tosca MA, Marseglia GL, et al. Asthma endotyping and biomarkers in childhood asthma. Pediatr Allergy Immunol Pulmonol. 2018;31:44–55.
38. Habib N, Pasha MA, Tang DD. Current understanding of asthma pathogenesis and biomarkers. Cells. 2022;11:2764.
39. Wang Z, Pianosi PT, Keogh KA, Zaiem F, Alsawas M, Alahdab F, et al. The diagnostic accuracy of fractional exhaled nitric oxide testing in asthma: a systematic review and meta-analyses. Mayo Clin Proc. 2018;93:191–8.
40. Horváth I, Hunt J, Barnes PJ, Alving K, Antczak A, Baraldi E, et al. Exhaled breath condensate: methodological recommendations and unresolved questions. Eur Respir J. 2005;26:523–48.

41. Kazani S, Planaguma A, Ono E, Bonini M, Zahid M, Marigowda G, et al. Exhaled breath condensate eicosanoid levels associate with asthma and its severity. J Allergy Clin Immunol. 2013;132:547–53.
42. Medrek SK, Parulekar AD, Hanania NA. Predictive biomarkers for asthma therapy. Curr Allergy Asthma Rep. 2017;17:69. https://doi.org/10.1007/s11882-017-0739-5.
43. di Palmo E, Cantarelli E, Catelli A, Ricci G, Gallucci M, Miniaci A, et al. The predictive role of biomarkers and genetics in childhood asthma exacerbations. Int J Mol Sci. 2021;22:4651.
44. Sahiner UM, Birben E, Erzurum S, Sackesen C, Kalayci Ö. Oxidative stress in asthma: part of the puzzle. Pediatr Allergy Immunol. 2018;29:789–800.
45. Bishopp A, Sathyamurthy R, Manney S, Webbster C, Krishna MT, Mansur AH. Biomarkers of oxidative stress and antioxidants in severe asthma: a prospective case-control study. Ann Allergy Asthma Immunol. 2017;118:445–51.
46. Maes T, Cobos FA, Schleich F, Sorbello V, Henket M, De Preter K, et al. Asthma inflammatory phenotypes show differential microRNA expression in sputum. J Allergy Clin Immunol. 2016;137:1433–46.
47. Midyat L, Gulen F, Karaca E, Ozkinay F, Tanac R, Demir E, et al. MicroRNA expression profiling in children with different asthma phenotypes. Pediatr Pulmonol. 2016;51:582–7.
48. Licari A, Brambilla I, Sacchi L, Marseglia G, Ciprandi G. Periostin, type 2 biomarker, is not associated with asthma control grade in asthmatic allergic children. Respir Med. 2019;151:118–20.
49. Licari A, Marseglia A, Caimmi S, Castagnoli R, Foiadelli T, Barberi S, et al. Omalizumab in children. Paediatr Drugs. 2014;16:491–502.
50. Bacharier LB, Jackson DJ. Biologics in the treatment of asthma in children and adolescents. J Allergy Clin Immunol. 2023;151:581–9.
51. Licari A, Castagnoli R, Marseglia A, Olivero F, Votto M, Ciprandi G, et al. Dupilumab to treat type 2 inflammatory diseases in children and adolescents. Paediatr Drugs. 2020;22:295–310.

Wheezing in Paediatric Patients

6

Giuliana Ferrante, Laura Venditto, Taulant Melengu, Beatrice Allena, Laura Tenero, Michele Piazza, and Piacentini Giorgio

Abstract

The prevalence of wheezing disorders in children younger than 6 years varies worldwide and appears to have increased during the last decade. It is estimated that about one in three children experiences wheezing during the first 3 years of life. One-third of preschoolers develop recurrent wheezing, defined as four or more episodes in the previous year. Many children with recurrent wheezing develop eosinophilic asthma, although only 40% of them will show recurrent wheezing later in childhood. Phenotyping preschool children with wheezing is essential to understanding the pathophysiology of the disease in order to provide effective management and treatment strategies. A symptom-based approach has been revealed to be inadequate and there is yet no consensus as to the appropriate way to manage preschool wheeze. Basic management requires the paediatrician to identify any underlying diagnosis and to establish empathetic communication with parents in order to decide whether to continue or not ineffective therapies.

Keywords

Asthma · Atopy · Diagnosis · Management Phenotype · Preschool · Treatment · Virus Respiratory infections · Wheezing

Test your learning and check your understanding of this book's contents: use the "Springer Nature Flashcards" app to access questions using ▶ https://sn.pub/nspbjm. To use the app, please follow the instructions in Chap. 1.

G. Ferrante (✉)
Department of Surgical Sciences, Dentistry, Gynaecology and Pediatrics, Pediatric Unit, University of Verona, Verona, Italy

Institute of Translational Pharmacology (IFT), National Research Council of Italy (CNR), Palermo, Italy
e-mail: giuliana.ferrante@univr.it

L. Venditto · T. Melengu · B. Allena
School of Pediatrics, University of Verona, Verona, Italy

L. Tenero
Pediatric Unit, University Hospital of Verona, Verona, Italy

M. Piazza
Department of Surgical Sciences, Dentistry, Gynaecology and Pediatrics, University of Verona, Verona, Italy

P. Giorgio
Department of Surgical Sciences, Dentistry, Gynaecology and Pediatrics, Pediatric Unit, University of Verona, Verona, Italy

C. Caffarelli, G. L. Marseglia (eds.), *Textbook of Pediatric Allergy*,
https://doi.org/10.1007/978-3-031-71283-8_6

6.1 Introduction

Wheeze represents a clinical sign resulting from different airway lumen disorders that lead to airflow limitation. It has been described as a high-pitched, continuous noise, usually associated with a prolonged expiratory phase. Depending on the level of obstruction (peripheral or central airways), it can be polyphonic or monophonic, respectively [1].

The prevalence of wheezing disorders in preschoolers, i.e. children younger than 6 years, varies worldwide and appears to have increased during the last decade [2]. It is estimated that about one in three children experiences wheezing during the first 3 years of life [3]. Most wheezing episodes are triggered by viral infections of the airways, and they involve 30–50% of preschool children [4]. Generally, such episodes are mild and transient. However, one-third of preschoolers develop recurrent wheezing, defined as four or more episodes in the previous year [5]. Recurrent wheezing has a significant impact on quality of life [6] as well as on healthcare resources [6]. Indeed, the economic burden of wheezing for the European Union is estimated at EUR 5.2 billion [7].

"Wheezing" should be considered an umbrella term for different diseases with diverse phenotypes [8]. The spectrum of disorders underlying wheezing in preschool age is wide and includes chronic suppurative lung diseases, chronic lung disease of prematurity, congenital airway abnormalities, airway tumours, foreign bodies and "preschool asthma" [9, 10]. Many children with recurrent wheezing develop eosinophilic asthma, although only 40% of them will show recurrent wheezing later in childhood [5]. Less is known about non-atopic or non-eosinophilic asthma. Namely, many children outgrow wheezing before school age. There is evidence that at least 60% of wheezy preschoolers will become symptom-free by age 6 years and the majority before adolescence [5]. However, this can only be ascertained in retrospect. The challenge is to identify preschoolers with asthma among those with other causes of wheezing, due to the lack of a clear definition of asthma and objective diagnostic tests in this age group [11]. Moreover, it is to point out that longitudinal cohort studies demonstrated that adolescents and adults with wheezing had a reduction in lung function before the age of 6 years compared to their peers who never had wheezing [12, 13].

Phenotyping preschool children with wheezing is therefore essential to understand the pathophysiology of the disease in order to provide effective management and treatment strategies. Indeed, a symptom-based approach has been revealed to be inadequate and there is yet no consensus as to the appropriate way to manage preschool wheeze.

6.2 Clinical Phenotypes in Preschool Wheezing

Preschool wheezing includes different diseases with different observable and measurable features (phenotypes). Each phenotype may be the result of different endotypes, clinical features and molecular pathways [8]. Over the last two decades, substantial effort has been devoted to understanding wheezing heterogeneity and several approaches have been used to categorize preschool wheezers.

The classification based on clinical features, proposed by the 2008 ERS task force, is based on triggers and symptoms. It simply divides wheezing into two clusters: "episodic viral wheezing" (EVW) and "multiple trigger wheezing" (MTW). The EVW occurs especially during autumn-winter seasons and presents with symptoms associated with viral respiratory tract infections, with healthy periods between episodes. Instead, the MTW may occur in every period of the year, with symptoms that are induced by heterogenous output triggers (passive smoke, allergens, cold and physical activity) [14].

This kind of classification may have limitations in clinical practice: it is based on the patient's characteristics at the time of examination that change over time and it does not consider that the two phenotypes may not fit clearly into either category. Indeed, they can show similarities and cover different endotypes, and they could change into one another [8].

The classification based on temporal patterns relies on the onset and the persistence of wheeze. The initial approach, using data on wheezing collected during the first six years of life in the *Tucson Children's Respiratory Study*, described four different wheezing patterns [5]:

1. Never wheeze (51.5%).
2. Transient early wheeze (20%), which occurs within the first three years of life and resolves by the sixth year, without lung function impairment. One manifestation of this pattern is bronchiolitis in the first year.
3. Late-onset wheeze (15%), which develops after three years of age and persists into childhood, is linked to atopy, and, in some studies, it is associated with reduced lung function and bronchial hyperresponsiveness.
4. Persistent wheeze (14%), which starts in early life, generally before three years of age, and also between 4–6 years, is strongly associated with atopy, high total immunoglobulin E (IgE) levels, early allergen sensitization and diminished lung function by the time of school age.

This finding was confirmed in several independent cohorts later. Subsequently, the methodology to classify wheezing phenotypes was extended to the use of unsupervised data-driven statistical approaches, apart from any preconceived bias of the clinician [15]. This approach allowed one to discover the existence of two further intermediate phenotypes, that drive a complete final classification [16]:

1. Never or infrequent wheeze.
2. Transient early wheeze, including preschool remitting and mid-childhood remitting wheeze (also called "prolonged early wheeze"). These two subgroups differed substantially in their association with allergic sensitization which resulted in being more commonly observed in children with mid-childhood remitting wheeze than in those with preschool remitting wheeze.
3. Late-onset wheeze, including school-age onset (intermediate wheeze, strongly associated with atopy) and late childhood onset wheeze.
4. Persistent wheezing, which is associated with the greatest impairment of lung function.

These wheeze phenotypes tend to share the same nomenclature, although they often differ substantially in terms of age of onset, temporal trajectory, distribution within a population and associated risk factors [17]. Furthermore, wheeze classes discovered using data-driven approaches do not present features actually observed in nature, so ideally should not be referred to as "phenotypes" (which means in theory "observable characteristics"). However, in the literature, they prefer to maintain the same nomenclature in all the studies [16].

The classification based on etiopathology identifies five different wheezing clusters [18]:

1. Atopic and eosinophilic (15%): type 2-high inflammation, with high total IgE, sensitization, high blood eosinophils, moderate rate of bacterial or viral detection
2. Infectious non-atopic (25%): low IgE levels, high bronchoalveolar lavage (BAL) neutrophils, high rate of bacterial and viral infection
3. Non-atopic and no infection (15%): low BAL neutrophils, low infection rate, low bacterial and viral detection
4. Structural abnormalities (20%): mainly airway malacia or laryngeal clefts, low IgE levels, and agranulocytic BAL
5. Aspiration/GERD (15%): microaspiration-associated late-onset wheeze, with a high rate of gastroesophageal reflux, little atopy and high BAL lipid-laden macrophages

Nonetheless, these classifications are not cumulative. For example, it has been shown that both EVW and MTW could have BAL eosinophilia or a normal BAL and atopy was not predictive of BAL findings. There was no relationship between EVW, MTW, and either blood eosinophils, atopic status or infection. Moreover, the pattern of wheezing could change spontaneously over time: EVW could persist beyond school age and MTW could be transient [9].

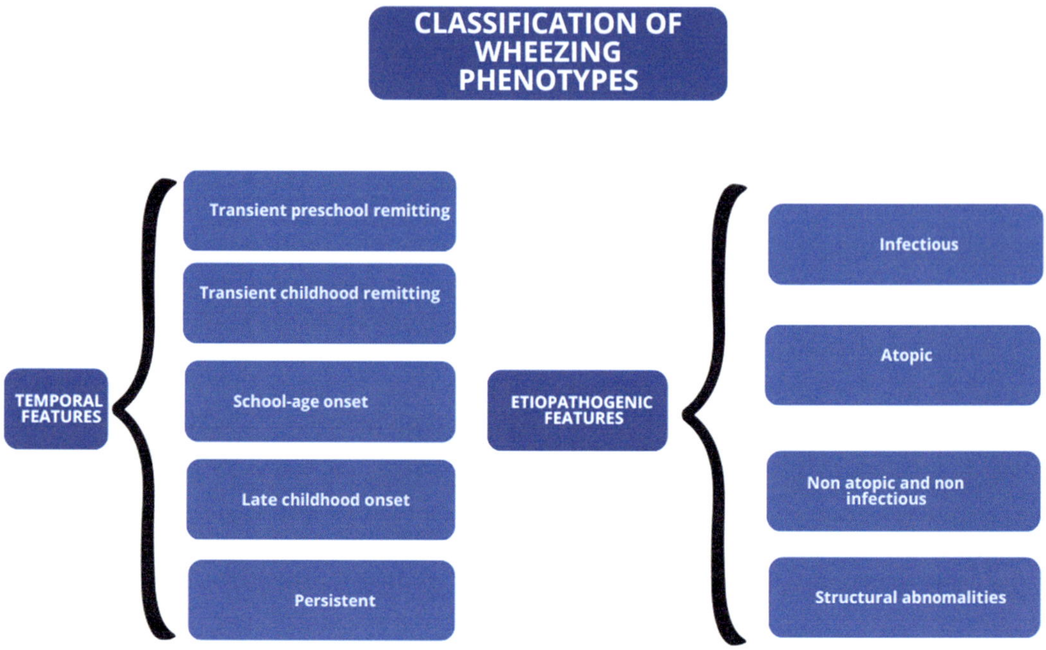

Fig. 6.1 Classification of wheezing based on temporal and etiopathogenic features

These inconsistencies between classifications may be explained by heterogeneous populations evaluated in different studies, different approaches for selecting observational features, and lack of uniformity in choosing type and number of variables [8].

To make the classifications of preschool wheezing reliable, we need consistent and reproducible phenotypes and to understand that clinical phenotypes are not statics [17].

Currently, investigations are ongoing to identify at-risk preschool children by phenotyping them according to asthma predictive indices. One of the most frequently used is the modified Asthma Predictive Index (mAPI), which includes four or more wheezing episodes during the last year, and at least one of the following main risk factors such as a parental history of asthma, doctor-diagnosed atopic dermatitis, sensitization to inhalant allergens, or two of the following minor risk factors such as sensitization to trophoallergens, >4% blood eosinophils or wheezing apart from cold [19].

Nonetheless, it is likely that more holistic indicators of wheezing are needed to describe individual trajectories and derive more homogenous phenotypes to facilitate better understanding of the natural history of the disease and allow for personalized treatment [16].

A simplified classification of wheezing based on temporal and ethiopathogenic features is proposed in Fig. 6.1.

6.3 Diagnosis and Differential Diagnosis

Since wheezing is a non-specific symptom, potentially caused by a variety of different conditions, the diagnostic approach in a preschool child should first confirm that the respiratory sound heard by the parents is actually a wheeze [20].

In this view, making the parents record their child while presenting wheezing could be a suitable option. A detailed anamnesis is then the key to making the right diagnosis and raising concerns, and usually, a negative physical examination when the child is unwell will be sufficient to exclude other underlying conditions, without warranting further diagnostic investigations. In fact, it should be noted that the majority of preschool children have a cough, for example, a wet cough after a viral cold lasting 1–2 weeks, as well as a gradually improving cough and wheeze after bronchiolitis are normal conditions that need only parent's reassurance [21].

Nevertheless, recurrent wheezing occurs in a large proportion of children 5-year-old or younger, typically with viral respiratory infections. The recognition that wheezing is the initial presentation of asthma even if quite difficult is important to start a treatment plan aimed at reducing short-term asthma-related complications since inhaled steroids do not produce a disease-modifying effect in this specific age range [22]. As suggested by Yang, in a child with acute wheezing and increased work of breathing, it is recommended to administer a trial of short-acting beta-agonists with or without oral steroids to observe the response [22]. If there is a clear improvement, and the child has experienced similar episodes in the past, a diagnosis of asthma may be considered. If the child presents a history of recurrent episodes of wheezing but not experiencing acute symptoms at the moment of the medical evaluation, the frequency and severity of reported symptoms should be taken into account. It could be reasonable to start a trial of inhaled steroids in case of a history of severe exacerbations, frequent symptoms, or previous need for oral steroids, emergency room visits or hospitalization; in case of response with improvement in the frequency and/or severity of symptoms, the diagnosis of asthma would be supported. However, if the symptoms are infrequent and mild, it is advisable to assess the child when symptomatic to better understand the nature of the wheezing.

For this purpose, the Global Initiative for Asthma (GINA) Strategy Report provides a strategy to diagnose asthma under 5 years of age [23]. In particular, the likelihood of an asthma diagnosis increases if children experience wheezing or coughing during activities such as exercise, laughing or crying, especially when there is no apparent respiratory infection. Additionally, the presence of allergic sensitization, eczema, allergic rhinitis, food allergy or a family history of asthma in first-degree relatives can also contribute to the likelihood of asthma. The response to controller treatment for 2–3 months or worsening of symptoms after the cessation can further support the diagnosis of asthma.

Nowadays, we lack lung function tests for preschool children to aid in the diagnosis of asthma. Multiple breath washout, spirometry and plethysmography have been demonstrated to not be sensitive for diagnosing mild asthmatic disease in young children [24], but new evidence suggests that impulse oscillometry [25] and forced oscillation technique (FOT) [26] could be considered. Specifically, FOT may be a useful tool to aid in diagnosing and managing asthma in preschool children (>2 years) [27], especially for children unable to perform spirometry, but the available reference values need to be validated in larger populations.

Fraction exhaled nitric oxide could become a tool to diagnose asthma in preschool wheezers since has been shown to predict allergic asthma among wheezy preschool children (cut-off > 35 ppb). Even if used at the moment only in research settings, in the future VOC profiling could help with the study and the monitoring of the preschool wheezing phenotypes [27]. Future approaches include structured light plethysmography and impedance pneumography; though promising, at the moment the evidence is scarce to recommend them in clinical practice [27].

Alternative potential causes for recurrent wheezing in preschool children need to be explored before starting any treatment. In fact, in a study [28] conducted in preschool children with persistent wheezing evaluated with flexible bronchoscopy, 34% had malacia disorders; this was confirmed later in another study [29] conducted on preschool children with steroid-refractory recurrent wheezing that 39% demonstrated structural abnormalities and 27% gastroesophageal reflux.

In fact, other potential causes for wheezing are recurrent viral respiratory infections, gastroesophageal reflux, unsafe swallowing with chronic aspiration, foreign body aspiration, suppurative lung diseases such as cystic fibrosis or primary ciliary dyskinesia, congenital anomalies (vascular rings or tracheo-bronchial stenosis),

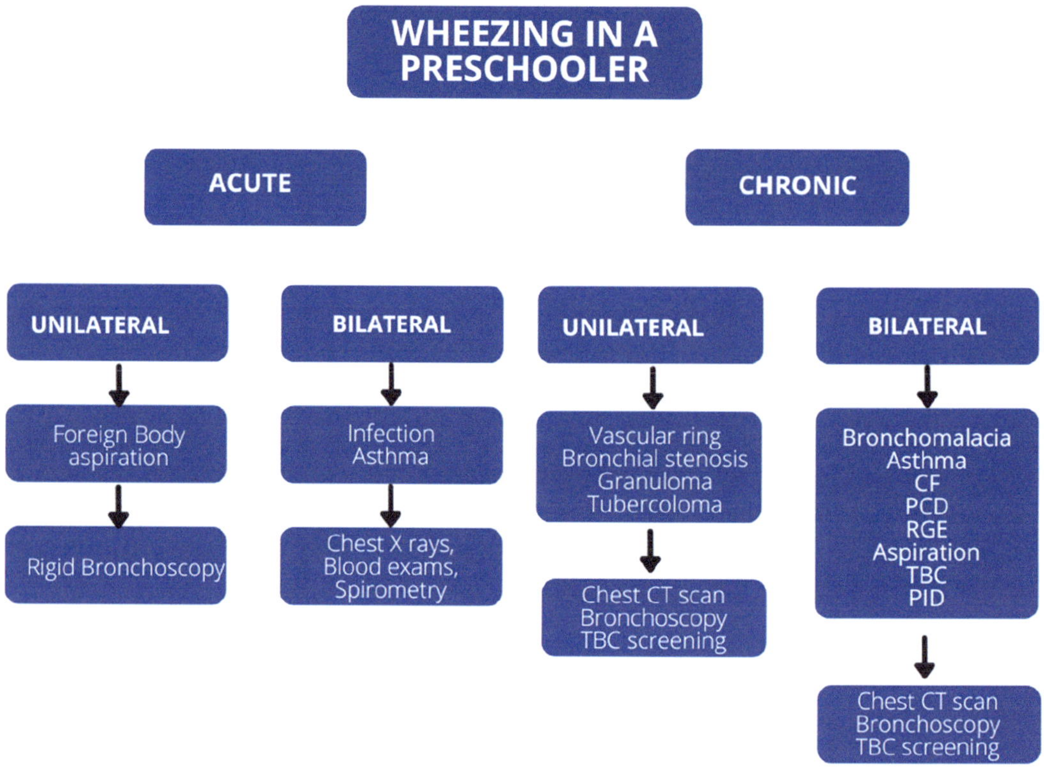

Fig. 6.2 Differential diagnosis of preschool wheezing. Modified by [30] Feleszko W, Jartti T, Bacharier LB. Current strategies for phenotyping and managing asthma in preschool children. Curr Opin Allergy Clin Immunol. 2022;22:107-114. doi: https://doi.org/10.1097/ACI.0000000000000819

airway compression by a tuberculoma, broncho-pulmonary dysplasia, nicotine exposure (tobacco or vapes), allergies, immune primitive disorders and congenital heart defects (Fig. 6.2) [18].

GINA suggests further investigations in case of onset of symptoms during the neonatal period, failure to thrive, continuous wheezing, symptoms not linked to typical triggers like viral respiratory infections, symptoms associated with vomiting, focal lung or cardiovascular signs, clubbing, hypoxemia while well, and lack of response to asthma treatment [23].

Table 6.1 summarizes the red flags in the clinical history and the examination that suggest other potential causes of wheezing [30].

In these cases, further investigations may be needed on the basis of clinical suspicion, for instance, skin prick test for aero-allergens or determination of serum-specific IgE, contrast-enhanced thorax CT, video fluoroscopy, pH study, sweat test, nasal brushing, micro laryngoscopy, bronchoscopy with broncho-lavage and microbiological culture. Bronchoscopy could be very useful in cases of severe wheezing and recurrent symptoms (despite high-dose inhaled steroids) to obtain clinically relevant information on structural abnormalities, eosinophilic airway inflammation, bacterial infection and GERD, but it should be performed by trained personnel [31].

Table 6.1 Red flags from history and physical examination that suggest possible diagnoses of wheezing

	Red flags	Possible diagnoses
History	Symptoms from the first day of life	Tracheomalacia, CF, PCD
	Sudden onset symptoms	Foreign body aspiration
	Chronic wet cough	CF, PCD, TBC, PID
	Cough after eating, being irritable while feeding, back arching, vomits	GERD
	Prematurity	Chronic lung disease of prematurity, bronchopulmonary dysplasia
	Recurrent chest infections	Tracheobronchomalacia, CF, PCD, PBB, PID, aspiration, GERD
	Persistent symptoms	Congenital defects as tracheobronchomalacia or vascular ring, foreign body aspiration
Physical examination	Clubbing	Heart defects, bronchiectasis, CF, PCD, chILD
	Weight loss	CF, TBC, chILD
	Failure to thrive	CF, IDP, chILD
	Chronic rhinitis and nasal polyps	CF, PCD
	Severe chest deformity	Jeune syndrome, lung hypoplasia, bronchial atresia
	Fixed, monophonic or asymmetric wheezing	Congenital defects such as tracheobronchomalacia or vascular ring, foreign body aspiration, granulomatosis, TBC

CF cystic fibrosis, *PCD* primary ciliary dyskinesia, *TBC* tuberculosis, *PID* primitive immunodeficiency, *GERD* gastroesophageal reflux disease, *PBB* protracted bacterial bronchitis, *chILD* interstitial lung disease of the childhood

6.4 Treatment

Reasons for initiation of pharmacotherapy in preschool children with wheezing could be the treatment of the present symptoms or prevention of progression to asthma. However, before any pharmacotherapy is started, any underlying diagnosis should be excluded and attention should be turned to environmental control. Exposure to passive smoking and vaping should be strictly avoided, and exposure to indoor and outdoor pollutants and aeroallergens should be minimized, especially in sensitized children [21].

There is no international consensus on any specific personalized treatment approach to preschool wheezing [21]. Anyway, certain phenotypes may respond to treatments differently, depending on the risk factors identified.

Short-acting beta-2-agonists (SABA) and anticholinergics (Ipratropium) represent the first-line treatment for managing acute attacks. Spacers with masks (or mouthpieces in children aged 3 years and over) are the preferred device through which administer drugs; a nebulizer is an alternative way to deliver medication [32].

If symptoms are frequent or severe, the child must be treated for current wheezing attacks and prevent future symptoms. Indeed, recurrent wheezing in preschool children can subsequently progress to asthma and deterioration of lung function [33]. Inhaled corticosteroids (ICS) have been suggested as the preferred initial treatment for preschool children at risk of asthma [34]. Indeed, ICS, administered continuously or intermittently, reduces the risk of virus-induced wheezing episodes [35]. Certain groups of children with wheezing seem to respond better to ICS, especially those sensitized to aeroallergens and with high peripheral eosinophilia [18].

Intermittent treatment may be considered for children with primarily viral-associated wheezing. However, it is to point out that administering high doses of ICS very often potentially affects the child's growth [36]. Children who have frequent symptoms not only associated with upper respiratory infections and those with severe exacerbations should be considered differently and may benefit from continuous therapy.

The effect of oral corticosteroids (OCS) on wheezing episodes in preschool children varies by degree of episode severity. OCS can be used to treat wheezy patients, in whom a short course of treatment (3–5 days) has been documented to be effective in reducing recurrent wheezing after a rhinovirus infection [37]. Generally, systemic steroids are indicated in extremely severe wheeze requiring admission to the hospital. Preschool children with acute wheeze not enough severe to require hospitalization do not need to be prescribed OCS [38].

Montelukast is the only leukotriene antagonist (LTRA) approved for preschool children and can be considered as a daily treatment to control wheezing symptoms in selected groups of patients. However, parents should be warned about the behavioural side effects, which have a prevalence of around 20% and can be very distressing [39]. A therapeutic trial should be discontinued in the absence of clear benefit.

A study on BAL of young children with recurrent wheeze demonstrated the predominance of neutrophilic inflammation suggesting bacterial infection [40]. Early administration of azithromycin reduces the risk of severe lower respiratory tract illnesses in these children, due to its antibiotic and anti-inflammatory properties [41]. The mechanism of azithromycin in wheezing remains uncertain and the main concern with its use is the potential emergence of macrolide-resistant organisms and the negative influence on gut microbiota. A trial can be considered in preschoolers with severe wheezing requiring intravenous treatment and oxygen [21].

A phenotype-directed treatment approach could be the following (Fig. 6.3).

- Children with intermittent viral-induced wheezing: for those with positive mAPI and features associated with a higher burden of disease (male gender, white race and greater baseline symptom frequency, need for recent ED care of hospitalization and/or evidence of sensitization to aeroallergen), daily low dose ICS would be the preferred approach. For those with positive mAPI and lower disease burden (females, non-white race, fewer symptoms, no recent ED or hospital care and absence of aeroallergen sensitization), an initial trial of high-dose intermittent ICS at the onset of upper respiratory infections symptoms is recommended. In children with negative mAPI, a trial of azithromycin started at the onset of respiratory tract infection symptoms is recommended [42].

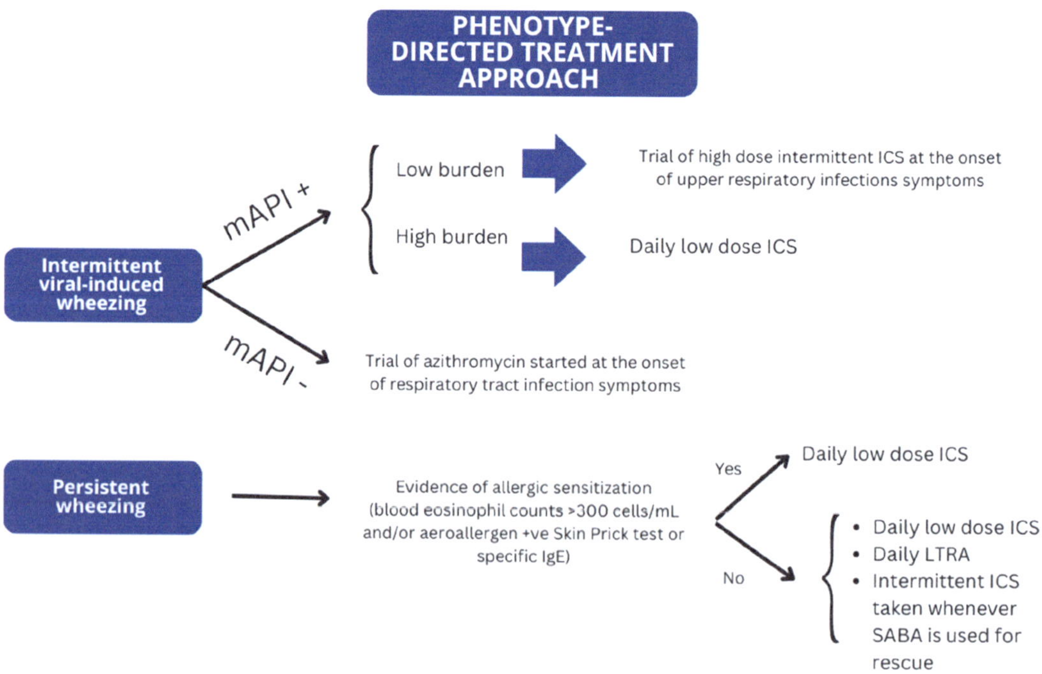

Fig. 6.3 Phenotype-directed treatment approach of preschool wheezing

– Children with persistent wheezing: for those with either blood eosinophil counts >300 cells/mL and/or aeroallergen sensitization daily low-dose ICS treatment would be the preferred approach; children without either feature may benefit from daily low-dose ICS, daily LTRA or intermittent ICS taken whenever SABA are used for rescue [35].

6.5 Conclusions

Preschool wheezing is a highly heterogeneous disease. To date, at least four to five distinct clusters have been identified, with different etiopathology and likely different responses to treatment. Apart from peripheral eosinophilia and allergic sensitization, we still cannot rely on objective features that could guide the assignment of a given patient to a certain phenotype. Therefore, we need to develop new biomarkers to characterize phenotypes/endotypes, particularly the "infectious" ones.

This approach could be particularly relevant for preventing asthma development in high-risk children but also for elucidating the role of biologic therapies targeting type 2 inflammation, with an emphasis on disease modification, as well as to identifying effective treatment strategies in those with non-atopic/non-eosinophilic pattern of inflammation. In this specific context, airway microbiome patterns may become useful to identify children who respond to antibiotic treatment.

The management of preschool wheezing in the next future must be moving towards personalized medicine, especially for reducing the overall burden of disease in children with severe symptoms. In the current state of things, basic management requires the paediatrician to identify any underlying diagnosis and to establish empathetic communication with parents in order to decide whether to continue or not ineffective therapies [18, 21].

Key Points

- The prevalence of preschool wheezing appears to have increased during the last decade
- "Wheezing" should be considered an umbrella term for different diseases with diverse phenotypes
- Many children with recurrent wheezing develop eosinophilic asthma
- There is no consensus as to the appropriate way to manage preschool wheeze
- Basic management requires the paediatrician to identify any underlying diagnosis and to establish empathetic communication with parents in order to guide the treatment
- Management of preschool wheezing in the future must be moving towards personalized medicine

Take-Home Messages

- Preschool wheezing is a highly heterogeneous disease.
- The spectrum of disorders underlying wheezing in preschool age is wide and includes chronic suppurative lung diseases, chronic lung disease of prematurity, congenital airway abnormalities, airway tumours, foreign bodies and "preschool asthma."
- Phenotyping preschool children with wheezing is essential to understand the pathophysiology of the disease in order to provide effective management and treatment strategies.
- We still cannot rely on objective features that could guide the assignment of a given patient to a certain phenotype,

(continued)

and we need to develop new biomarkers to characterize phenotypes/endotypes.

- Since wheezing is a non-specific symptom, the diagnostic approach in a preschool child should first confirm that the respiratory sound heard by the parents is actually a wheeze.
- Before any pharmacotherapy is started, any underlying diagnosis should be excluded and attention should be turned to environmental control.
- The paediatrician should establish an empathetic relationship with parents in order to decide whether to continue or not ineffective therapies.

References

1. Chatziparasidis G, Priftis KN, Bush A. Wheezing as a respiratory sound. In: Priftis K, Hadjileontiadis L, Everard M, editors. Breath sounds. Cham: Springer; 2018. p. 207–23.
2. Bloom CI, Franklin C, Bush A, Saglani S, Quint JK. Burden of preschool wheeze and progression to asthma in the UK: population-based cohort 2007 to 2017. J Allergy Clin Immunol. 2021;147:1949–58.
3. Bisgaard H, Szefler S. Prevalence of asthma-like symptoms in young children. Pediatr Pulmonol. 2007;42:723–8.
4. Henderson J, Granell R, Heron J, Sherriff A, Simpson A, Woodcock A, et al. Associations of wheezing phenotypes in the first 6 years of life with atopy, lung function and airway responsiveness in mid-childhood. Thorax. 2008;63:974–80.
5. Martinez FD, Wright AL, Taussig LM, Holberg CJ, Halonen M, Morgan WJ. Asthma and wheezing in the first six years of life. The Group Health Medical Associates. N Engl J Med. 1995;332:133–8.
6. Moorman JE, Akinbami LJ, Bailey CM, Zahran HS, King ME, Johnson CA, et al. National surveillance of asthma: United States, 2001–2010. Vital Health Stat. 2012;3:1–58.
7. van den Akker-van Marle ME, Bruil J, Detmar SB. Evaluation of cost of disease: assessing the burden to society of asthma in children in the European Union. Allergy. 2005;60:140–9.
8. Fainardi V, Santoro A, Caffarelli C. Preschool wheezing: trajectories and long-term treatment. Front Pediatr. 2020;8:240.
9. Guiddir T, Saint-Pierre P, Purenne-Denis E, Lambert N, Laoudi Y, Couderc R, et al. Neutrophilic steroid-refractory recurrent wheeze and eosinophilic steroid-refractory asthma in children. J Allergy Clin Immunol Pract. 2017;5:1351–61.
10. Bush A. Pathophysiological mechanisms of asthma. Front Pediatr. 2019;7:68.
11. Visness CM, Gebretsadik T, Jackson DJ, Biagini Myers J, Havstad S, Lemanske RF Jr, et al. Children's Respiratory and Environmental Workgroup. Asthma as an outcome: exploring multiple definitions of asthma across birth cohorts in the Environmental influences on Child Health Outcomes Children's Respiratory and Environmental Workgroup. J Allergy Clin Immunol. 2019;144:866–9.
12. Horak E, Lanigan A, Roberts M, Welsh L, Wilson J, Carlin JB, et al. Longitudinal study of childhood wheezy bronchitis and asthma: outcome at age 42. BMJ. 2003;326:422–3.
13. Phelan PD, Robertson CF, Olinsky A. The Melbourne Asthma Study: 1964–1999. J Allergy Clin Immunol. 2002;109:189–94.
14. Brand PL, Baraldi E, Bisgaard H, Boner AL, Castro-Rodriguez JA, Custovic A, et al. Definition, assessment and treatment of wheezing disorders in preschool children: an evidence-based approach. Eur Respir J. 2008;32:1096–110.
15. Collins SA, Pike KC, Inskip HM, Godfrey KM, Roberts G, Holloway JW, et al. Southampton Women's Survey Study Group. Validation of novel wheeze phenotypes using longitudinal airway function and atopic sensitization data in the first 6 years of life: evidence from the Southampton Women's survey. Pediatr Pulmonol. 2013;48:683–92.
16. Oksel C, Granell R, Haider S, Fontanella S, Simpson A, Turner S, STELAR Investigators, Breathing Together Investigators, et al. Distinguishing wheezing phenotypes from infancy to adolescence. a pooled analysis of five birth cohorts. Ann Am Thorac Soc. 2019;16:868–76.
17. Oksel C, Granell R, Mahmoud O, Custovic A, Henderson AJ, STELAR, Breathing Together Investigators. Causes of variability in latent phenotypes of childhood wheeze. J Allergy Clin Immunol. 2019;143:1783–90.
18. Feleszko W, Jartti T, Bacharier LB. Current strategies for phenotyping and managing asthma in preschool children. Curr Opin Allergy Clin Immunol. 2022;22:107–14.
19. Guilbert TW, Morgan WJ, Zeiger RS, Mauger DT, Boehmer SJ, Szefler SJ, et al. Long-term inhaled corticosteroids in preschool children at high risk for asthma. N Engl J Med. 2006;354:1985–97.
20. Cane RS, McKenzie SA. Parents' interpretations of children's respiratory symptoms on video. Arch Dis Child. 2001;84:31–4.
21. Bush A. Basic clinical management of preschool wheeze. Pediatr Allergy Immunol. 2023;34:e13988.

22. Yang CL, Gaffin JM, Radhakrishnan D. Question 3: can we diagnose asthma in children under the age of 5 years? Paediatr Respir Rev. 2019;29:25–30.
23. Reddel HK, Bacharier LB, Bateman ED, Brightling CE, Brusselle GG, Buhl R, et al. Global initiative for asthma strategy 2021: executive summary and rationale for key changes. Am J Respir Crit Care Med. 2022;205:17–35.
24. Arianto L, Hallas H, Stokholm J, Bønnelykke K, Bisgaard H, Chawes BL. Multiple breath washout for diagnosing asthma and persistent wheeze in young children. Ann Am Thorac Soc. 2019;16:599–605.
25. Burman J, Malmberg LP, Remes S, Jartti T, Pelkonen AS, Mäkelä MJ. Impulse oscillometry and free-running tests for diagnosing asthma and monitoring lung function in young children. Ann Allergy Asthma Immunol. 2021;127:326–33.
26. Boccaccino A, Peroni DG, Pietrobelli A, Piacentini GL, Aversano MP, Spinosa E, et al. Forced oscillometry is applicable to epidemiological settings to detect asthmatic children. Allergy Asthma Proc. 2007;28:170–3.
27. Elenius V, Chawes B, Malmberg PL, Adamiec A, Ruszczyński M, Feleszko W, EAACI Preschool Wheeze Task Force for Diagnostics of Preschool Wheeze, et al. Lung function testing and inflammation markers for wheezing preschool children: a systematic review for the EAACI Clinical Practice Recommendations on Diagnostics of Preschool Wheeze. Pediatr Allergy Immunol. 2021;32:501–13.
28. Cakir E, Ersu RH, Uyan ZS, Oktem S, Karadag B, Yapar O, et al. Flexible bronchoscopy as a valuable tool in the evaluation of persistent wheezing in children. Int J Pediatr Otorhinolaryngol. 2009;73:1666–8.
29. Teague WG, Lawrence MG, Williams S, Garrod AS, Froh D, Early SV, et al. Novel treatment-refractory preschool wheeze phenotypes identified by cluster analysis of lung lavage Constituents. J Allergy Clin Immunol Pract. 2021;9:2792–801
30. Bush A. Diagnosis of asthma in children under five. Prim Care Respir J. 2007;16:7–15.
31. Saglani S, Nicholson AG, Scallan M, Balfour-Lynn I, Rosenthal M, Payne DN, et al. Investigation of young children with severe recurrent wheeze: any clinical benefit? Eur Respir J. 2006;27:29–35.
32. Al-Shamrani A, Bagais K, Alenazi A, Alqwaiee M, Al-Harbi AS. Wheezing in children: Approaches to diagnosis and management. Int J Pediatr Adolesc Med. 2019;6:68–73.
33. Deliu M, Fontanella S, Haider S, Sperrin M, Geifman N, Murray C, et al. Longitudinal trajectories of severe wheeze exacerbations from infancy to school age and their association with early-life risk factors and late asthma outcomes. Clin Exp Allergy. 2020;50:315–24.
34. Beigelman A, Bacharier LB. Management of preschool children with recurrent wheezing: lessons from the NHLBI's Asthma Research Networks. J Allergy Clin Immunol Pract. 2016;4:1–8.
35. Fitzpatrick AM, Jackson DJ, Mauger DT, Boehmer SJ, Phipatanakul W, Sheehan WJ, et al. Individualized therapy for persistent asthma in young children. J Allergy Clin Immunol. 2016;138:1608–18.
36. Ducharme FM, Lemire C, Noya FJ, Davis GM, Alos N, Leblond H, et al. Preemptive use of high-dose fluticasone for virus-induced wheezing in young children. N Engl J Med. 2009;360:339–53.
37. Panickar J, Lakhanpaul M, Lambert PC, Kenia P, Stephenson T, Smyth A, et al. Oral prednisolone for preschool children with acute virus-induced wheezing. N Engl J Med. 2009;360:329–38.
38. Oommen A, Lambert PC, Grigg J. Efficacy of a short course of parent-initiated oral prednisolone for viral wheeze in children aged 1-5 years: randomised controlled trial. Lancet. 2003;362:1433–8.
39. Benard B, Bastien V, Vinet B, Yang R, Krajinovic M, Ducharme FM. Neuropsychiatric adverse drug reactions in children initiated on montelukast in real-life practice. Eur Respir J. 2017;50:1700148.
40. Schwerk N, Brinkmann F, Soudah B, Kabesch M, Hansen G. Wheeze in preschool age is associated with pulmonary bacterial infection and resolves after antibiotic therapy. PLoS One. 2011;6:e27913.
41. Jaffé A, Bush A. Anti-inflammatory effects of macrolides in lung disease. Pediatr Pulmonol. 2001;31:464–73.
42. Bacharier LB, Guilbert TW, Mauger DT, Boehmer S, Beigelman A, Fitzpatrick AM, et al. Early administration of azithromycin and prevention of severe lower respiratory tract illnesses in preschool children with a history of such illnesses: a randomized clinical trial. JAMA. 2015;314:2034–44.

Atopic Dermatitis in Children

7

Bianca Gragnoli, Giulia Tonini, Nunzia Maiello, Elena Galli, and Pasquale Comberiati

Abstract

Atopic dermatitis (AD) is a chronic-relapsing inflammatory skin disease that affects worldwide from 0.2% to 36% of the paediatric population. It is often associated with other atopic diseases such as rhinoconjunctivitis, asthma, and food allergy. The pathogenesis of the disease involves a combination of genetic factors, environmental influences, epidermal barrier dysfunctions, and immune dysregulation. Clinical manifestations are characterized by a typical age-related distribution, with pruritus as a main symptom. Infants usually present with acute exudative lesions localized on the cheeks, trunk, and limbs, that evolve during childhood and adolescence to chronic lichenified lesions that predominate on the flexural sites. This chapter aims to provide an overview of the epidemiology, pathogenesis, clinical features, diagnosis, complications, and social and economic impact of the disease, with a focus also on the current available treatments including behavioural, topical, and systemic therapies, with particular attention on biological drugs that recently improved greatly the prognosis of atopic dermatitis.

Keywords

Atopic dermatitis · Atopic march · Pruritus Lichenification · Filaggrin · Epidermal barrier Th2 · Th17 · Skin microbiota · AhR · Flexor surface · Impetiginization · Dupilumab Eosinophilia · Upadacitinib

Test your learning and check your understanding of this book's contents: use the "Springer Nature Flashcards" app to access questions using ▶ https://sn.pub/nspbjm. To use the app, please follow the instructions in Chap. 1.

B. Gragnoli · P. Comberiati
Department of Clinical and Experimental Medicine, Section of Paediatrics, University of Pisa, Pisa, Italy

G. Tonini
Unit of Dermatology, University of Pisa, Pisa, Italy

N. Maiello
Department of Woman, Child and Specialized Surgery, University of Campania "Luigi Vanvitelli", Naples, Italy

E. Galli (✉)
Pediatric Allergology Unit, Department of Pediatric Medicine, S. Pietro Hospital Fatebenefratelli, Rome, Italy
e-mail: galli.elena@fbfrm.it

C. Caffarelli, G. L. Marseglia (eds.), *Textbook of Pediatric Allergy*,
https://doi.org/10.1007/978-3-031-71283-8_7

7.1 Introduction

Atopic dermatitis (AD), also known as atopic eczema, is a chronic-relapsing inflammatory skin disease typical of the infant age, but that can also affect adolescents and adults [1]. There have been recent reports of cases of moderate-severe AD persisting into adulthood or with a very delayed onset [2]. AD is a polygenic skin disease that results from a combination of genetic susceptibility and environmental factors, giving rise to a wide range of clinical manifestations. It can frequently be associated with other atopic diseases such as asthma, rhinoconjunctivitis, and food allergy, which can follow AD in time or appear simultaneously. This model is called "atopic march", and it was proposed to describe the natural history of atopic diseases. AD often appears in the first infancy, and it is considered the first step of the atopic march. Therefore, increasing the understanding of the mechanisms that cause AD can represent a key point also in the prevention of other allergic diseases [3]. Primary care paediatricians have a fundamental role in the management of AD patients because almost 50% of children with AD are treated in primary care settings [4].

7.2 Social and Economic Impact

AD has a strong negative impact on the quality of life of both patients and caregivers. It has been found to have a bigger impact on health-related quality of life than other common chronic disorders, such as asthma and diabetes [5]. The impact of AD on physical health is mostly related to pruritus, scratching, pain, sleep disturbance, and impaired performance at school/work. Sleep disturbance has been detected in up to 60% of AD children, achieving 83% during exacerbation. Overall, sleep disorders are also observed during a remission phase or an apparent "well-being" status in AD patients as well as in AD patients' family members. In addition, AD poses a substantial impact on the psychosocial well-being of patients and their relatives. The psychological burden associated with AD includes behaviour problems, difficult social interactions, poor self-esteem, embarrassment for visible skin lesions, anxiety, depression, and attention deficit hyperactivity disorders. Parents can also be strongly burdened by the emotional weight of seeing their children suffering from the disease and by the lack of sleep [6].

AD poses a significant burden on health-care resources, although the exact economic and social costs of AD might be underestimated. One of the largest American studies estimated the costs for AD at 5.297 billion in 2015. However, it is difficult to assess the real economic impact because, in addition to the direct costs that are up to the patient, such as paying for the skin care treatment, there are also the indirect costs such as the time lost at school/work and those related to the psychological burden and social stigma. Moreover, in the last years, there has also been an increase in access to the emergency department because of AD, resulting in a higher financial burden [7]. A recent analysis showed that AD costs are comparable to those of diabetes and exceed those of asthma and other important chronic diseases [6].

7.3 Epidemiology

The prevalence of AD varies across countries. Several studies show that AD affects from 0.2% to 36% of the paediatric population worldwide [8]. A systematic review that analysed the prevalence of AD in different countries from 1990 to 2010 showed that the prevalence was about 5.1–10% in Australia and Mexico, and 10% in the UK, Nigeria, and South Africa [9]. In Italy, the prevalence is around 16.8% [10]. There is also a strong heterogeneity in the distribution of the disease in rural and industrialized environments. In particular, the prevalence of AD in low-income countries and rural areas is generally lower than in industrialized or high-income countries. This distribution underlines the important impact of lifestyle and environment on the natural history of the disease.

Several prospective cohort studies also showed a different prevalence and persistence of AD based on the age of onset:

- Early onset type: refers to AD occurring in the two first years of life. This is the most frequent type of AD. In 45% of cases AD develops during the first 6 months of life, in 60% of cases within the first 2 years, and roughly in 85% by the age of five [11]. Almost 70–80% of patients with early-onset AD show remission by adulthood, while 10–30% persist in the adult age.
- Late-onset type: it includes AD that begins after puberty.
- Senile-onset type: a rare subset of AD beginning after 60 years of age.

7.4 Etiopathogenesis

The underlying pathogenesis of AD combines a complex interplay of genetic background, environmental influences, immune dysregulation, impaired epidermal barrier, altered skin pH, and reduced microbiota diversity. However, the relative contribution of each of these components is yet to be determined.

7.4.1 Epidermal Barrier Dysfunction

The epidermis is composed of five layers: the stratum corneum (the most superficial one), the stratum lucidum, the stratum granulosum, the stratum spinosum, and the stratum basale.

The epidermis is a fundamental physical barrier to the penetration of microorganisms, but it represents also the first immunological defense, with its skin microbiome. The cutaneous barrier performs its protective function by preventing **trans-epidermal loss of water** (TEWL) and producing antimicrobial peptides, such as β2-, β3-defensins, RNA-ase-7, and cathelicidin (LL37) [12]. Filaggrin (FLG) is a keratin filament aggregating protein that acts as one of the most important components in the structure of the stratum corneum. FLG polymers are cleaved and dephosphorylated into monomers, which associate with keratin filaments to form the stratum corneum. Degradation products of filaggrin, such as urocanic acid and pyrrolidinocarboxylic acid, represent some of the most important natural components of the Natural Moisturizing Factor (NFM) [13] and they contribute to the hydration of the stratum corneum and the acidity of the skin's pH [14].

Patients with AD present an increase in TEWL, both in lesional and non-lesional skin, that increases the risk for early onset AD. Moreover, the level of TEWL is strongly related to the severity of the disease [15]. Epidermal barrier dysfunctions also increase the risk of epicutaneous sensitization to certain aero-allergens, which may represent the first step to the development of food and respiratory allergies.

Patients with AD often show alterations in the composition of the cutaneous barrier in terms of monounsaturated fatty acids, ceramides, and sphingosine. Furthermore, keratinocytes of patients with AD have been shown to produce pro-inflammatory cytokines, including GM-CSF, allarmines as thymic stromal lymphopoietin (TSLP), IL-33, IL-25, and some chemokines as RANTES and CCL5 (a potent chemokine in allergic inflammation, higher in skin lesions presenting with severe AD than mild AD), which condition the differentiation, activation, and chemotactic recall of cutaneous dendritic cells, determining inflammatory skin hyperactivity, also related with altered activator protein 1 (AP-1) activation [15]. Pro-inflammatory cytokines such as TSLP, IL-25, and IL-33 activate Th2 cells, which promote cytokine-associated inflammation (IL-4, IL-5 and IL-13), eosinophilia, and the production of immunoglobulin E (IgE) [16].

Below the stratum corneum, the tight junctions form a second barrier at the level of the stratum granulosum. Bioelectrical anomalies due to reduced levels of **claudin-1** (CLDN1), a fundamental adhesive protein in tight junctions, have been found in some patients with AD [17]. An inverse correlation between the expression of CLDN1 and total circulating eosinophils and IgE has been found in various studies, which suggests that a CLDN1 deficiency may be related to Th2 lymphocyte polarization [17].

7.4.2 Genetic Factors

The genetic pattern of AD is very complex and characterized by various polymorphisms. The mutations of filaggrin (FLG) act as a major driver in the process that leads to AD. The **filaggrin gene** (FLG) is located on chromosome 1q2 and encodes the protein filaggrin, which is the main structural protein of the stratum corneum. Those mutations are often related to early onset, increased severity, and persistence in the adulthood of the disease. Furthermore, FLG mutations determine an augmented risk of epicutaneous sensitization and consequent development of allergic diseases including asthma and rhinoconjunctivitis in patients with AD [18]. Among FLG mutations, the most common are R501X and 2282del4, which determine a complete loss of function of FLG [19]. Instead, other mutations lead to a decreased expression of FLG, resulting in reduced production of keratohyalin granules that cause important alterations in the stratum granulosum [20].

In addition to FLG gene mutation, there are alterations in the Th2 signalling pathway, upregulation of IL-4 and IL-13, and gain-of-function mutation of IL-4R IL-13R receptors [21]. Other associated mutations are observed in the expression of IL-31 and IL-33, STAT6, TSLP and IL-7R and TSLP receptors, interferon regulatory factor 2, and Toll-like receptor 2 (TLR2). Additionally, polymorphisms of the gene encoding the vitamin D receptor seem to play a role [22], along with polymorphisms of cytochrome P450 family 27 subfamily A [23].

7.4.3 Immune Dysregulation

With regard to immune abnormalities, AD is currently considered a biphasic T-cell-mediated disease. A **Th2** signal predominates in the acute phase, whereas a Th2 to Th1 switch promotes disease chronicity. Recent studies have proposed a significant role for IL-22-producing T cells and to a lesser extent IL-17-producing Th17 cells, in the initiation and maintenance of AD [24, 25]. Keratinocytes in AD patients also produce inflammatory cytokines such as IL1, IL-33, and thymic stromal lymphopoietin (TSLP). The latter plays a central role in activating the Th2 response through dendritic cells [26].

The pathogenesis of AD is strongly influenced by the expression of Th2 cytokines, in particular IL-4, IL-13, IL-31, and Th22 cytokines such as IL-22. **IL-4,** and **IL-13** are among the main mediators of AD. These cytokines increase *Staphylococcus aureus* (SA) adhesion to the skin, suppress filaggrin and β-3 defensin production, and alter IL-17 and IL-22 release from Th17 cells. IL-4 and IL-13 play an important role in chemokine production, dysfunction of the skin barrier, suppression of antimicrobial peptides, and allergic inflammation; they mediate signalling cascades through interaction with heterodimeric receptors including IL-13Rα1 and IL-4Rα, which, through JAK1 phosphorylation mediated by STAT6, create an overlapping mechanism that further amplifies the action of these interleukins [27]. Both IL-4 and IL-13 stimulate IgE production by plasma cells, B-cell differentiation, and Th2 cell development and differentiation [28]. They also contribute to the damage of keratinocytes and consequent dysfunction of the skin barrier by significantly reducing filaggrin expression, even in patients without a mutation in the FLG gene [29]. Loricrin and involucrin, which are important for epidermal integrity, are also downregulated by IL-13 and IL-4. Activation of the Th2 axis through IL-13 production can also increase tissue fibrosis by recruiting fibrocytes and fibroblasts to the inflammatory lesion [30]. Given the predominant role of IL-4 and IL-13 in the pathophysiology of AD, numerous studies have been conducted to identify therapeutic approaches aimed at inhibiting these cytokines.

IL-31 is another Th2 cytokine, highly expressed in lesional skin. Its production is increased by exposure to staphylococcal superantigens, underlining a strong relationship between SA colonization and pruritus, as IL-31 receptors are also located in dorsal root ganglia and cutaneous C nerve fibres [31].

7.4.4 Skin Dysbiosis

The alteration of the skin microbiome plays a catalytic role in immune dysregulation and skin barrier impairment. The skin of AD individuals frequently exhibits loss of bacterial diversity and overgrowth of the pathogenic bacteria SA. These bacteria can promote inflammation and AD flare-ups by causing direct proteolytic damage to the epidermal barrier and immune dysregulation. Also, in AD skin there is often a depletion of human antimicrobial peptides (AMPs) and commensal coagulase-negative staphylococci (CoNS), which could selectively inhibit SA through the production of bacteriocins/AMPs and autoinducing peptides (AIPs) [11]. In particular, staphylococcus epidermidis is one of the principal CoNS that predominates in the healthy microbiota, and helps tissue repair by binding TLR2 to keratinocytes and increases the production of IL-17 and INFγ from T lymphocytes [32].

Skin commensal microorganisms play a role in maintaining homeostasis by exfoliating the outermost layer of the SC using microbial enzymes and controlling its pH by metabolizing lipids such as sebum and free fatty acids [33]. Symbiotic skin microbiota activates the **aromatic hydrocarbon receptor** (AhR) of keratinocytes, and thus maintains the integrity of the barrier function [34]. CoNS inhibit the colonization of SA by producing antibiotics, phenol-soluble modulin γ and δ (PSMγ and PSMδ). Additionally, they inhibit the formation of SA biofilm by producing the serine protease glutamyl endopeptidase (Esp). Metabolites of tryptophan, derived from the skin microbiota, can activate AhR, thus inhibiting the production of TSLP by KC and improving the skin's epidermal barrier [35].

In turn, the activation of AHR upregulates AMPs. The innate immune responses of keratinocytes, such as the production of cytokines and chemokines, can also be dampened by AHR ligands, although this effect strongly depends on the ligand source, receptor activation duration, and local inflammatory cytokine environment [36]. The activation of AHR also controls sphingolipid synthesis through the regulation of serine-palmitoyl transferase, a critical enzyme for ceramide biosynthesis [37]. The loss of microbiome diversity, a characteristic of AD, can directly lead to defects in the skin barrier through AHR signalling [34].

SA is not a natural saprophyte of the skin. The increased production of alpha-toxin by SA induces cytotoxicity towards keratinocytes and polarizes T lymphocytes towards a Th2 response. At the same time, the production of δ-toxin induces mast cell degranulation and promotes allergic skin inflammation. An increased level of specific IgE for SA enterotoxins has been found in the skin of AD patients. Enterotoxins can induce the release of histamine and leukotrienes by basophils, and some SA enterotoxins also act as superantigens, directly activating T lymphocytes by activating their Vβ TCR. Furthermore, with the progressive deterioration of the integrity of the epidermal barrier, strains of SA that do not produce enterotoxins are replaced by strains that do, resulting in increased inflammation and itching induced by the direct action of some enterotoxins and cytokines produced by T lymphocytes activated by these antigens, particularly IL-31. A correlation has been found between the severity of AD and the density of SA colonization on lesions, whereas specific antibiotics against SA have been shown to improve the disease. Alterations in the skin barrier, particularly a deficiency in the production of ceramides, sphingosine, monounsaturated fatty acids, and antimicrobial peptides, facilitate SA colonization. Furthermore, the mutation of TLR-2, the main pattern recognition receptor for lipoteichoic acid expressed on SA cell membranes, reduces the production of IL-8, IL-1β, and TNF-α by monocytes and increases the amount of IL-6 and IL-12, facilitating the onset of skin inflammation.

7.4.5 Role of the Skin pH

Patients with AD have significantly elevated skin pH levels, both in involved and uninvolved skin. **High skin pH** level has a negative impact on antimicrobial defence, bacterial overgrowth, and barrier homeostasis, leading to altered lipid synthesis, increased protease activity, activation of PAR2, and itching [38, 39].

Skin acidification can occur through three mechanisms: the breakdown of phospholipids by secretory phospholipase A2, which releases free fatty acids, the transport of protons into the extracellular compartment via the sodium–hydrogen exchanger protein, and the catabolism of structural components of the stratum corneum, leading to the generation of free amino acids. Increased skin pH levels reduce also the epidermal barrier rejuvenation process and can affect the function of a serine protease (KLK5 and KLK7) causing hyperactivation of the pathway implicated in the desquamation and consequent thinning of the skin barrier [40].

7.5 Clinical Features

AD presents with a wide range of clinical manifestations, which show a typical **age-related distribution.**

- Infants (≤2 years) typically develop acute lesions characterized by itchy papules and vesicles with poorly defined erythema, initially involving the cheeks, with sparing of the central part of the face. These lesions often evolve with serous exudate, crusts, and forming large plaques. Other areas that may be affected by these skin lesions are the trunk, limbs, and rarely nappy area.
- In childhood (aged 2 years and older), AD is characterized by a reduction of the exudative component. The skin is often dry, the erythema is paler, and lichenified papules and plaques affect typically flexor surfaces, hands, feet, neck, and eyelids.
- Adolescents typically present with symmetrical papules and plaques, often associated with **lichenification** and excoriations, affecting flexural regions, face, neck, and distal extremities. In the case of important pruritus, also excoriations and scratching lesions can be found.
- In adults, atypical presentations such as portrait-like dermatitis, diffuse eczema, and erythrodermia can occur, in addition to the most frequent clinical phenotypes of flexural eczema, head and neck eczema, and hand eczema [41].

There are many clinical variants of AD, and some of them present with a typical pattern and localization. In the facial area, a site-specific manifestation of AD is cheilitis sicca, a typical eczema of the lips, with redness of the mucosa associated with fissurations and dryness. Eyelid eczema, characterized by lichenification, can be present as a single manifestation of AD especially in adolescents and adults. Another feature typical of childhood AD is ear eczema, presenting as an erythematous, scaling itchy lesion, localized in the retroarticular area or under the ear lobe. A typical feature of AD in adolescents is portrait dermatitis, in which eczema spreads from the head-neck area to the seborrheic areas of the trunk (upper third of the back and sternal region). This form has to be distinguished from seborrheic dermatitis. Some authors suggest the pathogenic role of Malassezia furfur in this variant of AD [42]. Juvenile plantar dermatosis is a common variant of atopic dermatitis in children, characterized by scaling and lichenified areas on the feet. Nummular lesions tend to develop on the extremities in children, they are shaped as discoid plaques with crusts.

Pruritus is a typical and disruptive symptom of AD. The skin of patients with AD is characterized by a strong hypersensitivity to stimuli that are harmless to other people who are not affected by the disease [43]. The scratching is exacerbated by many different stimuli such as pain, elevated temperature, or rubbing by clothing. Clinically it is a difficult symptom to control, also because it creates a vicious circle of scratching that leads to a worsening of the lesions. Moreover, it strongly affects the quality of life of the patients, particularly the sleep quality is strongly decreased [44].

7.6 Diagnosis

Diagnosis of AD is based on the typical morphology and distribution of the skin manifestations. Currently, there are no pathognomonic lesions or biomarkers to diagnose AD. For this reason, diagnostic criteria have been developed to assist with diagnosis. The most commonly used criteria are the Hanifin and Rajka criteria, and subsequent modifications, including the UK Working Party's Diagnostic Criteria for Atopic Dermatitis.

There are four major clinical features: pruritus, chronic-relapsing course, typical distribution, and family or personal history of atopy, associated with minor criteria as shown in Table 7.1. One of the most important minor criteria is the age of onset under 2 years.

The UK Working Party then reformulated the criteria in 1994 aimed at simplifying the diagnostic process for patients over 2 years of age [11]. This set of criteria includes only one major criterion, namely the presence of pruritic eczema in the last 12 months, which must be present for a diagnosis to be made. At least three other minor criteria must be associated [45].

Table 7.1 Diagnostic criteria for atopic dermatitis

Hanifin and Rajka Criteria (1980) (at least 3 major criteria + 3 minor criteria)	UK Working Party Criteria (1994) (the major criterion + at least 3 minor criteria)	Japanese guidelines for AD (2020) (all the three criteria)
Major criteria		
Pruritus	An itchy skin condition in the last 12 months	Pruritus
Typical morphology and distribution of lesions according to age		Typical morphology and distribution of lesions according to age
Chronic or chronic-relapsing course		Chronic or relapsing course
Positive family and/or personal history of atopic diseases		
Minor criteria		
Early onset age (<2 years)	Early onset age (<2 years)	
Objective clinical symptoms: Xerosis Ichtyosis/keratosis pilaris/palmar hyperlinearity Non-specific hand dermatitis Nipple eczema Cheilitis Perifollicular accentuation Pityriasis alba Anterior neck folds	Personal history of atopic disease	
Subjective clinical symptoms: Itch when sweating Intolerance to wool and lipid solvents	History of flexural involvement	
Immunological anomalies: Elevated serum IgE Skin prick test positivity Food intolerance	Dry skin in the last 12 months	
Recurrent skin infections	Visible flexural dermatitis	
Functional anomalies: Facial pallor/erythema White dermatographism Course influences by environmental/emotional factors		
Anomalies of eyes and eye areas: Recurrent conjunctivitis Dennies-Morgan infraorbital fold Keratoconus Anterior subcapsular cataract		

A breakthrough regarding the diagnostic criteria for AD has been observed following the publication of the updated 2020 Japanese Guidelines [46]. These guidelines were aimed at simplifying the diagnosis of AD and reducing the number of criteria. They consider only the presence of itching, typical morphology and distribution of lesions, and chronic or chronically remitting disease course as diagnostic criteria for AD, regardless of the severity of the disease. Conversely, in these new guidelines, age of onset and personal or family history of atopy or high levels of IgE are not considered fundamental criteria. Indeed, it has been found that at least 5–15% of atopic patients do not present high total IgE levels.

Choosing the best treatment is important to evaluate the clinical stage of AD. Many validated scores can help the physician in assessing the severity of the disease. The most widely used tool is the SCORing Atopic Dermatitis (**SCORAD**). It is based on the intensity of the skin lesions (60%), the size of the affected area (20%), and the patient's self-reported symptoms (20%).

- SCORAD >50 indicates severe AD.
- SCORAD 25–50 indicates moderate AD.
- SCORAD <25 indicates mild AD [47].

The Patient-Oriented Scoring Atopic Dermatitis index (**POSCORAD**) is a more recent variant [48]. POSCORAD was developed by the European Task Force on Atopic Dermatitis and introduced in 2011. It represents a self-evaluation tool that helps the patient and the family to understand and manage the disease.

Another score, used to assess the severity of AD, is the Eczema Area Severity Index (**EASI**), recommended by the Harmonising Outcome Measures for Eczema (HOME), an international group composed of various professionals in the field dedicated to standardizing outcomes of clinical research on atopic dermatitis. The EASI assesses the clinical signs of disease, assigning points only to visible lesions, giving equal weight to both the intensity and extent of the lesion, without taking into account the subjective symptoms of atopic dermatitis. For this reason, it is always paired with the evaluation of other scores such as the Numeric Rating Scale (NRS) for itch and sleep and the Dermatology Life Quality Index (DLQI). AD is considered moderate-severe when the EASI score is >16–20.

7.6.1 Differential Diagnosis

The differential diagnosis of AD includes infections, infestations, immunodeficiencies, autoimmune diseases, and other chronic dermatosis. Infant AD, in the first months of life, is often associated with **seborrheic dermatitis**. Another mimic is **scabies**, which in infants can affect the whole body. Scabies can usually be differentiated by the presence of crusted papules, the involvement of the armpits and diaper area, and the presence of vesicles or pustules on the hands and feet. Children and adolescents without a personal or family history of allergies or without an adequate response to treatment for AD, who present with a rash resembling eczema, should have a detailed medical history taken and consider patch testing to determine if they have allergic contact dermatitis. Other possible differential diagnoses are shown in Table 7.2.

7.6.2 Complications

The most common complication of AD is represented by bacterial and viral infections. In particular, the **impetiginization** of AD lesions is very frequent, and it is linked to the vast colonization of SA on the skin, which can also lead to an exacerbation of the disease. The colonization of the skin by herpes simplex virus, known as eczema herpeticum, represents a rare complication. It consists of the rapid spread of a herpes simplex virus infection over the skin affected by AD, in particular, on the trunk, head, and neck. AD represents also a risk factor for the development of widespread Molluscum contagiosum, more likely in children. Ocular complications, such as **atopic keratoconjunctivitis** or vernal conjunctivitis, are also frequent. Rarer ocular complications include subcapsular cataracts, in particular anterior cataracts and keratoconus.

Table 7.2 Differential diagnosis of atopic dermatitis

Differential diagnosis of atopic dermatitis
Chronic dermatoses
Seborrheic dermatitis
Contact dermatitis
Psoriasis
Infections and infestations
Scabies
HTLV-1-associated dermatitis
Chronic or neonatal mucocutaneous candidiasis
Impetigo
Primary immunodeficiencies
Hyper IgE syndrome
Wiskott–Aldrich syndrome
DiGeorge syndrome
IPEX (immune dysregulation, polyendocrinopathy, enteropathy, X-linked)
X-linked hypogammaglobulinemia
Common variable immunodeficiency
Ataxia telangiectasia
Metabolic or genetic disorders
Keratosis pilaris
Phenylketonuria
Acrodermatitis enteropathica
Pellagra
Riboflavin deficiency
Autoimmune disorders
Dermatomyositis
Lupus erythematosus
Dermatitis herpetiformis

7.7 Treatment

The treatment of AD is still not definitive and varies with the specificity of the patient. The treatment aims to improve the skin state, reduce itching, promote remission, and prevent complications.

The treatment differs based on the clinical variant and severity of the disease. The basic non-pharmacologic therapy for patients with AD includes behavioural education programmes, the use of emollients and bath oils, and avoiding clinically significant allergens.

Generally, topical treatments such as emollients, corticosteroids, and topical calcineurin inhibitors are used as first-line treatment for mild forms and as adjuvants in more severe forms. In the latter, when topical therapy alone is not sufficient, phototherapy and the use of systemic drugs may be added.

7.7.1 Skin Care

Skincare is defined as careful and daily attention to the restoration of the altered skin barrier using specific emollients and detergents [49]. It has a strength of recommendation A and level of evidence I. It is important to restore the architecture of the skin to maintain adequate hydration, a good balance between the production and desquamation of corneocytes, and a balanced lipid layers composition.

Correct cleansing is essential to eliminate sebaceous secretions, environmental contaminants, and tissue debris [49]. It has to be performed daily, only for 10 min, with warm water (not hot) and with substances that do not impair the hydrolipidic film. The homeostasis of the SC is of primary importance, that is why aggressive detergents are not recommended, and at the same time, water alone is not appropriate to eliminate lipophilic substances.

Daily use of moisturizers is fundamental in the management of AD. They reduce TEWL, itching, and xerosis. Recently, products with an ideal ratio of ceramide–cholesterol–saturated fatty acid ratio of 3:1:1 have been created. They are known as third-generation emollient barrier repairers (Emollients plus) and represent an excellent nutritional blend [50]. **Emollients plus** have an acid pH and they can penetrate the skin and restore its structure and function. Moreover, active ingredients that have specific anti-inflammatory, antipruritic, and antibacterial properties can be added to dermatological cosmetics, to improve clinical symptoms and decrease the need for corticosteroids. A novel therapeutic approach involves the manipulation of the altered skin microbiome by using extracts from non-pathogenic gram-negative bacteria that act as pre-probiotics and symbiotics to balance or modulate the immune system [51].

7.7.2 Topical Corticosteroids (TCSs)

Topical corticosteroids (TCS) are considered the first-line treatment of AD [52, 53]. Many randomized controlled trials have demonstrated their effectiveness also in reducing itching. When used correctly, TCSs have also shown an excellent safety profile. TCSs have broad anti-inflammatory effects achieved through specific receptor binding on adaptive immune cells, which inhibits the release of pro-inflammatory cytokines. To obtain the best results, it is necessary to consider the type of the molecule, the treatment site, the stage of AD, and the length of treatment. The potency classification of available topical corticosteroids is shown in Table 7.3. Normally, applying TCSs once daily at night is recommended. For acute forms, a high-power TCS for a short period followed by a switch to less potent preparations is preferred.

TCS should be chosen in the early stages of treatment, specifically to control the acute inflammatory phase. In case of frequent exacerbations, a proactive approach, such as applying TCS once or twice a week at the location of exacerbation, even when there is no injury present, is recommended to reduce the number of relapses. It is safe to administer an average monthly dose of 15 gr of medium-high potency TCS to a newborn,

Table 7.3 Potency classification of topical corticosteroids (from Patrizi et al. 2023)

Group/potency	Active ingredient	Vehicle	Concentration (%)
Group I—mild	Hydrocortisone	Cream	0.5
	Hydrocortisone acetate	Cream	0.5
Group II—moderate	Aclomethasone dipropionate		
	Clobethasone butyrate	Cream	0.5
	Dexamethasone sodium phosphate	Ointment	0.2
	Dexamethasone valerate	Cream	0.1
	Desonide		
	Fluocortinbutylester		
	Hydrocortisone butyrate	Cream, cream hydrophilic, emulsion, cutaneous solution, ointment	0.1
Group III—potent	Beclomethasone dipropionate	Cream	0.025
	Betamethasone benzonate	Cream	0.025
		Cream, skin emulsion, gel	0.1
	Beclomethasone dipropionate	Cutaneous solution	0.05
		cream, skin emulsion, ointment	0.1
	Betamethasone dipropionate	Cream, cutaneous solution, ointment	0.05
	Budesonide	Cream, oinment	0.025
	Deoxymethasone	emulsion	0.25
	Diflucortolone valerate	Cream, cream hydrophobic, cutaneous solution, ointment	0.1
		Cream hydrophobic, ointment	0.3
	Diflucortone valerianate		
	Fluocinolone acetonide	Cream	0.025
		cutaneous solution	0.01
	Fluocinonide	Cream, gel, cutaneous solution	0.05
	Fluocortolone pivalate/caproate	Cream hydrophobic	0.25
		Cream	0.25
	Fluticasone propionate	Oinment	0.005
		Cream	0.05
	Methylprednisolone aceponate	Cream, cream hydrophobic, emulsion, cutaneous solution ointment	0.1
	Mometasone furoate	Cream, cutaneous solution, ointment	0.1
	Prednicarbato	Cream	0.25
Group IV—very potent	Alcinonide	Cream	0.1
	Clobetasol propionate	Oinment	0.05

30 gr to a child, and 60–90 gr to an adult. Unfortunately, the fear of corticosteroids, known as "**corticosteroid phobia**," it is very common and it is still a significant obstacle to the use of TCSs. It is crucial to explain the different types of TCSs available, as well as when and how to use these medications, and reassure patients of their excellent safety profile.

7.7.3 Topical Calcineurin Inhibitors (TCIs)

Tacrolimus is derived from the bacterium *Streptomyces tsubaensis* and pimecrolimus is the chemical derivate of *Ascomycin*. They are the two TCIs used in the topical treatment of AD approved respectively in 2000 and 2001 as a second-line treatment of AD. Short- and long-term efficacy of tacrolimus and pimecrolimus, in children over 2 years old and adults, has been demonstrated by several studies [54]. **Tacrolimus** ointment is recommended for moderate to severe cases, using the 0.03% formulation for patients aged 2–15 years and the 0.1% formulation for patients 16 years and older. **Pimecrolimus** cream 1% is indicated for mild to moderate cases from 2 years of age. The treatment involves twice-daily applications for 2–3 weeks, followed by an evening application until the lesions resolve. TCIs can cause a burning sensation, warmth, tingling, and transient worsening of AD, especially if applied to acutely inflamed skin; therefore, acute lesions should be initially treated with corticosteroids, and then a subsequent switch to TCIs should be evaluated. TCIs are particularly recommended for sensitive skin areas (eyelids, folds, and anogenital area). Actually, in comparison to TCS, their high molecular weight (822 Da) only permits limited penetration into healthy skin, thereby maintaining the formation of tight junctions (TJs) [55]. A possible TCI-TCS combination scheme involves the use of TCIs on sensitive skin areas, as none of the TCIs induce cutaneous atrophy [56], and TCS in other affected areas. The use of TCIs is not associated with the development of lymphoma or melanoma or other malignancies from photoexposure; in any case, appropriate sun protection is indicated in patients on treatment. TCIs are not associated with glaucoma or cataracts. The proactive use of tacrolimus twice a week seems to reduce recurrences. TCIs have also been found to be effective in controlling itching in AD, as long as the eczema does not disappear.

7.7.4 Wet Wrap Therapy

Wet wrap therapy can be useful in severe atopic AD or during important reactivations of the disease. The procedure is based on the application of TCS, sometimes mixed with emollients, associated with an inner wet layer and outer dry layer of cotton gauge, left in place for several hours (8–24 h) per day, for a maximum of 2 weeks. The treatment aims to increase the penetration of TCS, reduce scratching, and increase the hydration of the skin.

7.7.5 Topical Antibiotics

AD represents a risk factor for the development of secondary bacterial infections. SA and *Streptococcus pyogenes* are the most common bacteria involved. In case of superinfection, it is mandatory to act with an antibiotical therapy. In particular, **mupirocin** and **fusidic acid** are considered the most suitable topical antibiotics. The duration of the treatment should be limited in time, normally it requires 2–3 applications per day for 7–10 days. Mupirocin is not indicated in children <1 year of age because of the lack of studies in this age group [57]. It is common to find also nasal colonization by SA associated with the recurrence of superinfections. In this case, intranasal therapy with mupirocin (2 applications a day for 5 days) can be used [58].

7.7.6 Systemic Antibiotics

Systemic antibiotics should be used, in combination with topical therapy, only if the bacterial superinfection affects more than 2% of the skin surface [58] and there is a strong tendency to relapse. The most used antibiotics are first- and second-generation cephalosporins, such as cephalexine. In case of strong impetiginization also amoxicillin–clavulanate or fluoroquinolones could be used. In the suspect of colonization by methicillin-resistant *Staphylococcus aureus* (MRSA) it is possible to perform a skin swab, and the treatment is based on clindamycin or trimethoprim-sulphamethoxazole.

7.7.7 Systemic Corticosteroids

Oral corticosteroids have a clear anti-inflammatory activity, but they are not recommended in patients with AD [59]. They rapidly reduce the skin inflammation on acute lesions of AD, but at the same time they do not act positively on skin barrier alterations and they have various systemic side effects. In particular, they can lead to immunosuppression, hypertension, osteoporosis, weight gain, and in children growth retardation [60]. Moreover, they can cause a rebound effect after the suspension of the therapy and they have a poor efficacy on itching and pain. For this reason, CSs should be administered only in serious cases with difficult symptom control and for a limited period. One of the most used treatment schemes is methylprednisolone 0.5 mg/kg/die for 1–2 weeks.

7.7.8 Phototherapy

Phototherapy is a second-line therapy, used in patients with a moderate or relapsing form of AD resistant to TCs and/or TCIs. It can be used also in children aged >12 years [61], because it leads to an improvement in skin lesions, itching, and quality of sleep. UV rays act on the skin with immunosuppressive, immunomodulatory, and anti-inflammatory effects. In particular, they induce apoptosis [62] in inflammatory cells, inhibit Langerhans cells, and reduce cytokine production. Additionally, UV rays also influence the skin microbiota, reducing colonization by SA [63]. In the paediatric age, NB-UVB is considered the safer option [58]. The most common side effects are xerosis, sunburn, and erythema. Co-treatment with TCS and emollients should be considered in the initial phases to prevent exacerbations. New treatment frontiers, such as excimer laser 308 nm or blue spectrum visible light therapy [64], could expand therapeutic options, but they have not yet been thoroughly investigated for use in patients with AD. All UV treatments ultimately expose patients to the risk of developing skin ageing and skin cancer. To reduce this risk, the combination with TCIs is recommended [61].

7.7.9 Systemic Immunosuppressants

Systemic immunosuppressants are sometimes used in adults, but due to their important side effects and difficult management, they are less and less chosen as treatment.

Cyclosporin A belongs to the calcineurin inhibitors family. It is an oral immunosuppressant, currently used as an off-label therapy in children with moderate to severe AD [65]. It shows a quick and good response profile, with a low incidence of side effects [66]. The dosage range is 2.5–5 mg/kg/day. Among the side effects it is important to include nephrotoxicity, infections, headache, hypertension, and tremor.

Methotrexate is an antimetabolite that acts as an inhibitor of folate synthesis. It has been studied in adult AD and it is currently used as an off-label second-line therapy in children, particularly if a long-lasting treatment is needed [67]. The major side effects are liver toxicity and teratogenic effects, while stomatitis, nausea, and vomiting are reversible and dose-related effects.

Other immunosuppressants used in the treatment of AD are **azathioprine** and **mycophenolate mofetil**. Azathioprine is a purine analogue while mycophenolate mofetil inhibits the inosine monophosphatase dehydrogenase they both act by reducing the proliferation of T lymphocytes, through different mechanisms. They are both rarely used as a second-line off-label treatment in children.

7.7.10 Biological Drugs

Given the central role of IL-4 and 13 in the pathophysiology of atopic dermatitis, numerous biologic drugs targeting these cytokines are currently in development. The first to be approved by the FDA was **dupilumab**, a drug demonstrating great clinical success and efficacy. It is a fully human IgG4κ monoclonal antibody that targets IL-4Rα, blocking both IL-4 and IL-13 signalling pathways through type 2 receptors, and also blocking IL-4 signalling through type 1 receptors.

Two other IL-13-targeting antibodies, tralokinumab and lebrikizumab, are currently in clinical trials. **Tralokinumab** is an IgG4λ monoclonal antibody that inhibits IL-13 binding to IL-13Rα1 and α2 receptors, blocking type 2 signalling, and interfering with IL-13 regulation mediated by IL-13Rα2 receptors. **Lebrikizumab**, a humanized IgG4κ monoclonal antibody, binds soluble IL-13 with high affinity but on a different epitope than tralokinumab. It blocks the formation of the IL-13R1α/IL-4Rα heterodimer but does not prevent IL-13 binding to the IL-13Rα2 receptor. These three drugs have been evaluated in both monotherapy and combination therapy for moderate to severe atopic dermatitis patients. However, comparisons between studies are difficult due to variations in methods, population, and the duration of treatment. While these drugs have shown clinical efficacy, long-term safety studies are still lacking, although there have been no indications of increased risk for serious complications such as infections, tumours, or cardiovascular events.

7.7.11 Dupilumab

In clinical studies on AD, treatment with dupilumab has been associated with a decrease in type 2 immune biomarker concentrations such as thymus and activation-regulated chemokine (TARC/CCL17), serum total IgE, and allergen-specific IgE compared to baseline. Additionally, treatment with dupilumab has been observed to reduce lactate dehydrogenase (LDH), a biomarker associated with the activity and severity of atopic dermatitis. Numerous studies have shown that even after 4 weeks of monotherapy treatment, dupilumab results in a rapid and significant improvement in clinical and pathophysiological parameters with minimal side effects. Improvement in skin lesions, itching, and quality of life becomes evident as early as two weeks into treatment. The efficacy and safety of dupilumab as monotherapy and in combination with topical corticosteroids were evaluated in three pivotal, randomized, double-blind, placebo-controlled trials (LIBERTY AD SOLO 1, LIBERTY AD SOLO 2, and LIBERTY AD CHRONOS) conducted on 2119 patients aged 18 years or older with moderate to severe atopic dermatitis defined by Investigator's Global Assessment score of ≥3, Eczema Area and Severity Index score of ≥16, and a minimum body surface area involvement of 10%. Eligible patients enrolled in the three studies had demonstrated an inadequate response to topical therapy [68–70].

The drug's safety is very good, with the most common adverse reactions being injection site reactions, conjunctivitis, blepharitis, and oral herpes. Very rare cases of serum sickness like illness have been reported in the development programme for atopic dermatitis. Recently, the drug's indication has been extended to adolescent patients over the age of 12. Dupilumab should be combined with emollients and, if necessary, with topical anti-inflammatory drugs. In 2020, a Phase 3 study demonstrated the safety and efficacy of dupilumab also in adolescents (aged 12–17 years) with moderate-severe AD, not adequately controlled by topical therapy [71].

*The approved dosage for the drug, in this age group, differs according to weight, as shown in * The dose may be increased to 200 mg every 2 weeks in patients weighing 15 kg to <60 kg.*

More recently Dupilumab was approved also in children aged 6–11 years old with severe AD. The phase 3 study LIBERTY AD PEDS, a randomized double-blind, placebo-controlled trial, demonstrated the efficacy and safety of this drug also in this group of age [72]. *The dosage scheme is visible in * The dose may be increased to 200 mg every 2 weeks in patients weighing 15 kg to <60 kg.*

Table 7.4. This biological drug was demonstrated to significantly reduce the EASI from baseline values. Moreover, it also reduces itching and the burden of anxiety and depression reported by both parents and children, improving quality of life.

Table 7.4 Recommended dose of dupilumab for paediatric atopic dermatitis

Bodyweight	Starting dose	Subsequent doses
Adolescents between the ages of 12 and 17		
<60 kg	400 mg (two 200 mg injections)	200 mg every 2 weeks
60 kg or more	600 mg (two 300 mg injections)	300 mg every 2 weeks
Children between the ages of 6 and 11		
15 to <60 kg	300 mg (one 300 mg injection) on day 1, followed by 300 mg on day 15	300 mg every 4 weeks [a], starting 4 weeks after the day 15 dose
60 kg or more	600 mg (two 300 mg injections)	300 mg every 2 weeks

[a]The dose may be increased to 200 mg every 2 weeks in patients weighing 15 kg to <60 kg

There are also recent studies that investigate the efficacy and safety of dupilumab in children from 6 months of age to 6 years. In particular, a phase 3 study demonstrated that dupilumab significantly improved atopic dermatitis signs and symptoms versus placebo in children younger than 6 years. Dupilumab was well tolerated and showed an acceptable safety profile, similar to results in older children and adults [73]. The use of dupilumab in this group of ages has been approved by EMA in March 2023.

7.7.12 JAK Inhibitors for AD: Upadacitinib

Janus kinases (JAKs) are intracellular tyrosine kinases acting as dimers in many signalling processes of cytokines receptors, in particular with the JAK-STAT pathway. The Janus kinases are divided into four families: JAK 1, JAK 2, JAK 3, and TYK2. They play a key role in both adaptative and innate immunity and that is the reason why they represent a good target for the treatment of inflammatory diseases. In particular, they seem to be an appropriate target in AD because of the numerous inflammatory cytokines (i.e. IL-4, IL-13, IL-31, and IL-22) that are activated by the JAK pathway and that are involved in the pathogenesis of AD [74, 75].

Upadacitinib is an oral, selective, and reversible JAK inhibitor, in particular, it acts on the JAK 1 pathway. It was developed to improve the safety of the treatment and at the same time reduce the side effects related to the inhibition of JAK 2 and JAK 3 [76]. At present time upadacitinib has been approved, also by the EMA, for the treatment of various diseases (i.e. ankylosing spondyloarthritis and moderate to severe ulcerative colitis) including moderate to severe AD in adults and adolescents older than 12 years who are candidates to systemic therapy. Patients must weigh >30 kg, and the dosage for adolescents (12–18 years) is 15 mg once a day. The most frequent side effects during the treatment are acne, upper respiratory tract infections, headache, blood creatine phosphokinase increase, and oral herpes [77]. Upadacitinib can be used with or without topical corticosteroids. Discontinuation of upadacitinib treatment should be considered in all patients who show no evidence of therapeutic benefit after 12 weeks of treatment [78].

Before starting the treatment, the immunological profile of the patient must be evaluated, as well as vaccinations, blood cell count, lipidic profile, and hepatic profile. Also screening for TBC and other infections (i.e. HIV, HCV, and HBV) has to be performed, along with a chest X-ray and a 12-lead electrocardiogram. In animal studies, upadacitinib has been shown to induce foetal teratogenic effects [79].

From double-blind randomized controlled phase 3 trials (Measure Up1 and Measure Up2), upadacitinib demonstrated to have a good security profile, and it has demonstrated superior efficacy in the treatment of AD compared to placebo [80, 81] and also to dupilumab [82, 83].

Key Points

- AD is a common chronic-relapsing inflammatory skin disease typical of the infant age and is often linked to other allergic disorders such as asthma,

(continued)

allergic rhinoconjunctivitis, and food allergies.
- It is a polygenic skin disease that results from a combination of genetic susceptibility and environmental factors, giving rise to a wide range of clinical manifestations.
- It is also associated with a higher susceptibility to skin infections, particularly from *Staphylococcus aureus*.
- Intense itching represents one of the main symptoms.
- Clinical manifestations show a typical age-related distribution.
- Taking a proactive approach to management is recommended, which includes regularly using moisturizers and using anti-inflammatory treatments to control the inflammation. For more severe cases, targeted immunomodulatory therapy is available.

Take-Home Messages

- AD is a common inflammatory skin disease, typical of the paediatric population.
- Epidermal barrier dysfunctions play a crucial role in the pathogenesis of AD along with genetic factors and immune dysregulation.
- Th2 polarization, with the production of many cytokines such as IL-4, IL-13, and IL-31, contributes to maintaining the inflammation status, both on lesional and non-lesional skin.
- Skin dysbiosis is another fundamental feature of AD, leading directly to skin barrier defects through different signalling pathways, including the one of AhR.
- In infants, AD manifests as an acute inflammation with the involvement of the cheeks, scalp, and outer parts of the limbs, later it shifts to chronic inflammation with lichenification and a preference for the skin folds.
- The diagnosis is based on the clinical presentation. Over the years the guidelines for the diagnosis of AD have been simplified, reducing the criteria to only three: pruritus, typical morphology, and distribution of lesions according to age and chronic-relapsing course.
- The treatment of AD has the aim of improving skin state, reducing itching, and promoting remission of the disease.
- Daily skin care is a milestone of the treatment of AD, along with topical corticosteroids, which are considered the first-line treatment.
- Topical calcineurin inhibitors can help the management of AD, in particular, in sensitive skin areas (eyelids, folds, and anogenital area).
- Biological drugs, such as dupilumab, demonstrated great clinical success and efficacy. Dupilumab is a fully human IgG4 k monoclonal antibody. It targets IL-4Ralfa, blocking both IL-4 and IL-13 signalling pathways, and silencing Th2 inflammation.
- Upadacitinib represents a new important therapeutical option, also in the paediatric population. It is an oral, selective, and reversible JAK 1 inhibitor. It acts by inhibiting the JAK pathway, which activates numerous inflammatory cytokines (i.e. IL-4, IL-13, IL-31, and IL-22) that are involved in the pathogenesis of AD.

References

1. Sidbury R, Davis DM, Cohen DE, Cordoro KM, Berger TG, Bergman JN, et al. Guidelines of care for the management of atopic dermatitis: section 3. Management and treatment with phototherapy and systemic agents. J Am Acad Dermatol. 2014;71:327–49.

2. Silvestre Salvador JF, Romero-Pérez D, Encabo-Durán B. Atopic dermatitis in adults: a diagnostic challenge. J Invest Allergol Clin Immunol. 2017;27:78–88.
3. Maiello N, Comberiati P, Giannetti A, Ricci G, Carello R, Galli E. New directions in understanding atopic march starting from atopic dermatitis. Children. 2022;9:450.
4. Yang EJ, Sekhon S, Sanchez IM, Beck KM, Bhutani T. Recent developments in atopic dermatitis. Pediatrics. 2018;142:e20181102.
5. Beattie PE, Lewis-Jones MS. A comparative study of impairment of quality of life in children with skin disease and children with other chronic childhood diseases. Br J Dermatol. 2006;155:145–51.
6. Drucker AM, Wang AR, Li WQ, Sevetson E, Block JK, Qureshi AA. The burden of atopic dermatitis: summary of a report for the National Eczema Association. J Invest Dermatol. 2017;137:26–30.
7. Kwa L, Silverberg JI. Financial burden of emergency department visits for atopic dermatitis in the United States. J Am Acad Dermatol. 2018;79:443–47.
8. Bylund S, Von Kobyletzki LB, Svalstedt M, Svensson Å. Prevalence and incidence of atopic dermatitis: a systematic review. Acta Dermato-Venereol. 2020;100:adv00160.
9. Silverberg JI. Public health burden and epidemiology of atopic dermatitis. Dermatol Clin. 2017;35:283–9.
10. Cantarutti A, Donà D, Visentin F, Borgia E, Scamarcia A, Cantarutti L, et al. Epidemiology of frequently occurring skin diseases in Italian children from 2006 to 2012: a retrospective, population-based study. Pediatr Dermatol. 2015;32:668–78.
11. Galli E, Cinicola B, Carello R, Caimmi S, Brindisi G, De Castro G, Zicari AM,et al. Atopic dermatitis. Acta Biomed. 2020;91(11-S):e2020011.
12. Fabbri P. Immunità & cute. Le dermatosi a patogenesi immunologica. Lingomed, Milano, Italy, 2012.
13. Kim Y, Lim KM. Skin barrier dysfunction and filaggrin. Arch Pharm Res. 2021;44:36–48.
14. Kim J, Kim BE, Leung DYM. Pathophysiology of atopic dermatitis: clinical implications. Allergy Asthma Proc. 2019;40:84–92.
15. Gupta J, Grube E, Ericksen MB, Stevenson MD, Lucky AW, Sheth AP, et al. Intrinsically defective skin barrier function in children with atopic dermatitis correlates with disease severity. J Allergy Clin Immunol. 2008;121:725–30.
16. Tsakok T, Woolf R, Smith CH, Weidinger S, Flohr C. Atopic dermatitis: the skin barrier and beyond. Br J Dermatol. 2019;180:464–74.
17. De Benedetto A, Rafaels NM, McGirt LY, Ivanov AI, Georas SN, Cheadle C, et al. Tight junction defects in patients with atopic dermatitis. J Allergy Clin Immunol. 2011;27:773–86.e1–7.
18. Irvine AD, McLean WHI, Leung DYM. Filaggrin mutations associated with skin and allergic diseases. N Engl J Med. 2011;365:1315–27.
19. Palmer CNA, Irvine AD, Terron-Kwiatkowski A, Zhao Y, Liao H, Lee SP,et al. Common loss-of-function variants of the epidermal barrier protein filaggrin are a major predisposing factor for atopic dermatitis. Nat Genet. 2006;38:441–6.
20. David Boothe W, Tarbox JA, Tarbox MB. Atopic dermatitis: pathophysiology. Adv Exp Med Biol. 2017;1027:21–37.
21. Namkung JH, Lee JE, Kim E, Kim HJ, Seo EY, Jang HY, et al. Association of polymorphisms in genes encoding IL-4, IL-13 and their receptors with atopic dermatitis in a Korean population. Exp Dermatol. 2011;20:915–9.
22. Heine G, Hoefer N, Franke A, Nöthling U, Schumann RR, Hamann L, et al. Association of vitamin D receptor gene polymorphisms with severe atopic dermatitis in adults. Br J Dermatol. 2013;168:855–8.
23. Suzuki H, Makino Y, Nagata M, Furuta J, Enomoto H, Hirota T,et al. A rare variant in CYP27A1 and its association with atopic dermatitis with high serum total IgE. Allergy Eur J Allergy Clin Immunol. 2016;71:1486–9.
24. Esaki H, Brunner PM, Renert-Yuval Y, Czarnowicki T, Huynh T, Tran G, et al. Early-onset pediatric atopic dermatitis is TH2 but also TH17 polarized in skin. J Allergy Clin Immunol. 2016;138:1639–51.
25. Brunner PM, Israel A, Zhang N, Leonard A, Wen HC, Huynh T, et al. Early-onset pediatric atopic dermatitis is characterized by TH2/TH17/TH22-centered inflammation and lipid alterations. J Allergy Clin Immunol. 2018;141:2094–106.
26. Liu YJ. Thymic stromal lymphopoietin: master switch for allergic inflammation. J Exp Med. 2006;203:269–73.
27. Moyle M, Cevikbas F, Harden JL, Guttman-Yassky E. Understanding the immune landscape in atopic dermatitis: the era of biologics and emerging therapeutic approaches. Exp Dermatol. 2019;28:756–68.
28. Silverberg JI, Kantor R. The role of interleukins 4 and/or 13 in the pathophysiology and treatment of atopic dermatitis. Dermatol Clin. 2017;35:327–34.
29. Howell MD, Kim BE, Gao P, Grant AV, Boguniewicz M, DeBenedetto A, et al. Cytokine modulation of atopic dermatitis filaggrin skin expression. J Allergy Clin Immunol. 2009;124(3 Suppl 2):R7–R12.
30. Oh M-H, Oh SY, Yu J, Myers AC, Leonard WJ, Liu YJ, et al. IL-13 Induces skin fibrosis in atopic dermatitis by thymic stromal lymphopoietin. J Immunol. 2011;186:7232–42.
31. Sonkoly E, Muller A, Lauerma AI, Pivarcsi A, Soto H, Kemeny L,et al. IL-31: a new link between T cells and pruritus in atopic skin inflammation. J Allergy Clin Immunol. 2006;117:411–17.
32. Paller AS, Kong HH, Seed P, Naik S, Scharschmidt TC, Gallo RL,et al. The microbiome in patients with atopic dermatitis. J Allergy Clin Immunol. 2019;143:1660.
33. Ito Y, Amagai M. Controlling skin microbiome as a new bacteriotherapy for inflammatory skin diseases. Inflamm Regen. 2022;42:26.
34. Uberoi A, Bartow-McKenney C, Zheng Q, Flowers L, Campbell A, Knight SAB, et al. Commensal microbiota regulates skin barrier function and repair via

signaling through the aryl hydrocarbon receptor. Cell Host Microbe. 2021;29:1235–48.
35. Yu J, Luo Y, Zhu Z, Zhou Y, Sun L, Gao J, et al. A tryptophan metabolite of the skin microbiota attenuates inflammation in patients with atopic dermatitis through the aryl hydrocarbon receptor. J Allergy Clin Immunol. 2019;143:2108–119.
36. van den Bogaard EH, Perdew GH. The Enigma of AHR activation in the skin: interplay among ligands, metabolism, and bioavailability. J Invest Dermatol. 2021;141:1385–8.
37. Majumder S, Kono M, Lee YT, Byrnes C, Li C, Tuymetova G, et al. A genome-wide CRISPR/Cas9 screen reveals that the aryl hydrocarbon receptor stimulates sphingolipid levels. J Biol Chem. 2020;295:4341–9.
38. Danby SG, Cork MJ. PH in atopic dermatitis. Curr Probl Dermatol. 2018;54:95–107.
39. Alam MJ, Xie L, Yap YA, Marques FZ, Robert R. Manipulating microbiota to treat atopic dermatitis: functions and therapies. Pathogens. 2022;11:642.
40. Lee HJ, Lee SH. Epidermal permeability barrier defects and barrier repair therapy in atopic dermatitis. Allergy Asthma Immunol Res. 2014;6:276–87.
41. Napolitano M, Fabbrocini G, Martora F, Genco L, Noto M, Patruno C. Children atopic dermatitis: diagnosis, mimics, overlaps, and therapeutic implication. Dermatol Ther. 2022;35:e15901.
42. Bayrou O, Pecquet C, Flahault A, Artigou C, Abuaf N, Leynadier F. Head and neck atopic dermatitis and Malassezia-furfur-specific IgE antibodies. Dermatology. 2005;211:107–13.
43. Akiyama T, Carstens E. Neural processing of itch. Neuroscience. 2013;250:697–14.
44. Tominaga M, Takamori K. Peripheral itch sensitization in atopic dermatitis. Allergol Int. 2022;71:265–77.
45. Williams HC, Burney PG, Hay RJ, Archer CB, Shipley MJ, Hunter JJ, et al. The U.K. Working Party's diagnostic criteria for atopic dermatitis. I. Derivation of a minimum set of discriminators for atopic dermatitis. Br J Dermatol. 1994;131:383–96.
46. Katoh N, Ohya Y, Ikeda M, Ebihara T, Katayama I, Saeki H,et al. Japanese guidelines for atopic dermatitis 2020. Allergol Int. 2020;69:356–69.
47. Torres T, Ferreira EO, Gonçalo M, Mendes-Bastos P, Selores M, Filipe P. Update on atopic dermatitis. Acta Medica Port. 2019;32:606–13.
48. Coutanceau C, Stalder JF. Analysis of correlations between patient-oriented SCORAD (PO-SCORAD) and other assessment scores of atopic dermatitis severity and quality of life. Dermatology. 2014;229:248–55.
49. Maiello N, Galli E, Carello R, Fantò M. Lo skin care nel bambino con dermatite atopica. Immunologia e allergologia pediatrica 2019:3;598–605.
50. Elias PM. Primary role of barrier dysfunction in the pathogenesis of atopic dermatitis. Exp Dermatol. 2018;27:847–51.
51. Glatz M, Jo JH, Kennedy EA, Polley EC, Segre JA, Simpson EL,et al. Emollient use alters skin barrier and microbes in infants at risk for developing atopic dermatitis. PLoS One. 2018;13:e0192443.
52. Galli E, Neri I, Ricci G, Baldo E, Barone M, Belloni Fortina A,et al. Consensus conference on clinical management of pediatric atopic dermatitis. Italian J Pediatr. 2016;42:26.
53. Chiricozzi A, Belloni Fortina A, Galli E, Girolomoni G, Neri I, Ricci G, et al. Current therapeutic paradigm in pediatric atopic dermatitis: practical guidance from a national expert panel. Allergol Immunopathol. 2019;47:194–206.
54. Cury Martins J, Martins C, Aoki V, Gois AFT, Ishii HA, da Silva EMK. Topical tacrolimus for atopic dermatitis. Cochrane Database Syst Rev. 2015;2015:CD009864.
55. Lee SE, Choi Y, Kim SE, Noh EB, Kim SC. Differential effects of topical corticosteroid and calcineurin inhibitor on the epidermal tight junction. Exp Dermatol. 2013;22:59–61.
56. Reitamo S, Rissanen J, Remitz A, Granlund H, Erkko P, Elg P, et al. Tacrolimus ointment does not affect collagen synthesis: Results of a single-center randomized trial. J Invest Dermatol. 1998;111:396–8.
57. Rangel SM, Paller AS. Bacterial colonization, overgrowth, and superinfection in atopic dermatitis. Clin Dermatol. 2018;36:641–7.
58. Galli E, Fortina AB, Ricci G, Maiello N, Neri I, Baldo E, et al. Narrative review on the management of moderate-severe atopic dermatitis in pediatric age of the Italian Society of Pediatric Allergology and Immunology (SIAIP), of the Italian Society of Pediatric Dermatology (SIDerP) and of the Italian Society of Pediatr. Ital J Pediatr. 2022;48:95.
59. Yu SH, Drucker AM, Lebwohl M, Silverberg JI. A systematic review of the safety and efficacy of systemic corticosteroids in atopic dermatitis. J Am Acad Dermatol. 2018;78:733–40.
60. Drucker AM, Eyerich K, de Bruin-Weller MS, Thyssen JP, Spuls PI, Irvine AD, et al. Use of systemic corticosteroids for atopic dermatitis: International Eczema Council consensus statement. Br J Dermatol. 2018;178:768–75.
61. Wollenberg A, Christen-Zäch S, Taieb A, Paul C, Thyssen JP, de Bruin-Weller M, et al. ETFAD/EADV Eczema task force 2020 position paper on diagnosis and treatment of atopic dermatitis in adults and children. J Eur Acad Dermatol Venereol. 2020;34:2717–44.
62. Morita A, Krutmann J. Ultraviolet a radiation-induced apoptosis. Methods Enzymol. 2000;319:302–9.
63. Dotterud LK, Wilsgaard T, Vorland LH, Falk ES. The effect of UVB radiation on skin microbiota in patients with atopic dermatitis and healthy controls. Int J Circumpolar Health. 2008;67:254–60.
64. Becker D, Langer E, Seemann M, Seemann G, Fell I, Saloga J, et al. Clinical efficacy of blue light full body irradiation as treatment option for severe atopic dermatitis. PLoS One. 2011;6:e20566.
65. Lansang P, Bergman JN, Landells I, Ramien ML, Lansang P. Approach to the assessment and man-

agement of pediatric patients with atopic dermatitis: a consensus document. Section IV: consensus statements on the assessment and management of pediatric atopic dermatitis. J Cutan Med Surg. 2019;23(5_suppl):3S–11S.
66. Hernández-Martín A, Noguera-Morel L, Bernardino-Cuesta B, Torrelo A, Pérez-Martin MA, Aparicio-López C, et al. Cyclosporine A for severe atopic dermatitis in children. efficacy and safety in a retrospective study of 63 patients. J Eur Acad Dermatol Venereol. 2017;31:837–42.
67. Anderson K, Putterman E, Rogers RS, Patel D, Treat JR, Castelo-Soccio L. Treatment of severe pediatric atopic dermatitis with methotrexate: a retrospective review. Pediatr Dermatol. 2019;36:298–302.
68. Thaçi D, Simpson EL, Deleuran M, Kataoka Y, Chen Z, Gadkari A, et al. Efficacy and safety of dupilumab monotherapy in adults with moderate-to-severe atopic dermatitis: a pooled analysis of two phase 3 randomized trials (LIBERTY AD SOLO 1 and LIBERTY AD SOLO 2). J Dermatol Sci. 2019;94:266–75.
69. Thomson J, Wernham AGH, Williams HC. Long-term management of moderate-to-severe atopic dermatitis with dupilumab and concomitant topical corticosteroids (LIBERTY AD CHRONOS): a critical appraisal. Br J Dermatol. 2018;178:897–902.
70. Rohner MH, Thormann K, Cazzaniga S, Yousefi S, Simon HU, Schlapbach C, et al. Dupilumab reduces inflammation and restores the skin barrier in patients with atopic dermatitis. Allergy: Eur. J Allergy Clin Immunol. 2021;76:1268–70.
71. Simpson EL, Paller AS, Siegfried EC, Boguniewicz M, Sher L, Gooderham MJ, et al. Efficacy and safety of dupilumab in adolescents with uncontrolled moderate to severe atopic dermatitis: a phase 3 randomized clinical trial. JAMA Dermatol. 2020;156:44–56.
72. Paller AS, Siegfried EC, Thaçi D, Wollenberg A, Cork MJ, Arkwright PD, et al. Efficacy and safety of dupilumab with concomitant topical corticosteroids in children 6 to 11 years old with severe atopic dermatitis: a randomized, double-blinded, placebo-controlled phase 3 trial. J Am Acad Dermatol. 2020;84:230.
73. Paller AS, Simpson EL, Siegfried EC, Cork MJ, Wollenberg A, Arkwright PD, et al. Dupilumab in children aged 6 months to younger than 6 years with uncontrolled atopic dermatitis: a randomised, double-blind, placebo-controlled, phase 3 trial. Lancet. 2022;400:908–19.
74. Clark JD, Flanagan ME, Telliez JB. Discovery and development of Janus kinase (JAK) inhibitors for inflammatory diseases. J Med Chem. 2014;57:5023–38.
75. Leung DYM, Guttman-Yassky E. Deciphering the complexities of atopic dermatitis: Shifting paradigms in treatment approaches. J Allergy Clin Immunol. 2014;134:769–79.
76. Guttman-Yassky E, , Thaçi D, Pangan AL, Hong HC, Papp KA, Reich K, et al. Upadacitinib in adults with moderate to severe atopic dermatitis: 16-week results from a randomized, placebo-controlled trial. J Allergy Clin Immunol. 2020;145:877–84.
77. Guttman-Yassky E, Thyssen JP, Silverberg JI, Papp KA, Paller AS, Weidinger S, et al. Safety of upadacitinib in moderate-to-severe atopic dermatitis: an integrated analysis of phase 3 studies. J Allergy Clin Immunol. 2023;151:172–81.
78. https://www.ema.europa.eu/en/documents/product-information/rinvoq-epar-product-information_en.pdf.
79. https://www.accessdata.fda.gov/drugsatfda_docs/label/2019/211675s000lbl.pdf.
80. Guttman-Yassky E, Teixeira HD, Simpson EL, Papp KA, Pangan AL, Blauvelt A, et al. Once-daily upadacitinib versus placebo in adolescents and adults with moderate-to-severe atopic dermatitis (measure up 1 and measure up 2): results from two replicate double-blind, randomised controlled phase 3 trials. Lancet. 2021;397:2151–68.
81. Simpson EL, Papp KA, Blauvelt A, Chu CY, Hong HC, Katoh N,et al. Efficacy and Safety of upadacitinib in patients with moderate to severe atopic dermatitis: analysis of follow-up data from the measure up 1 and measure up 2 randomized clinical trials. JAMA Dermatol. 2022;158:404–13.
82. Reich K, Teixeira HD, de Bruin-Weller M, Bieber T, Soong W, Kabashima K, et al. Safety and efficacy of upadacitinib in combination with topical corticosteroids in adolescents and adults with moderate-to-severe atopic dermatitis (AD Up): results from a randomised, double-blind, placebo-controlled, phase 3 trial. Lancet. 2021;398:746.
83. Blauvelt A, , Teixeira HD, Simpson EL, Costanzo A, De Bruin-Weller M, Barbarot S, et al. Efficacy and safety of upadacitinib vs dupilumab in adults with moderate-to-severe atopic dermatitis: a randomized clinical trial. JAMA Dermatol. 2021;157:1047–55.

Allergic Conjunctivitis in Children

8

Cristiana Indolfi, Giulio Dinardo, Angela Klain, and Michele Miraglia del Giudice

Abstract

Allergic conjunctivitis (AC) is a common condition affecting both children and adults and that can significantly affect quality of life. The European Academy of Allergy and Clinical Immunology's Ocular Allergy group has revised the classification of allergic conjunctivitis to differentiate between two types of ocular surface hypersensitivity disorders: ocular allergy and ocular non-allergic hypersensitivity. The former can be IgE-mediated or non-IgE-mediated and includes seasonal allergic conjunctivitis, perennial allergic conjunctivitis, vernal keratoconjunctivitis and atopic keratoconjunctivitis. The latter is classified as non-allergic and includes various conditions like giant papillary conjunctivitis and irritative conjunctivitis. The diagnosis of AC is mainly clinical, with the presence of tearing, itching, redness and oedema indicating the condition. A slit-lamp examination is recommended to rule out corneal involvement and other types of conjunctivitis. Allergy tests, such as skin prick tests and serum-specific IgE determination, can help identify potential triggering agents. Environmental prevention is fundamental in reducing exposure to these agents. Non-specific treatments, such as cold compress and lacrimal substitutes, can alleviate symptoms, while drug therapy targets different phases of the allergic reaction.

Keywords

Ocular inflammatory pathologies · Allergic conjunctivitis · Children · Classification Aeroallergens · Vernal conjunctivitis · Atopic keratoconjunctivitis · Giant papillary conjunctivitis · Contact blepharoconjunctivitis

Test your learning and check your understanding of this book's contents: use the "Springer Nature Flashcards" app to access questions using ▶ https://sn.pub/nspbjm. To use the app, please follow the instructions in Chap. 1.

8.1 Introduction

Allergic conjunctivitis (AC) refers to a group of heterogeneous ocular inflammatory pathologies that affect the conjunctiva, eyelids and cornea [1]. AC is children's most common non-infectious conjunctivitis and shares pathophysiology similar to other allergic conditions. Numerous factors

C. Indolfi · G. Dinardo (✉) · A. Klain
M. Miraglia del Giudice
Department of Woman, Child and of General and Specialized Surgery, University of Campania Luigi Vanvitelli, Naples, Italy

C. Caffarelli, G. L. Marseglia (eds.), *Textbook of Pediatric Allergy*,
https://doi.org/10.1007/978-3-031-71283-8_8

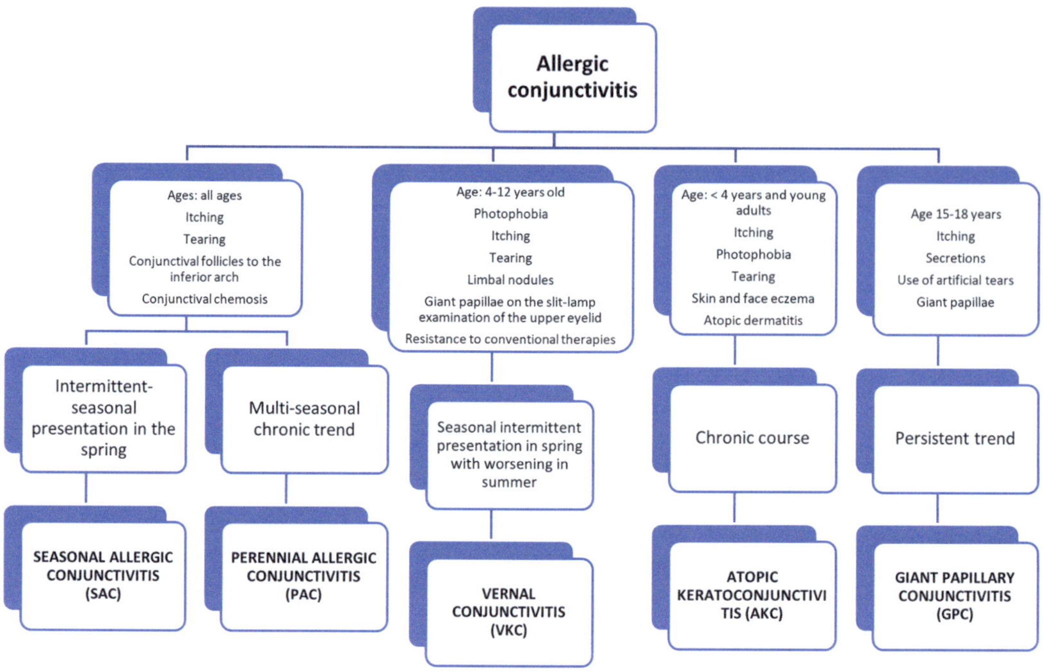

Fig. 8.1 Classification of allergic conjunctivitis in children and adolescents

are involved in the allergic ocular response: the main causes are represented by specific allergens in the air (e.g. pollen, mites, animal hair, chemical allergens and food allergens) and other factors that may contribute to amplifying the allergic reaction are non-specific factors (quality of the tear film, pollutants and dry cold air) [2]. AC is a very frequent condition, affecting about 30% of the general population [3], with a prevalence of up to 25% in children (Fig. 8.1) [4]. AC may coexist with other allergic diseases including allergic rhinitis (AR) (leading to a common disorder called rhinoconjunctivitis), asthma and atopic dermatitis [5]. Furthermore, AC negatively affects health-related quality of life (QOL) for children and their parents [6, 7].

8.2 Pathogenesis of Allergic Conjunctivitis

The main characteristics of allergic patients are the increased and persistent production of immunoglobulin E (IgEs), the preferential expansion of T helper 2 (Th2) lymphocytes and the facilitated release of pro-inflammatory mediators by mast cells and basophils [8]. AC develops since the eye is in direct contact with the outside environment, resulting in aeroallergens quickly melting in the tear film and provoking a type I immune reaction. The sensitization to an immunogenic substance is represented by the uptake of antigens by macrophages, dendritic cells or other cells belonging to the antigen-presenting cells (APC) system. These cells process the antigens and expose them on the surface in the form of peptides associated with class II histocompatibility molecules. Class II molecules bind allergenic peptides to form a stable complex that is recognized by specific T cell receptors. When an allergic person is exposed to an allergen, pro-inflammatory cytokines including IL-3, IL-4, IL-5 and IL-13 are released by Th2 cells and they may induce the release of immunoglobulin E (IgEs) by B cells. IgEs bind to the mast cell membrane and the subsequent cross-linking by their respective allergens triggers mast cell degranulation and the release of preformed mediators, including histamine, tryptase, leukotrienes and prostaglandins [9]. The preformed and newly produced mediators are directly responsible for vasodilation, vascular permeability and the onset of different symptoms, including redness, pruritus, chemosis, tearing and papillary response. This initial stage of an allergic reaction begins immediately after exposure to the allergens and lasts 20–30 min. The late phase of an allergic reaction begins a few hours later with the invasion of inflammatory cells, such as eosinophils, which release substances that exacerbate inflammation and draw in other immune cells, which feeds the cycle of inflammation [2]. AC can be triggered as a result of direct contact with antigens (airborne or topically applied substances), inhalation or ingestion, and it may be accompanied by symptoms of more severe allergic reactions. The most common symptoms have been listened below:

- Red, itchy eyes.
- Profuse watery discharge.
- Conjunctival oedema.

Children frequently wipe their eyes, which worsens the situation.

8.3 Classification

The European Academy of Allergy and Clinical Immunology's (EAACI) Ocular Allergy group has revised the classification of allergic conjunctivitis to distinguish between two types of ocular surface hypersensitivity disorders: ocular allergy or ocular non-allergic hypersensitivity. The first type can be caused by either IgE-mediated or non-IgE-mediated mechanisms. IgE-mediated ocular allergy encompasses seasonal allergic conjunctivitis (SAC), perennial allergic conjunctivitis (PAC), vernal keratoconjunctivitis (VKC) and atopic keratoconjunctivitis (AKC). On the other hand, non-IgE-mediated forms include contact blepharoconjunctivitis (CBC), VKC and AKC. The second type of eye hypersensitivity is classified as non-allergic and encompasses a variety of conditions, including giant papillary conjunctivitis (GPC), irritative conjunctivitis, irritative blepharitis and other mixed or borderline forms. Both IgE and non-IgE mediated pathways have been implicated in the pathogenesis of VKC and AKC. The most prevalent types of allergic conjunctivitis, its clinical manifestation and care, and potential future treatments are discussed in the sections that follow (Table 8.1) [2, 10].

8.3.1 Seasonal Allergic Conjunctivitis (SAC)

Seasonal allergic conjunctivitis (SAC), called hay fever conjunctivitis as well, is the most prevalent form of allergic conjunctivitis, accounting for more than half of all cases (Fig. 8.2). As suggested by its name, SAC is characterized by seasonal symptoms related to specific aeroallergens. SAC is an IgE-mediated allergic reaction, often accompanied by rhinitis, which is more prevalent in the spring and fall when pollen levels are high. The most characteristic symptom is sporadic itching, but redness of the conjunctiva, eyelid swelling, tearing and small papillary hypertrophy of the tarsal conjunctiva are also common but non-specific signs. Symptoms are frequently bilateral but not necessarily symmetric in terms of degree of involvement and come and go depending on the patient's exposure to the allergen(s). A precise medical history, followed by allergy testing, can identify specific sensitization [2, 10].

Key Point Box

Seasonal allergic conjunctivitis (SAC) is the most prevalent form of allergic conjunctivitis.

8.3.2 Perennial Allergic Conjunctivitis (PAC)

Perennial allergic conjunctivitis (PAC) is an IgE-mediated reaction to allergens present throughout the year. PAC is usually caused by indoor airborne antigens, such as dust mites, animal dander,

Table 8.1 Characteristics of the allergic conjunctivitis

	Mediating process	Timeframe of manifestation	Background	Signs	Clinical manifestations
Seasonal allergic conjunctivitis (SAC)	Pollen IgE-mediated	Seasonal recurrence	Atopic Children/adults	Conjunctival hyperemia	Intense itching, redness of the conjunctiva, watery discharge
Perennial allergic conjunctivitis (PAC)	Dust mites, animal dander IgE-mediated	Perennial with seasonal recurrence	Atopic Children/adults	Conjunctival hyperemia	Intense itching, redness of the conjunctiva, watery discharge
Vernal keratoconjunctivitis (VKC)	IgE- and non-IgE-mediated	Typically seen in spring/summer, may persist year-round in warmer regions	School-aged or prepubertal children ± atopic Male > Female	Severe photophobia Giant papillae Horner-Trantas dots	Intense itching, photophobia Cobblestone-like appearance of superior tarsal conjunctiva or limbal with Horner-Trantas dots
Atopic keratoconjunctivitis (AKC)	IgE- and non-IgE-mediated	Long-term condition with periodic flare-ups	Adult (30–50 years) atopic	Atopic dermatitis Punctate keratitis Hertoghe's sign	Eyelid eczema, Dennie-Morgan lines, Hertoghe's sign, intense itching
Giant papillary conjunctivitis (GPC)	Non-allergic	Removing the precipitating factor resolves the symptoms	Contact lenses, postoperative sutures, ocular prostheses	Use of contact lenses	Tarsal conjunctiva with giant papillae. Itching, sensation of a foreign object in the eye

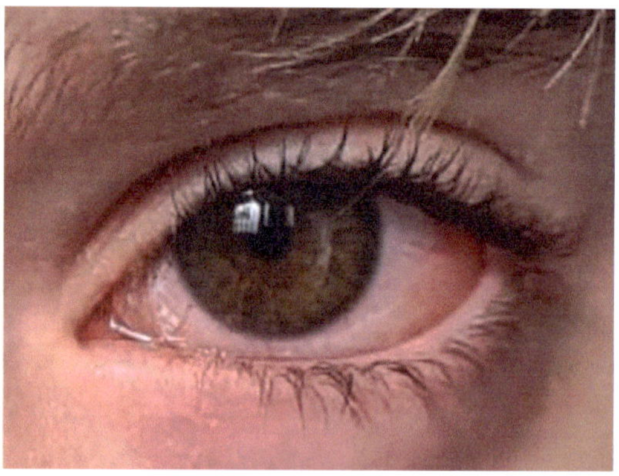

Fig. 8.2 Allergic conjunctivitis

moulds or due to multiple sensitizations. PAC is characterized by the same signs and symptoms as SAC, but it is a chronic condition with persistent, frequently mild symptoms, aggravated by prolonged exposure to allergens and exacerbated by non-specific irritating factors. Although neither SAC nor PAC alters the cornea, they have a large socioeconomic impact and have a considerable influence on the patient's quality of life [2, 10, 11].

8.3.3 Vernal Keratoconjunctivitis (VKC)

Vernal keratoconjunctivitis (VKC) is a persistent and severe form of ocular allergy that usually affects children and young adults in tropical or mild/warm climates [12]. It is a bilateral chronic inflammatory disorder that typically involves the upper tarsal or limbal conjunctiva (Fig. 8.3).

VKC typically affects boys between 4 and 12 years of age (male-to-female ratio, 3:1) and often resolves after puberty. There are between 1.2 and 10.6 incidences per 10,000 people in Europe [13]. Type 1 (IgE-dependent) and type (IgE-independent) immunological pathogenic pathways are responsible for causing VKC [14].

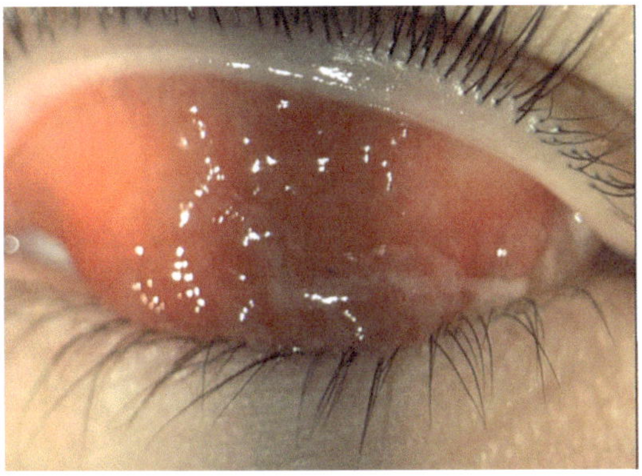

Fig. 8.3 Vernal keratoconjunctivitis (*Courtesy F. Mori*)

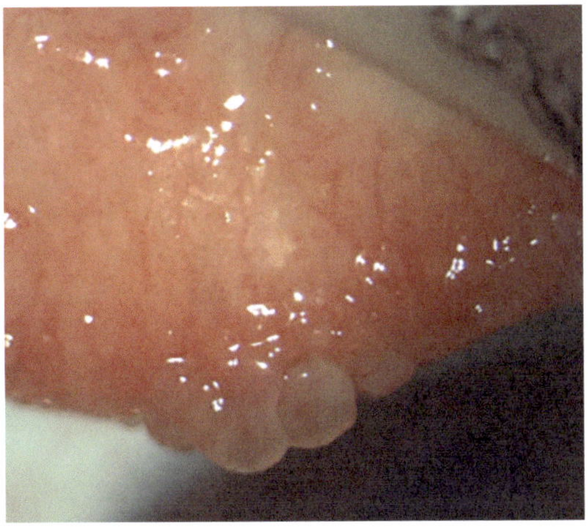

Fig. 8.4 Vernal keratoconjunctivitis cobblestone-like hypertrophic papillae (*Courtesy F. Mori*)

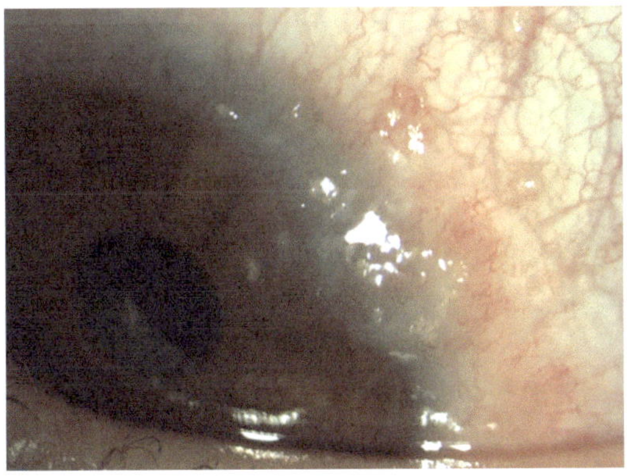

Fig. 8.5 Vernal keratoconjunctivitis limbal form (*Courtesy F. Mori*)

The IgE-mediated mechanism explains only 50% of patients' severity and clinical course of the disease, which is related to T-cell-mediated responses, eosinophil infiltration, activation and non-specific hyper-reactivity. The increased number of activated CD4+ T lymphocytes and typical Th2 cells found in patients with VKC point to a type 4 hypersensitivity reaction [15]. Typical symptoms of VKC include intense itching, tearing and photophobia. Disease exacerbation can be triggered by allergen re-exposure or more frequently by non-specific stimuli, such as sunlight, wind and dust [2]. Vernal keratoconjunctivitis (VKC) can manifest in two forms: the tarsal form and the limbal form. The tarsal form is more common in Western countries, in this type there are irregularly sized hypertrophic papillae (>1 mm) that give the tarsal surface a "cobblestone-like" appearance surrounded by mucus strings/goblets (Fig. 8.4). Asymmetric tarsal involvement is common.

The limbal form is more common in subtropical countries, in this type there are transient, multiple limbal or conjunctival gelatinous yellow-grey infiltrates, accompanied by white points or deposits known as Horner-Trantas dots (representing degenerating eosinophils and epithelial cell debris) and thickened and opacified limbal papillae that may appear for 360° (Fig. 8.5). The presence of punctate keratitis, epithelial macroerosions, ulcers and plaques are indicative of corneal involvement, which may result in varying degrees of scarring even after resolution [2, 10, 11].

Key Point Box

Vernal keratoconjunctivitis (VKC) is a bilateral chronic inflammatory disorder that typically involves the upper tarsal or limbal conjunctiva.

8.3.4 Atopic Keratoconjunctivitis (AKC)

Atopic keratoconjunctivitis (AKC) is a persistent inflammatory, bilateral condition that involves the eyelids, conjunctiva and possibly the cornea, and can be defined as the ocular manifestation of atopic dermatitis. AKC is more common in males with a peak of prevalence in patients between the ages of 30 and 50 with a personal or family history of atopic disorders. AKC affects 25–42% of people with atopic dermatitis and often begins in young people and persists until the fifth decade of life [2].

Pathogenesis is mediated by IgE-, Th2- and Th1-mediated pathways. Typical AKC manifestations can occur in patients without definitive skin involvement. The main sign of patients with AKC is an eczematous lesion of the eyelid that has a tendency to thicken, indurate and fissure [10].

Eyelid eczema can cause a range of symptoms including hyperpigmentation of the eyelids (known as panda eyes), oedema that causes horizontal creases of the eyelids (Dennie-Morgan lines) and the absence of the lateral end of the eyebrows (known as Hertoghe's sign). The inferior fornix and palpebral conjunctiva are the predominant sites of conjunctival redness and chemosis and sometimes even Horner-Trantas dots in the limbus, especially in more acute phases. The involvement of the cornea can range from superficial punctate keratitis to corneal ulcers, corneal scarring and pannus, and it tends to follow the involvement of the conjunctiva and palpebra. Patients with AKC complain of severe itching most of the year, which is usually more severe during the winter months and in colder climates [2]. AKC may be associated with *Staphylococcus aureus* colonization of the eyelid and meibomian gland dysfunction. Similar to VKC, the limbus and cornea can be involved [10].

Key Point Box

Atopic keratoconjunctivitis (AKC) is a persistent inflammatory, bilateral condition that involves the eyelids, conjunctiva and possibly the cornea, and can be defined as the ocular manifestation of atopic dermatitis.

8.3.5 Giant Papillary Conjunctivitis (GPC)

Giant papillary conjunctivitis (GPC) is a form of hypersensitivity-induced inflammation of the tarsal conjunctiva caused by non-allergic hypersensitivity. The aetiology and pathology of large papillary conjunctivitis are not thoroughly known. Its occurrence is often linked to the use of contact lenses, especially soft lenses, as well as ocular prostheses, postoperative sutures and scleral buckles [10].

GPC is characterized by the infiltration of various types of immune cells, such as basophils, eosinophils, plasma cells and lymphocytes. According to clinical data, it could be caused by a combination of mechanical damage and hypersensitivity to antigenic proteins that were left on the surface of the prosthesis, sutures or contact lens. Although GPC may be asymptomatic in its early stages, slit lamp examination can reveal initial signs.

The symptoms of GPC typically include itching, a sensation of a foreign object in the eye, discharge that may be watery or mucous, slight redness of the conjunctiva and the formation of papillary reactions on the upper tarsal conjunctiva. Patients may also experience Trantas' dots, limbal infiltration, and bulbar conjunctival hyperemia and oedema. Additionally, soft contact lens wearers have a higher chance (around 5–10%) of developing upper tarsal papillary hypertrophy, which is characterized by a cobblestone-like appearance, while this occurs in 3–4% of hard contact lens wearers [11]. The treatment consists mostly on removing the lenses or any mechanical cause and administering local anti-inflammatory medicines; the prognosis is favourable.

8.3.6 Contact Blepharoconjunctivitis (CBC)

Contact blepharoconjunctivitis (CBC) refers to an allergic or irritant response that occurs when various substances come into contact with either the skin of the eyelid or the conjunctival sac. The patients develop an inflammation of the palpebral skin and conjunctiva. The most noticeable symptoms of CBC include itchiness and a burning sensation in the eyelids. The condition is typically identified by the presence of swelling, redness of the eyelid skin, eczema, redness of the conjunctiva and the formation of papillae [2, 10].

8.4 Diagnosis

The diagnosis of AC is basically clinical. In the presence of tearing, itching, redness and oedema, the diagnosis is straightforward. It is recommended to perform a slit-lamp examination when conjunctivitis is isolated to make sure the cornea is unaffected and there are no giant papillae on the tarsal conjunctiva, superficial punctate keratitis, vernal ulcers or plaques. Allergy tests (skin prick test, serum-specific IgE determination and conjunctival provocation test) can help in the aetiological diagnosis for identifying possible triggering agents. Consultation with an allergy specialist is important to allow the guidance of environmental hygiene, a part of the treatment and for the management of other types of allergic conditions, such as AR [16, 17]. The ophthalmologist is in charge of making the ultimate determination about any other types of ACs besides SAC and PAC.

8.5 Treatment

In every allergic patient, the first therapeutic intervention is to reduce environmental exposure to triggering factors. Environmental prevention is fundamental, both in the forms of SAC in which the patient must be instructed to keep away as much as possible from contact with pollen, and in PACs where it is essential to perform remediation of one's home to reduce the levels of dust mites and animal hair [2].

Key Point Box

In the treatment of allergic conjunctivitis, the first therapeutic intervention is to reduce environmental exposure to triggering factors.

Non-specific treatments, including the use of a cold compress and lacrimal substitutes, are useful to alleviate symptoms. Drug therapy is instead aimed at intervening in the different phases of the allergic reaction (Fig. 8.6). The main treatments in AC in children are represented by

- Local antihistamines and mast cell stabilizers.
- Local steroids.
- Oral antihistamines (in case of multiple allergies).
  - Pharmacologic treatment of AC involves the use of topic dual-activity agents (antihistamines and mast cell stabilizers), such as ketotifen and opalatadine, which may be sufficient for mild cases [18]. These molecules are non-competitive and selective antagonists of histamine H1 receptors, but they also act as a membrane stabilizer at the mast cell level. Compared with either topical antihistamines (such as levocabastine, pheniramine maleate and azelastine) or mast cell stabilizers (nedocromil sodium, lodoxamide and pemirolast), topical dual-activity agents are generally clinically superior due to both symptom/sign relief and tolerability [19]. These drugs are now considered first-line treatment in AC and they are free of side effects. These are used to ameliorate symptoms but may be augmented by other treatments (e.g. local steroids) when the signs are also significant or if the presentation is more than just mild.
  - Oral antihistamines, such as fexofenadine, cetirizine or hydroxyzine, can be very helpful, especially if other areas of the body (e.g. ears, nose and throat) are affected by allergies. Due to their anticholinergic effects and capacity to pass the blood–brain barrier, oral first-generation antihistamines should be avoided [20]. Antihistamines of the second generation are recommended over those of the first generation because they have a lower tendency to pass the blood–brain barrier and have fewer anticholinergic side effects [21]. In the presence of conjunctivitis alone, it is recommended to use topical antihistamines because of their faster onset of action (3–15 min) and a bet-

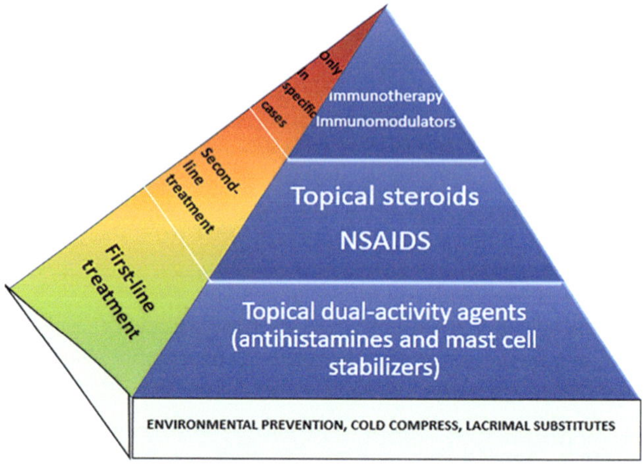

Fig. 8.6 Allergic conjunctivitis treatment algorithm (Adaptation from Dupuis 2020) [7]

ter safety profile due to less systemic absorption than oral antihistamines since they directly target the ocular tissues [22].

- Corticosteroid-based eye drops have more powerful anti-inflammatory effects. However, they should be used for short-term treatment (5–7 days), and carefully monitored by an ophthalmologist because they could cause an increase in intraocular pressure (glaucoma), cataracts and an increased risk of eye infections [23].
- Topical non-steroidal anti-inflammatory medications are rarely used due to their inconsistent tolerance. Topical NSAIDs are generally used short-term, as an add-on to a topical antihistamine or dual-action agent [17]. Systemic anti-inflammatory medications are administered only in rare instances and in certain circumstances.
- In situations with SAC or PAC where symptomatic treatment is insufficient to guarantee a good quality of life, the allergist may recommend allergen immunotherapy, particularly when the involvement of a specific allergen has been explicitly documented. Either sublingual immunotherapy (SLIT) or subcutaneous immunotherapy (SCIT) improves clinically and immunologically ocular symptoms [24, 25].
- Topical immunosuppressants can be used in those with chronic cell-mediated inflammation such as VKC and AKC. In severe forms, cyclosporine concentrated at 1–2% in eye drops is prescribed in cases of keratoconjunctivitis as a steroid-sparing treatment. [26] Also, the use of tacrolimus ointment is under study in children refractory to conventional treatment of vernal keratoconjunctivitis [27].
- Biological drugs against IgE, IL-5, IL-4 and IL-13 have dramatically improved recent treatment outcomes in allergic diseases including asthma, rhinitis and atopic dermatitis. However, these drugs have not been approved for ocular allergic diseases, also because various adverse ocular symptoms have been observed in clinical trials [28].

Take-Home Messages

- AC is a common condition that affects up to 25% of children. It often occurs in association with other allergic diseases such as rhinitis, asthma or atopic dermatitis.
- The most prevalent type of AC in children is the seasonal form.
- The most common symptoms are tearing, itching, redness and oedema.
- The diagnosis of AC is primarily clinical, based on personal detailed history and ocular examination. It is important to perform a slit-lamp examination to rule out corneal involvement and an allergy test to identify the responsible causative agents.

(continued)

- The differential diagnosis must be placed by comparing other less common conditions such as vernal keratoconjunctivitis (VKC), atopic keratoconjunctivitis (AKC), contact blepharoconjunctivitis (CBC) and giant papillary conjunctivitis (GPC).
- The first preventive and therapeutic approach is based on the avoidance of the causative agent.
- Drug treatments include the use of topical dual-activity agents (antihistamines and mast cell stabilizers), oral antihistamines, topical corticosteroids, topical non-steroidal anti-inflammatory drugs, immunotherapy and immunomodulators for cell-mediated AC. Other treatments such as biological drugs are being investigated to assess their safety and therapeutic effects in both adults and children.

References

1. Abelson MB, Shetty S, Korchak M, Butrus SI, Smith LM. Advances in pharmacotherapy for allergic conjunctivitis. Expert Opin Pharmacother. 2015;16:1219–31.
2. Villegas BV, Benitez-Del-castillo JM. Current knowledge in allergic conjunctivitis. Turkish J Ophthalmol. 2021;51:45–54.
3. Kausar A, Akhtar N, Akbar N. Epidemiological aspects of allergic conjunctivitis. J Ayub Med Coll Abbottabad. 2022;34:135–40.
4. Fauquert JL. Diagnosing and managing allergic conjunctivitis in childhood: the allergist's perspective. Pediatr Allergy Immunol. 2019;30:405–14.
5. Chong-Neto HJ, Rosario C, Leonardi A, Filho NAR. Ocular allergy in children and adolescents. Allergol Immunopathol (Madr). 2022;50:30–6.
6. Zhang SY, Li J, Liu R, Lao HY, Fan Z, Jin L, Liang L, Liu Y. Association of allergic conjunctivitis with health-related quality of life in children and their parents. JAMA Ophthalmol. 2021;139:830–7.
7. Del Giudice MM, Marseglia A, Leonardi S, La Rosa M, Salpietro C, Brunese FP, et al. Allergic rhinitis and quality of life in children. Int J Immunopathol Pharmacol. 2011;24:25–8.
8. Del Giudice MM, Allegorico A, Marseglia GL, Martelli A, Calvani M, Cardinale F, et al. Allergic rhinoconjunctivitis. Acta Biomed. 2020;91:1–3.
9. Dupuis P, Prokopich CL, Hynes A, Kim H. A contemporary look at allergic conjunctivitis. Allergy Asthma Clin Immunol. 2020;516:5.
10. Leonardi A, Bogacka E, Fauquert JL, Kowalski ML, Groblewska A, Jedrzejczak-Czechowicz M, et al. Ocular allergy: recognizing and diagnosing hypersensitivity disorders of the ocular surface. Allergy. 2012;67:1327–37.
11. Bielory L. Allergic and immunologic disorders of the eye. Part II: ocular allergy. J Allergy Clin Immunol. 2000;106:1019–32.
12. Ghiglioni DG, Zicari AM, Parisi GF, Marchese G, Indolfi C, Diaferio L, et al. Vernal keratoconjunctivitis: an update. Eur J Ophthalmol. 2021;31:2828–42.
13. La Rosa M, Lionetti E, Reibaldi M, Russo A, Longo A, Leonardi S, et al. Allergic conjunctivitis: a comprehensive review of the literature. Ital J Pediatr. 2013;39:18.
14. Brindisi G, Cinicola B, Anania C, De Castro G, Nebbioso M, Miraglia Del Giudice M, et al. Vernal keratoconjunctivitis: state of art and update on treatment. Acta Biomed. 2021;92:e2021517.
15. Addis H, Jeng BH. Vernal keratoconjunctivitis. Clin Ophthalmol. 2018;12:119–23.
16. Vazirani J, Shukla S, Chhawchharia R, Sahu S, Gokhale N, Basu S. Allergic conjunctivitis in children: current understanding and future perspectives. Curr Opin Allergy Clin Immunol. 2020;20:507–15.
17. Fauquert JL, Jedrzejczak-Czechowicz M, Rondon C, Calder V, Silva D, Kvenshagen BK, et al. Conjunctival allergen provocation test: guidelines for daily practice. Allergy. 2017;72:43–54.
18. Ben-Eli H, Solomon A. Topical antihistamines, mast cell stabilizers, and dual-action agents in ocular allergy: current trends. Curr Opin Allergy Clin Immunol. 2018;18:411–6.
19. Leonardi A, Silva D, Perez Formigo D, Bozkurt B, Sharma V, Allegri P, et al. Management of ocular allergy. Allergy. 2019;74:1611–30.
20. Corsico AG, Leonardi S, Licari A, Marseglia G, Miraglia Del Giudice M, Peroni DG, et al. Focus on the cetirizine use in clinical practice: a reappraisal 30 years later. Multidiscip Respir Med. 2019;14:40.
21. Parisi GF, Leonardi S, Ciprandi G, Corsico A, Licari A, Miraglia del Giudice M, et al. Antihistamines in children and adolescents: a practical update. Allergol Immunopathol (Madr). 2020;48:753–62.
22. Simons FER, Simons KJ. Histamine and H1-antihistamines: celebrating a century of progress. J Allergy Clin Immunol. 2011;128;1139–1150.
23. Iordache A, Boruga M, Mușat O, Jipa DA, Tătaru CP, Mușat GC. Relationship between allergic rhinitis and allergic conjunctivitis (allergic rhinoconjunctivitis)—review. Rom J Ophthalmol. 2022;66:8–12.

24. Calderon MA, Penagos M, Sheikh A, Canonica GW, Durham SR. Sublingual immunotherapy for allergic conjunctivitis: cochrane systematic review and meta-analysis. Clin Exp Allergy. 2011;41:1263–72.
25. Del Giudice MM, Licari A, Brambilla I, Tosca MA, Ciprandi G. Allergen immunotherapy in pediatric asthma: a pragmatic point of view. Children (Basel). 2020;7:58.
26. Leonardi A. Management of vernal keratoconjunctivitis. Ophthalmol Ther. 2013;2:73–88.
27. Fiorentini SF, Khurram D. Therapeutic effects of topical 0.03% Tacrolimus ointment in children with refractory vernal keratoconjunctivitis in Middle East. Saudi J Ophthalmol. 2019;33:117.
28. Fukuda K, Kishimoto T, Sumi T, Yamashiro K, Ebihara N. Biologics for allergy: therapeutic potential for ocular allergic diseases and adverse effects on the eye. Allergol Int. 2023;72:234–44.

9 Allergic Rhinitis in the Child

Anna Maria Zicari, Giulia Brindisi, Alessandra Gori, and Marzia Duse

Abstract

Allergic rhinitis (AR) is a widespread respiratory condition in children characterized by nasal inflammation triggered by exposure to allergens. It has a global prevalence and is often associated with other atopic diseases. Genetic factors influence the development of AR. It involves a complex immune response that produces allergen-specific IgE antibodies, resulting in the inflammation and activation of immune cells.

Children with AR experienced nasal symptoms such as sneezing, itching, congestion, and rhinorrhea. These symptoms can significantly impact their daily activities, sleep, and cognitive function. Additionally, AR may manifest with extra-nasal symptoms, including itchy or watery eyes, allergic conjunctivitis, and dark circles under the eyes.

Diagnosing AR in children involves a thorough medical history, physical examination, skin prick tests, and allergen-specific IgE testing that can identify the specific allergens causing the allergic reaction. Objective measures such as rhinomanometry, nasal nitric oxide measurement, nasal eosinophilia, and nasal provocation tests may be used in specific cases to provide further diagnostic information. The management of AR in children focuses on three main approaches: allergen avoidance, pharmacotherapy, and allergen immunotherapy. Strategies to minimize exposure to allergens are essential in reducing symptoms. Pharmacotherapy options include intranasal corticosteroids, oral antihistamines, nasal antihistamines, and leukotriene receptor antagonists. In severe cases, short-term systemic corticosteroids may be prescribed. Allergen immunotherapy, administered through injections or sublingual tablets, can help desensitize children to specific allergens and provide long-term relief. Early recognition, accurate diagnosis, and appropriate management are crucial for effectively managing AR in children, improving their quality of life, and preventing complications. By combining allergen avoidance, pharmacotherapy, and immunotherapy, healthcare professionals can successfully control AR symptoms in children.

Keywords

Allergic rhinitis · Atopy · Asthma
Antihistamines · Intranasal corticosteroids
Allergen immunotherapy · Environmental control measures · Quality of Life
Component-resolved diagnosis · Allergic conjunctivitis · Persistent · Intermittent

A. M. Zicari (✉) · G. Brindisi · A. Gori · M. Duse
Department of Mother and Child and Urological Sciences, La Sapienza University, Rome, Italy
e-mail: annamaria.zicari@uniroma1.it; marzia.duse@fondazione.uniroma1.it

C. Caffarelli, G. L. Marseglia (eds.), *Textbook of Pediatric Allergy*,
https://doi.org/10.1007/978-3-031-71283-8_9

Test your learning and check your understanding of this book's contents: use the "Springer Nature Flashcards" app to access questions using ▶ https://sn.pub/nspbjm. To use the app, please follow the instructions in Chap. 1.

Key Points

- **Definition**: Allergic rhinitis is an inflammatory condition of the nasal passages triggered by exposure to allergens such as pollen, dust mites, pet dander, or mold spores. Intermittent AR is characterized by symptoms for <4 days per week or <4 consecutive weeks. Persistent AR is characterized by symptoms occurring more than 4 days per week for at least four consecutive weeks.
- **Prevalence**: Allergic rhinitis is a common condition, especially in children, affecting up to 40% of the pediatric population.
- **Symptoms**: Common symptoms include sneezing, runny nose, nasal congestion, itching of the nose or eyes, and watery eyes. These symptoms may be intermittent or persist year-round and stratified into mild and moderate–severe.
- **Risk Factors**: Various factors contribute to developing allergic rhinitis in children. Genetic predisposition, air pollution, tobacco smoke exposure, and early exposure to inhalant and food allergens are the mains called into question.
- **Pathogenesis**: **Nasal epithelial cells respond to environmental allergens by producing alarmins such as IL-25, IL-33, and thymic stromal lymphopoietin**. Alarmins activate dendritic cells, T cells, and type 2 innate lymphoid cells crucial in Th2-related diseases like AR. Th2 cells release cytokines like IL-4, IL-5, and IL-13, which activate B cells and initiate IgE production. Plasma cells produce specific IgE antibodies, which bind to FcεRI receptors on mast cells and basophils. Crosslinking of IgE on these cells leads to degranulation and the release of inflammatory mediators, causing the symptoms of AR.
- **Diagnosis**: Diagnosis is typically based on the child's medical history, symptoms, and physical examination. Skin prick tests or specific IgE sampling are the first level of allergological investigation. Component-Resolved Diagnosis may be performed to identify specific allergens causing the symptoms. Functional respiratory tests provide information about the degree of inflammation and nasal obstruction.
- **Impact on Quality of Life**: Allergic rhinitis can significantly affect a child's quality of life, leading to impaired sleep, reduced concentration at school, and decreased participation in physical activities.
- **Comorbidities**: Allergic rhinitis is associated with an increased risk of developing other allergic conditions, such as conjunctivitis and asthma. It is essential to monitor and manage these comorbidities simultaneously.
- **Treatment Options**: Management of allergic rhinitis involves symptomatic therapy, including allergen avoidance and pharmacotherapy. Treatment options include antihistamines, intranasal corticosteroids, nasal decongestants (short-term use), and allergen immunotherapy, the only disease-modifying treatment able to change the allergic rhinitis natural history.
- **Long-Term Outlook**: Allergic rhinitis may be a chronic condition. Effective management can help control symp-

(continued)

toms, improve quality of life, and minimize the risk of complications. Parents and caregivers must work closely with healthcare professionals to develop an individualized treatment plan that addresses the child's specific needs and aims to provide optimal symptom control and relief.

9.1 Introduction

Certain conditions can profoundly impact a child's well-being and development in pediatric health. Among these, allergic rhinitis (AR) stands as a prevalent and often underestimated respiratory disorder that affects a significant number of children worldwide. As we delve into this focus chapter, we will shine a light on the intricate nuances of allergic rhinitis in children, revealing its far-reaching implications and exploring avenues for improved understanding and management.

Picture a vibrant playground filled with the laughter and joyous energy of children at play. Nevertheless, for some, this idyllic scene is marred by incessant typical symptoms like sneezing, itchy eyes, and nasal congestion. Allergic rhinitis, a condition often dismissed as mere seasonal discomfort, may transform this youthful exuberance into a struggle against persistent symptoms that can cast a shadow on a child's daily life.

Traditionally, AR was considered a nasal airway disease. However, the unified airway theory now views it as part of a systemic allergic response. Conditions like asthma and atopic dermatitis share a common underlying pathology. AR is classically categorized as seasonal or perennial. However, that is changing because some cases exhibit both. Alongside nasal symptoms, patients may experience allergic conjunctivitis, nonproductive cough, Eustachian tube dysfunction, and chronic sinusitis [1].

In this chapter, we embark on a journey to uncover the unique dimensions of allergic rhinitis in children, recognizing its prevalence and shedding light on its significant impact on their physical health, emotional well-being, academic performance, and overall quality of life. We will navigate the intricate web of risk factors contributing to its development, explore the intersection between allergic rhinitis and other allergic conditions, and delve into the challenges children and their families face as they grapple with this often-misunderstood respiratory ailment.

Moreover, we shall examine the crucial role of early intervention and effective management strategies in alleviating the burden of allergic rhinitis in children. From exploring the potential of allergen avoidance to the use of pharmacological interventions tailored for pediatric patients, we will venture into the realm of prevention and treatment, seeking to empower healthcare professionals with the knowledge and facilities to improve the quality of life for these young individuals.

As we embark on this chapter, let us recognize the immense importance of revealing the complexity surrounding allergic rhinitis pathogenesis in children. By deepening our understanding of this condition, we can pave the way for early identification, timely intervention, and care, ensuring that every child can revel in the joys of childhood unencumbered by the burdensome symptoms of allergic rhinitis.

9.2 Definition

Allergic rhinitis (AR) is a type 1 hypersensitivity response mediated by immunoglobulin E (IgE) in the nasal mucosa [2]. It occurs when a sensitized individual is exposed to allergens, leading to characteristic clinical manifestations, including anterior and posterior rhinorrhea, nasal congestion, itching, and sneezing. AR is highly prevalent and can have substantial physical consequences and persistent symptoms [3]. Furthermore, its close association with asthma supports the unified airway theory, which suggests that upper and lower airway inflammation share underlying pathophysiological mechanisms [4]. It is important to note that the definition of

AR can vary among published studies, with some considering it a sensitization to allergens. AR is rare in infants and typically emerges in school-age children. Due to the gradual development of sensitization, it is unlikely to manifest before age 2. This timing is likely due to the rapid evolution of the immune system during early childhood [5]. AR often arises from an exaggerated response of T helper (Th)-2 lymphocytes and the initiation of a systemic IgE-driven reaction, which can dominate a child's immune system until it reaches full maturity. Therefore, a more detailed clarification is required. Atopic diseases encompass a variety of interconnected conditions that manifest as diverse clinical phenotypes, varying from involving single organs to multi-system disorders [6]. Indeed, although patients with allergic diseases, including AR, are sensitized by default, not all patients with allergic sensitization may show symptoms of allergic disease. In addition, sensitization may not correlate with the severity of AR [7–10]. On the other side, other patients may suffer from an entire range of symptoms associated with multi-morbidity [11]. Against that background, improved methods to assess sensitization, distinguishing clinically significant, and using established diagnostic measures can enhance the precision of diagnostic correctness and the ability to anticipate symptom persistence. Presently, component-resolved diagnostics (CRD), as we will explore subsequently, stands as the most precise means of verifying clinical allergy and might provide insights into the mechanisms underlying the occurrence and severity of allergic respiratory conditions [12].

Thus, in general, exposure to allergens may prompt allergen-specific IgE (sIgE) production in the atopic individual. Subsequent exposure triggers both early and late-stage reactions, leading to the clinical manifestations of AR. The early-stage reaction typically occurs minutes after the sensitized allergen's re-introduction, producing a rapid onset of nasal itching, congestion, and rhinorrhea. The late-stage reaction often occurs during the 4- to 8-h period after allergen re-introduction and results in congestion, hyposmia, increased anterior and posterior rhinorrhea, and nasal hyper-responsiveness [1]. The proposals outlined by Allergic Rhinitis and its Impact on Asthma (ARIA) have classified allergic rhinitis (AR) based on its presumed cause and the timing of its occurrence. Traditionally, AR has been divided into two categories: seasonal, also known as hay fever, and perennial. Seasonal AR is typically associated with outdoor allergens, such as pollen, and tends to occur during periods of high pollen counts. On the other hand, perennial AR is linked to indoor allergens like house dust mites (HDM), insects, and animal dander and is generally present throughout the year [13]. It is important to note that the classification of seasonal versus perennial AR can sometimes be complex. For instance, seasonal AR might persist for longer durations due to the effects of climate change, leading to prolonged periods of elevated pollen counts. Seasonal AR might also extend across multiple seasons due to polysensitization. Similarly, manifestations of perennial allergy may not be constant throughout the entire year. This is especially applicable to individuals allergic to HDM, who might exhibit mild or intermittent moderate/severe AR. Air pollution can also influence variations in allergen sensitivity, resulting in fluctuations in symptom severity based on location and air quality [6]. Considering these complexities, ARIA introduced an alternative classification based on the duration and persistence of symptoms. Intermittent AR involves symptoms occurring for <4 days per week or lasting for <4 consecutive weeks. Persistent AR entails symptoms happening more than 4 days per week and persisting for at least four consecutive weeks. Importantly, the prior categories of seasonal and perennial AR do not align with the new classification of intermittent/persistent AR, as they represent distinct levels of disease stratification. Therefore, intermittent and persistent AR are not interchangeable with seasonal and perennial classifications. Additionally, ARIA's guidelines suggest a severity classification (mild and moderate-severe) based on the impact of these symptoms (Fig. 9.1). AR can lead to problematic symptoms such as disrupted sleep, limitations in daily activities, leisure or sports engagement, hindered school or work performance, or troublesome symptoms. AR is categorized as mild if

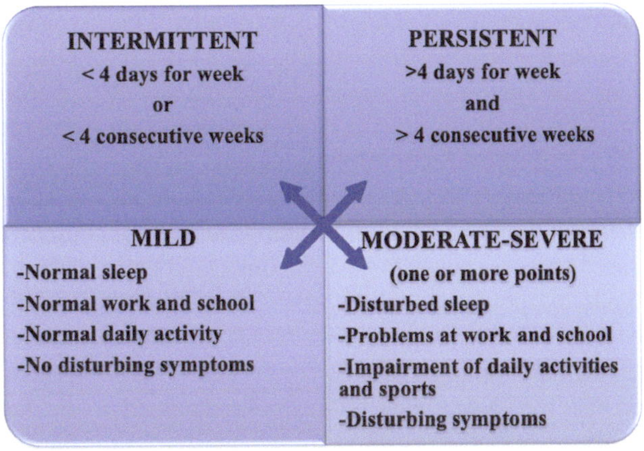

Fig. 9.1 ARIA classification of allergic rhinitis according to the duration of its symptoms, intermittent or persistent, or, according to the severity of the symptoms, mild or moderate–severe (adapted from Allergo J Int 2019; 28: 255–276)

none of these consequences occur. Conversely, it is classified as moderate–severe if one or more of these symptoms are present [14, 15].

9.3 Epidemiology

The epidemiology of allergic rhinitis in children is a topic of significant concern and interest for recognizing its prevalence, risk factors, and potential preventive measures to alleviate its burden due to its substantial impact on the pediatric population.

Epidemiological studies have consistently shown that AR is rising among children, and approximately 10–20% of children globally experience it. The prevalence rates tend to vary depending on geographic location, with higher rates observed in urban areas and developed countries due to increased exposure to allergens, changes in lifestyle factors, and environmental influences [2, 16].

In more detail, the prevalence of AR has increased globally, and in adults it varies widely across studies, with an approximate range of 5–50%. Certainly, also different diagnostic criteria and definitions of AR contribute to the variations in prevalence estimates [2]. Indeed, AR diagnosed by physicians might potentially provide lower prevalence estimates in comparison to assessments based on questionnaires or reactions from allergy tests. Incorporating allergen testing or employing ICD codes from databases could also result in disparate prevalence figures. Furthermore, the prevalence of AR is subject to fluctuations over time; certain studies note an escalation in prevalence across years, whereas others document a decline [6]. The majority of AR symptoms emerge prior to the age of 20, reaching their zenith between 20 and 40 years of age, and subsequently tapering off gradually [17, 18]. Geographic location plays a significant role in AR prevalence, with variations observed between countries and even within regions of the same country. Climate change can impact AR prevalence by altering environmental exposures by lengthening pollen seasons and increasing pollen counts. The prevalence of perennial AR may be higher in urban settings and colder climates, while latitude can influence both perennial and seasonal AR patterns. Understanding the geographic and climatic influences on AR prevalence is essential for better management and treatment strategies [6].

Studies on the incidence and prevalence of AR in children have shown that symptoms can manifest as early as 12 months. Incidence rates in children show a peak age at diagnosis between 24 and 29 months [19]. In a study involving 18-month-old atopic children, a prevalence estimate of 9.1% was determined for symptoms consistent with AR. A longitudinal study conducted in Germany suggested that clinically significant AR typically emerges after two periods of seasonal allergen exposure, with no cases diagnosed by the age of 1. The remission rate of AR in children is relatively modest, as reported at 12% in a study encompassing children aged 4–8 [20, 21]. The majority of studies investigating AR prevalence in children are cross-sectional, with the International Study of Asthma and Allergies in Childhood (ISAAC) studies being notable for their extensive scope. Epidemiological surveys based on questionnaires have encompassed hundreds of thousands of children across diverse countries. The mean prevalence of AR was found to be 8.5% among 6–7-year-olds and 14.6% among 13–14-year-olds [20–23]. Regional disparities were noted, with a lower prevalence in the Indian subcontinent and a higher prevalence in Latin America. Various other studies conducted in countries such as Costa Rica, Japan, the United Arab Emirates, Nigeria, Brazil, and Ecuador have reported differing prevalence rates [6]. The prevalence of AR generally rises with age up to young adulthood. However, it is important to consider the limitations of questionnaire-based investigations, as variations in responder education and disparities in researcher definitions of AR could impact prevalence estimates. Different approaches to measuring point prevalence and lifetime prevalence of AR can also lead to divergent outcomes. On the whole, the available evidence points toward an increasing prevalence of AR in children, although recent data suggest that this upward trend might not persist in the future. The drivers influencing AR prevalence are complex and multifactorial [6].

9.4 Predisposing Factors

Various factors contribute to the development of allergic rhinitis in children. According to the latest literature data, here we will examine the causative role of what appear to be the most significant determinants. Genetic predisposition holds a prominent role, with children having a family history of allergic diseases displaying an increased likelihood of developing the condition. Twin studies have indicated that genetic factors contribute significantly, accounting for up to 70–80% of the variability in susceptibility to AR [24, 25]. However, the hereditary effect is not solely attributable to a single gene or polymorphism; rather, multiple genes and their variations interact to influence the initiation, persistence, and severity of the disease [6]. The latest genome-wide association studies (GWASs) have identified various single nucleotide polymorphisms associated with AR. For example, LRRC32, which regulates T-cell function, has been linked to AR, asthma, and other allergy-related conditions. GWASs have also unveiled common genetic mechanisms between AR and other allergic diseases, with an overlap in susceptibility loci for sensitization and self-reported allergies. More extensive investigations have both reaffirmed many previously identified AR susceptibility loci and unveiled novel ones, such as IL7R and CXCR5 [26]. In parallel, the candidate gene approach, which focuses on genes with established relevance to disease biology, has contributed to AR research. This approach has consistently identified several genes, aligning with findings from genome-wide association studies. Genes associated with antigen presentation, pathogen recognition, interleukin signaling, and proinflammatory signaling have been implicated in AR [6, 24]. These revelations deepen our comprehension of AR's genetic underpinnings and underscore potential avenues for future research and therapeutic interventions. Furthermore, epigenetic mechanisms, which involve alterations in gene expression without changing the DNA sequence, have been proposed as a bridge between genetic and environmental factors in AR. Recent studies have illuminated associations between DNA methylation, influenced by risk factors such as tobacco smoking and exposure to air pollution, and AR along with related outcomes. However, whether these epigenetic changes contribute causally to AR development or function as exposure markers remains uncertain [24, 25].

It is imperative for forthcoming research to explore the role of epigenetics in AR and elucidate the functional rationale behind the connection among genetic variants, environmental exposures, and the onset of the disease. Air pollution, characterized by the contamination of the environment through diverse agents (chemical, physical, or biological), has undergone comprehensive scrutiny regarding its implications for human health. The intricate relationship between air pollution and AR necessitates a thorough comprehension. Initial evidence suggested minimal or inconsequential links between air pollutants and AR onset. Nevertheless, recent investigations have unveiled a positive correlation between air pollution and AR [6]. Elevated levels of pollutants such as PM, ozone, nitrogen dioxide (NO_2), and sulfur dioxide (SO_2) were found to correspond with the augmented prevalence and severity of AR. Children subjected to heightened air pollutant levels displayed an increased susceptibility to developing AR. Thus, the findings revealed a positive link between air pollution and the prevalence of allergic rhinitis. And highlighted geographical region and economic status as potential factors that could potentially modify this association: the impact of air pollutants exhibited greater significance and magnitude in developing nations compared to developed ones, excluding PM10 [26]. The understanding of air pollution's influence on AR severity has notably advanced in recent times. The "Impact of Air Pollution on Sleep, Asthma and Rhinitis" (POLLAR) initiative was introduced to assess the interplay between sleep disorders, air pollution, and AR, utilizing machine learning techniques. Strategies for addressing AR symptoms induced by pollution have been consolidated in a consensus paper [27].

Air pollution affects countries worldwide, and comprehending its repercussions on AR and the spectrum of noncommunicable diseases (NCDs) characteristic of the modern era is vital for crafting effective prevention and management strategies. Numerous studies have investigated the connection between exposure to tobacco smoke and allergic rhinitis (AR). Although the majority of prospective cohort studies and systematic reviews have failed to establish a link between active or passive tobacco smoke and AR, contradictory findings have emerged. Some studies propose a potential protective influence of tobacco smoke against AR development, while others indicate adverse effects on bronchial epithelial barrier function, leading to heightened allergen penetration [6]. Nicotine, a component of tobacco smoke, has demonstrated immunosuppressive properties by dampening type 2 immune responses [28]. Recent meta-analyses have delved into the impact of tobacco smoke on AR. One such analysis suggested that smoking might decrease AR risk, while another revealed that maternal passive smoking during pregnancy raised the likelihood of offspring developing AR. Concerning maternal smoking during pregnancy, no significant association was observed with increased rhinoconjunctivitis in childhood and adolescence. However, among children who developed AR, maternal smoking of ten or more cigarettes per day during pregnancy correlated with persistent rhinoconjunctivitis [29, 30]. The effects of electronic cigarettes and heated tobacco products on AR are also gaining attention. A survey study indicated that current smokers of traditional tobacco cigarettes faced a higher risk of AR compared to users of heated tobacco products and electronic cigarettes [6, 31, 32]. In conclusion, although the majority of investigations suggest no direct link between tobacco smoke exposure and AR, conflicting outcomes hint at a potential protective aspect of tobacco smoke. Nonetheless, considering the substantial evidence of tobacco smoke's detrimental impact on human health, efforts toward smoking cessation and the establishment of smoke-free environments are imperative to enhance public health and alleviate the burden of various tobacco-related ailments. Further research is necessary to comprehensively comprehend the effects of tobacco and emerging smoking products on AR development, even though the ultimate goal remains a world free from such necessities.

The connection between early allergen exposure and its role as a predisposing factor in the development of AR remains unsettled. Allergen exposures during early life that are identified as significant risk factors for AR at age six are often found to lose significance by age 12 or beyond [6]. Notably, there is no established link between early mite exposure and AR. Some studies propose a dose–response curve resembling a bell shape, implying that both very low and very high exposures might potentially have protective effects. Exposure levels below 2 mg of dust mite allergen per gram of house dust have been suggested as a "safe" threshold for averting primary allergic diseases in atopic children. It is important, however, to consider that the risk of allergic disease during childhood might also be influenced by mono- versus polysensitization at an early stage [33]. On the other hand, it has been established that the development of pollen sensitization in early life is associated with the later emergence of AR in childhood. Subsequent to initial pollen sensitization in children, there is a gradual rise in the level and number of pollen sensitizations. The percentage of new AR cases increases gradually from ages 3 to 12, at an approximate annual rate of 2%. With the alterations in the environment due to global warming, such as extended pollination seasons, it is anticipated that pollen sensitization in young children will escalate, leading to heightened rates of AR in adolescence and adulthood. A more promising avenue of research might involve focusing on early-life sensitization rather than solely on pollen exposure. Sensitization to specific allergenic molecules in early childhood more accurately predicts the development of AR in later years. Notably, higher levels of specific allergens and multiple pathogenesis-related class 10 allergens at a young age are indicative of AR development in adolescence. Conducting longitudinal pollen studies is intricate due to the year-to-year fluctuations in pollen counts and the challenges in controlling a young child's level of exposure. Hence, in early childhood, component-resolved diagnostics could potentially serve as the most effective tool for foreseeing pollen-induced AR in later life [6, 34, 35]. In contrast, recent studies with stronger evidence have demonstrated that early-life exposure to fungal allergens or dampness presents a risk factor for AR, even though a clear dose–response relationship is not yet precisely defined. Regarding early-life exposure to animal-derived allergens, making evidence-based recommendations on the protective effect of such exposure to cats and dogs remains a challenge [6]. The exact mechanism underpinning the effects of pet exposure on AR remains uncertain. However, it is suggested that environmental exposure could potentially impact the risk of AR based on the stage of immune system development. In summation, while definitive recommendations are challenging to provide regarding childhood exposure to pets and its connection to AR, it is suggested that early exposure within the first year of life might reduce the risk.

9.5 Pathogenesis

Our comprehension of the pathogenesis of allergic rhinitis (AR) has progressed to acknowledge the significant roles played by the nasal innate immune response in tandem with the well-established IgE-driven mechanisms. The initial line of defense against inhaled allergens and irritants resides in the nasal epithelium. However, disruptions to its barrier function can permit allergen penetration into local tissues, perpetuating persistent inflammation. Nevertheless, the precise role of epithelial barrier dysfunction in AR development is still under investigation [36]. Nasal epithelial cells express pattern recognition receptors known as Toll-like receptors (TLRs) and respond to environmental molecules by generating alarmins such as IL-25, IL-33, and Thymic stromal lymphopoietin (TSLP). These alarmins stimulate dendritic cells, T cells, and type 2 innate lymphoid cells (ILC2s), which are pivotal in Th2-associated conditions like AR. Upon activation by cytokines released by epithelial cells, ILC2s produce type 2 cytokines like IL-5 and IL-13 [37–39]. Diverse forms of inflammation manifest at different stages of AR, with the prevalence of a type 2 immune response being the most typical. This type of response involves Th2 cells, M2 macrophages, eosinophils, and, in addition, ILC2s. However, alternative patterns, featuring mixed type 2 and type 3, or even type 1 inflammation, can arise based on factors such as allergen protease activity and environmental circumstances. The process of endotyping, which classifies patients according to their distinct inflammatory patterns, emerges as essential for personalized medicine in AR [6]. Cellular interactions play a crucial role: IL-33 acts upon type 2 ILCs, prompting mast cell degranulation; IL-25 influences Th2 cells and ILC2s; and TSLP triggers the activation of dendritic cells. Allergen-specific CD4+ T cells oversee various facets of the allergic response, including IgE production, eosinophilia, and type 2 inflammation. Dendritic cells and basophils also assume pivotal roles in initiating and amplifying the Th2 response. Exposure to allergens increases the count of ILC2s in peripheral blood and nasal mucosa. Significantly, the therapeutic efficacy of intranasal corticosteroids (INCS) treatment is seen to reduce the increase in ILC2s, underscoring the critical role of ILC2s in the inflammatory cascade. Furthermore, ILC2s contribute to the permeability of the epithelial barrier through IL-13. Innovative therapies targeting the innate immune system, such as anti-IL-13 treatment and allergen immunotherapy (AIT), hold promise in alleviating AR symptoms and enhancing clinical outcomes. Notably, AIT has demonstrated a reduction in ILC2s and an increase in IL-10-producing ILCs in the peripheral blood of AR patients, aligning with improved clinical parameters. B and plasma cells produce IgE locally in AR, contributing to the expansion of circulating memory B cells. Eosinophils and mast cells exert pivotal roles in the early and late phases of allergic responses, driving inflammation, tissue remodeling, and the accumulation of inflammatory cells. Consequently, both innate and effector mechanisms contribute to allergic diseases, with a pronounced Th2 bias observed in AR mucosa. Regulatory T cells (Tregs) play a crucial role in controlling AR development by suppressing other immune cells. The balance between effector and regulatory cell types plays a pivotal role in dictating the occurrence of an allergic response. Other cell types, including regulatory B cells and Th17 cells, could also influence AR [37–40]. As highlighted earlier, allergic rhinitis is also rooted in the adaptive immune system and the generation of specific IgE antibodies. The adaptive immune response can be simplified into T-helper (Th) cell response types: Th1, Th2, and Th17. The Th1 response is protective against intracellular pathogens, the Th17 response is defensive against bacteria and fungi, and the Th2 response is geared toward defense against parasites [36]. In the context of AR, the release of alarmins and other molecules triggers the recruitment of inflammatory cells and fosters Th2 polarization. Upon exposure to an allergen, dendritic cells process and present it to naïve helper T cells, which then differentiate into allergen-specific Th2 cells. These Th2 cells release cytokines like IL-4, IL-5, and IL-13, stimulating B cells and initiating IgE production. Plasma cells then produce specific IgE antibodies, which attach to FcεRI receptors on mast cells and basophils. Crosslinking of IgE on these cells leads to degranulation and the release of inflammatory mediators, manifesting as the symptomatic manifestations of AR [37–40]. Traditionally, AR was conceived as a result of systemic immune responses that give rise to systemic IgE production. This systemic reactivity is exemplified by the cutaneous reaction observed in skin testing. In sum, comprehending the immunologic cascade and the role of IgE receptors in allergic diseases like AR provides insights into the underlying mechanisms and potential targets for therapeutic interventions. In recent years, substantial strides have been made in understanding the immunologic processes initiated by IgE receptor activation. Three types of IgE receptors exist: FcεRI, FcεRII (CD23), and FcεRIII. FcεRI, present on mast cells and basophils, triggering degranulation and cytokine production. Dendritic cells and macrophages also possess FcεRI, facilitating antigen processing and presentation. FcεRII is found in macrophages and epithelial cells, enabling the uptake of IgE antigen complexes. FcεRIII is found in B cells and regulates IgE production and antigen processing [2, 6]. The emphasis here is on the sequence of events ensuing FcεRI activation. When antigens bind, or better yet, crosslink two IgE/FcεRI complexes, mast cells and basophils are activated, leading to degranulation and the release of diverse mediators like histamine, leukotrienes, and platelet-activating factors. This process marks the early allergic response, resulting in vasodilation, edema, and bronchoconstriction. The β and γ subunits of FcεRI incorporate the immunoreceptor tyrosine-based activation motif (ITAM). Following receptor stimulation, ITAM undergoes phosphorylation and activates the tyrosine kinase Syk, a key player in mast cell activation, degranulation, and the production of chemokines, cytokines, and lipid mediators. Following FcεRI stimulation, mast cells undergo de novo gene transcription, leading to the upregulation of numerous genes encoding cell surface molecules, cytokines/chemokines, signaling molecules, and enzymes. Simultaneously, specific genes associated with signal transduction, apoptosis, and cell proliferation are downregulated. Crosslinking FcεRI through antigen-bound IgE initiates the activation of transcription factors like STAT-5, NFAT, AP-1, NF-κB, and EGR-2, leading to the upregulation of genes linked to FcεRI expression. This process culminates in the production and release of cytokines and chemokines that attract inflammatory cells, including eosinophils, basophils, neutrophils, macrophages, and T cells. This late allergic response contributes to airway inflammation, hyperresponsiveness, airway remodeling, and mucus hypersecretion [2, 6, 37]. Separately, it is important to acknowledge Local Allergic Rhinitis (LAR). While systemic allergen sensitization can be detected through serum in vitro or allergy skin tests, these methods do not directly provide insights into the immune response within the target organ. Recent research lends support to the notion of local IgE production, particularly in the context of a condition known as local allergic rhinitis (LAR). LAR is characterized by allergic nasal symptoms in patients who test negative in systemic allergy tests. However, positive nasal provocation testing (NPT) and the detection of nasal sIgE or positive basophil activation tests (BAT) indicate a localized allergic response in these individuals. LAR's prevalence is approximately 26% in Mediterranean countries (Portugal, Spain, Italy, and Greece) and 7–10% in Asian countries (China and Korea). LAR might affect around 47% of children previously classified as having nonallergic rhinitis. Environmental factors, including humidity, temperature, and pollution, are linked to a higher incidence of LAR. However, the conversion rate to systemic detection of allergen sensitivity, the development of asthma, or worsening clinical progression is low, occurring in about 3% of cases [6, 38–40]. Local IgE production has been demonstrated in allergic rhinitis (AR) and LAR patients. In LAR, nasal secretions have been observed to contain sIgE following natural or controlled allergen exposure through NPT, even during nonexposure periods. It is believed that in LAR individuals, sIgE produced at the mucosal level might be sufficient to sensitize nasal effector cells without reaching skin mast cells or becoming detectable in the bloodstream. The immunopathology of local sIgE production in LAR is yet to be comprehensively understood. Flow cytometry analysis of nasal lavage confirms a nasal IgE-mediated inflammatory response in LAR patients, marked by increased eosinophils, basophils, mast cells, CD3+ and CD4+ T cells, local sIgE, and proinflammatory mediators such as tryptase and eosinophil cationic protein (ECP) during exposure to aeroallergens. NPT studies have unveiled distinct immediate/early and late phases of the allergic response in LAR. For these patients, nasal mucosal reactions to administered allergens primarily occur through IgE-coated mast cells and basophil stimulation. This step triggers the secretion of various substances that contribute to inflammation, sIgE production, and eosinophil activation. Subsequently, serum IL-5 levels increase, and IL-5 is transported to the lungs, increasing exhaled nitric oxide (NO) and bronchial hyperreactivity. Studies have also shown that sIgE produced in the nasal mucosa of LAR patients sensitized to specific allergens can bind to the high-affinity FcεRI receptor on basophils. The mechanism of basophil activation in LAR appears to be linked to sIgE, as evidenced by BAT experiments with wortmannin pretreatment, which reversed positive outcomes when wortmannin was introduced, suggesting that basophils may be the initial target cells for locally produced sIgE, subsequently transported from the site of inflammation (nasal mucosa) to the general circulation [6, 38–40].

In conclusion, it is essential to recognize that sensory neurons, axonal reflexes, and neurotransmitters exert influence over the pathophysiology of AR. The trigeminal sensory, sympathetic, and parasympathetic nervous systems work in unison to regulate processes in the upper airway mucosa and provide protection against allergens. The trigeminal nerve, responsible for innervating the nasal cavity, consists of nociceptive fibers that can be stimulated by physical and chemical triggers, including inflammatory mediators such as bradykinin, histamine, acetylcholine, and capsaicin. These mediators activate sensory neurons via Transient Receptor Potential (TRP) ion channels, inducing hyperexcitability of neurons in AR patients. Changes in TRP channels lead to sustained hyperexcitability, affecting stimulation thresholds and membrane potentials. The depolarization of nociceptive channels on sensory nerves results in the release of neuropeptides such as substance P, Calcitonin Gene-Related Peptide (CGRP), and neurokinin-A. These neuropeptides interact with receptors in the nasal epithelium, glands, and blood vessels, prompting glandular secretion, increased vascular permeability, edema, vasodilation, and the activation of inflammatory cells. Substance P and CGRP also activate mast cells, initiating the release of histamine and other inflammatory mediators, further fueling the hypersensitivity reaction. Neurokinin A, another neuropeptide, contributes to increased vascular permeability, vasodilation, bronchial smooth muscle contraction, mucus secretion, mast cell degranulation, and leukocyte activation. In AR patients, neuropeptides and inflammatory mediators are notably elevated, leading to the peripheral sensitization of nerve fibers and potentially central sensitization. Neural growth factor (NGF), released by mast cells and eosinophils, contributes to nasal hyperresponsiveness and heightened neuropeptide levels. Clinical trials exploring novel therapies targeting these pathways, such as bradykinin antagonists and TRP channel blockers, have not yielded successful outcomes in seasonal AR [6, 41, 42]. Overall, the pathophysiology of AR involves an intricate interplay among diverse immune cells, cytokines, inflammatory mediators, and neural mechanisms, underscoring the multifaceted nature of the disease.

9.6 Principal Associated Conditions

Allergic rhinitis can considerably impact children's physical and emotional well-being. The persistent and bothersome symptoms can disrupt sleep patterns, leading to fatigue and reduced cognitive function, which may affect academic performance. Children with allergic rhinitis may experience irritability, mood swings, and decreased participation in physical activities. Additionally, allergic rhinitis is often associated with other allergic conditions, such as asthma or atopic dermatitis, which may further complicate the child's health and quality of life.

9.6.1 Quality of Life (QoL)

The consistent body of evidence underscores that individuals with allergic rhinitis (AR) consistently exhibit diminished overall quality of life (QoL), both in general and in relation to their specific condition, in comparison to those without AR. Treatments encompassing intranasal corticosteroids (INCS), oral antihistamines, and allergen immunotherapy (AIT) have yielded enhancements in the QoL of AR patients [6]. The adoption of disease-specific QoL measures, such as the Rhinoconjunctivitis Quality of Life Questionnaire (RQLQ) and the Sino-Nasal Outcome Test (SNOT-22), has gained prominence and contributes invaluable insights into the impact of AR on QoL [43]. Objective assessments, including olfaction tests, have also proven to be beneficial in evaluating QoL among AR patients. However, some studies continue to rely on unvalidated methodologies for QoL assessment, resulting in challenges when comparing findings across different studies. There remains a paucity of direct comparisons between AR treatments with regard to their effects on QoL, with only a limited number of studies focusing on the distinctions between monotherapy and combination therapy. Emerging evidence is shedding light on the influence of AR not only on the QoL of children but also on that of their parents, highlighting the necessity for a comprehensive evaluation encompassing both populations. Long-term follow-up investigations indicate that AIT leads to sustained improvements in QoL when compared to placebo. Furthermore, seasonal variations in QoL have been observed, with QoL deteriorating during allergen-exposure seasons and improving outside those periods. It is of paramount importance to comprehend the impact of AR on QoL and to assess the efficacy of interventions in ameliorating well-being [6]. Further research is imperative to establish more comprehensive and standardized methodologies for evaluating QoL in AR, particularly when studying children and comparing diverse treatment modalities. By addressing the repercussions of AR on QoL, healthcare providers can tailor treatments and interventions more effectively, thereby enhancing the overall health and well-being of individuals grappling with AR.

9.6.2 Sleep Disturbance

Allergic rhinitis (AR) has a notable correlation with sleep disruptions in both the adult and pediatric populations. Numerous studies have extensively investigated this connection, and the prevailing consensus indicates that AR has an adverse impact on sleep quality, while effective AR treatment tends to mitigate sleep disturbances. Nevertheless, the strength of the evidence can vary, with more robust and conclusive data available for adults in comparison to children. In the case of adults, a substantial body of evidence underscores the detrimental effect of AR on sleep quality. This has been demonstrated through subjective assessments encompassing daytime sleepiness, sleep quality, and symptom reporting, all evaluated using well-validated measurement tools. In children, although the quality of available data is somewhat lower, it does point toward an association between AR and sleep disruptions. These disturbances manifest as heightened snoring, sleep-disordered breathing (SDB), and obstructive sleep apnea (OSA). However, the findings are not consistently uniform; certain studies indicate that while AR may be prevalent among those with OSA, it might not significantly influence the severity of the condition. Moreover, AR has emerged as a recognized risk factor for the exacerbation of OSA-related quality of life following adenotonsillectomy, along with an elevated susceptibility to nocturnal enuresis. Research examining the evolution of nasal inflammation over time has established a link between alterations in nasal cytokine levels and changes in polysomnogram (PSG) outcomes. The PSG parameters and sleep disturbances of AR patients tend to worsen during symptomatic periods or peak allergen seasons. In adults, the impact of AR on PSG parameters varies based on different study findings. Treatment of AR, particularly through the use of intranasal corticosteroids (INCS) or a combination of INCS and montelukast, has been linked to improvements in sleep quality, daytime sleepiness, sinonasal symptoms, and overall quality of life. Additionally, AR treatment has shown promise in enhancing compliance with continuous positive airway pressure (CPAP) therapy. Notably, addressing AR through treatment has been associated with a reduction in sleep fragmentation and snoring tendencies, thereby contributing positively to sleep patterns [6, 44].

9.6.3 Asthma

Extensive epidemiological investigations revealed that as many as 30% of individuals diagnosed with allergic rhinitis (AR) go on to develop asthma. Notably, persistent AR is linked with a notably higher risk of asthma development compared to intermittent AR. Remarkably, the Children's Respiratory Study uncovered that the likelihood of asthma emergence doubles by the age of 11 in cases where AR is diagnosed during infancy. This risk factor for asthma remains significant across both childhood and adulthood, irrespective of whether patients exhibit atopic or nonatopic characteristics. A pivotal shared risk factor between these two conditions is aeroallergen sensitization, with the majority of inhaled allergens contributing to hyperresponsiveness in both the nasal and bronchial passages. Moreover, there exists a potential mechanistic link involving common genetic polymorphisms and perturbed circulating microRNAs. Growing evidence suggests that exposure to air pollutants from traffic sources might elevate the risk of developing both AR and asthma; however, further comprehensive studies are warranted to establish concrete conclusions in this regard. Likewise, the independent effect of cigarette smoking on increasing asthma risk among AR patients is a subject requiring further validation through additional research. When it comes to treatment strategies, a body of evidence supports the positive impacts of diverse AR therapies on the management of both AR and asthma. Treatments such as intranasal corticosteroids (INCS), intranasal antihistamines, oral antihistamines, leukotriene receptor antagonists (LTRAs), and allergen immunotherapy (AIT) have shown beneficial effects on both conditions. Particularly, AIT holds promise in altering the allergic inflammation seen in AR and asthma. Rigorous prospective randomized trials and comprehensive systematic reviews have been conducted to minimize biases and provide robust evidence in this domain [6, 45]. In summation, a substantial and compelling association links AR and asthma, and a range of factors such as allergen sensitization, genetic influences, exposure to traffic-related air pollutants, and smoking might contribute to the emergence of asthma in individuals grappling with AR. The approaches to AR treatment have demonstrated advantages in the management of both AR and asthma, underscoring the interconnectedness of these two conditions within the shared airway system.

9.6.4 Adenoid Hypertrophy

Children with adenoid hypertrophy (AH) and allergic rhinitis (AR) may experience similar symptoms, such as nasal obstruction and rhinorrhea. Adenoids, which commonly enlarge during preschool years, typically regress during puberty. Studies examining the relationship between AH and allergic sensitization draw from two populations. The first includes allergic children assessed for AH, which has shown a higher prevalence than nonallergic controls. The second population consists of children suspected of AH who are assessed for allergic sensitization. The studies that indicated these observations yielded mixed results. Some report a negative association between allergy sensitization and adenoid volume, while others find a positive association between AH with AR and mold sensitivity [6]. Immunologic evidence suggests allergic physiology in the adenoid tissue, including a higher Th17/Treg ratio in children with AR, Th1, and Th2 gene expression in the adenoid tissue of children with AH and AR, and increased tissue eosinophilia and markers of Th2 inflammation in children with AH and AR compared to AH alone. Local allergic sensitization has also been observed in children testing negative for systemic allergen sensitization [46].

The use of INCS has demonstrated effectiveness in reducing nasal obstruction in AH, independent of allergy. However, the impact of INCS on adenoid size reduction remains unclear. Some studies suggest that AR may be a risk factor for refractory nasal symptoms after adenoidectomy [6].

In summary, AH is more common in allergic children compared to nonallergic controls. The association between allergic sensitivity and AH in children referred for nasal obstruction is inconsistent, possibly due to age and symptom presentation differences. Further research is needed to understand better the relationship between AH, AR, and allergic sensitization in children.

9.6.5 Conjunctivitis

The accurate determination of the prevalence of allergic conjunctivitis (AC) is intricate due to a range of factors. Diverse studies employ varying definitions of AC and assessment questionnaires, often failing to distinguish between AC and symptoms of allergic rhinitis (AR). It is widely acknowledged that AC is frequently considered a secondary manifestation of AR. Moreover, a more comprehensive characterization of AR and AC phenotypes within study samples is warranted. Many prevalence investigations rely on subjective questionnaires, lacking objective evidence of allergic sensitization. Despite grappling with these challenges, there is a notable burden of AC linked to AR. Research has indicated the prevalence of concurrent AR and AC, with global rates showing variability. The occurrence of ocular allergy symptoms in allergic children has been documented as notably high. The correlation between AR and AC has been observed across various age groups, encompassing adolescents and young children [6].

The ISAAC studies, a comprehensive global study series on allergic disorders, have offered valuable insights into the relationship between AR and AC. These investigations have highlighted the frequent connection between itchy/watery eyes and AR symptoms, impacting a substantial portion of children affected by AR. Across different regions, global prevalence studies have showcased an escalating prevalence of allergic rhinoconjunctivitis, albeit with regional disparities. Ocular allergy symptoms might be underreported due to symptom variability and a predominant focus on nonocular allergy symptoms [20]. Despite the established toll of AC on quality of life, it often goes unnoticed and undertreated, unless the cases are severe. Ocular allergy symptoms significantly compromise the quality of life linked to AR and frequently motivate individuals to seek allergy treatment [6]. When evaluating patients with AR, it is imperative to examine and address ocular symptoms.

9.7 Diagnosis

The diagnosis of AR is primarily made by the anamnesis, physical examination, and, finally, specific laboratory and functional tests.

Based on the anamnesis, it is possible to investigate the possible presence of familiarity, the onset of allergic symptoms, their characterization, and any associated comorbidities such as asthma [6, 47].

The physical examination makes it possible to detect the child's general condition and, particularly, the characteristic signs of AR through anterior rhinoscopy. It allows us to visualize the signs of inflammation at the level of the nasal mucosa, such as hyperemia or pallor, the presence of serous and mucous secretions, and hypertrophy of the inferior nasal turbinates.

Suppose the rhinoscopic examination is performed with a fiberoptic endoscope. In that case, it is possible, in addition to detecting the characteristics of the nasal mucosa, also inspect the nasal cavities as a whole and therefore highlight anatomical, infectious, or reactive conditions often associated with AR (septum deviation and hypertrophy of the turbinates, polyposis, inflammation of the paranasal sinuses, and adenoid hypertrophy) [3, 48].

Regarding the first level diagnostic tests, skin prick tests (SPT) can be carried out, representing an effective method for highlighting any sensitization toward the suspected allergens.

SPTs, in association with the clinical history and physical examination, confirm the diagnosis of AR, helping with the differential diagnosis of nonallergic rhinitis. Other complementary tests are specific IgE (sIgE) and molecular diagnostics (component-resolved diagnosis—CRD). As regard other second-level diagnostic tests, it is possible to carry out a functional evaluation of the degree of nasal obstruction by performing active anterior rhinomanometry (AAR), an evaluation of the extent of allergic inflammation by measuring nitric oxide nose (nFeNO), and finally the evaluation of cellularity through nasal cytology and nasal local IgE.

9.7.1 Skin Prick Test (SPT)

SPTs are detectable by easy applicability, high sensitivity and specificity, good compliance, immediacy of the result, and low economic cost. For the execution of the SPT, drops of allergenic extracts are placed on the intact skin at the level of the flying surface of the forearm. Subsequently, with a disposable sterile lancet, the skin is pricked at every single drop of allergen to allow it to penetrate the superficial layers of the dermis. The reaction is read after 15–20 min, evaluating the degree of response concerning the wheal, which is considered positive when it has a diameter of at least 3 mm. The execution of the test also requires the application of a positive control represented by histamine and a negative control represented by the physiological solution [49].

The limitations of SPTs are represented by the considerable variability of the response, which depends not only on the type of allergenic extract used, but also on the type of lancet, the skill and precision of the operator, and the pharmacological therapy in progress.

Furthermore, while they represent an irreplaceable diagnostic tool capable of reproducing an IgE-mediated reaction in vivo, they are unable to provide a quantitative estimate of IgE. For this reason, it is helpful to perform another first-level test, represented by the quantitative dosage of specific serum IgE, indicated or in case of discrepancy between the anamnesis and the skin tests, in children with extensive atopic dermatitis or dermatographism or who are taking antihistamines. All these conditions can modify the skin's reaction to the allergenic extract, thus invalidating the reliability of the test [49, 50].

9.7.2 Specific IgE (sIgE)

The most frequently used method for determining specific serum IgE is the ImmunoCAP Fluorescence Enzyme Immuno Assay.

It is based on detecting IgE antibodies labeled with a fluorescent enzyme, which reacts with the patient's specific IgE. After incubation of the patient's serum with the anti-IgE antibodies, they bind to the patient's specific IgE, forming a complex. IgE antibodies that have no aggregate form are subsequently washed off. The fluorescence measurement is proportional to the IgE concentration in the analyzed serum. Finally, calibration curves are analyzed to evaluate the test results where the individual dosages of specific IgE are expressed in concentrations. The test positivity cut-off is >0.35 KU/L. Similarly, to SPTs, the results of specific IgE vary according to the extract and the method used; therefore, they are not comparable. Furthermore, another limitation is represented by the possibility of obtaining false-positive or negative results in the presence of high levels of total IgE (>2000 IU/L), low levels of specific IgE concerning total IgE, local production of specific IgE, their absence in the circulation, and low presence of the allergen in the extract used [50, 51].

9.7.3 Component-Resolved Diagnosis (CRD)

Both SPTs and specific IgE dosage do not allow to establish, in a patient showing an allergic polysensitization, whether it is due to a co-sensitization (sensitization to distinct and unique molecules of different allergenic sources) or to a mechanism of cross-reactivity (sensitization to various allergenic sources containing homologous molecules). Hence, there is need to resort to second-level diagnostic tests aimed at recognizing the epitopes of individual allergens, paving the way for molecular allergology. The specific molecular dosages relating to the individual allergens to which the subject is sensitized represent the primary second-level laboratory investigations [52].

In recent years, several allergens have been identified, cloned, and sequenced. Many of these are currently available in molecular diagnostics routinely performed in many centers using microarrays (ImmunoCAP ISAC, Thermo Fosher Scientific, Sweden) and microarrays (ALEX, MADx, Austria) methods, or singleplex (ImmunoCAP), in the form of recombined or natural allergens. The former are obtained thanks to recombinant DNA technology (e.g., rPhl p 1) by introducing the DNA encoding the allergen into a host organism. The latter is obtained by biochemical purification starting from the biological source (e.g., nPhl p. 4). Adequately complete panels of recombinant molecules have a sensitivity >70% in mimicking the allergic source.

The allergenic molecules are divided into "genuine," accurate markers of a given source and into "panallergens," proteins shared by allergenic sources also taxonomically unrelated to each other, responsible for apparent polysensitizations in tests performed with extracts [53].

Among the markers of cross-reactivity, some are commonly referred to as "panallergens," underlining the ubiquitous distribution of these molecules in nature. Panallergens include the group of profilins, polcalcins, and nonspecific lipid transport proteins (nsLTPs). In conclusion, the identification of panallergens has allowed the development of a new concept of diagnosis in the allergy field, the component-resolved diagnosis (CRD) or molecular diagnostics, identifying the markers of primary sensitization and those of cross-reactivity and thus allows distinguishing between true and false polysensitization [54].

9.7.4 Anterior Active Rhinomanometry (AAR)

AAR is a noninvasive method to study objectively and reproducibly nasal airflow and resistance at a pressure of 150 Pa. The values obtained are then compared with the height-dependent ones, adapting the pediatric values of the nasal flow reported in the literature [55, 56].

The AAR is an easy-to-perform exam in which the child is asked to breathe with his mouth closed spontaneously after positioning a face mask hermetically placed on the face and after alternately occluding the nostrils using a nasal toggle. The face mask is connected to a rhinomanometer and to a computer with a flowmeter, which allows measuring the air flows (in cm^3/s) separately at the level of the right nostril and left nostril at pressures of 75, 100, 150, and 300 Pa, both inspiration and expiration. The results obtained are interpreted considering the inspiratory nasal flows at 150 Pa, compared with the height-dependent pediatric reference values reported in the literature [56, 57].

The data obtained are graphically represented by the software on a system of Cartesian axes and a sinusoidal oscillogram, allowing the inspiratory and expiratory nasal resistances to be visualized separately for each nasal cavity (Fig. 9.2) [55, 56].

Nasal obstruction can be classified into five groups: very severe if mean airflow values are <44% of expected; severe if the values are between 44% and 54%; moderate if the values are between 55% and 65%; mild if the values are between 66% and 76%; and absent if the values are >76% (10.1002/ppul.10066).

Through AAR, two tests can be performed: one is the nasal provocation test (NAPT) with the aero-allergen and the other one is the decongestion test.

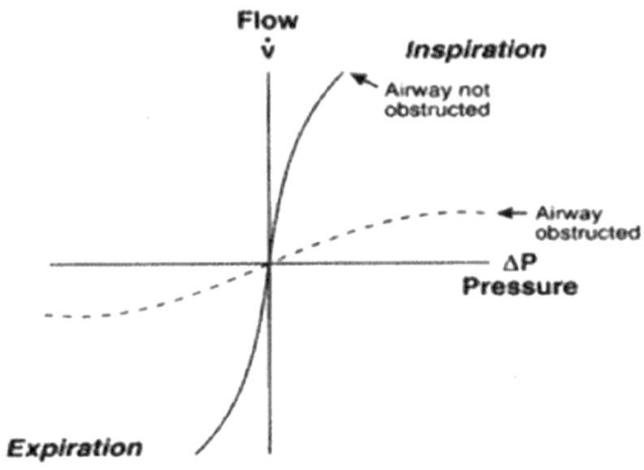

Fig. 9.2 Graphic representation of the results obtained at the rhinomanometric examination

NAPT requires the nasal instillation of the allergen; however, nonspecific hyper-reactivity must be ruled out by the nasal administration of lactose [39].

Then, after the lactose test, 40 units of the suspected allergen extract are instilled in each nostril; 30 min after the insufflation of this extract, another AAR is performed. NAPT is considered positive if there has been an increase in nasal resistance of at least 50% compared to the baseline value in at least one of the two nostrils. This procedure can be repeated twice, 30 min apart if there is a negative NAPT result at the first nasal instillation of the suspected allergen [58].

NAPT is useful for the diagnosis of local allergic rhinitis (LAR), where there is the positivity of the NAPT to single or multiple aeroallergens (10.2500/ajra.2016.30.4352) (10.2500/aap.2020.41.200063).

Instead, the nasal decongestion test provides additional information on nasal obstruction, using a sympathetic alpha mimetic such as naphazoline nitrate nasal spray (Rinazine® 100 mg/100 ml), one puff in each nostril. After 15 min, an AAR post-decongestion is repeated to evaluate the modification of the nasal airflow [40, 58].

The decongestion test is used for the differential diagnosis between AR, in which after the decongestion test, the nasal flow improves concerning obstructive anatomical conditions, such as septal deviations, adenotonsillar hypertrophy, and nasal polyps in which after decongestion test there is no improvement in nasal airflow.

9.7.5 Nasal Nitric Oxide (nFeNO)

The determination of nFeNO, a marker of eosinophilic inflammation, synthesized by epithelial cells of the nasal mucosa, has shown utility in disease monitoring [59]. Measured using the nFeNO technique exhaled through a fixed flow hermetic face mask connected to an analyzer (Medisoft nFeNO analyzer), according to American Thoracic Society/European Respiratory Society (ERS/ATS) recommendations. For each maneuver during inspiration, a total lung capacity, subjects inhale through the nose from a NO-free air analyzer and then exhale via disposable nosepieces at a constant flow of 350 mL/s for 60 s [59].

9.7.6 Nasal Cytology

Nasal cytology is an advantageous method in the clinical and diagnostic field for a precise definition of allergic and nonallergic rhinopathies.

It allows the detection of the cellular variations of an epithelium exposed to physicochemical irritations or acute and chronic inflammation. In particular, nasal cytology has clarified the physio-pathological mechanisms underlying AR and identified new nosological entities such as noninfectious and nonallergic rhinitis.

The material of the rhino cytological smear is taken by scraping the superficial layer of the cen tral portion of the inferior nasal turbinate of both choanae, using a special curette, subsequently fixed in the air, stained with the May Grunwald-Giemsa technique, and analyzed under an optical microscope with magnification 1000x with a percentage estimation of cellularity in at least 50 microscopic fields.

The patient affected by AR presents an infiltrate of immunophlogistic cells such as eosinophils, neutrophils, lymphocytes, and mast cells with important signs of eosinophilic-mast cell degranulation.

In the case of minimally persistent inflammation, the rhino-cystogram is characterized by infiltration of neutrophils and only minimally of eosinophils [60, 61].

9.7.7 Local Nasal IgE

The research of specific nasal IgE is a noninvasive procedure, highly specific (>90%) but not very sensitive (22–40%) due to the possible post-washing dilution (operator-dependent procedure) [39].

Each patient underwent nasal washing with 10 ml of saline solution following the method of Naclerio et al. [62].

Subsequently, samples of approximately 1.5 mL of nasal wash are subjected to centrifugation with a reduction of 50% of the initial volume, and then the samples are stored at −80 °C until final analysis. Nasal sIgE is determined using the ImmunoCAP method Fluorescence Enzyme immunoassay with a positivity cut-off value set at 0.35 AU/mL [39].

9.8 Therapy

In daily practice, most patients with AR receive health education and allergen avoidance measures and are treated with symptomatic medications, including oral antihistamines and intranasal corticosteroids, in line with guidelines and criteria for AR and its impact on asthma (ARIA) [63].

Identifying the trigger that causes rhinitis can help establish avoidance measures to control symptoms; however, the ubiquity of many allergenic sources is often a difficult practice to follow.

Alongside environmental prevention, some simple measures, such as maintaining proper cleaning of the nasal cavities, are of great use in alleviating AR symptoms in children and improving the functionality of the nasal mucosa. Nasal washings with physiological and/or hypertonic saline solution facilitate the removal of any allergens, irritants, and mucous secretions [64].

As regard the drug therapy of AR, the ARIA guidelines recommend a stepwise therapeutic approach based on the severity and frequency of symptoms [65].

However, symptomatic treatment cannot prevent the natural progression of AR toward clinical worsening and the development of allergic comorbidities such as asthma and new sensitizations over time. Currently, allergen-specific immunotherapy (AIT) is available, the only viable strategy for modulating the immune system with a possible effect on allergic symptoms [63].

The mainstay drugs for AR therapy in childhood are oral antihistamines and topical nasal corticosteroids.

9.8.1 Antihistamines

Antihistamines, defined as inverse agonists of H1 histamine receptor, determine the downregulation of allergic inflammation, which can occur either directly, through the blockade of H1 receptors on nerve endings and small vessels, or indirectly, through the blockade of intracellular signal transduction mediated by nuclear factor NF-kB, by reducing the transcription of genes involved in antigen presentation and the expression of proinflammatory cytokines, adhesion molecules, and chemotactic factors. The anti-H1 antihistamines are functionally classified into two groups, the first- and second-generation molecules, and are indicated for treating all forms of AR [66].

Some pharmacological characteristics of these molecules significantly limit the use of first-generation H1 antihistamine drugs in treating AR. The first-generation H1 antihistamines can cross the blood–brain barrier and cause sedatives, thus reducing the child's alertness and attention. They are poorly selective for the receptor and are also able to bind other nonhistamine receptors such as serotonergic, cholinergic, and alpha-adrenergic ones, causing not only the sedative effect but also dry mouth, nausea, vomiting, diarrhea, constipation, anorexia, pollakiuria, dysuria, urinary retention, and increased appetite. The route of administration of first-generation H1 antihistamines can be either oral or systemic [66].

Different formulations for the second-generation molecules are available for systemic use (drops, syrup, and tablets) and topical nasal use. Given their low lipophilicity, these molecules almost lack the ability to cross the blood–brain barrier at ordinary doses of use. This characteristic leads to minimal or absent sedative, antiserotonin, and anticholinergic effects to the advantage of tolerability and compliance. Furthermore, the binding of the new antihistamines with the H1 receptor is more stable and persistent, so administrations can be more dilated over time with a once-daily administration [67].

Some latest-generation drugs are able to exert an allergic anti-inflammatory action through [68]

- Inhibition of the production of proinflammatory cytokines (e.g., IL-4, IL-13, and chemokines) and the release, in addition to histamine, of other preformed or newly formed mediators by mast cells and basophils.
- Reduction of the recruitment of eosinophils in the chronic phase of the allergic inflammatory process.
- Reduction of the increased expression of membrane receptors at the level of nasal epithelial cells and vascular endothelium, in particular, the leukocyte adhesion molecule ICAM-1.

A single dose of 2.5 mg should be used in children weighing between 10 and 25 kg, while a dose of 5 mg could be used in children weighing more [69].

According to age, Desloratadina 1.25 mg once a day between 2 and 5 years of age, 2.5 mg once a day between 6 and 12 years, and 5 mg once a day between 13 and 18 years. For Levocitirizine 1.25 mg twice a day between 2 and 5 years of age, 5 mg once a day between 6 and 12 years, and 5 mg once a day between 13 and 18 years [70, 71].

Their use in subjects affected by AR is particularly effective in controlling irritative symptoms, mainly mediated by the action of histamine, i.e. itching, tearing, and watery rhinorrhea. The benefit of nasal congestion is minor and, therefore, on the obstructive type symptoms, which are instead the prerogative of treatment with topical corticosteroids. In seasonal AR, antihistamine treatment should be started before pollination to allow the drug to saturate the H1 receptors. This treatment should be continued for the entire duration of pollination in order to block the receptors on the mast cells. In persistent AR, the antihistamine treatment should instead be modulated based on the clinical symptoms and has a dual target: controlling the persistent minimal inflammation of the nasal mucosa, reducing the inflammatory infiltrate, and, at the same time, the expression of the adhesion molecules 68).

9.8.2 Nasal Corticosteroids

Nasal corticosteroids are indicated in the treatment of both mild and moderately severe persistent AR and moderately severe intermittent AR. They noticeably reduce all rhinitis symptoms and, in particular, evidence of nasal obstruction, with better-documented efficacy than antihistamines (10.1177/0194599814561600).

The dosage is 200 mcg/die, 2 puffs for each nostril above 12 years of age, and 100 mcg/die 1 puff for each nostril under 12 years of age.

The mechanism of action of steroids provides, through the interaction with specific receptors, two types of effects [72]:

- The genomic effect, mediated by the intracellular receptor, which occurs over hours and/or days and consists of the activation or repression at the nuclear level of multiple genes involved in the inflammatory process.
- The nongenomic effect, triggered by the link with receptors present on the membrane cell or in the cytoplasm, which is mediated by the rapid activation of second intracellular messengers and is responsible for vasoconstriction at the level of the nasal mucosa; such an effect is also attributable to the rapidity of action of these drugs, which can be seen in about 6–7 h from their administration.

Steroids exert their anti-inflammatory action on the nasal mucosa with different mechanisms:

- Limit uptake and antigenic processing by Langerhans cells.
- Reduce the number of Langerhans cells.
- Reduce the number and survival of eosinophils in the lamina propria.
- Limit the influx of basophils and mast cells into the nasal mucosa and limit the number of T lymphocytes in the epithelium.
- Reduce the expression of IL-4 mRNA, limiting the switch of B-lymphocytes and the consequent synthesis of IgE, but also the expression of IL-3, IL-5, and IL-13.
- Limit the release of mediators, both preformed and newly generated.
- Inhibits the seasonal increase of specific IgE.

The new-generation corticosteroids have more excellent fat solubility than the pre-existing molecules. This characteristic allows an increased and more rapid absorption at the level of the nasal mucosa, more permanent in the absorbent tissue, more remarkable ability to reach the cytosolic receptor for steroids, less bioavailability, i.e., less circulating drug and fewer systemic side effects.

However, topical corticosteroid therapy can cause nosebleeds, dryness of the mucosa, and a tendency to crust, if it is a question of transient side effects that are negligible with the use of more recently introduced preparations. As far as the systemic effects are concerned, the possibility has been studied that, if administered in the long term, they can influence growth by acting on the hypothalamic-pituitary axis through the ingested, absorbed, and circulating portion. However, this eventuality has been reduced by clinical studies conducted with some molecules, which have demonstrated good long-term tolerability at the recommended doses, even in the pediatric age [50].

As regards the other drugs envisaged by the ARIA guidelines, there is no evidence of superior efficacy compared to nasal steroids. Nasal decongestants are contraindicated and cannot be used in children under 12 years of age; therefore, they are not the drugs currently used in pediatric AR. See the box plot below for the summary of ARIA guidelines recommendations:

Summary of Aria Guidelines Recommendation

- Oral or nasal antihistamines are less effective than nasal steroids in symptom control. However, some patients with mild/moderate disorder prefer oral medications to those intranasal.

(continued)

- The comparison between oral and nasal antihistamines remains uncertain between the guidelines. There are currently no clear indications.
- In patients with severe AR, nasal steroids remain the first-line treatment, even if the effect is delayed.
- The combination of oral antihistamine and non-nasal steroid is more effective than nasal steroid alone.
- All recommended drugs are considered safe at dosage recommended.
- First-generation antihistamines are sedatives, and should not be used, as well as topical or systemic vasoconstrictors for periods longer than 10 days.

9.8.3 Allergen Immunotherapy (AIT)

Specific allergen immunotherapy (AIT) represents the only possible curative approach to allergic pathologies through a specific antigen immunological mechanism of action, allowing the modification of the natural history of the disease and obtaining a reduction or remission of symptoms [73].

Systematic reviews of the literature and meta-analyses have shown that in patients with AR, AIT if prescribed and practised correctly, reduces chronic inflammation, symptoms, and use of pharmacotherapy and consequently improves the quality of life of these children after discontinuation of treatment.

From the first treatment performed more than 100 years ago by Noon, AIT has evolved in all its aspects: allergens used, vehicles, adjuvants, administration routes, and therapeutic schemes [74].

AIT consists of administering, in progressively increasing doses, purified extracts of single or multiple allergens in order to progressively reduce the body's immunological reactivity to the allergens to which it is sensitized, obtaining an immunological tolerance.

A first induction phase, in which the allergen is administered in increasing doses until the maximum dose is reached, is followed by a second maintenance phase in which a constant dose of allergen is administered, represented by the maximum therapeutic dose [75].

AIT acts on the immune system in the early stages of the response to the allergen and restores the balance between Th1 and Th2 lymphocytes, which, as it is known, is unbalanced toward the Th2 phenotype in allergic patients. Among the main effects of this immunological mechanism, there is the reduction of allergen-specific IgE, the induction of allergen-specific IgG class antibodies that block the allergen-induced activation of immunocompetent cells, and the reduction of cytokine synthesis Th2, which favor the development of the allergic reaction.

AIT also increases the activity and proliferation of regulatory T lymphocytes (Tregs), which are responsible for tolerance to allergens [76].

In detail, once the allergen has entered the body, it is captured by Langerhans cells and transported to the lymph nodes, where it stimulates the formation of specific allergen IgG and Th1 and Treg lymphocytes for increased IL-10 synthesis.

Allergen-specific IgG competes with IgE for allergen binding, blocking the allergic reaction, inhibiting IgE-mediated degranulation of mast and basophil cells, and presentation of the allergen to T cells, thereby reducing the number of switch cells allergen-specific memory B [77].

Treg lymphocytes interact by a contact mechanism by interaction between two counter-receptors: CTLA-4 and TGF-β, expressed on their surface, and CD28 and TGF-β type II receptor (TβRII), expressed on the surface of target cells. The interaction between TGF-β and TβRII blocks the synthesis of IL-2, a cytokine responsible for the proliferation and differentiation of T lymphocytes. It thus modifies the immunological phenotype of the allergic subject in favor of a Th1-type phenotype [78].

Given the complexity of the immunological mechanism of action of the AIT, the effect of its administration on symptoms is not immediate but requires medium–long treatment times, from 3 to 5 years in total.

Although the conventional routes of administration are subcutaneous (SCIT) and sublingual (SLIT) or oral, other routes of administration are currently being tested, such as the epicutaneous and intralymphatic routes [79, 80]. Due to the possibility of administering it outside the hospital environment, without medical supervision, and for better compliance by the child, SLIT has become increasingly used in daily clinical practice, especially in the pediatric age group.

In the treatment of AR, according to the EAACI (European Academy of Allergy and Clinical Immunology) guidelines, AIT should be considered in the presence: moderate–severe symptoms of AR in association or not with symptoms of allergic conjunctivitis or in the presence of symptoms milder when the patient wants to benefit from the long-term effects of AIT both in terms of improvement of symptoms and prevention of comorbidities; inadequate symptom control despite systemic antihistamine and/or topical corticosteroid therapy, environmental prophylaxis, and/or the presence of significant pharmacotherapy side effects [81].

Contraindications to treatment are

- Absolute in case of uncontrolled or severe asthma, the presence of systemic autoimmune diseases, and malignant neoplasms in progress.
- Related in case of controlled asthma, beta-blocker therapy, severe cardiovascular pathologies, systemic autoimmune diseases in remission or specific organs, severe psychiatric disorders, reduced adherence to therapy, primary and secondary immunodeficiencies, and history of severe adverse reactions to AIT.

Regarding side effects, AIT is a safe and well-tolerated treatment. Most of the adverse reactions reported are localized and resolve spontaneously and in a short time without the need for any intervention.

In SLIT, adverse reactions occur in 10–15% of patients and are divided into [82]:

- Local: itching and burning sensation of the oral mucosa, lip edema, tongue swelling, and peri palpebral angioedema.
- Systemic: generalized urticaria, nausea, anaphylaxis, abdominal pain, and bronchospasm.

No fatal reactions have ever been reported.

As far as SCIT is concerned, the most provoking reactions are [83]:

- Local: erythema and swelling at the injection site.
- Systemic: sporadic reported cases of anaphylaxis and fatal adverse events.

For this reason, the first administration of AIT should occur in a protected environment (hospital), with doctors capable of recognizing, documenting, and treating any reactions in the most appropriate way.

Recent studies have shown that AIT has a fundamental role in improving patients' clinical symptoms and a decisive effect in modifying the evolution of the molecular allergenic profile and, with it, the course of the disease.

Therefore, AIT may modify the progression of allergic sensitization profiles, the so-called "molecular spreading." In other words, the sequential development of the IgE response mediated toward distinct, noncross-reactive molecules but came from the same allergen, starting from only the allergenic molecule defined as "initiator" [52].

Early initiation with AIT in the preclinical window could even prevent molecular spread by blocking the increase in IgE in preschool children with only a positive family history, perhaps preventing the onset of AR or delaying the onset of the disease, or finally, making, in case of development of the same, the mildest symptoms. This type of intervention is defined as "resolved component prophylaxis," similar to the "resolved component therapy" concept.

In conclusion, the use of allergological molecular diagnostics (CRD) and AIT in the last decade is growing increasingly, paving the way for precision allergology. Therefore, it becomes increasingly important to identify the phenotype of the individual disease in order to personalize the therapeutic choices for each individual patient after having early identified the initiator molecule of the allergic response [35, 84, 85] .

Take-Home Messages

- Allergic rhinitis is a common condition characterized by nasal inflammation triggered by allergens.
- Symptoms include sneezing, runny nose, nasal congestion, and itching of the nose or eyes.
- Allergic rhinitis can significantly impact a person's quality of life, affecting sleep, concentration, and daily activities.
- Diagnosis involves evaluating symptoms, medical history, and may include allergy testing.
- Management includes allergen avoidance, medications (antihistamines and nasal corticosteroids), and allergen immunotherapy.
- Environmental control measures can help reduce exposure to allergens.
- Allergic rhinitis may be associated with other allergic conditions, such as asthma, atopic dermatitis, and conjunctivitis.
- Long-term management can help control symptoms, improve quality of life, and minimize complications.
- Individualized treatment plans should be developed with healthcare professionals to address specific needs.
- Education and awareness about triggers, treatment options, and self-management are key for effectively managing allergic rhinitis.

References

1. Akhouri S, House SA. Allergic rhinitis. In: StatPearls. Treasure Island (FL): StatPearls Publishing; 2023. [cited 2023 Aug 23]. Available from: http://www.ncbi.nlm.nih.gov/books/NBK538186/.
2. Nur Husna SM, Tan HTT, Md Shukri N, Mohd Ashari NS, Wong KK. Allergic rhinitis: a clinical and pathophysiological overview. Front Med. 2022;9:874114.
3. Bousquet J, Anto JM, Bachert C, Baiardini I, Bosnic-Anticevich S, Walter Canonica G, et al. Allergic rhinitis. Nat Rev Dis Primer. 2020;6:1–17.
4. Kanda A, Kondo K, Hosaka N, Kobayashi Y, Bui DV, Yun Y, et al. Eosinophilic upper airway inflammation in a murine model using an adoptive transfer system induces hyposmia and epithelial layer injury with convex lesions. Med Sci Basel Switz. 2019;7:E22.
5. Hill DA, Spergel JM. The atopic march: critical evidence and clinical relevance. Ann Allergy Asthma Immunol Off Publ Am Coll Allergy Asthma Immunol. 2018;120:131–7.
6. Wise SK, Damask C, Roland LT, Ebert C, Levy JM, Lin S, et al. International consensus statement on allergy and rhinology: allergic rhinitis – 2023. Int Forum Allergy Rhinol. 2023;13:293–859.
7. Custovic A, Custovic D, Kljaić Bukvić B, Fontanella S, Haider S. Atopic phenotypes and their implication in the atopic march. Expert Rev Clin Immunol. 2020;16:873–81.
8. Oksel C, Custovic A. Development of allergic sensitization and its relevance to paediatric asthma. Curr Opin Allergy Clin Immunol. 2018;18:109.
9. Shtessel M, Tversky J. Reliability of allergy skin testing. Ann Allergy Asthma Immunol. 2018;120:80–3.
10. Migueres M, Dávila I, Frati F, Azpeitia A, Jeanpetit Y, Lhéritier-Barrand M, et al. Types of sensitization to aeroallergens: definitions, prevalences and impact on the diagnosis and treatment of allergic respiratory disease. Clin Transl Allergy. 2014;4:16.
11. Testera-Montes A, Salas M, Palomares F, Ariza A, Torres MJ, Rondón C, et al. Local respiratory allergy: from rhinitis phenotype to disease spectrum. Front Immunol. 2021;12:691964.
12. Eiringhaus K, Renz H, Matricardi P, Skevaki C. Component-resolved diagnosis in allergic rhinitis and asthma. J Appl Lab Med. 2019;3:883–98.
13. Bousquet J, van Cauwenberge P, Khaltaev N. Allergic rhinitis and its impact on asthma. J Allergy Clin Immunol. 2001;108:S147–334.
14. Bousquet J, Annesi-Maesano I, Carat F, Léger D, Rugina M, Pribil C, et al. Characteristics of intermittent and persistent allergic rhinitis: DREAMS study group. Clin Exp Allergy. 2005;35:728–32.
15. Bauchau V, Durham SR. Epidemiological characterization of the intermittent and persistent types of allergic rhinitis. Allergy. 2005;60:350–3.
16. Licari A, Magri P, De Silvestri A, Giannetti A, Indolfi C, Mori F, et al. Epidemiology of allergic rhinitis in children: a systematic review and meta-analysis. J Allergy Clin Immunol Pract. 2023;11:2547–56.
17. Skoner DP. Allergic rhinitis: definition, epidemiology, pathophysiology, detection, and diagnosis. J Allergy Clin Immunol. 2001;108(1 Suppl):S2–8.
18. Wheatley LM, Togias A. Clinical practice. Allergic rhinitis. N Engl J Med. 2015;372:456–63.
19. Hill DA, Grundmeier RW, Ram G, Spergel JM. The epidemiologic characteristics of healthcare provider-diagnosed eczema, asthma, allergic rhinitis, and food allergy in children: a retrospective cohort study. BMC Pediatr. 2016;16:133.
20. Aït-Khaled N, Pearce N, Anderson HR, Ellwood P, Montefort S, Shah J, et al. Global map of the preva-

lence of symptoms of rhinoconjunctivitis in children: The International Study of Asthma and Allergies in Childhood (ISAAC) Phase Three. Allergy. 2009;64:123–48.

21. Björkstén B, Clayton T, Ellwood P, Stewart A, Strachan D, Phase III Study Group TI. Worldwide time trends for symptoms of rhinitis and conjunctivitis: Phase III of the International Study of Asthma and Allergies in Childhood. Pediatr Allergy Immunol. 2008;19:110–24.
22. Mallol J, Crane J, von Mutius E, Odhiambo J, Keil U, Stewart A. The International Study of Asthma and Allergies in Childhood (ISAAC) phase three: a global synthesis. Allergol Immunopathol (Madr). 2013;41:73–85.
23. Strachan D, Sibbald B, Weiland S, Ait-Khaled N, Anabwani G, Anderson HR, et al. Worldwide variations in prevalence of symptoms of allergic rhinoconjunctivitis in children: the International Study of Asthma and Allergies in Childhood (ISAAC). Pediatr Allergy Immunol. 1997;8:161–8.
24. Choi BY, Han M, Kwak JW, Kim TH. Genetics and epigenetics in allergic rhinitis. Genes. 2021;12:2004.
25. Karmaus W, Ziyab AH, Mukherjee N. Chapter 19: Epigenetics of allergic diseases allergies, eczema, asthma, and rhinitis. In: Tollefsbol TO, editor. Epigenetics in human disease. 2nd ed. Academic Press; 2018. p. 573–606. [cited 2023 Aug 23]. (Translational Epigenetics; vol. 6). Available from: https://www.sciencedirect.com/science/article/pii/B9780128122150000194.
26. Li S, Wu W, Wang G, Zhang X, Guo Q, Wang B, et al. Association between exposure to air pollution and risk of allergic rhinitis: a systematic review and meta-analysis. Environ Res. 2022;205:112472.
27. Bousquet J, Anto JM, Annesi-Maesano I, Dedeu T, Dupas E, Pépin JL, et al. POLLAR: Impact of air Pollution on Asthma and Rhinitis. A European Institute of Innovation and Technology Health (EIT Health) project. Clin Transl Allergy. 2018;8:36.
28. Kim HH, Lee CS, Yu SD, Lee JS, Chang JY, Jeon JM, et al. Near-road exposure and impact of air pollution on allergic diseases in elementary school children: a cross-sectional study. Yonsei Med J. 2016;57:698–713.
29. Skaaby T, Taylor AE, Jacobsen RK, Paternoster L, Thuesen BH, Ahluwalia TS, et al. Investigating the causal effect of smoking on hay fever and asthma: a Mendelian randomization meta-analysis in the CARTA consortium. Sci Rep. 2017;7:2224.
30. Zhou Y, Chen J, Dong Y, Shen J, Tian M, Yang Y, Song L, Li J. Maternal tobacco exposure during pregnancy and allergic rhinitis in offspring: A systematic review and meta-analysis. Medicine (Baltimore). 2021 ;100:e26986. https://journals.lww.com/md-journal/fulltext/2021/08270/maternal_tobacco_exposure_during_pregnancy_and.16.aspx.
31. Chung SJ, Kim BK, Oh JH, Shim JS, Chang YS, Cho SH, et al. Novel tobacco products including electronic cigarette and heated tobacco products increase risk of allergic rhinitis and asthma in adolescents: analysis of Korean youth survey. Allergy. 2020;75:1640–8.
32. Bousquet J, Bachert C, Alexander LC, Leone FT. Hypothesis: may e-cigarette smoking boost the allergic epidemic? Clin Transl Allergy. 2016;6:40.
33. Kuehr J, Frischer T, Meinert R, Barth R, Forster J, Schrauba S, et al. Mite allergen exposure is a risk for the incidence of specific sensitization. J Allergy Clin Immunol. 1994;94:44–52.
34. Scadding GK, Smith PK, Blaiss M, Roberts G, Hellings PW, Gevaert P, et al. Allergic rhinitis in childhood and the new EUFOREA algorithm. Front Allergy. 2021:2:706589.
35. Hatzler L, Panetta V, Lau S, Wagner P, Bergmann RL, Illi S, et al. Molecular spreading and predictive value of preclinical IgE response to Phleum pratense in children with hay fever. J Allergy Clin Immunol. 2012;130:894–901.
36. Gu ZW, Wang YX, Cao ZW. Neutralization of interleukin-17 suppresses allergic rhinitis symptoms by downregulating Th2 and Th17 responses and upregulating the Treg response. Oncotarget. 2017;8:22361–9.
37. Poole JA, Rosenwasser LJ. The role of Immunoglobulin E and immune inflammation: implications in allergic rhinitis. Curr Allergy Asthma Rep. 2005;5:252–8.
38. Mortada MM, Kurowski M. Challenges in local allergic rhinitis diagnosis, management, and research: current concepts and future perspectives. Medicina (Mex). 2023;59:929.
39. Rondón C, Canto G, Blanca M. Local allergic rhinitis: a new entity, characterization and further studies. Curr Opin Allergy Clin Immunol. 2010;10:1–7.
40. Zicari AM, Occasi F, Di Fraia M, Mainiero F, Porzia A, Galandrini R, et al. Local allergic rhinitis in children: novel diagnostic features and potential biomarkers. Am J Rhinol Allergy. 2016;30:329–34.
41. Mandhane SN, Shah JH, Thennati R. Allergic rhinitis: an update on disease, present treatments and future prospects. Int Immunopharmacol. 2011;11:1646–62.
42. Kim D, Baraniuk JN. Neural aspects of allergic rhinitis. Curr Opin Otolaryngol Head Neck Surg. 2007;15:268–73.
43. Passali FM, Passali GC, Passali D, Ciprandi G. Smell impairment in patients with allergic rhinitis. Int Forum Allergy Rhinol. 2021;11:1031–2.
44. Liu J, Zhang X, Zhao Y, Wang Y. The association between allergic rhinitis and sleep: a systematic review and meta-analysis of observational studies. Bhatt GC, editor. PLoS ONE. 2020;15:e0228533.
45. Acevedo-Prado A, Seoane-Pillado T, López-Silvarrey-Varela A, Salgado FJ, Cruz MJ, Faraldo-Garcia A, et al. Association of rhinitis with asthma prevalence and severity. Sci Rep. 2022;12:6389.
46. Masieri S, Trabattoni D, Incorvaia C, De Luca MC, Dell'Albani I, Leo G, Fet al. A role for Waldeyer's ring in immunological response to allergens. Curr Med Res Opin 2023;30:303–6.

47. De Vittori V, Pacilio A, Indinnimeo L, Marazzato M, De Castro G, Brindisi G, et al. When asthma and rhinitis coexist, could rhinitis reduce asthma control in children? Allergy Asthma Proc. 2019;40:210.
48. Siddiqui Z, Walker A, Pirwani M, Tahiri M, Syed I. Allergic rhinitis: diagnosis and management. Br J Hosp Med. 2022;83:1–9.
49. Frati F, Incorvaia C, Cavaliere C, Di Cara G, Marcucci F, Esposito S, et al. The skin prick test. J Biol Regul Homeost Agents. 2018;32(1 Suppl. 1):19–24.
50. Seidman MD, Gurgel RK, Lin SY, Schwartz SR, Baroody FM, Bonner JR, et al. Clinical practice guideline: allergic rhinitis. Otolaryngol Neck Surg. 2015;152(Suppl. 1);S1–43.
51. Van Hage M, Hamsten C, Valenta R. ImmunoCAP assays: pros and cons in allergology. J Allergy Clin Immunol. 2017;140:974–7.
52. Dramburg S, Matricardi PM. Molecular diagnosis of allergy: the pediatric perspective. Front Pediatr. 2019;7:369.
53. Wyler DK, Wyler SM. Mastocytoma of the rear limb of a dog. Mod Vet Pract. 1980;61:439–41.
54. Matricardi PM, Kleine-Tebbe J, Hoffmann HJ, Valenta R, Hilger C, Hofmaier S, et al. EAACI molecular allergology user's guide. Pediatr Allergy Immunol. 2016;27:1–250.
55. Zapletal A, Chalupová J. Nasal airflow and resistance measured by active anterior rhinomanometry in healthy children and adolescents: Rhinomanometry in Healthy Children. Pediatr Pulmonol. 2002;33:174–80.
56. Cilluffo G, Zicari AM, Ferrante G, Malizia V, Fasola S, Duse M, et al. Assessing repeatability and reproducibility of Anterior Active Rhinomanometry (AAR) in children. BMC Med Res Methodol. 2020;20:86.
57. Brindisi G, Marazzato M, Brunetti F, Castro G, Loffredo L, Carnevale R, et al. Allergic rhinitis, microbiota and passive smoke in children: a pilot study. Licari A, editor. Pediatr Allergy Immunol. 2022;33(S27):22–6.
58. Schiavi L, Brindisi G, De Castro G, De Vittori V, Loffredo L, Spalice A, et al. Nasal reactivity evaluation in children with allergic rhinitis receiving grass pollen sublingual immunotherapy. Allergy Asthma Proc. 2020;41(5):357–62.
59. Brindisi G, De Vittori V, De Nola R, Di Mauro A, De Castro G, Baldassarre ME, et al. The role of nasal nitric oxide and anterior active rhinomanometry in the diagnosis of allergic rhinitis and asthma: a message for pediatric clinical practice. J Asthma Allergy. 2021;14:265–74.
60. Gelardi M, Iannuzzi L, Quaranta N, Landi M, Passalacqua G. NASAL cytology: practical aspects and clinical relevance. Clin Exp Allergy. 2016;46:785–92.
61. Gelardi M, Cavaliere C, Jannuzzi L. Nasal cytology. J Biol Regul Homeost Agents. 2018;32(1 Suppl. 1):37–40.
62. Naclerio RM, Creticos PS, Norman PS, Lichtenstein LM. Mediator release after nasal airway challenge with allergen. Am Rev Respir Dis. 1986;134:1102.
63. Brożek JL, Bousquet J, Agache I, Agarwal A, Bachert C, Bosnic-Anticevich S, et al. Allergic Rhinitis and its Impact on Asthma (ARIA) guidelines—2016 revision. J Allergy Clin Immunol. 2017;140:950–8.
64. Head K, Snidvongs K, Glew S, Scadding G, Schilder AG, Philpott C, et al. Saline irrigation for allergic rhinitis. Cochrane ENT Group, editor. Cochrane Database Syst Rev. 2017;6:CD012597.
65. Bousquet J, Schünemann HJ, Togias A, Bachert C, Erhola M, Hellings PW, et al. Next-generation Allergic Rhinitis and Its Impact on Asthma (ARIA) guidelines for allergic rhinitis based on Grading of Recommendations Assessment, Development and Evaluation (GRADE) and real-world evidence. J Allergy Clin Immunol. 2020;145:70–80.e3.
66. Church MK, Maurer M, Simons FER, Bindslev-Jensen C, Van Cauwenberge P, Bousquet J, et al. Risk of first-generation H 1-antihistamines: a GA 2 LEN position paper. Allergy. 2010;65:459–66.
67. Licari A, Ciprandi G, Marseglia A, Castagnoli R, Barberi S, Caimmi S, et al. Current recommendations and emerging options for the treatment of allergic rhinitis. Expert Rev Clin Immunol. 2014;10:1337–47.
68. Fitzsimons R, Van Der Poel LA, Thornhill W, Du Toit G, Shah N, Brough HA. Antihistamine use in children. Arch Dis Child Educ Pract Ed. 2015;100:122–31.
69. Potter P, Maspero JF, Vermeulen J, Barkai L, Németh I, Baillieau RA, et al. Rupatadine oral solution in children with persistent allergic rhinitis: A randomized, double-blind, placebo-controlled study. Pediatr Allergy Immunol. 2013;24:144–50.
70. Murdoch D, Goa KL, Keam SJ. Desloratadine: an update of its efficacy in the management of allergic disorders. Drugs. 2003;63:2051–77.
71. Hair PI, Scott LJ. Levocetirizine: a review of its use in the management of allergic rhinitis and skin allergies. Drugs. 2006;66:973–96.
72. Sastre J, Mosges R. Local and systemic safety of intranasal corticosteroids. J Investig Allergol Clin Immunol. 2012;22:1–12.
73. Alvaro-Lozano M, Akdis CA, Akdis M, Alviani C, Angier E, Arasi S, et al. Allergen immunotherapy in children user's guide. Pediatr Allergy Immunol. 2020;31(S25):1–101.
74. Dworetzky M, Cohen SG, Frankland AW. The allergy archives. J Allergy Clin Immunol. 2003;111:1142–50.
75. Incorvaia C, Al-Ahmad M, Ansotegui IJ, Arasi S, Bachert C, Bos C, et al. Personalized medicine for allergy treatment: allergen immunotherapy still a unique and unmatched model. Allergy. 2021;76:1041–52.
76. Ciprandi G, Marseglia GL, Castagnoli R, Valsecchi C, Tagliacarne C, Caimmi S, et al. From IgE to clinical trials of allergic rhinitis. Expert Rev Clin Immunol. 2015;11:1321–33.
77. James LK, Till SJ. Potential mechanisms for IgG4 inhibition of immediate hypersensitivity reactions. Curr Allergy Asthma Rep. 2016;16:23.
78. Rolland J, Prickett S, Gardner L, O'Hehir R. T cell targeted strategies for improved efficacy and safety

of specific immunotherapy for allergic disease. Anti-Inflamm Anti-Allergy Agents Med Chem. 2013;12:201–22.

79. Muraro A, Roberts G, Halken S, Agache I, Angier E, Fernandez-Rivas M, et al. EAACI guidelines on allergen immunotherapy: executive statement. Allergy. 2018;73:739–43.
80. Bousquet J, Pfaar O, Agache I, Bedbrook A, Akdis CA, Canonica GW, et al. ARIA-EAACI care pathways for allergen immunotherapy in respiratory allergy. Clin Transl Allergy. 2021;11:e12014.
81. Roberts G, Pfaar O, Akdis CA, Ansotegui IJ, Durham SR, Gerth Van Wijk R, et al. EAACI guidelines on allergen immunotherapy: allergic rhinoconjunctivitis. Allergy. 2018;73:765–98.
82. Ai T, Zhang P, Luo R, Fan Y, Xia W, Wang L. Effectiveness of sublingual immunotherapy with house dust mite drops in asthmatic children at different ages. Front Pediatr. 2023;11:1170860.
83. Lin J, Kong Y, Chen H, Zhu M, Lv Q, Xu B, et al. Effects of acupuncture on obstructive sleep apnea-hypopnea syndrome: a meta-analysis. Res Nurs Health. 2023;46:220–35.
84. Cipriani F, Tripodi S, Panetta V, Perna S, Potapova E, Dondi A, et al. Early molecular biomarkers predicting the evolution of allergic rhinitis and its comorbidities: a longitudinal multicenter study of a patient cohort. Pediatr Allergy Immunol. 2019;30:325–34.
85. Matricardi PM. Molecular profile clustering of IgE responses and potential implications for specific immunotherapy. Curr Opin Allergy Clin Immunol. 2013;13:438–45.

10 Hymenoptera Venom Allergy in Children

Mattia Giovannini, Francesca Mori, and Elio Novembre

Abstract

Hymenoptera are taxonomically classified into different families: Apidae, including honeybees (*Apis mellifera*) and bumblebees (*Bombus*), *Vespidae*. The latter include subfamilies: Vespinae (wasps, including hornets, dolichovespules, and vespules) and Polistinae (paper wasp).

Hymenoptera venom hypersensitivity can be associated with both nonimmunological and immunological (IgE- or non-IgE-mediated) mechanisms. Several types of reactions are possible: toxic, unusual local, large local, and systemic.

An accurate clinical history and the correct use of skin and in vitro tests are crucial to properly diagnose Hymenoptera venom allergy. The in vitro tests comprise the dosage of specific serum IgE to venom extracts and to allergenic molecules. In complex diagnoses, Basophil Activation Tests and CAP inhibition can also be employed. Facing a systemic reaction, in order to exclude mastocytosis, a basal tryptase measurement should be carried out.

Based on the current guidelines, in case of anaphylaxis during the acute phase of an allergic reaction to Hymenoptera stings, signs and symptoms shall be tackled with adrenaline as the first-line treatment as well as corticosteroids and antihistamines as subsequent lines of treatment.

After a systemic reaction, the treatment for patients with hypersensitivity to Hymenoptera venom is based on venom immunotherapy (VIT), as there is no guarantee that subjects will not be stung again. In such cases, the venom is identified after a thorough allergological work-up. Both accelerated and conventional VIT administration protocols, performed in an adequate environment, have proved to be safe and effective.

In patients with a previous episode of Hymenoptera venom anaphylaxis, preventing a second episode is essential. Early therapy and environmental protection measures must be enforced. It is important to avoid risky behaviors and insect-inhabited places.

Keywords

Hymenoptera · Venom · Allergy · Children · Pediatrics

M. Giovannini (✉)
Allergy Unit, Meyer Children's Hospital IRCCS, Florence, Italy

Department of Health Sciences, University of Florence, Florence, Italy

F. Mori
Allergy Unit, Meyer Children's Hospital IRCCS, Florence, Italy
e-mail: francesca.mori@meyer.it

E. Novembre
Department of Health Sciences, University of Florence, Florence, Italy
e-mail: elio.novembre@unifi.it

C. Caffarelli, G. L. Marseglia (eds.), *Textbook of Pediatric Allergy*,
https://doi.org/10.1007/978-3-031-71283-8_10

Abbreviations

BAT	Basophil activation test
EMA	European Medicines Agency
LLRs	Large local reactions
sIgE	Specific IgE
SPTs	Skin prick tests
SRs	Systemic reactions
VIT	Venom immunotherapy

Test your learning and check your understanding of this book's contents: use the "Springer Nature Flashcards" app to access questions using ▶ https://sn.pub/nspbjm. To use the app, please follow the instructions in Chap. 1.

10.1 Stinging Hymenoptera and Their Allergens

Hymenoptera venom allergy is included among the main causes of mortality and morbidity in both pediatric age and adulthood [1]. Hymenoptera are taxonomically classified into different families: *Apidae*, including honeybees (*Apis mellifera*) and bumblebees (Bombus), *Vespidae*. The latter includes subfamilies *Vespinae* (wasps, including hornets, dolichovespules, and vespules) and *Polistinae* (paper wasp) [2]. Finally, ants also belong to the order Hymenoptera [3].

Hymenoptera usually stings to protect their hives and nests from predators or for defense [1]. Their venom includes the allergens causing Hymenoptera venom allergy.

Among Hymenoptera, only honeybees leave both the poison sac and the serrated stinger into the stung subject's skin, consequently eviscerating themselves to death [4]. Instead, yellow jackets can sting multiple times and have smooth stingers [5]. Different species of Hymenoptera release different amounts of venom with a sting. Such amounts can also vary within the same species [4, 6, 7] (Table 10.1).

Recognizing the type of Hymenoptera after being stung by one is not always possible [1]. Yet, it is crucial to identify it to perform a proper diagnostic therapeutic process [1]. In particular, in 73% of cases, the type of Hymenoptera is identified through an entomological notice board in an allergy visit [1]. Moreover, knowing their specific features, such as positioning and nest appearance, can help determine the species involved. Specifically, *Vespa*, *Dolichovespula,* and *Vespula* generally prefer underground environments to make their nests up. Hornets opt for hollow trees, whereas, finally, *Polistes* often seek shelter for nests under roof coverings [1].

Table 10.1 Quantity of venom released during a sting and characteristics of the main Hymenoptera; modified from [1]

Hymenoptera	Characteristics	Venom/sting
Honeybees	Herbivore; hive defense; stocky body covered with hair; 1–1.5 cm; serrated sting	50–140 mcg
Bumblebees	Nonaggressive; used for pollination of plants in greenhouses (they do not need to see the sun for orientation); massive body, hairy, black with streaks, white or reddish spot at the end of the abdomen; 2–3 cm; smooth sting	10–31 mcg
Yellow jackets	Aggressive, carnivorous: insect eater; attracted by food: meat, fish, and sugary substances; truncated abdomen (crossed shield), yellow with black streaks; 1.5–2 cm; smooth sting	1.7–3.1 mcg
Hornets	Moderate aggression, night flyer; massive yellow, black, and rusty body; 2.5–3.5 cm; smooth sting	Venom dry weight poison sac 260 mcg
Paper wasps	Moderate aggression; tapered body with ogival abdomen, black with yellow stripes, thin legs; 1–1.7 cm	4.2–17 mcg

Table 10.2 Studies on the epidemiology of reactions to Hymenoptera stings in children and potential association with atopic predisposition

Authors, year	Country	Number of patients	Hymenoptera sting history	Atopy	Prevalence LLR	Prevalence MSR	Prevalence SSR
Novembre et al. (1998) (questionnaire + SPT) [8]	Italy (Florence)	1175	228 (19.4%)	Related	224 (19.06%)	4 (0.34%)	
Graif et al., 2006 [10] (questionnaire)	Israel (Tel Aviv)	10,021	5624 (56.3%)	Related	1156 (11.5%)	654 (6.5%)	250 (2.5%)
Jennings et al. (2010) (questionnaire) [11]	Ireland (Cork)	4112	1544 (37.5%)	Related	90 (2.2%)	53 (1.3%)	8 (0.2%)
Quercia et al. (2014) [9] (questionnaire)	Italy (Ravenna)	1035	173 (16.7%)		9 (0.9%)	5 (0.5%)	1 (0.01%)

LLR large local reactions, *MSR* mild systemic reactions, *SPT* skin prick test, *SSR* moderate to severe systemic sting reactions

10.2 Epidemiology

According to an Italian study [8], 3.7% of children are sensitized to Hymenoptera venom. The prevalence of large local reactions (LLRs) varies from 0.9% in Italy to 11.5% in Israel. Instead, systemic reactions (SRs) in the same countries range between, respectively, <1% and 6.5% [9, 10]. According to a questionnaire-based study carried out in Israel, moderate to severe SRs account for 2.5% of cases. Data concerning the epidemiology of pediatric reactions to Hymenoptera stings are available in Table 10.2.

Twenty percentage of the general anaphylaxis among children is represented by systemic anaphylactic reactions associated with Hymenoptera venom [12], with fatal cases reported starting from the age of 5 [13].

10.3 Clinical Presentation and Pathogenesis

Hymenoptera venom hypersensitivity can be associated with both nonimmunological and immunological (IgE- or non-IgE-mediated) mechanisms. Several types of reactions are possible: toxic, unusual toxic [14–16], unusual [14], local, large local, and systemic.

10.3.1 Local Reactions

Generally, after an insect sting, nonallergic subjects report local reactions such as erythema, edema, and pain around the puncture spot. Except for occasional, small peri-lesional reactions detectable for a few days, lesions settle within 24 h.

10.3.2 LLRs

In LLRs, edema endures for more than 24 h. Starting from the puncture site, it then spreads through a diameter >10 cm. Other frequent clinical manifestations include headache, fever, asthenia, and loco-regional lymphangitis and/or lymphadenopathies. The positivity rates for skin prick tests (SPTs) and serum-specific IgE (sIgE) for Hymenoptera venom are, respectively, 70–90% and 26–50%. Clinical aspects and in vivo and vitro examinations suggest mostly an IgE-mediated reaction, in some cases a cell-mediated response or a combination of both [5].

10.3.3 SRs

Different immunological mechanisms, such as the activation of complement mediated by IgG-venom complexes, may determine SRs (anaphylaxis and nonanaphylaxis). Such reactions are mainly IgE mediated and involving, for example, the skin and mucous membranes, gastrointestinal system, cardiovascular system, respiratory system, and nervous system [5].

Clinical manifestations often are noticeable a few minutes or a few hours after the sting. Currently, from a diagnostic perspective, anaphylaxis from Hymenoptera venom and other etiologies follow the criteria stated in the guidelines. Instead, several classifications have been developed in time to define the grade of severity of SRs [17]. More than 60% of SRs in children are described as limited to the skin and mild, whereas adults suffer from cardiovascular or respiratory manifestations in 70% of cases [18].

10.4 Diagnosis

Confirming the pathogenesis, classifying the reaction type, and identifying the stinging insect are the factors leading to an accurate diagnosis, which also requires a preliminary proper medical history. Recognizing the insect through the entomological notice board is just as important [5, 19].

When only local reactions are involved, the diagnosis is merely clinical, and running allergological tests is discretionary [1]. Instead, with suspected SRs, the latter need to be performed, including, for instance, skin tests (i.e., SPTs and intradermal tests) and/or searching for sIgE so as to identify the Hymenoptera species concerned. Still, a so-called "refractory" period occurs after the massive release of mediators of the allergic response during the acute reaction [5]. That is why, in order to avoid false negatives, such tests should be carried out 2–4 weeks after acute adverse reaction.

10.4.1 Skin Tests

According to the guidelines, SPTs should be the first diagnostic step, followed by intradermal tests as a second diagnostic level in case of a negative result. Only expert personnel in a setting equipped for any reactions shall run these tests [5, 19].

The concentration for SPTs is 100 μg/ml. Starting with very low concentrations is obligatory in case of intradermal reactions, in agreement with the clinical manifestations suffered by the patient. The usual concentrations range from 0.001 to a maximum of 1 μg/ml [5]. Nonetheless, as children demonstrate less skin sensitivity, higher concentrations (0.1 mg/ml) have been suggested from the beginning in order to speed up the process [20].

Intradermal tests consist in injecting 0.02 ml of the allergenic extract into the dermis, which provokes a wheal of about 3 mm in diameter. About 15–20 min should pass before reading the results. If the diameter of the wheal obtained is double the diameter of the initial wheal or increases by at least 3 mm in the mean diameter, the test is considered positive [19, 21]. This kind of test is also recommended even in the event of a positive SPT to accurately define the cutaneous endpoint, which is beneficial in follow-ups and particularly to assess the efficacy of any specific immunotherapy (venom immunotherapy, VIT) [1, 22].

10.4.2 Dosage of sIgE

Serum venom-IgE can be measured through different diagnostic—usually immunoenzymatic—techniques. Serological tests using whole extracts are generally less sensitive than skin tests, whereas up to 20% of patients with positive skin tests can result negative to in vitro tests to detect sIgE against whole venom extract. On the other side, in vitro tests can result positive in about 10% of patients with negative skin tests. That is why running both tests is recommended in the guidelines [5, 19].

The result of either in vivo or in vitro diagnostic tests is not associated with the severity of a reaction. The highest positivity of the tests has been identified in subjects with LLRs, while approximately 25% of patients who suffered from an SR have negative SPT or positive intradermal tests only at a concentration of 1 μg/ml [5]. It is not always possible to detect sIgE after a fatal reaction to Hymenoptera stings [23]; yet, in such cases, the possibility of mast cell diseases has not been taken into consideration, but they often present negative skin tests and sIgE dosages [24].

sIgE to molecular allergens of the Hymenoptera venom are accessible and beneficial, especially for complex diagnoses [25]. Measuring total IgE can help properly interpret the result of sIgE, particularly so when the levels are very low [25].

10.4.3 Complex Diagnoses

Searching for species-specific molecular allergens (Apidae: Api m 1, Api m 2, Api m 3, Api m 5, Api m 10; Vespidae: Ves v 1, Ves v 5; Polistinae: Pol d 5) may be extremely helpful in patients with a possible history of clinically manifest IgE-mediated allergy and positive test results for both Vespidae and Apidae venom or Vespidae and Polistinae venom. Yet, a careful clinical history to recognize the insect that has most probably caused the reaction must also be taken into account. sIgE to cross-reactive molecular allergens such as Cross-Reactive Carbohydrate Determinants (CDDs) may support to distinguish genuine sensitization from co-sensitization cases [25, 26]. As a consequence, allergy specialists may rely on molecular allergology to choose the most adequate venom for VIT, this way avoiding unsuitable treatments with double venoms in some cases [27].

In cases of both negative skin tests and sIgE and suggestive clinical history as well as in cases of double positivity and molecular allergens tests with inconclusive results, performing Basophil Activation Tests (BATs) [1, 28] is recommended. The suitability of BATs for diagnosis in subjects with negative sIgE and skin tests and mast cell disorders is disputed [29, 30].

In order to evaluate how many sIgE (initially dosed to bind a specific venom) can bind to another venom with which the serum of the patient is previously incubated, CAP inhibition [31, 32] can be used. Yet, such test has some downsides in terms of costs and the difficulty to interpret results and requires highly qualified centers.

Basal serum basal tryptase should be dosed in case of an SR, as adult patients with high baseline tryptase levels and/or mast cell diseases are at remarkably higher risk of developing severe Hymenoptera sting reactions [33, 34]. A study has shown that the pediatric basal tryptase cutoff to predict a higher risk of severe reactions to Hymenoptera venom is 4.8 mcg/L [35].

For their unethical nature, their possible risk, and their low negative predictive value, sting challenges with live insects are no longer recommended to diagnose adverse reactions to venom [36].

10.5 Management

Based on the current guidelines, in case of anaphylaxis during the acute phase of an allergic reaction to Hymenoptera stings, signs and symptoms can be tackled with adrenaline as the first-line treatment as well as, e.g., corticosteroids and antihistamines as subsequent lines of treatment [37]. Specifically, when discharged from emergency care, pediatric patients with anaphylaxis to Hymenoptera venom should be adequately taught how to recognize and manage future allergic reactions (Table 10.3).

Considering its life-threatening potential, whenever Hymenoptera stings result in emergency treatments for suspected anaphylaxis, patients should be referred to specialists (possibly age-appropriate) who are trained and competent to investigate, diagnose, and monitor Hymenoptera venom allergy properly. Patients who may need VIT are also appropriately referred to allergist immunologists. On the contrary, patients with a negative clinical history should not be investigated, as venom sensitization may occur without a clinical meaning.

Patients with a history of LLR may undergo SPTs, intradermal tests, and in vitro tests such as sIgE determination at the clinician's discretion in particular cases. For instance, patients who are likely to be stung again with sizable and recurrent LLRs may benefit from immunotherapy [1].

Adrenaline should be provided to all children with a clinical history of anaphylaxis, while for LLRs (even more so after one single episode) and

Table 10.3 Information that should be provided before discharge from emergency care for severe reactions to Hymenoptera stings

Information/action	Expected response
Description of signs and symptoms of anaphylaxis	Prompt recognition of a future anaphylactic event
Information about the risk of biphasic anaphylaxis	Suspect a subsequent severe event after complete recovery of clinical manifestations and correct management of first reaction
Individualized avoidance measures	Prevent future stings by considering factors such as patient's age, activity, occupation, hobbies, residential conditions, access to medical care, and personal anxiety level
Training on the use of adrenaline autoinjectors	Correct adrenaline administration using autoinjectors
Referral to a specialist	Correct diagnosis, management (personalized action plan), and follow-up
Contact for educational programs or patients' associations	Training of caregivers (e.g., school staff)

cases of mere cutaneous systemic involvement, no unanimous consensus has been acknowledged on the constant prescription of adrenaline autoinjectors [18]. The latter should also be prescribed specifically for pediatric patients with high elevated baseline serum levels of tryptase or mast cell disorders and SRs to Hymenoptera venom, even in concomitance with VIT [37]. Concerning this, among children undergoing VIT, adrenaline autoinjectors should be provided specifically in the presence of risk factors due to incomplete clinical protection, such as severe honeybee allergy, lack of sting protection during VIT, adverse reactions during immunotherapy, and very severe onset reaction (Table 10.4).

Among several measures, the European Medicines Agency (EMA) has recently suggested the prescription of two adrenaline autoinjectors for patients at risk for anaphylaxis. Based on all the available data, the EMA confirmed intramuscular administration to be the best route for getting a quick response when treating anaphylaxis [38, 39].

Table 10.4 Indications to prescription of adrenaline autoinjectors[b]; modified from [1]

Children with previous systemic reaction or with large local reaction and high risk of re-stings (e.g., children of beekeepers) before immunotherapy
Patients with a history of large local reactions at risk of multiple stings (e.g., children of beekeepers)
Patients with a history of only one large local reaction, as the risk of more severe reactions in the event of a new sting cannot be excluded[a]
Children undergoing immunotherapy who, in the maintenance or discontinuation phase, are still at risk of incomplete clinical protection (e.g., severe honeybee allergy, lack of protection demonstrated by new Hymenoptera stings during immunotherapy, adverse reactions during immunotherapy, and very serious reactions at onset)
Children with high tryptase levels and a history of systemic Hymenoptera reactions, regardless of immunotherapy

[a]However, in case of repeated, large local reactions, prescribing an adrenaline autoinjector is not necessary, as the risk of systemic reactions is very low

[b]Among patients to be prescribed two adrenaline autoinjectors, consider, e.g., uncontrolled asthmatics (asthma is a risk factor for fatal anaphylaxis), obese patients (i.e., risk of underdosing), patients living far from a hospital, patients with mastocytosis, and patients with a history of severe systemic reactions who have required multiple doses of adrenaline

10.6 VIT

After an SR, the treatment for patients with hypersensitivity to Hymenoptera venom is based on VIT, as there is no guarantee that subjects will not be stung again. In such cases, the venom is identified after a thorough allergological work-up [40–42].

This kind of therapy lasts 3–5 years, including an induction and a maintenance phase, and consists of a subcutaneous injection between the elbow and the shoulder. In VIT, increasing doses are administered, starting from 0.001 to 0.1 mcg of the selected venom, up to a maximum dosage of 100 mcg, which is advisable for all Hymenoptera.

During the first year, the maintenance dose should be administered every 4 weeks. In the following years, the interval should be increased to 6–8 weeks. In particular cases, e.g., in patients likely to be stung again—such as beekeepers' children—or with systemic re-sting reactions during VIT, a higher maintenance dose of 200 mcg may be considered [43]. According to some pediatric studies, even a lower maintenance dose (50 mcg) appears effective [44, 45]. Different types of VIT protocols exist [46]. The choice must rely on both clinical and organizational factors such as the severity of the previous reactions and the type of allergen used [47].

The indications for performing VIT are shown in Table 10.5.

SRs involving not only the skin are the key factors to opt for VIT in pediatric age, as the development of future, more important reactions seems unlikely in patients with only cutaneous SRs. In these cases, VIT is determined only by the presence of risk factors. The indications for carrying VIT out do not include generally LLRs or random sensitization to Hymenoptera venom (e.g., following allergy multiplex tests) in patients with no clinical history of SRs [43]. Conversely, the presence of severe and recurrent LLRs can justify the use of VIT [1].

According to the guidelines [43], children up to the age of 5 are unlikely to suffer SRs after a Hymenoptera sting. However, in these cases, VIT can be prescribed based on criteria like risk factors of future SRs and clinical manifestations. VIT is generally a useful treatment to lower the risk of new SRs, as proved by the comparison with untreated patients [43, 48]. Its use is beneficial in 77–84% of honeybee allergy cases and in 91–96% of wasp allergy cases [49–53].

Table 10.5 Indications for VIT; modified from [1]

Systemic skin reaction in the presence of risk factors[a] with documented sensitization through positive allergy tests (skin tests and/or serum-specific IgE)
Systemic reaction involving other systems than the skin with documented sensitization through positive allergy tests (skin tests and/or serum-specific IgE)
Systemic reaction in patients with clonal mast cell disease with documented sensitization by positive allergy tests (skin tests and/or serum-specific IgE)

[a]E.g., risk of exposure (increased sting risk, as in children of beekeepers), distance from a first aid point, and compromised quality of life (e.g., excessive anxiety in the child or their parents)

VIT has equally proved to be safe, seeing that most of the local adverse reactions take place at the injection site. Low rates of LLRs and contained rates (4–6%) of SRs were also reported in the latest pediatric studies, the latter occurring more frequently with honeybee venom in the build-up phase [54–56]. LLRs that are sometimes not even reported were described, and the studies mainly focused on reporting systemic ones.

Even lifelong VIT can be recommended in patients with clonal mast cell disorders [1], although no data on the long-term protection of VIT beyond 15 years are currently available.

While following up with patients undergoing immunotherapy, sensitization should be monitored by running allergy tests (skin tests and sIgE) 3 and 5 years after the therapy started and after every new sting. At the end of the VIT, a control visit should be scheduled every time a new puncture occurs and at each appointment arranged to prescribe adrenaline with the performance of the therapeutic education session [1]. After each single dose is administered, the patient should be kept under observation for at least 1 h. The administration must be carried out with the necessary safety measures to exclude possible—though rare—severe adverse reactions [19].

10.7 Prevention

In patients with a previous episode of Hymenoptera venom anaphylaxis, preventing a second episode is essential. Early therapy and environmental protection measures must be enforced. It is important to avoid risky behaviors and insect-inhabited places. The risk of suffering new Hymenoptera stings can be substantially lowered through prevention and prompt referral to an allergist for correct diagnosis and proper follow-up [57]. In addition, treating new stings properly is crucial in susceptible subjects [58] (Table 10.6).

Patients allergic to Hymenoptera sting should receive detailed written information and be explained how to avoid future stings. An emergency medical kit including, e.g., antihistamines, steroids and, above all, adrenaline

Table 10.6 Actions to be taken in case of Hymenoptera puncture in patients at risk for anaphylaxis

Check the time immediately, as it is useful to evaluate the onset of clinical manifestations
Leave the scene of the accident as quickly—though cautiously—as possible
In the event of a honeybee sting, remove the sting immediately, preferably with a magnetic card or similar
In case signs and symptoms appear, take the necessary emergency medications, as personalized treatment plan
If you are alone, try to reach an inhabited place or a first aid as soon as possible; report your condition and position to the emergency medical service at the initial clinical manifestations. If you are in a company, immediately inform those around you and start the previous procedures together
Own a plate or form with identification notes indicating the allergic condition

autoinjectors, when needed, should be provided, together with practical, clear demonstration supervised by a qualified nurse or a doctor [59]. Allergic patients must be made aware of the possibility of undergoing VIT, as it is the only treatment that can improve their quality of life and modifying the natural history of the disease. Considering its low-cost nature, patients should always be educated on how to avoid future stings as a preventive measure. Several recommendations have been proposed, which can potentially minimize the risk of re-sting, based on the current knowledge of Hymenoptera's habitats and living conditions [58].

Take-Home Messages

- Hymenoptera are taxonomically classified into different families: Apidae, including honeybees (*Apis mellifera*) and bumblebees (Bombus), Vespidae. The latter includes subfamilies: Vespinae (wasps, including hornets, dolichovespules, and vespules) and Polistinae (paper wasp).
- Hymenoptera venom hypersensitivity can be associated with both nonimmunological and immunological (IgE- or non-IgE-mediated) mechanisms. Several types of reactions are possible: toxic, unusual local, large local, and systemic.
- An accurate clinical history and the correct use of skin and in vitro tests are crucial to properly diagnose Hymenoptera venom allergy. The in vitro tests comprise the dosage of specific serum IgE to venom extracts and to allergenic molecules. In complex diagnoses, Basophil Activation Tests and CAP inhibition can also be employed. Facing a systemic reaction, in order to exclude mastocytosis, a basal tryptase measurement should be carried out.
- Based on the current guidelines, in case of anaphylaxis during the acute phase of an allergic reaction to Hymenoptera stings, signs and symptoms shall be tackled with adrenaline as a first-line treatment as well as corticosteroids and antihistamines as subsequent lines of treatment.
- After a systemic reaction, the treatment for patients with hypersensitivity to Hymenoptera venom is based on venom immunotherapy (VIT), as there is no guarantee that subjects will not be stung again. In such cases, the venom is identified after a thorough allergological work-up. Both accelerated and conventional VIT administration protocols, performed in an adequate environment, have proved to be safe and effective.
- In patients with a previous episode of Hymenoptera venom anaphylaxis, preventing a second episode is essential. Early therapy and environmental protection measures must be enforced. It is important to avoid risky behaviors and insect-inhabited places.

Acknowledgments Not applicable.

Material in the Electronic Repository Not applicable.

Ethic Statement Not applicable.

Data Sharing and Data Accessibility Not applicable.

Conflicts of Interests The authors declare that they have no conflict of interest to disclose in relation to this paper.

Financial Support This research did not receive any specific grant from funding agencies in the public, commercial, or nonprofit sectors.

Author Contributions MG and EN conceptualized the work. MG and EN acquired the data and drafted the initial manuscript. MG, FM, and EN analyzed the data and reviewed the manuscript. All authors have read and agreed to the published version of the manuscript.

References

1. Bilò M, Pravettoni V, Bignardi D, Bonadonna P, Mauro M, Novembre E, et al. Hymenoptera venom allergy: management of children and adults in clinical practice. J Investig Allergol Clin Immunol. 2019;29:180–205.
2. Severino MG, Campi P, Macchia D, Manfredi M, Turillazzi S, Spadolini I,et al. European Polistes venom allergy. Allergy. 2006;61:860–3.
3. Caplan EL, Ford JL, Young PF, Ownby DR. Fire ants represent an important risk for anaphylaxis among residents of an endemic region. J Allergy Clin Immunol. 2003;111:1274–7.
4. Hoffman DR, Jacobson RS. Allergens in hymenoptera venom XII: how much protein is in a sting? Ann Allergy. 1984;52:276–8.
5. Bilo BM, Rueff F, Mosbech H, Bonifazi F, Oude-Elberink JNG. Diagnosis of Hymenoptera venom allergy. Allergy. 2005;60:1339–49.
6. Schumacher M, Tveten M, Egen N. Rate and quantity of delivery of venom from honeybee stings. J Allergy Clin Immunol. 1994;93:831–5.
7. Pecoraro L, Giovannini M, Mori F, Saretta F, Barni S, Castagnoli R, et al. Immunotherapy for Hymenoptera venom allergy compared with real-life stings: are we doing our best? Clin Exp Allergy. 2021;51:209–11.
8. Novembre C, Bernardini V, Ingargiola L, Vierucci. Epidemiology of insect venom sensitivity in children and its correlation to clinical and atopic features. Clin Exp Allergy. 1998;28:834–8.
9. Quercia O, Incorvaia C, Marseglia GL, Puccinelli P, Dell'albani I, Emiliani F, Frati F, Stefanini GF. Prevalence and incidence of reactions to insect stings in children: a reappraisal. Minerva Pediatr. 2014;66:257–60.
10. Graif Y, Romanozelekha O, Livne I, Green M, Shohat T. Allergic reactions to insect stings: results from a national survey of 10,000 junior high school children in Israel. J Allergy Clin Immunol. 2006;117:1435–9.
11. Jennings A, Duggan E, Perry IJ, Hourihane JO. Epidemiology of allergic reactions to hymenoptera stings in Irish school children. Pediatr Allergy Immunol. 2010;21:1166–70.
12. Worm M, Moneret-Vautrin A, Scherer K, Lang R, Fernandez-Rivas M, Cardona V, et al. First European data from the network of severe allergic reactions (NORA). Allergy. 2014;69:1397–404.
13. Pouessel G, Tanno LK, Claverie C, Lejeune S, Labreuche J, Dorkenoo A, et al. Fatal anaphylaxis in children in France: analysis of national data. Pediatr Allergy Immunol. 2018;29:101–4.
14. Castagnoli R, Giovannini M, Mori F, Barni S, Pecoraro L, Arasi S, et al. Unusual reactions to hymenoptera stings: current knowledge and unmet needs in the pediatric population. Front Med (Lausanne). 2021;8:717290.
15. Fitzgerald KT, Flood AA. Hymenoptera stings. Clin Tech Small Anim Pract. 2006;21:194–204.
16. Bresolin NL, Carvalho FC, Goes JC, Fernandes V, Barotto AM. Acute renal failure following massive attack by Africanized bee stings. Pediatr Nephrol. 2002;17:625–7.
17. Simons FER, Ardusso LRF, Bilò MB, El-Gamal YM, Ledford DK, Ring J, Sanchez-Borges M, et al. World Allergy Organization anaphylaxis guidelines: summary. J Allergy Clin Immunol. 2011;127:587–593.e22.
18. Bilò MB, Cichocka-Jarosz E, Pumphrey R, Oude-Elberink JN, Lange J, Jakob T, et al. Self-medication of anaphylactic reactions due to Hymenoptera stings-an EAACI Task Force Consensus Statement. Allergy. 2016;71:931–43.
19. Krishna MT, Ewan PW, Diwakar L, Durham SR, Frew AJ, Leech SC, et al. Diagnosis and management of hymenoptera venom allergy: British Society for Allergy and Clinical Immunology (BSACI) guidelines. Clin Exp Allergy. 2011;41:1201–20.
20. Cichocka-Jarosz E, Stobiecki M, Brzyski P, Rogatko I, Nittner-Marszalska M, Sztefko K, et al. Simplification of intradermal skin testing in Hymenoptera venom allergic children. Ann Allergy Asthma Immunol. 2017;118:326–32.
21. Chiriac AM, Bousquet J, Demoly P. In vivo methods for the study and diagnosis of allergy. In: Middleton's allergy. Elsevier; 2014. p. 1119–32.
22. Corallino M, Nico A, Kourtis G, Caiaffa MF, Macchia L. Skin testing technique and precision in stinging insect allergy. J Clin Nurs. 2007;16:1256–64.
23. Hoffman DR. Fatal reactions to hymenoptera stings. Allergy Asthma Proc. 2003;24:123–7.
24. Bonadonna P, Perbellini O, Passalacqua G, Caruso B, Colarossi S, Dal Fior D, et al. Clonal mast cell disorders in patients with systemic reactions to Hymenoptera stings and increased serum tryptase levels. J Allergy Clin Immunol. 2009;123:680–6.
25. Matricardi PM, Kleine-Tebbe J, Hoffmann HJ, Valenta R, Hilger C, Hofmaier S, et al. EAACI molecular allergology user's guide. Pediatr Allergy Immunol. 2016;27:1–250.

26. Müller UR, Johansen N, Petersen AB, Fromberg-Nielsen J, Haeberli G. Hymenoptera venom allergy: analysis of double positivity to honey bee and *Vespula* venom by estimation of IgE antibodies to species-specific major allergens Api m1 and Ves v5. Allergy. 2009;64:543–8.
27. Sturm GJ, Biló MB, Bonadonna P, Hemmer W, Caruso B, Bokanovic D, et al. Ves v 5 can establish the diagnosis in patients without detectable specific IgE to wasp venom and a possible north-south difference in Api m 1 sensitization in Europe. J Allergy Clin Immunol. 2012;130:817.
28. Balzer L, Pennino D, Blank S, Seismann H, Darsow U, Schnedler M, et al. Basophil activation test using recombinant allergens: highly specific diagnostic method complementing routine tests in wasp venom allergy. PLoS One. 2014;9:e108619.
29. Bonadonna P, Zanotti R, Melioli G, Antonini F, Romano I, Lenzi L, et al. The role of basophil activation test in special populations with mastocytosis and reactions to hymenoptera sting. Allergy. 2012;67:962–5.
30. Stoevesandt J, Sturm GJ, Bonadonna P, Oude Elberink JNG, Trautmann A. Risk factors and indicators of severe systemic insect sting reactions. Allergy. 2020;75:535–45.
31. Savi E, Peveri S, Makri E, Pravettoni V, Incorvaia C. Comparing the ability of molecular diagnosis and CAP-inhibition in identifying the really causative venom in patients with positive tests to Vespula and Polistes species. Clin Mol Allergy. 2016;14:3.
32. Quercia O, Cova V, Martini M, Cortellini G, Murzilli F, Bignardi D, et al. CAP-inhibition, molecular diagnostics, and total IgE in the evaluation of polistes and vespula double sensitization. Int Arch Allergy Immunol. 2018;177:365–9.
33. Ruëff F, Przybilla B, Biló MB, Müller U, Scheipl F, Aberer W, et al. Predictors of severe systemic anaphylactic reactions in patients with Hymenoptera venom allergy: importance of baseline serum tryptase—a study of the European Academy of Allergology and Clinical Immunology Interest Group on Insect Venom Hypersensitivity. J Allergy Clin Immunol. 2009;124:1047–54.
34. Bonadonna P, Bonifacio M, Lombardo C, Zanotti R. Hymenoptera allergy and mast cell activation syndromes. Curr Allergy Asthma Rep. 2016;16:5.
35. Yavuz ST, Sackesen C, Sahiner UM, Buyuktiryaki B, Arik Yilmaz E, et al. Importance of serum basal tryptase levels in children with insect venom allergy. Allergy. 2013;68:386–91.
36. Ruëff F, Przybilla B, Müller U, Mosbech H. The sting challenge test in Hymenoptera venom allergy position paper of the subcommittee on Insect Venom Allergy of the European Academy of Allergology and Clinical Immunology. Allergy. 1996;51:216–25.
37. Muraro A, Roberts G, Worm M, Bilò MB, Brockow K, Fernández Rivas M, et al. Anaphylaxis: guidelines from the European Academy of Allergy and Clinical Immunology. Allergy. 2014;69:1026–45.
38. Lieberman P, Nicklas RA, Randolph C, Oppenheimer J, Bernstein D, Bernstein J, et al. Anaphylaxis—a practice parameter update 2015. Ann Allergy Asthma Immunol. 2015;115:341–84.
39. EMA Adrenaline auto-injectors. https://www.ema.europa.eu/en/medicines/human/referrals/adrenaline-auto-injectors.
40. Dhami S, Nurmatov U, Varga E-M, Sturm G, Muraro A, Akdis CA, et al. Allergen immunotherapy for insect venom allergy: protocol for a systematic review. Clin Transl Allergy. 2015;6:6.
41. Sahiner UM, Durham SR. Hymenoptera venom allergy: how does venom immunotherapy prevent anaphylaxis from Bee and wasp stings? Front Immunol. 2019;10:1959.
42. Valentine MD, Schuberth KC, Kagey-Sobotka A, Graft DF, Kwiterovich KA, Szklo M, et al. The value of immunotherapy with venom in children with allergy to insect stings. N Engl J Med. 1990;323:1601–3.
43. Sturm GJ, Varga E-M, Roberts G, Mosbech H, Bilò MB, Akdis CA, et al. EAACI guidelines on allergen immunotherapy: Hymenoptera venom allergy. Allergy. 2018;73:744–64.
44. Konstantinou GN, Manoussakis E, Douladiris N, Hatziioannou A, Giavi S, Saxoni-Papageorgiou P, et al. A 5-year venom immunotherapy protocol with 50 µg maintenance dose: safety and efficacy in school children. Pediatr Allergy Immunol. 2011;22:393–7.
45. Houliston L, Nolan R, Noble V, Pascoe E, Hobday J, Loh R,et al. Honeybee venom immunotherapy in children using a 50-µg maintenance dose. J Allergy Clin Immunol. 2011;127:98–9.
46. Saretta F, Giovannini M, Pessina B, Barni S, Liccioli G, Sarti L, et al. Venom Immunotherapy protocols in the pediatric population: how to choose? Frontiers in Pediatrics. 2023;11:1192081.
47. Fiedler C, Miehe U, Treudler R, Kiess W, Prenzel F. Long-term follow-up of children after venom immunotherapy: low adherence to anaphylaxis guidelines. Int Arch Allergy Immunol. 2017;172:167–72.
48. Dhami S, Zaman H, Varga E-M, Sturm GJ, Muraro A, Akdis CA, et al. Allergen immunotherapy for insect venom allergy: a systematic review and meta-analysis. Allergy. 2017;72:342–65.
49. Ruëff F, Przybilla B, Biló MB, Müller U, Scheipl F, Seitz MJ, et al. Clinical effectiveness of hymenoptera venom immunotherapy: a prospective observational multicenter study of the European Academy of Allergology and Clinical Immunology Interest Group on Insect Venom Hypersensitivity. PLoS One. 2013;8:e63233.
50. Macchia D, Cortellini G, Mauro M, Meucci E, Quercia O, Manfredi M, et al. Vespa crabro immunotherapy versus Vespula-venom immunotherapy in Vespa crabro allergy: a comparison study in field re-stings. World Allergy Org J. 2018;11:3.
51. Hunt KJ, Valentine MD, Sobotka AK, Benton AW, Amodio FJ, Lichtenstein LM. A controlled trial of immunotherapy in insect hypersensitivity. N Engl J Med. 1978;299:157–61.

52. Muller U, Helbling A, Berchtold E. Immunotherapy with honeybee venom and yellow jacket venom is different regarding efficacy and safety. J Allergy Clin Immunol. 1992;89:529–35.
53. Ruëff F, Vos B, Oude Elberink J, Bender A, Chatelain R, Dugas-Breit S, et al. Predictors of clinical effectiveness of Hymenoptera venom immunotherapy. Clin Exp Allergy. 2014;44:736–46.
54. Gür Çetinkaya P, Esenboğa S, Uysal Soyer Ö, Tuncer A, Şekerel BE, Şahiner ÜM. Subcutaneous venom immunotherapy in children. Ann Allergy Asthma Immunol. 2018;120:424–8.
55. Steiss J-O, Jödicke B, Lindemann H. A modified ultrarush insect venom immunotherapy protocol for children. Allergy Asthma Proc. 2006;27:148–50.
56. Nittner-Marszalska M, Cichocka-Jarosz E, Małaczyńska T, Kraluk B, Rosiek-Biegus M, Kosinska M, et al. Safety of ultrarush venom immunotherapy: comparison between children and adults. J Investig Allergol Clin Immunol. 2016;26:20–47.
57. Bonifazi F, Jutel M, Bilo BM, Birnbaum J, Muller U. Prevention and treatment of hymenoptera venom allergy: guidelines for clinical practice. Allergy. 2005;60:1459–70.
58. Clark S, Camargo CA. Emergency treatment and prevention of insect-sting anaphylaxis. Curr Opin Allergy Clin Immunol. 2006;6:279–83.
59. El Turki A, Smith H, Llewellyn C, Jones CJ. A systematic review of patients', parents' and healthcare professionals' adrenaline auto-injector administration techniques. Emerg Med J. 2017;34:403–16.

11 Anaphylaxis

Calvani Mauro and Decimo Fabio

Abstract

Anaphylaxis is a rapid-onset systemic hypersensitivity reaction that can have a potentially fatal outcome. It is caused by the release of preformed mediators and de novo synthesis of mediators from mast cells and basophils, typically mediated by IgE. In childhood, the most common triggers for anaphylactic reactions are foods, followed by drugs. Clinical manifestations may occur with certain evocative symptoms preceding the onset of the classic symptoms, which affect the skin or mucosa, respiratory system, gastrointestinal system, cardiovascular system, and may contribute to the onset of neurological symptoms.

The diagnosis of anaphylaxis is based on clinical criteria. Treatment involves promptly recognizing the signs and symptoms of an anaphylactic reaction and rapidly administering intramuscular adrenaline, which is the preferred first-choice drug due to its speed and effectiveness. Auto-injectors are preferable for easy use in patients who have received appropriate training. Antihistamines are only useful in treating skin symptoms, such as hives and itching. Corticosteroids are recommended for treating shock and asthma, along with inhaled beta-2-agonists.

It is important to note that after the initial medical intervention, anaphylactic reactions often require immediate hospitalization to optimize therapy and monitoring. This is necessary to assess any protracted or biphasic response that, although infrequent, can still pose a life-threatening risk to the patient.

Keywords

Anaphylaxis · IgE-mediated allergy · Childhood · Food allergy · Life-threatening systemic allergic reaction · Biphasic reactions · Plasma tryptase assay · Intramuscolar adrenaline · Autoinjector · Antihistamines · Corticosteroids · Beta-2 short agonists · Hospital observation · Long term management · Behavioral strategies

Test your learning and check your understanding of this book's contents: use the "Springer Nature Flashcards" app to access questions using ▶ https://sn.pub/nspbjm. To use the app, please follow the instructions in Chap. 1.

C. Mauro (✉)
Operative Unit of Pediatrics, S. Camillo-Forlanini Hospital, Rome, Italy

D. Fabio
Department of Woman, Child and of General and Specialized Surgery, University of Campania "Luigi Vanvitelli", Naples, Italy
e-mail: fabio.decimo@unicampania.it

C. Caffarelli, G. L. Marseglia (eds.), *Textbook of Pediatric Allergy*,
https://doi.org/10.1007/978-3-031-71283-8_11

11.1 Introduction

Anaphylaxis is a severe, life-threatening systemic allergic reaction that occurs suddenly after contact with an allergy-causing substance and that may have a wide range of clinical manifestations [1].

11.2 Anaphylaxis Triggers (Causes, Elicitors, or Inducers)

In pediatric age, foods represent the main triggers, followed by drugs. The foods most commonly involved are milk, eggs, fish, peanuts, and nuts in early life; and wheat, cereals, and shellfish in young adults [2]. Among drugs, the most common culprits are betalactam antibiotics and non-steroidal anti-inflammatory drugs (NSAIDs) [3]. Hymenoptera venom is also among the agents able to cause anaphylactic reactions. In some cases, the presence of more than one trigger is necessary for the allergic reaction, while one trigger alone is tolerated. This rare condition is called summation anaphylaxis (SA) [4]. Hidden allergens (such as sulfite, spices, dust mite allergen, mislabeled or undeclared known food allergens, food additive carmine powder, and psyllium), inhalation or contact aeroallergens, alpha-gal anaphylaxis, catamenial anaphylaxis, undifferentiated somatoform anaphylaxis are other less frequent causes of anaphylaxis. Cholinergic urticaria and cold urticaria sometimes can evolve into anaphylaxis. Finally, idiopathic anaphylaxis (IA) refers to anaphylaxis without a discernible cause after completion of an appropriate diagnostic evaluation [5].

11.3 Underlying Mechanisms

Most anaphylaxis reactions are due to the IgE-mediated mechanism. It is triggered by the interaction of an allergen (usually a protein) with the allergen-specific IgE/high-affinity receptor (FcεRI) complex expressed on effector cells, particularly mast cells and basophils, with subsequent release of preformed and de novo synthesis of mediators and cytokines responsible of clinical manifestations [6–8].

IgE-mediated anaphylaxis should be differentiated from other mechanism [9], also characterized by immediate systemic reactions, which may be immunologic and nonimmunologic. In immunologic mechanisms, the involved agents act through an IgG-mediated pathogenetic mechanism, complement activation (anaphylatoxins, C3a, C5a), and immune complexes formation exerting a direct action on mast cells and basophils. They are generally induced by immunoglobulin G (IgG) infusion (e.g., in children with immunodeficiency), contrast agents, NSAIDs, dextrans, and biologic drugs.

Physical exertion, stress, infection, heat, cold, sunlight, NSAIDs, and alcohol are able to contribute to the development of an allergic reaction to anaphylaxis with nonimmunologic mechanisms [10].

11.4 Epidemiology

Defining the epidemiology of anaphylaxis is challenging due to several factors including: (a) variations in the definition used in different studies; (b) differences in study populations (hospitalized patients, emergency room admissions, specialist clinics, general pediatric populations, populations covered by private insurance, general population, etc.); (c) issues with underdiagnosis and overdiagnosis; (d) individuals affected by anaphylaxis may not always seek medical attention; and (e) ICD9 codes do not include a separate category for anaphylaxis without shock.

Despite these challenges, there seems to be an increasing incidence and prevalence of anaphylaxis over the past 10–20 years. It remains uncertain whether this increase is due to a genuine rise in anaphylactic reactions or improved recognition of clinical manifestations by healthcare providers [11].

Recent data show wide variation in the global incidence of anaphylaxis in children, ranging from 50 to 112 episodes per 100,000 individuals per year, with a prevalence of 0.3–3.1% [12–14]. In Europe, the estimated incidence among children ranges from 1 to 761 cases per 100,000 individuals per year, with over a quarter of anaphylaxis cases occurring before the age of 18, and the most affected age group being 0–4 years old. A retrospective study conducted in the United States found a 101% increase in emergency department admissions for anaphylaxis between 2005 and 2014, along with a 37.6% increase in hospitalizations for the same reason. Similar upward trends have been observed in Europe, the United Kingdom, and Australia, with Australia having the highest hospitalization rate for anaphylaxis [13, 15].

However, the overall mortality rate from anaphylaxis remains relatively stable, with fatal outcomes estimated at approximately 0.5–1% among hospitalized anaphylaxis cases [16].

Data on fatal anaphylaxis in children are limited and vary across regions. In the United Kingdom, where a national registry for fatal anaphylaxis has been established since 1992, the mortality rate has more than halved in the past 20 years [17]. In a U.S. study, a total of 2458 anaphylaxis-related deaths were reported between 1999 and 2010. Among individuals aged 19 years or younger, 22.6% of anaphylaxis-related deaths were attributed to food ingestion, with the highest proportion (52.4%) of these deaths occurring in outpatient facilities. Furthermore, in the same age group, 3.4% of the deaths were associated with drug reactions, and the majority of these cases (58.6%) took place in inpatient facilities [18]. Similar findings have been observed in France and Australia [19, 20].

Overall, although anaphylaxis is relatively common, deaths from anaphylaxis are fortunately rare, particularly in the first years of life, with a mortality rate of less than 1 death per million inhabitants per year [8]. Factors associated with a higher risk of fatal anaphylaxis triggered by food ingestion include adolescence, previous reaction history, peanut and tree nut allergies, bronchial asthma, and the absence of skin symptoms.

11.5 Definition and Clinical Criteria for Anaphylaxis

Defining anaphylaxis is challenging due to its diverse clinical manifestations and underlying pathophysiological mechanisms. As a result, there is no internationally standardized definition, and it has evolved over time, with ongoing discussions and updates.

Previously, a consensus definition of anaphylaxis was "a serious allergic reaction that can lead to death," [1] confirmed by the International Consensus on Anaphylaxis [21]. Afterward, other guidelines have proposed different definitions. The European Academy of Allergy and Clinical Immunology (EAACI) defines anaphylaxis as "a life-threatening reaction characterized by the acute onset of symptoms involving various organ systems, requiring immediate medical intervention" [22]. The Australasian Society of Clinical Immunology and Allergy (ASCIA) Guideline defines anaphylaxis as "an acute onset illness with typical skin features (urticarial rash or erythema/flushing and/or angioedema), along with involvement of the respiratory and/or cardiovascular system and/or persistent severe gastrointestinal symptoms. It also includes any acute onset of hypotension or bronchospasm or upper airway obstruction where anaphylaxis is considered possible, even in the absence of typical skin features" [23]. The World Allergy Organization (WAO) defines anaphylaxis as "a serious systemic hypersensitivity reaction that usually has a rapid onset and may cause death" [10]. Common elements in the different definitions of anaphylaxis are: (a) being a consequence of an allergic reaction or hypersensitivity, (b) having an acute or rapid onset compared to exposure to the trigger, (c) being a systemic reaction involving multiple organs or systems, and (d) being life-threatening.

However, there are exceptions to these points. In some cases, anaphylaxis may develop "later," as seen in delayed anaphylaxis to red meat [24] or summation anaphylaxis [4]. Additionally, anaphylaxis may not always manifest as a systemic reaction, as suggested by the previous definition from the ASCIA.

11.6 Clinical Presentation

Symptoms of food anaphylaxis may develop within seconds to a few hours after the ingestion of a food allergen, with most reactions developing within the first hour. A "metallic" taste in the mouth, a tingling sensation, itching, a burning sensation in the hands and/or feet, an anogenital region, or feelings of anxiety, and/or disorientation are reported as part of prodromal symptoms of anaphylaxis. These symptoms may precede the onset of more classic symptoms affecting the skin, respiratory system, gastrointestinal system, and cardiovascular system.

The skin and mucosal tissue are commonly involved in anaphylaxis, leading to the appearance of erythema, hives, itching, and, in some cases, generalized urticaria with angioedema. The respiratory tract is frequently affected, with symptoms ranging from sneezing, nasal discharge, and obstruction to coughing, wheezing, and laryngeal stridor, eventually leading to significant breathing difficulties. Asthma is more commonly seen in children who already have asthma and is a risk factor for fatal outcomes, particularly in childhood, whereas cardiovascular impairment is a more frequent cause of death for anaphylaxis in adults.

Gastrointestinal symptoms may start with oral itching and/or burning of the tongue, followed by abdominal pain, nausea, vomiting, or diarrhea. Although gastrointestinal symptoms are not life-threatening, they can be associated with cardiovascular impairment, possibly due to increased intestinal permeability and fluid loss, as well as diarrhea [2].

Initial cardiovascular involvement may be challenging for parents to detect, as it presents with tachycardia, which may be followed by hypotension, arrhythmias, or bradycardia.

Cardiac and respiratory involvement contributes to the onset of neurological symptoms, such as worsening malaise, decreased reactivity, agitation in younger children, and even loss of consciousness. Headache may occur following the resolution of the event.

11.7 Clinical Diagnosis of Anaphylaxis

The essential clinical criteria for making a correct diagnosis of anaphylaxis have evolved over time and are still being discussed and updated. In 2006, the National Institute of Allergy and Infectious Disease and Food Allergy and Anaphylaxis Network proposed a universally accepted definition of anaphylaxis and established clinical criteria that would accurately identify cases of anaphylaxis [1]. Their aim is to provide healthcare practitioners on how to accurately recognize anaphylaxis symptoms, avoiding overtreatment for mild reactions while ensuring timely pharmacological intervention for reactions that pose a small risk of progressing into a life-threatening form. It has been demonstrated that these criteria have a diagnostic accuracy of up to 95% [3] (see Table 11.1).

Recently, the WAO Anaphylaxis Committee [10] reviewed and modified these criteria to simplify them. The updated criteria consist of two main criteria:

1. Acute onset of an illness (within minutes to several hours) with simultaneous involvement of the skin, mucosal tissue, or both, along with at least one of the following: (a) respiratory compromise, (b) reduced blood pressure or associated symptoms of organ dysfunction, and (c) severe gastrointestinal symptoms.
2. Acute onset of hypotension, bronchospasm, or laryngeal involvement following exposure to a known or highly probable allergen for that patient (within minutes to several hours), even in the absence of typical skin involvement.

However, these modified criteria have not yet been validated.

Table 11.1 Clinical criteria indicative of anaphylaxis (from Sampson HA et al. 2006, modified)

Anaphylaxis is highly probable in the presence of one of the following criteria:
1. Acute onset (minutes to several hours) of a clinical presentation involving the skin and/or mucosal tissue (e.g., generalized urticaria, itching or flushing, swollen lips, tongue, or uvula)
And at least one of the following:
(a) respiratory impairment (e.g., dyspnea, wheezing-bronchospasm, stridor, reduced PEF, hypoxemia)
(b) blood pressure decrease or symptoms of organ dysfunction (e.g., hypotonia-collapse, syncope, incontinence)
2. Two or more of the following clinical presentations that occur suddenly after exposure to a likely allergen or other trigger for that patient (minutes to a few hours):
(a) clinical presentation involving the skin and/or mucosal tissue (e.g., generalized urticaria, itching or flushing, swelling of lips, tongue, or uvula)
(b) respiratory impairment (e.g., dyspnea, wheezing-bronchospasm, stridor, reduced PEF, and hypoxemia)
(c) blood pressure decrease or symptoms of organ dysfunction (e.g., hypotonia-collapse, syncope, and incontinence)
(d) gastrointestinal tract symptoms (e.g., abdominal cramps and vomiting)
3. Blood pressure decreases after exposure to a known allergen for that patient or another anaphylaxis trigger (minutes to several hours)

11.8 Diagnostic Tests in Acute Anaphylaxis

Diagnosis of anaphylaxis is primarily based on the clinical history and recent exposure to the triggering allergen and biomarkers have no role in acute management. However, certain laboratory tests, such as tryptase, histamine, chymase, carboxypeptidase A3, dipeptidyl peptidase I (DPPI), basogranulin, CCL-2, and platelet-activating factor (PAF), collected during or immediately after the acute event on serum, plasma, and possibly urine, can support the clinical diagnosis, aid in differential diagnosis, and confirm the diagnosis in cases of fatal outcomes [25].

Up to now, the only test suggested to be used is the plasma tryptase assay, which detects the enzyme released by mast cells, a central cell in the allergic reaction. Two forms of tryptase can be detected: mature tryptase and total tryptase. While the exact biological function of tryptase is not fully defined, a rapid increase in serum or plasma levels indicates mast cell involvement in the observed clinical manifestation [26]. Serum levels start to rise 5 min after the onset of anaphylaxis symptoms, peak between 30 and 90 min, and remain elevated for several hours in cases of substantial increases due to the half-life of approximately 2 h.

Normal values of total tryptase range between 1 and 11.4 ng/ml (with a mean value of 3–5 ng/ml), with slightly higher levels in infants compared to children and adults [27]. Conversely, serum levels of mature tryptase are not detectable in healthy individuals who have never experienced anaphylaxis (<1 ng/ml).

Therefore, it is recommended to measure tryptase levels between 30 min and 2 h after the onset of the reaction (although elevated values may persist for longer) and compare them with measurements taken at least 24 h after complete resolution of symptoms, even when acute-phase levels are within normal limits. These measurements are crucial for a correct differential diagnosis, distinguishing anaphylaxis from other conditions such as mast cell disorders and hereditary alpha-tryptasemia, which are characterized by elevated basal tryptase levels that do not decrease within a few hours like in anaphylaxis.

In this regard, a "consensus" on mast cell activation disorders, including mast cell activation syndromes, suggested in 2010 that an acute serum level of total tryptase, obtained between half an hour and 2 h after the onset of the reaction, should be at least 20% higher than the basal tryptase level + 2 ng/ml to indicate mast cell activation syndrome and anaphylaxis [28].

However, it is important to note the following:

- Measurement of tryptase levels should not delay the administration of adrenaline if necessary.
- The increase in tryptase levels does not occur in all patients with anaphylaxis, and a failure to find elevated tryptase levels does not rule out the event, especially if samples are collected more than 4 h after the onset of the episode or in the absence of hypotension.
- The most significant increases in tryptase levels have been observed after drug-induced anaphylaxis.
- The increase in tryptase levels correlates with the severity of hypotension during anaphylaxis but not with skin, respiratory, or gastrointestinal signs or symptoms [29].

Regarding histamine, a biogenic amine found in mast cells and basophils, increased levels of plasma or urinary histamine can support the diagnosis of anaphylaxis, although normal levels do not rule it out. After its release, the majority of free histamine is quickly metabolized into other metabolites (methylhistamine and methylimidazole acetic acid) that are excreted in urine and can be detected in certain laboratories. Thus, although plasma histamine assays have higher sensitivity than tryptase, their usefulness in clinical practice is limited due to the short half-life of histamine [10, 22].

11.9 Differential Diagnosis of Anaphylaxis

When making a diagnosis of anaphylaxis, it is necessary to consider and exclude other potential diagnoses [22], including, depending on the main symptoms presented:

- *Involvement of the skin or mucosal tissue:* chronic remittent or physical urticaria and angioedema.
- *Respiratory diseases:* acute laryngotracheitis, laryngeal, tracheal, or bronchial obstruction (e.g., foreign substances, intermittent laryngeal obstruction or vocal cord dysfunction), and status asthmaticus (without involvement of other organs).
- *Cardiovascular diseases:* vasovagal syncope and cardiac arrhythmias.
- *Pharmacological or toxic reactions:* scombroid fish poisoning.
- *Neuropsychiatric diseases:* hyperventilation syndrome, anxiety and panic disorder, and somatoform disorder (e.g., psychogenic dyspnea).
- *Endocrinological diseases:* hypoglycemia, thyrotoxic crisis, carcinoid syndrome, vasointestinal polypeptide tumors, and pheochromocytoma.

11.10 Prompt Initial Treatment of Anaphylaxis

At the onset of allergic reactions, it is impossible to predict whether the reaction will progress to anaphylaxis and potentially lead to death within minutes or resolve spontaneously. Therefore, the prompt administration of intramuscular adrenaline (epinephrine) is the primary treatment approach. Additionally, placing the patient in a supine position with elevated legs (anti-shock position) helps redistribute circulating blood volume and enhances perfusion to vital organs. If there is no difficulty in breathing, the patient can be placed in the Trendelenburg position. It is important not to raise the patient. Keeping the patient flat improves venous blood return to the heart, while an upright position may impede blood return, leading to inadequate circulation and low blood pressure [23]. Seek assistance and continuously monitor vital signs, including cardiac and respiratory activity as well as blood pressure, while ensuring open airways.

In cases of anaphylaxis resulting from insect bites or drug/vaccine injections, apply a tourniquet above the injection site and release it for 1 min every 3 min to slow down the absorption of the substance.

Adrenaline is crucial in the treatment of anaphylaxis. All guidelines recommend the intramuscular administration of adrenaline as the first-line drug. The recommended dose is 0.01 mg/kg of a 1:1000 (1 mg/ml) solution, up to a maximum of 0.5 mg in adults and 0.3 mg in children, injected into the anterolateral thigh. A

Table 11.2 Dosing of available epinephrine autoinjectors in Italy

Brand	Dose	Needle length	Expiry (months)
Chenpen©	**150** mcg (for children15–30 kg) **300** mcg (for children > 30 kg) **500** mcg (for >50 kg—authorized only for adults)	10 ± 1.5 mm 10 ± 1.5 mm 10 ± 1.5 mm	21–24
Fastjekt©	**150** mcg (for children 15–30 kg) **300** mcg (for children > 30 kg)	16 mm 16 mm	19–20
Jekt©	**150** mcg (for children 15–30 kg) **300** mcg (for children > 30 kg)	13 mm 15 mm	18

Epinephrine doses may need to be repeated every 5–15 min
Epinephrine autoinjectors should be kept at 20–25 °C

second dose may be repeated after 5–15 min if the response to the initial injection is inadequate [30]. The specific dosing for available autoinjector devices in Italy is outlined in Table 11.2.

It should be administered early once symptoms of anaphylaxis have been recognized or suspected [30] because it is the drug that acts most quickly on all pathways of anaphylaxis. Its clinical effects include inducing vasoconstriction, bronchodilation, reduced mucosal edema, increased inotropy, and chronotropy. Epinephrine also downregulates the continued release of mediators of anaphylaxis, such as PGE2, from mast cells and circulating basophils [31].

There are no absolute contraindications to the use of adrenaline for anaphylaxis. Serious adverse effects are very rare when epinephrine is administered at the appropriate intramuscular dose. In cases of anaphylaxis with hemodynamic compromise, intravenous (IV) crystalloid fluids should be infused. Anaphylactic shock occurs due to a profound reduction in venous tone and fluid extravasation, so adrenaline may not be effective without restoring circulatory volume.

Parenteral administration of glucagon may be used in patients with anaphylaxis who do not respond optimally to adrenaline, particularly in patients taking beta-blockers, although there is limited evidence supporting its use [10].

According to recent guidelines, antihistamines are considered a second- or third-line intervention and should not be used as the initial emergency treatment for airway/breathing/circulation problems, as their effect has only been demonstrated in relieving skin symptoms. Their onset of action is approximately 30 min after administration, with a peak effect after 1–2 h. Antihistamines are unable to stabilize or prevent mast cell degranulation, nor do they prevent the appearance of respiratory and/or cardiovascular symptoms or a biphasic reaction. Their use must not delay the management of respiratory or cardiovascular symptoms of anaphylaxis, which requires the use of adrenaline and IV fluids.

Glucocorticoids are commonly used in the treatment of anaphylaxis, although there is no evidence supporting their effectiveness in the acute phase due to their relatively slow onset of action. Therefore, their administration is recommended as a second- or third-line treatment for anaphylaxis. A recent Canadian study involving 3498 cases of anaphylaxis, both prospectively and retrospectively, showed that the administration of steroids before arrival at the hospital was associated with an increased risk of intensive care unit admissions, with an odds ratio of 2.84 (95% CI 1.5–6.97), after correcting for several confounding factors [32].

Thus, it was suggested that steroids should not be used in the acute phase but only in cases of shock, anaphylaxis refractory to 2 doses of adrenaline, and uncontrolled asthma [33].

Beta-2 agonists (such as salbutamol) may be useful as adjunct treatment for lower respiratory symptoms caused by anaphylaxis, following initial treatment with IM adrenaline in the presence of persistent respiratory symptoms. They can be administered using metered-dose inhaler devices with a spacer or aerosol. However, they should not be used, even parenterally, as an alternative to further parenteral treatment with adrenaline [33].

Following an episode of anaphylaxis, even if the symptoms have subsided, it is necessary to observe the patient since in 3–20% of cases, symptoms can reoccur without re-exposure to the allergen (biphasic reaction), in a completely

Table 11.3 Duration of hospital observation after an episode of anaphylaxis in the different recent Guidelines or Position Papers

ASCIA Guideline (2020) [23]	Observe the patient for at least 4 h after the last dose of adrenaline. Relapse protracted and/or biphasic reactions may occur. Overnight observation is strongly recommended if they: (a) had severe or protracted anaphylaxis (e.g., required repeated doses of adrenaline or IV fluid resuscitation), OR (b) have a history of severe/protracted anaphylaxis, OR (c) have other concomitant illness (e.g. severe asthma, history of arrhythmia, systemic mastocytosis), OR (d) live alone or are remote from medical care, OR (e) present for medical care late in the evening
WAO Guidance Anaphylaxis 2020 [10]	Around half of biphasic reactions occur within the first 6–12 h following reaction. Patients with anaphylaxis need to be observed: this is important especially in severe reactions and those requiring multiple doses of epinephrine
Anaphylaxis—A 2020 Practice Parameter Update [30]	For patients without severe risk features, discharge after a 1-h asymptomatic observation may be reasonable. If the clinical impression is that a patient has a higher risk of biphasic reaction (i.e., 17% or greater) or risk factors for anaphylaxis fatality (e.g., cardiovascular comorbidity, lack of access to epinephrine, lack of access to emergency medical services (EMS), poor self-management skills), then extended observation of up to 6 h or longer (including hospital admission) may be appropriate
European Resuscitation Council. Evidence update for the treatment of anaphylaxis. (2021) [33]	(a) Consider fast-track discharge (after 2 h observation from resolution of anaphylaxis) if: a good response (within 5–10 min) to a single dose of adrenaline given within 30 min of onset of reaction AND complete resolution of symptoms AND the patient already has unused adrenaline auto-injectors (AAI) and has been trained how to use them AND there is adequate supervision following discharge (a) Minimum 6 h observation after resolution of symptoms recommended if: 2 doses of IM adrenaline needed to treat reaction OR previous biphasic reaction (c) Observation for at least 12 h following resolution of symptoms if any one of the following: (1) severe reaction requiring >2 doses of adrenaline (2) patient has severe asthma or reaction involved severe respiratory compromise (3) possibility of continuing absorption of allergen, e.g., slow release medicines (4) patient presents late at night, or may not be able to respond to any deterioration (5) patients in areas where access
EAACI Guidelines: Anaphylaxis (2021 update) [22]	The task force suggests that they are monitored for 6–8 h with respiratory compromise and at least 12–24 h with hypotension. Before discharge, assess the risk of future reactions and prescribe adrenaline autoinjectors to those at risk of recurrence. However, the duration of observation may be extended in the presence of certain risk factors, such as severe asthma, evening or nighttime presentation, limited access to emergency care, previous history of biphasic reactions, multi-organ involvement, severe respiratory component, or the need for multiple doses of epinephrine for initial treatment

unpredictable manner. Although biphasic anaphylaxis can occur within 72 h, a systematic review of 27 studies showed that approximately half of the episodes of biphasic anaphylaxis occur after 10–11 h [34]. However, there is no consensus in the literature regarding the duration of observation after an episode of anaphylaxis.

Different guidelines recommend varying durations of hospital observation following an episode of anaphylaxis. The duration ranges from 1 h in patients without severe symptoms or regression of symptoms to 12 h or more in patients with severe reactions requiring 2 or more doses of adrenaline (see Table 11.3).

11.11 Long-term Management of Anaphylaxis

The primary objective of long-term management of anaphylaxis is the prevention and treatment of future episodes. In this context, the EAACI guidelines offer recommendations regarding the prescription of adrenaline auto-injectors for patients at risk of developing anaphylaxis, based on anamnestic evidence of specific allergen involvement or individual predisposition [22]. Additionally, these guidelines differentiate between absolute and relative recommendations (see Table 11.4), emphasizing that in cases of relative recommendations, the prescription of adrenaline should be carefully evaluated if more than one of the listed conditions is present in the same patient.

Table 11.4 Absolute and relative indications for adrenaline prescription in pediatric age—(modified from Muraro A et al. 2022)

Absolute and relative indications to adrenaline prescription on pediatric age
1. Absolute indications
• Previous food, latex, or aeroallergens anaphylaxis
• Previous exercise-induced anaphylaxis
• Previous idiopathic anaphylaxis
• Concomitant persistent uncontrolled or moderate-severe asthma or concomitant food allergy[a]
• Hymenoptera venom allergy in patients with more extensive involvement than muco-cutaneous alone or at high risk of re-exposure
• During and after immunotherapy for hymenoptera venom in patients with more extensive than muco-cutaneous reactions alone and risk of re-exposure
• Systemic mastocytosis with severe skin involvement (>50%) and increased serum tryptase level (>20 ng/ml) and with bullous form in the first 3 years of life
2. Relative indications
• Previous mild to moderate reaction to foods[a] known to be associated with anaphylactic reactions in own geographic area
• Adolescents with mild-to-moderate allergic food reactions[a]
• Distant from hospital or frequent international travels in case of mild-moderate food, hymenoptera venom, latex, or aeroallergens reactions
• Previous mild-to-moderate reaction to small amounts of food[a]
• Patients with hymenoptera venom allergy or drug allergy with more extensive involvement than muco-cutaneous alone and concomitant cardiovascular disease
• Oral food immunotherapy

[a]Except for "pollen food syndrome" unless positive history of systemic symptoms

There are differences in guidelines regarding the prescription of adrenaline in patients with IgE-mediated food allergies in the absence of anaphylaxis. The NIAID expert panel [35] recommends adrenaline prescription for all cases of IgE-mediated food allergy due to the unpredictable occurrence of severe reactions. The EAACI and BSACI guidelines [22, 36] instead suggest prescription only in cases of reported anaphylaxis or mild reactions to small food amounts.

Recently, the European Medicines Agency (EMA) [37] and the EAACI guidelines [22] have highlighted the option of prescribing two auto-injectors per patient in case of occasional risk of failure to administer the auto-injector due to technical issues, inappropriate administration site, or the potential need for two successive doses of adrenaline, which can occur in up to 10% of anaphylaxis cases [38].

However, this remains a controversial issue [39]. The EAACI, in agreement with other authors [40], emphasizes that prescribing two auto-injectors may reduce patient availability in carrying both devices and increase related costs.

It should be noted that during an anaphylactic reaction, the real problem lies not in the lack of a sufficient number of auto-injectors, but rather in having them available and not using them in a timely and appropriate manner. Therefore, it is crucial to provide patients, parents, and individuals who care for at-risk individuals (such as babysitters and school staff) [41] with a personalized treatment plan for proper symptom management. Additionally, qualified personnel should provide structured and comprehensive training, including precise instructions on recognizing anaphylaxis symptoms, situations requiring adrenaline administration, and proper auto-injector usage [22, 42, 43]. Up to now, this training process is often inadequate. Some authors have noted that despite visual and verbal instructions from trained personnel and the provision of a written action plan, only half of patients with recurrent anaphylaxis are able to recognize symptoms and correctly use the adrenaline auto-injector [42, 44].

It has been observed that most cases of fatal food anaphylaxis occur in the adolescent-young adult age group [45, 46]. However, only 10% of college students at risk of food anaphylaxis carry the adrenaline auto-injector at all times. This can be attributed to a tendency in this age group to evade medical supervision and reject their at-risk status, as they often remain asymptomatic for extended periods [42].

Therefore, in all individuals at risk of anaphylaxis, even if they have been asymptomatic for a long time, it is essential to consistently implement useful behavioral strategies to avoid triggers and promptly manage emergencies. However, this inevitably places a significant psychological burden on both the patients themselves and their family members, leading to constant anxiety, stress, and significant impacts on their quality of life.

Lastly, there is a need to improve anaphylaxis management guidelines in school settings. Food-related anaphylaxis occurs more frequently in schools than in any other community setting, necessitating educational support and the development of appropriate protocols for managing at-risk individuals [22, 42, 47].

11.12 Summary

In conclusion, anaphylaxis is a rapid-onset systemic hypersensitivity reaction that can have potentially fatal outcomes. Although anaphylaxis is relatively common, death from anaphylaxis is fortunately rare in children. At the onset of allergic reactions, it is impossible to predict the course of the reaction, whether it will progress into anaphylaxis with a potentially rapid and severe outcome, or if the patient will respond promptly to treatment or recover spontaneously. Thus, the prompt administration of intramuscular adrenaline remains the cornerstone of treatment.

Key Points

- Anaphylaxis is a rapid-onset systemic reaction, with possible, although rare, fatal outcome.
- Diagnosis of anaphylaxis is mainly based on clinical criteria.
- The rapid administration of intramuscular adrenaline is the first choice treatment.
- Antihistamines and corticosteroids are considered second- and third-line interventions.
- The long-term management of anaphylaxis is prevention and the treatment of new episodes.

References

1. Sampson HA, Muñoz-Furlong A, Campbell RL, Adkinson NF Jr, Bock SA, Branum A, et al. Second symposium on the definition and management of anaphylaxis: summary report—second National Institute of Allergy and Infectious Disease/Food Allergy and Anaphylaxis Network symposium. Ann Emerg Med. 2006;47:373–80.
2. Calvani M, Cardinale F, Martelli A, Muraro A, Pucci N, Savino F, et al. Risk factors for severe pediatric food anaphylaxis in Italy. Pediatr Allergy Immunol. 2011;22:813–9.
3. Poowuttikul P, Seth D. Anaphylaxis in children and adolescents. Pediatr Clin N Am. 2019;66:995–1005.
4. Calvani M, Anania C, Cuomo B, D'Auria E, Decimo F, Indirli GC, et al. Summation anaphylaxis: a challenging diagnosis. Pediatr Allergy Immunol. 2020;31(Suppl. 26):33–5.
5. Calvani M. Update on idiopathic anaphylaxis. Pediatr Allergy Immunol. 2022;33(Suppl. 27):52–3.
6. Galli SJ, Tsai M. IgE and mast cells in allergic disease. Nat Med. 2012;18:693–704.
7. Brown SGA, Stone SF, Fatovich DM, Burrows SA, Holdgate A, Celenza A, et al. Anaphylaxis: clinical patterns, mediator release, and severity. J Allergy Clin Immunol. 2013;132:1141–9.

8. Mikhail I, Stukus DR, Prince BT. Fatal anaphylaxis: epidemiology and risk factors. Curr Allergy Asthma Rep. 2021;21:28.
9. Simons FER, Ardusso LRF, Bilò MB, El-Gamal YM, Ledford DK, Ring J, et al. World allergy organization guidelines for the assessment and management of anaphylaxis. World Allergy Organ J. 2011;4:13–37.
10. Cardona V, Ansotegui IJ, Ebisawa M, El-Gamal Y, Fernandez Rivas M, Fineman S, et al. World allergy organization anaphylaxis guidance 2020. World Allergy Organ J. 2020;13:100472.
11. Bagos-Estevez AG, Ledford DK. Anaphylaxis: definition, epidemiology, diagnostic challenges, grading system. Immunol Allergy Clin N Am. 2022;42:1–11.
12. Pattanaik D, Lieberman P, Lieberman J, Pongdee T, Keene AT. The changing face of anaphylaxis in adults and adolescents. Ann Allergy Asthma Immunol. 2018;121:594–7.
13. Motosue MS, Li JT, Campbell RL. Anaphylaxis: epidemiology and differential diagnosis. Immunol Allergy Clin N Am. 2022;42:13–25.
14. Tejedor Alonso MA, Moro Moro M, Múgica García MV. Epidemiology of anaphylaxis. Clin Exp Allergy. 2015;45:1027–39.
15. Turner PJ, Campbell DE, Motosue MS, Campbell RL. Global trends in anaphylaxis epidemiology and clinical implications. J Allergy Clin Immunol Pract. 2020;8:1169–76.
16. Turner PJ, DunnGalvin A, Hourihane JOB. The Emperor has no symptoms: the risks of a blanket approach to using epinephrine autoinjectors for all allergic reactions. J Allergy Clin Immunol Pract. 2016;4:1143–6.
17. Baseggio Conrado A, Ierodiakonou D, Gowland MH, Boyle RJ, Turner PJ. Food anaphylaxis in the United Kingdom: analysis of national data, 1998–2018. BMJ. 2021;372:n251.
18. Jerschow E, Lin RY, Scaperotti MM, McGinn AP. Fatal anaphylaxis in the United States, 1999–2010: temporal patterns and demographic associations. J Allergy Clin Immunol. 2014;134:1318–28.
19. Mullins RJ, Wainstein BK, Barnes EH, Liew WK, Campbell DE. Increases in anaphylaxis fatalities in Australia from 1997 to 2013. Clin Exp Allergy. 2016;46:1099–110.
20. Pouessel G, Claverie C, Labreuche J, Dorkenoo A, Renaudin JM, Eb M, et al. Fatal anaphylaxis in France: analysis of national anaphylaxis data, 1979–2011. J Allergy Clin Immunol. 2017;140:610–2.
21. Simons FER, Ardusso LR, Bilò MB, Cardona V, Ebisawa M, El-Gamal YM, et al. International consensus on (ICON) anaphylaxis. World Allergy Organ J. 2014;7:9.
22. Muraro A, Worm M, Alviani C, Cardona V, DunnGalvin A, Garvey LH, et al. EAACI guidelines: Anaphylaxis (2021 update). Allergy. 2022;77:357–77.
23. Australian Society of Clinical Immunology and Allergy (ASCIA) (2020) Guideline for the acute management of anaphylaxis. https://www.allergy.org.au/hp/papers/acutemanagement-of-anaphylaxis-guidelines
24. Commins SP, Satinover SM, Hosen J, Mozena J, Borish L, Lewis BD, et al. Delayed anaphylaxis, angioedema, or urticaria after consumption of red meat in patients with IgE antibodies specific for galactose-alpha-1,3-galactose. J Allergy Clin Immunol. 2009;123:426–33.
25. Beck SC, Wilding T, Buka RJ, Baretto RL, Huissoon AP, Krishna MT. Biomarkers in human anaphylaxis: a critical appraisal of current evidence and perspectives. Front Immunol. 2019;10:494.
26. Schwartz LB. Diagnostic value of tryptase in anaphylaxis and mastocytosis. Immunol Allergy Clin N Am. 2006;26:451–63.
27. Sahiner UM, Yavuz ST, Buyuktiryaki B, Cavkaytar O, Arik Yilmaz E, Tuncer A, et al. Serum basal tryptase levels in healthy children: correlation between age and gender. Allergy Asthma Proc. 2014;35:404–8.
28. Valent P, Akin C, Arock M, Brockow K, Butterfield JH, Carter MC, et al. Definitions, criteria and global classification of mast cell disorders with special reference to mast cell activation syndromes: a consensus proposal. Int Arch Allergy Immunol. 2012;157:215–25.
29. Schwartz LB, Yunginger JW, Bokhari R, Bokhari R, Dull D. Time course of appearance and disappearance of human mast cell tryptase in the circulation after anaphylaxis. J Clin Invest. 1989;83:1551–5.
30. Shaker MS, Wallace DV, Golden DBK, Oppenheimer J, Bernstein JA, Campbell RL, et al. Anaphylaxis-a 2020 practice parameter update, systematic review, and Grading of Recommendations, Assessment, Development and Evaluation (GRADE) analysis. J Allergy Clin Immunol. 2020;145:1082–123.
31. Vadas P, Perelman B. Effect of epinephrine on platelet-activating factor-stimulated human vascular smooth muscle cells. J Allergy Clin Immunol. 2012;129:1329–33.
32. Gabrielli S, Clarke A, Morris J, Eisman H, Gravel J, Enarson P, et al. Evaluation of prehospital management in a Canadian emergency department ana phylaxis cohort. J Allergy Clin Immunol Pract. 2019;7:2232–2238.e3.
33. Dodd A, Hughes A, Sargant N, Whyte AF, Soar J, Turner PJ. Evidence update for the treatment of anaphylaxis. Resuscitation. 2021;163:86–96.
34. Liu X, Lee S, Lohse CM, Hardy CT, Campbell RL. Biphasic reactions in emergency department anaphylaxis patients: a prospective cohort study. J Allergy Clin Immunol Pract. 2020;8:1230–8.
35. Boyce JA, Assa'd A, Burks AW, et al. Guidelines for the diagnosis and management of food allergy in the United States: report of the NIAID-sponsored expert panel. J Allergy Clin Immunol. 2010;126(6 Suppl):S1–58.
36. Jones C. Allergy UK, a national patient organisation, response to the BSACI guideline: prescribing an adrenaline auto-injector. Clin Exp Allergy. 2016;46:1619–20.
37. European Medicines Agency. Adrenaline Auto-injectors. In: https://www.ema.europa.eu/en/medicines/human/referrals/adrenaline-auto-injectors.

38. Patel N, Chong KW, Yip AYG, Ierodiakonou D, Bartra J, Boyle RJ, et al. Use of multiple epinephrine doses in anaphylaxis: a systematic review and meta-analysis. J Allergy Clin Immunol. 2021;148:1307–15.
39. Dribin TE, Waserman S, Turner PJ. Who needs epinephrine? Anaphylaxis, autoinjectors, and parachutes. J Allergy Clin Immunol Pract. 2023;11:1036–46.
40. Shaker M, Turner PJ, Greenhawt M. A cost-effectiveness analysis of epinephrine autoinjector risk stratification for patients with food allergy-one epinephrine autoinjector or two? J Allergy Clin Immunol Pract. 2021;9:2440–51.
41. Tiyyagura GK, Arnold L, Cone DC, Langhan M. Pediatric anaphylaxis management in the prehospital setting. Prehosp Emerg Care. 2014;18:46–51.
42. Brockow K, Schallmayer S, Beyer K, Biedermann T, Fischer J, Gebert N, et al. Effects of a structured educational intervention on knowledge and emergency management in patients at risk for anaphylaxis. Allergy. 2015;70:227–35.
43. Fernandez-Mendez F, Saez-Gallego NM, Barcala-Furelos R, Abelairas-Gomez C, Padron-Cabo A, Perez-Ferreiros A, et al. Learning and treatment of anaphylaxis by laypeople: a simulation study using pupilar technology. Biomed Res Int. 2017; 2017:9837508.
44. Mullins RJ. Anaphylaxis: risk factors for recurrence. Clin Exp Allergy. 2003;33:1033–40.
45. Bock SA, Muoz-Furlong A, Sampson HA. Fatalities due to anaphylactic reactions to foods. J Allergy Clin Immunol. 2001;107:191–3.
46. Bock SA, Muñoz-Furlong A, Sampson HA. Further fatalities caused by anaphylactic reactions to food, 2001–2006. J Allergy Clin Immunol. 2007;119:1016–8.
47. Portnoy JM, Shroba J. Managing food allergies in schools. Curr Allergy Asthma Rep. 2014;14:1–7.

12 Drug Allergy in Children

Silvia Maria Elena Caimmi, Paolo Triggiano,
and Carlo Caffarelli

Abstract

Drug allergies constitute a significant healthcare concern because of their frequency and the entity of their manifestations, ranging from mild skin rashes to life-threatening anaphylaxis. This chapter provides an overview of drug allergy epidemiology, mechanisms, diagnosis, and management strategies. The development of drug allergies involves complex immunological processes. Drugs can act as haptens, binding in various ways to endogenous proteins and triggering an immune response that involves the activation of several immune cells, resulting in the release of inflammatory mediators such as histamine. Genetic predisposition and prior sensitization play pivotal roles in determining individual susceptibility to drug allergy. Accurate diagnosis is therefore essential to evaluate drug discontinuation. Patient history, combined with diagnostic tools such as skin tests, in vitro tests, and drug provocation tests, represents the crucial step of the allergological workup. However, the diagnostic tools may have limitations, necessitating careful interpretation by experienced clinicians. When identified, the cornerstone of drug allergy management lies in the avoidance of the implicated drug and the use of alternative medications. When that is not possible, drug desensitization protocols have proved to be an effective strategy. In conclusion, drug allergies are intricate immune responses that can lead to various clinical manifestations. Understanding the underlying mechanisms, precise diagnosis, and effective management are essential for providing optimal patient care. Collaborative efforts between clinicians, researchers, and patients are needed to address this challenge and to enhance our ability to prevent and manage drug hypersensitivity reactions effectively.

Test your learning and check your understanding of this book's contents: use the "Springer Nature Flashcards" app to access questions using ▶ https://sn.pub/nspbjm. To use the app, please follow the instructions in Chap. 1.

S. M. E. Caimmi (✉) · P. Triggiano
UOC Pediatria, Fondazione IRCCS Policlinico San Matteo, Pavia, Italy
e-mail: silviamaria.caimmi@unipv.it

C. Caffarelli
Clinica Pediatrica, Azienda Ospedaliero-Universitaria, Department of Medicine and Surgery, Università di Parma, Parma, Italy

C. Caffarelli, G. L. Marseglia (eds.), *Textbook of Pediatric Allergy*,
https://doi.org/10.1007/978-3-031-71283-8_12

12.1 Introduction

Adverse drug reactions (ADRs) are a response to a noxious and unintended medicine and are generally classified by the European Academy for Allergy and Clinical Immunology (EAACI) group into two types [1]. Type A reactions are exaggerated responses to drugs' normal pharmacological actions when administered at the standard therapeutic dose. Type B reactions are unpredictable responses based on known pharmacological actions of the drug. Both reactions are dose-independent. Type B reactions, however, can be potentially life-threatening and may warrant a change in the treatment. Drug hypersensitivity reaction (DHR) may be defined as an adverse drug reaction (ADR), to an otherwise safe and effective therapeutic agent, that is immunologically mediated [2]. DHRs represent a relevant clinical field due to their frequency and potential severity. In the last decades, immunological research revealed the underlying mechanism of this type of reaction, enabling better diagnosis and case management. However, DHRs remain not preventable, causing 3–5% of hospitalizations [3]. The presentation is heterogeneous, including multiple forms of allergic, pharmacologic, and pseudoallergic reactions to medication that result from an exaggerated immunologic or inflammatory response [4]. Coombs and Gell's classification is no longer suitable to realize all possible DHRs since it defines the phenotypes (i.e., the clinical manifestations) of DHRs but not all different pathogenic mechanisms (endotypes). In addition, Coombs and Gell's classification does not include the more recently discovered pseudoallergic reactions (PARs) [5]. In the pediatric age, there are many diagnoses of drug allergy that are not confirmed by an accurate allergy workup. An incorrect diagnosis leads to negative consequences on the quality of medical care since the patient is left without the first-choice drug. Furthermore, it has been demonstrated that antibiotic allergic labels limit their use and increase microbial antibiotic resistance. This generates significant socioeconomic indirect costs and supports the necessity of evidence-based allergy workup and delabeling. In this chapter, we will outline the most recent advancements in the epidemiology, classification, clinical presentation, and management of DHRs.

12.2 Epidemiology

ADRs globally account for 3–6% of hospital admissions, occurring in 10–15% of hospitalized patients and up to 25% of outpatients [6]. DHRs are approximately less than 10% of all ADRs, representing 1–2% of all admissions and 3–5% of hospitalized patients [7]. Nevertheless, the true incidence of drug allergy is not known, mainly because most epidemiologic studies report ADRs rather than drug allergy. Moreover, children are frequently misdiagnosed as being "allergic" to a medication. They carry this label into adulthood if no accurate allergic workup is performed.

12.2.1 Risk Factors

Among all the patients treated with a given drug, DHRs occur only in a small percentage of the cases. This predisposition could be explained both by genetic and environmental factors. Even though the development of DHR is impossible to predict, factors that increase its likelihood have been identified. These factors can be divided into drug-related and patient-related. Drug-related factors include the nature of the drug, the degree of exposure (dose, duration, and frequency of administration), the route of administration, and cross-sensitization. Among the patient-related factors, age, sex and genetic factors such as acetylation status and human leukocyte antigen (HLA) type, concurrent medical illnesses such as EBV infection, HIV, and asthma, and previous drug reaction, as well as multiple allergy syndrome have been observed [6]. The combination of these factors may allow the onset of a DHR.

12.2.1.1 Drug-Related Factors

Nature of the Drug

The drug features that increase its immunogenicity and subsequently, its potential to elicit DHRs involve the ability to act as a hapten, a prohapten, or to bind covalently to immune receptors [8]. Based on this, some classes of drugs such as antibiotics and analgesics tend to be associated with a higher frequency of drug allergies [9].

Degree of Exposure

Although rigorous studies on this subject are lacking, intermittent and repeated administration appears to favor DHRs more than uninterrupted and prolonged treatment [6].

Route of Administration

Topical application is associated with an increased risk of sensitization, especially on inflamed skin. The parenteral route appears to be more sensitizing than oral administration despite systematic studies on this issue are lacking [6].

Cross-Sensitization

Once sensitization to a given drug occurs, reactions to drugs that present a similar chemical structure or that produce similar metabolites may occur. Some examples are cross-reactions among phenothiazine derivatives or, even if rare, between beta-lactam (BL) drugs [9].

12.2.1.2 Patient-Related Factors

Age and Sex

Concerning the age groups, it is unclear if DHRs are actually less frequent in children than in adults, due to multiple biases such as the discrepancy between self-reported ADR and proved DHR, lack of accurate allergic workup, and multiple drug regimens, mainly in geriatric patients. It has been suggested that DHRs are less frequent and less severe in children and elderly because of immaturity and involution of their immune systems, respectively [10]. However, patients aged >65 years present an increased risk of severe reactions such as anaphylactic shock [11]. With regard to sex, females appear more likely to develop drug allergies than males [12] after puberty [13]. This difference may be explained by different hormonal interactions with immune cells and epigenetic factors. However, it may also depend on higher drug consumption in women compared to men [6]. Furthermore, there are no differences in manifestations and mortality [14]. Consequently, the selection of a drug cannot be based on sex.

Genetics

HLA class I (HLA A, HLA B, and HLA C) molecules are ubiquitous intracellular antigens to CD8+ cytotoxic T cells. HLA class II (HLA DP, HLA DQ, and HLA DR) molecules are found on the immune cells, and they present extracellular antigens to CD4+ helper T cells. It has been suggested that the features of this presentation of drug-derived antigen from the major histocompatibility complex (MHC) play a key role in the development of drug hypersensitivity [15]. There is a strong association between the haplotype HLA-DRB1*07:01-HLA-DQB1*02:02-DQA1*02:01 and immediate hypersensitivity to asparaginase and between HLADRB1*07:01 and polyethyleneglycol in asparaginase. Immediate penicillin hypersensitivity reactions have been associated with HLA-DRB1*10:01 and HLA-B*55:01. The HLA haplotypes carrying a higher risk of delayed DHR associated with a given drug vary according to the geographical area are depicted in Table 12.1.

Table 12.1 HLA haplotypes associated with severe delayed hypersensitivity reactions [6]

HLA	Population	DHR
B*15:02	Han Chinese, Thai, Indian	SJS/TEN for carbamazepine
A*31:01	Northern Europe	MPE, DRESS, SJS/TEN for carbamazepine
B*57:01	Caucasians	Severe hypersensitivity for abacavir
B*58:01	Han Chinese, Caucasians	SJS/TEN, DRESS for allopurinol
B*13:01	Chinese, Papuans/Australian, Aboriginals	DRESS for dapsone
B*57:01	European	Liver injury from flucloxacillin

SJS Steven-Johnson syndrome, *TEN* toxic epidermal necrolysis, *MPE* maculopapular exanthema, *DRESS* drug reaction with eosinophilia and systemic symptoms

Concurrent Medical Illness

A concurrent illness may affect the immunologic response to drugs by altering metabolic pathways. For example, in conditions with impairment of cellular hypersensitivity (e.g., sarcoidosis), exanthems, and contact dermatitis are less likely to occur, whereas in immunodeficiency, such as hypogammaglobulinemia, antibody-mediated allergy is rare [6]. The underlying disease also may imply an increased exposure to high doses of the drug, as it occurs in cystic fibrosis patients, who present a higher incidence of beta-lactam allergy [16]. Similarly, patients with HIV and AIDS frequently present DHRs to cotrimoxazole. It is unclear whether this increased likelihood of developing DHRs is due to predisposition or frequent use of the drugs [6]. With regard to chemotherapeutic agents, it has been reported that several factors, such as disease severity, histological type, cumulative dose, and past drug allergies, increase the risk of DHRs. Finally, infections appear to be associated with DHRs. Maculopapular rashes arise commonly in patients with Epstein-Barr virus or picornavirus infection after amoxicillin administration [17]. The role of human herpesvirus-6 in the drug reaction with eosinophilia and systemic symptoms/drug-induced hypersensitivity reaction (DRESS/DIHS) is also well-known. Its reactivation induces proinflammatory cytokines that induce the reaction through cross-reaction of expanded $CD8^+$ T cells with the administered drug [18].

Previous Drug Exposure

DHR to a certain drug may increase the likelihood of developing sensitivity to other drugs. So, particular attention is necessary in this group of patients [7]. Additionally, it is worth noticing that even if IgE-mediated reactions generally require previous exposure to a given drug, anaphylaxis may develop upon first exposure to neuromuscular blocking agents after previous intake of products that contain pholcodine such as cough syrup [19].

Multiple Drug Hypersensitivity Syndrome (MDHS)

MDHS is defined as confirmed drug hypersensitivity to at least two chemically and pharmacologically unrelated drugs. It was first described in 1989 by Sullivan at al. as a distinct clinical entity that differs from cross-reactivity (due to structural similarities, common metabolic pathways, or pharmacological mechanisms), flare-up reactions (exacerbation of an existing DHR by the early switch of therapy to a novel drug), or multiple drug intolerance syndrome (ADR to ≥3 classes of chemically unrelated drugs without proven immunologic mechanism). The epidemiology of MDHS is not defined because data are mostly based only on history, without skin testing and drug provocation test (DPT) which are mandatory for confirming the diagnosis. A major study enveloped in Montpellier demonstrated a prevalence of 0.5% in 9250 patients explored by allergy workup [20]. A variety of drugs were considered, the most common being antibiotics and nonsteroidal anti-inflammatory drugs (NSAIDs). Some of the risk factors reported are female, comorbidities, old age, chronic urticaria or angioedema, intolerance to NSAIDs, DRESS, patients affected by LES or HIV disease, history of asthma or atopy, and intermittent treatments. The mechanisms for developing MDHS are not fully understood. IgE-mediated activation of mast-cells and basophils seems to play a key role. It has also been suggested that a certain group of CD4+T cells is critical in reducing the threshold for activation by drugs. Gex-Collet et al. suggested three types of MDHS in nonimmediate reactions: simultaneous, sequential, and distant MDHS. In the first type, multiple sensitizations occur against drugs given at the same time. In the second type, multiple sensitizations develop to drugs given for the same episode, but in a staggered manner. Finally, in the third type, the symptoms of a new DHR can also appear years apart, when the initial DHR has disappeared. It is important to recall that skin testing and DPT are mandatory for confirming the diagnosis. It is also possible that MDHS is under-detected [21].

12.3 Mechanisms

Depending on the involved mechanism, DHRs can be classified as allergic and nonallergic. The allergic reactions are mediated by a specific immune response to a drug that acts as a hapten, while nonallergic reactions include all the reactions without an underlying demonstrated immune mechanism. Historically immune-mediated DHRs are included in the Coombs and Gell's classification. According to a more recent classification [22], the mechanism involved in each reaction could be determined by how drugs interact with the immune system. The interactions could be divided into antibody-mediated and T-cell-mediated (Table 12.2). Immediate type I reactions are mediated by drug-specific IgE antibodies with the involvement of Th2 cells and B cells. Delayed type IV reactions are mediated by specific TH1, TH2, and cytotoxic T cells to drugs. Further delayed reactions are type II, mediated by IgG and type III, and by immunocomplexes and complement.

There are several mechanisms by which T cells involved in type I or IV reactions are stimulated by drugs [23]. Hapten concept: haptens are chemically reactive small compounds (<1 KDa) that bind to proteins/peptides and modify them covalently. Haptens may covalently bind to cellular proteins, transmitting a danger signal, which stimulates the innate immune system. Haptens may also form neoantigens. The hapten-protein complexes are processed and then presented to T cells.

Pro-hapten concept: Pro-haptens cannot form a covalent bond until being metabolized and converted into a chemically reactive compound. Pharmacologic interaction with *immune receptors (PI) concept*: A chemically inert drug, or its metabolite, even if unable to covalently bind to proteins, may be able to "fit" to some immune receptors (T-cell receptor or HLA), enhancing the binding with the antigen, bypassing its processing, and thus activating, under certain circumstances, immune cells which then expand and cause inflammatory reactions of different types.

The non-covalent binding of a drug or its metabolite may also provoke a structural alteration of the HLA binding region which prevents the recognition of self-peptide, resulting in autoimmune reactions. This mechanism has been described as the *altered self-repertoire concept* [24].

Besides the above-mentioned mechanisms, in the last decades, PARs, nonimmune mediate reactions, have been described. PARs are IgE-independent, do not require previous sensitization, are not specific, and globally seem to account for two-thirds of DHRs. Immediate PARs are clinically indistinguishable from immune-mediated reactions [25]. The underlying pathogenetic mechanisms of PARs can involve the complement system's activation with the generation of C3a and C5a anaphylatoxins, which bind to complement receptors on mast cells (*complement activation-related pseudoallergy* (CARPA)), i.e., by contrast, dyes. Another mechanism is the off-target occupation of receptors such as Mas-related G-protein receptor (MRGPRX2) on the surface mast cells by neuromuscular blocking agents (NMBAs) and fluoroquinolones [6]. Mechanisms also include cytokine storm-like reactions with cytokine release from T cells, macrophages, and monocytes, i.e., by chemotherapy, monoclonal antibodies, or COX-1 over-inhibition by nonsteroidal anti-inflammatory drugs. Mixed type I and cytokine storm-like reactions can occur with chemotherapy and monoclonal antibodies.

12.4 Clinical Pictures

DHRs could be immediate and delayed. The immediate DHRs, mostly IgE-mediated or pseudoallergic, generally occur within 1 h, but in some cases before 6 h, from the intake of the culprit drug. Immediate reactions may present with urticaria/angioedema [6], bronchospasm, or anaphylaxis, a potentially life-threatening multisystem reaction classically characterized by urticaria, pruritus, or generalized flushing, accompanied by systemic involvement with throat tightness, dyspnea, back pain, nausea, vomiting, diarrhea, and hypotension. In pediatric settings, urticaria, vomiting, and laryngeal edema are the most prevalent manifestations [26]. The intravenous and intramuscular routes usually determine more rapid and severe reactions, compared with the oral one [27]. Symptoms due to cytokine storm-like reactions comprise fever,

Table 12.2 Adapted from Khan, David A et al. "Cephalosporin allergy: current understanding and future challenges"

	Type of immunologic reaction						
	Antibody-mediated			T-cell-mediated			
	Type I	Type II	Type III	Type IVa	Type IVb	Type IVc	Type IVd
Immune reactant	IgE	IgG	IgG	IFN-γ, TNFα (Th1 cells)	IL-4/13, IL-5 (Th2 cells)	Perforin/ granzyme 8 (CTL)	CXCL8, GM-CSF (T-cell)
Antigen	Soluble antigen	Cell- or matrix-associated antigens	Soluble antigens	Antigen presented by cells or direct T-cell stimulation	Antigen presented by cells or direct T-cell stimulation	Cell-associated antigen or directed T-cell stimulation	Soluble antigen presented by cell or direct T-cell stimulation
Effector	Mast cell activation	FcR+ cells (phagocytes, NK cells)	FcR+ cells, complement	Macrophage activation	Eosinophils	T-cells	Neutrophils
Example of hypersensitivity reaction	Urticaria, angioedema, bronchospasm, anaphylaxis, e.g., beta lactams	Hemolytic anemia, thrombocytopenia, e.g., beta-lactams, rifampin, sulfa antibiotics	Serum sickness, hypersensitivity vasculitis, Arthus reaction e.g., beta-lactams, sulfa antibiotics, minocycline	Tuberculin reaction, contact dermatitis (with IVc)	DRESS, maculopapular exanthema with eosinophilia	SJS/TEN, bulbous exanthema and fixed drug eruption, hepatitis	AGEP, Behçet's disease

chills, nausea, pain, headache, malaise, and then collapse and desaturation. Reactions due to CARPA present hypotension and oxygen desaturation. The delayed hypersensitivity reactions, which are cell-mediated, arise after 6 h from the last administration (from 2 to 5 days on average) [3]. The delayed reactions can be noncutaneous or cutaneous. Organ-specific delayed drug reactions that frequently occur without skin signs include cytopenia, hepatitis, enterocolitis, interstitial nephritis, and vasculitis. Cutaneous delayed manifestations (Table 12.3) are further rationally divided into mild and severe reactions.

12.4.1 Mild Cutaneous Delayed Allergic Reactions (MCAR)

12.4.1.1 Maculo-Papular Exanthema (MPE)

The characteristic lesions are erythematous macules and infiltrated papules, occasionally itchy, that may be widespread with different degrees of confluence. The trunk and proximal extremities usually are the most affected regions, with a symmetrical distribution, while mucosae are generally spared. Desquamation is common in the resolution phase [3, 6]. MPE represents the most frequent DHR and usually occurs 5–7 days after the start of the culprit drug (ranging from 4 to 14 days) [6]. However, in the case of a previous sensitization to the drug, the lesions can appear in a few hours, reaching the maximal extension within 1 or 2 days. The eruption usually disappears after 7–14 days after the culprit drug discontinuation [3]. It seems nevertheless worthy of note that the majority of MPE occur during infections and are not due to drugs (even if viral infection may impact DHRs, as described before). Thus, drug discontinuation can be avoided when limited cutaneous involvement is associated with clear signs of viral infections, and it is possible to follow the patient. Since MPE can be the first manifestation of a severe cutaneous allergic reaction (SCAR), a close follow-up of the patient must be ensured (see below) [3].

12.4.1.2 Erythema Multiforme (EM)

The main features of this type of MCAR are erythematous to violaceous macules which can evolve into targetoid plaque with a peripheral ring of erythema and central duskiness evolving

Table 12.3 Main manifestations of late immune-mediated adverse reaction to drugs

	Mild			Severe		
Entity	MPE	EM	SSLR	AGEP	SJS/TEN	DRESS
Median delay (days)	5–7	2–3	5–10	2	10–14	14–42
Typical skin lesions	Erythematous macules, infiltrated papules	Erythematous to violaceous macules	Urticarial-type lesions	Pustules on erythematous, edematous skin	Painful erythematous macules	MPE
Skin detachment	No	Possible	No	Rare	Frequent	Rare
Distribution	Symmetrical	Symmetrical, acral	Start in the flexures, then generalized	Widespread	Widespread	Widespread
Most affected regions (or % of body surface)	Trunk and proximal extremities	Extremities, hands, feet	Skin and joints	Folds and flexural areas	<10% and > 30% of skin surface, respectively	>50% of body surface
Mucosal involvement	Rare	Common	No	No	Frequent, severe	Possible, mild
Systemic involvement	No	Possible	Possible	Usually not	Yes	Yes

MPE maculopapular exanthema, *EM* erythema multiforme, *SSLR* serum sickness-like reaction, *SJS* Steven-Johnson syndrome, *TEN* toxic epidermal necrolysis, *DRESS* drug reaction with eosinophilia and systemic symptoms in epidermal necrosis. A progression to vesiculation or blistering is also possible [28]. The distribution is normally symmetrical, with variable mucosal involvement. Mucosal involvement when present predominantly affects the oral mucosa and lips. In cases with extensive mucosal involvement, mycoplasma pneumonia-induced rash and mucositis (MIRM), SJS, and TEN represent possible differential diagnoses (3). Fever and malaise can be associated [29]. EM normally recovers over 2–3 weeks. Recurrences have been rarely described [30].

Fixed drug eruption (FDE): FDE is an erythematous to violaceous plaque that may have a bullous central part that always appears at the same site after re-exposure to the culprit drug [6]. Pruritus or burning sensation can be associated [31]. The plaques can be unique or, more rarely, multiple and can affect any mucosal or cutaneous surface. The lesion usually arises within a week from drug exposure and resolves within a few days, resulting in a circumscribed hyperpigmentation that may persist for months or years [32]. In case of re-exposure, a flare at the same site occurs within 1–8 h [33].

12.4.1.3 Serum Sickness-Like Reaction (SSLR)

SSLR is an acute inflammatory condition affecting predominantly children. Even if pathophysiology remains unclear, drugs are considered the main trigger. Different from the serum-sickness, SSSLR is not associated with antigen-antibody complex formation, and blood concentrations of the complement system are usually normal. The main characteristics are represented by the development of skin rash and joint inflammation with or without fever, usually preceded by exposure to a drug. Some theories consider the possibility that drugs, or their metabolites, may act as haptens and bind plasma proteins which subsequently induce an abnormal immunologic response, while another theory suggests that drug metabolites by themselves have a direct toxic effect on the lymphocytes of affected patients. The most common drugs associated with this condition are BLs, especially cefaclor and amoxicillin, and a great variety of other drugs such as sulfonamide antibiotics, anticancer agents, anticonvulsants, anti-inflammatory agents, griseofulvin, metronidazole, bupropion, and more recently biologic agents such as rituximab, infliximab, and efalizumab, among others [34].

12.4.2 Severe Cutaneous Delayed Allergic Reactions (SCAR)

12.4.2.1 Acute Generalized Exanthematous Pustulosis (AGEP)

Acute generalized exanthematous pustulosis (AGEP) is a rare SCAR caused by drugs in >90% of cases, with a reported incidence in children of 1–5 cases per million [35]. It is characterized by the onset of sterile, nonfollicular, and small pustules on erythematous and edematous skin, starting from folds. Then, flexural areas of extremities are involved. Localization at the face, trunk, and extremities is also possible. Fever, neutrophilia, and peripheral blood eosinophilia are present in one-third of patients. Nonfollicular subcorneal and/or intracorneal pustules are the most relevant histopathological features. Mucous membranes are not affected. AGEP is associated with antibiotics (especially beta-lactams, quinolones, macrolides, and sulfonamides) and more rarely with antiepileptics (e.g., carbamazepine), hydroxychloroquine, diltiazem, and acetaminophen [36]. Viral and bacterial infections, CMV, EBV, parvovirus B19, and streptococcus, among others, have been frequently reported as precipitant factors [3]. Diagnostic criteria for AGEP were established by an international committee, the European Study of Severe Cutaneous Adverse Reactions (EuroSCAR). AGEP usually appears after 48 h from culprit drug exposure. The involvement of drug-specific T cells in the pathomechanism can be confirmed by positive skin patch tests and lymphocyte transformation tests. After the elimination of the causative drug, pustules usually spontaneously disappear in a few days with desquamation, and the reaction fully resolves within 15 days. Internal organs are not usually involved [37, 38] Generally, it is self-limited, and no systemic treatment is required although oral corticosteroid may be helpful in some individuals.

12.4.2.2 Steven-Johnson Syndrome/Toxic Epidermal Necrolysis (SJS/TEN)

SJS/TEN is a severe, potentially fatal, and immune-mediated pathology, which is generally triggered by drugs. The incidence is 1–5 cases per million people. It is considered to be a single disease with a wide spectrum of symptoms. The distinguishing element between the two clinical pictures is given by the cutaneous extension involvement. In SJS, the skin area involved is less than 10%, whereas in TEN, it is more than 30%. When the skin involvement is between 10 and 30%, it is denominated SJS/TEN overlap [39]. Fever, dysphagia, and ocular pruritus often occur 1–7 days before cutaneous involvement. The skin manifestations initially present as painful erythematous roundish macules, that can sequentially assume a target shape, and show confluence in larger blisters, leading to skin detachment [6]. All the body surfaces can be affected and mucous membranes included. Systemic involvement is present in over 90% of cases presenting as primary or as a complication of skin detachment (e.g., infections, sepsis, and electrolyte imbalance). After skin, the most affected organ is the eye. In approximately 85% of cases, conjunctival hyperemia, palpebral edema, and photophobia occur [3]. The mortality associated with severe TEN is approximately 30%, but >50% in the elderly and immunocompromised populations [38]. In children aged under 5 years, it is associated with a higher mortality rate, and short-term morbidity includes ocular, respiratory, gastrointestinal, and genito-urinary complications, as well as mucositis and sepsis. Given the necrotizing nature of lesions, in the long term, the disease can result in permanent atrophic-cicatricial lesions at different sites, including skin, eyes, esophagus, and bronchi [40]. Drugs are the most prevalent cause of SJS/TEN. In children, among more than 100 culprit drugs, anticonvulsants (phenobarbital, lamotrigine, and carbamazepine) are the most common, followed by antibiotics (particularly sulfonamides, BLs, trimethoprim-sulfamethoxazole, and azithromycin), NSAIDs, paracetamol, and chemotherapeutic agents [41, 42]. The disease usually appears within 2 weeks after drug intake, but longer intervals of up to 8 weeks have been reported. Given the frequent systemic involvement, upon the suspicion of SJS/TEN, close monitoring of vital parameters is required, in addition to the suspected drug discontinuation. Other causative agents of SJS/TEN are influenza virus, EBV, HHV-6, HHV-7, parvovirus, adenovirus, coxsackie, mycoplasma, and some chemical industrial compounds. In 20% of cases, the causative agent remains unknown, and recurrences in children are described [43]. Differential diagnosis includes MCAR (especially those with extensive mucosal involvement), DRESS (see below), AGEP (for the rare cases with mucous membrane involvement), and staphylococcal scalded skin syndrome [44].

12.4.2.3 DRESS

Another rare but severe and potentially fatal SCAR is DRESS, a pathological entity occurring between 0.1 and 1 out of 1000 drug exposures [45], in which both visceral and cutaneous involvement is present. Fever, malaise, and lymphadenopathy are mostly present. In the peripheral blood, eosinophilia, leukocytosis, transaminase elevation, and atypical lymphocytes are frequently detected [6]. A complex interaction between genetic predisposition, immunological response, metabolic impairment, and herpetic virus reactivation is supposed to stand at the base of this disease [46]. From the clinical point of view, an MPE is the most frequent presentation sign (89% of cases), preceding or accompanying fever (present in 96% of cases) and malaise [45]. MPE generally involves more than 50% of the body surface, and in half of the cases, it is associated with facial edema. The exanthema can persist for months after the culprit drug discontinuation. Mucous membranes, especially oral and conjunctival, can be affected, even if in a milder and less necrotic form than in SJS/TEN [47]. The systemic involvement affects more frequently the liver, with lesions that may in some cases progress to diffuse necrosis and fulminant hepatitis. Myocarditis, pancreatitis, pneumonia, nephritis, and arthritis are less common [46]. In both children and adults, the mortality rate is around 5% [48]. The main long-term sequelae are hypothyroidism, diabetes, and liver insufficiency, which occur globally in 10.8% of cases [45]. The most frequent causative drugs are the aromatic anticonvulsants (carbamazepine, phenytoin, lamotrigine, and phenobarbital). More rarely, NSAIDs, sulfasalazine, and other drugs can be implicated [46]. The interval between assumption and DHR ranges normally from 2 to 6 weeks, but longer periods of up to 3.5 months are described [46]. Considering the clinical presentation, frequently aspecific, and some pediatric conditions–such as Kawasaki disease and lymphoma—that can mimic it, the SCAR-J diagnostic criteria have been proposed [49]. The diagnosis is confirmed by the presence of all seven criteria (typical DIHS) or the first five (atypical DIHS):

1. Maculopapular rash developing ≥3 weeks after starting therapy with a limited number of drugs
2. Prolonged clinical symptoms 2 weeks after discontinuation of the suspected drug
3. Fever (≥38 °C)
4. Liver abnormalities (alanine aminotransferase [ALT] ≥ 100 U/L)
5. Leukocyte abnormalities (at least one present)[a]
    (a) Leukocytosis (>11 × 10^9/L)
    (b) Atypical lymphocytosis (>5%)
    (c) Eosinophilia (>1.5 × 10^9/L)
6. Lymphadenopathy
7. Human herpes virus (HHV)–6 reactivation

[a]This can be replaced by other organ involvement, such as renal involvement

12.4.3 Drug-Induced Enterocolitis Syndrome (DIES)

Drug-induced enterocolitis syndrome (DIES) is an inflammatory condition of the gastrointestinal tract primarily affecting pediatric patients. This condition is a rare form of non-IgE-mediated allergy described for the first time in 2014. Few patients have been reported in the literature so far, with more than 70% of cases in pediatric settings. The main triggers are amoxicillin or amoxicillin-clavulanic acid, along with pantoprazole and paracetamol, specifying that beta-lactam antibiotic therapy alone accounts for more than half of the cases. This could be explained through the hypothesis of the alteration of the intestinal immune system balance provoked by these drugs as a trigger of inflammatory response and subsequent enterocolitis [50]. Ingestion of the triggering drug activates the immune system, leading to the production and release of inflammatory mediators such as cytokines and chemokines, probably following a T cell-driven mechanism. These mediators can cause a systemic response characterized by vasodilation, increased vascular permeability, and hypotension, ultimately resulting in shock. Mechanisms leading to shock in non-IgE-mediated forms of DIES are associated with a systemic and inflammatory immune response [51]. Common clinical manifestations of DIES in children include severe vomiting, diarrhea, extreme lethargy, and pallor. The diagnosis of DIES is based on diagnostic criteria that include both major and minor criteria as shown in Table 12.4.

To establish the diagnosis of DIES in pediatric patients, it is necessary to fulfil both major criteria and at least three minor criteria. Accurate assessment of the patient's clinical history, exclusion of other causes of enterocolitis, and supportive findings aid in the diagnosis. Laboratory findings that can support the diagnosis of this new pathological entity are neutrophilic leukocytosis and the increase in the methemoglobin, with normal tryptase dosage and negative allergy tests. Currently, the diagnosis of DIES primarily depends on clinical diagnostic criteria and is occasionally confirmed by a DPT which appears to be the only test useful for validating or excluding DIES and to evaluate the tolerance of related and unrelated compounds [52]. DIES, such as food protein enterocolitis syndrome (FPIES), which recognizes milk, soy, rice, meat, eggs, and fish as triggers, manifests itself as a non-IgE-mediated reaction, with a wide range of gastrointestinal and systemic symptoms. Like in FPIES, intravenous fluid and antiemetics (i.e., ondansetron) for the treatment of vomiting appear to be effective, while the benefit of adrenaline appears unclear [53, 54].

Table 12.4 Major and minor diagnostic criteria of DIES

Major criteria	Minor criteria
1. Vomiting between the first and the fourth hour after exposure to a suspected drug	1. Diarrhea in 24 h (usually 5–10 h)
2. Resolution of vomiting upon drug discontinuation	2. Repetitive vomiting
	3. Lethargy
	4. Pallor
	5. Emergency department visit
	6. Intravenous fluid support
	7. Hypotension
	8. Hypothermia

12.5 Diagnosis

The diagnostic workup usually starts with the clinical history including the type of reaction, the response to treatment, and the time interval between drug exposure and symptom development and between clinical manifestations and testing. Both in vivo and in vitro diagnostic tests are used. Skin prick test (SPT) is useful for IgE-mediated reactions, intradermal test (IDT), immediate DHR (immediate reading) or delayed DHR (delayed reading), and patch test, for both delayed and contact reactions. Unfortunately, the diagnostic accuracy of skin tests for most drugs is uncertain. Skin testing can be helpful for immediate reactions, while the value for delayed reactions is unclear. Among in vitro tests for immediate reactions, drug-specific IgE levels and the concentration of mediators such as tryptase are the most used. The basophil activation test (BAT) that measures the expression of CD63 and/or CD203c in basophils incubated with the suspected drug and the lymphocyte transformation tests have been shown which might be useful in the diagnosis of T-cell-mediated delayed hypersensitivity reactions. However, validated commercial assays are lacking. DPT (or drug challenge) represents the gold standard for identifying patients who tolerate a drug. The aim is to show tolerance instead of eliciting a reaction [54]. It is performed both for immediate and delayed reactions. DPT consists of administering the culprit drug at a therapeutic dose as a single step or with incremental dose escalation at fixed intervals, generally reaching a cumulative dose equal to a daily standard weight-adjusted dose. Dose escalation may follow a two-step challenge with administration of 10%–25% of the therapeutic dose followed by administration of the remaining dose 20–30 min later or a three-step protocol, 1/10, 2/10, and 7/10 of the full dose every 60 min. Reactions during DPT are potentially life-threatening. So, this procedure must be performed under strict medical supervision and with resuscitative equipment available [6]. The drug challenge is contraindicated in SCARs, other skin reactions (autoimmune, generalized fixed bullous eruption, and Sweet's syndrome), vasculitis, organ-specific reactions, and anaphylaxis. The choice of tests depends not only on whether the reaction was suspected to be IgE or non-IgE mediated but also on the compound class.

12.5.1 BLs

The drugs belonging to this class structurally share the central BL ring and differ in the side chain. The side chain represents the more immunogenically active part of the compound. Cross-reactivity between penicillins and cephalosporin is linked to the R1 group/side chains. There is evidence [54] that there is high risk of cross-reaction for cefaclor, cefadroxil, cefprozil, and cephalexin and a lower risk for cefazolin, cefuroxime, cefixime, cefotaxime, ceftriaxone, ceftazidime, cefpodoxime, ceftibuten, and cefepime, irrespective of their generation. Therefore, in patients with penicillin allergy, a non-cross-reactive cephalosporin can be routinely administered without previous testing [54]. Cross-reactivity between penicillins or cephalosporin and carbapenems is low. So, a carbapenem may be routinely given to patients with a history of penicillin/cephalosporin allergy without prior investigations [54]. Monobactam usually represents a safe option in the case of allergy to both penicillins and cephalosporines except for those with ceftazidime allergy, which shares a side chain with aztreonam [55]. Larger trials are warranted to ascertain whether in patients with SCARs due to a BL an alternative BL is tolerated. The panel of reagents for skin testing includes major and minor determinants of penicillin (e.g., PPL and MDM), amoxicillin, and any other suspected BLs [56]. The diagnostic workup begins from SPT and, if negative, IDT, with a reading after 20' [57]. Highest nonirritating concentrations recommended for both prick and intradermal testing with beta-lactams are as follows [56]: benzylpenicilloyl-poly-L-lysine, 6.0×10^{-5} mol/L; benzylpenicilloyl-octa-L-lysine, 8.64×10^{-5} mol/L; sodium benzylpenilloate, 1.5 $\times 10^{-3}$ mol/L; benzylpenicillin, 10,000 IU/mL; amoxicillin and other semi-synthetic penicillins, 20 mg/mL; cefepime, 2 mg/mL; other cephalosporins, 20 mg/mL; clavulanic acid, 20 mg/mL; aztreonam, 2 mg/mL; Imipenem-cilastin, 0.5–0.5 mg/mL; and meropenem and ertapenem, 1 mg/mL. In patients with anaphylaxis or severe cutaneous reactions, dilute concentrations of the reagents starting from 1/1000 or 1/100 should be used. Skin tests are endowed with a relatively high diagnostic value in immediate reactions although the positive predictive value has not been clearly ascertained. The rate of patients with a history of BL allergy with positive skin tests ranges from 7% to 76% [58]. Specific IgE assays are marketed for amoxicillin, ampicillin, penicilloyl G and V, and cefaclor. Specific IgE has a lower sensitivity than skin tests (12.5–25%) with good specificity (83–100%). BAT has a sensitivity of around 50% and a specificity between 89 and 97%. Recent studies report that between 8.4% and 30.7% of patients who resulted negative for these tests do react to DPT [58]. In vitro tests should be initially performed in case of an immediate severe reaction, with the aim of reducing the risk of immediate reaction during skin testing. In anaphylaxis, the acute tryptase assay may be useful to confirm the diagnosis. The accuracy of detecting IgE-mediated sensitization decreases over time for both skin tests and in vitro tests, so it is advisable to undertake the diagnostic procedure after a time interval of 3–6 weeks after the reaction [56]. Many studies show that DPT is safe and reliable, even with the administration of a single therapeutic dose; some authors suggest continuing administration for 5 days to improve the diagnostic performance of the test and the family's belief that the drug is tolerated [56]. In patients with SCAR, it is recommended to first perform the patch test (6 months after the reaction) and if there is a negative result, to continue the workup with the IDT at the maximal dilution, whereas DPT is contraindicated [57].

12.5.2 Non-BL Antibiotics

In children, among non-BL antibiotics, sulfonamides and macrolides are the drugs that more frequently trigger DHR [59]. Regarding macrolides, one study showed that azithromycin is more allergenic than clarithromycin in children [60]. For these drugs, the usefulness of skin tests is controversial, with sensitivity varying from 0% to 75% depending on the case series. So, skin testing with nonirritating concentrations should be limited to patients with severe anaphylactic reactions or with an unclear clinical history. Otherwise, patients should proceed directly to DPT [56]. Sulfonamides are mostly associated with MCAR such as MPE but may also be responsible for SCAR. In the assessment of delayed DHRs, IDT and patch testing are associated with low sensitivity but higher specificity. So, the direct challenge remains the gold standard for the diagnosis of hypersensitivity to sulfonamides [61]. Vancomycin, a glycopeptide widely used in children, frequently causes the so-called "red man syndrome," an infusion reaction whose severity can vary from the appearance of rash and itching to bronchospasm and hypotension. This syndrome appears to be related to direct activation of the MRGPR X2 receptor. IgE-mediated reactions to vancomycin are rare, and skin tests can result in false positives. Therefore, the management is based on either slowing the rate of administration or desensitization, in the moderate and severe reactions, respectively [62]. IgE-mediated and delayed allergic reactions to aminoglycosides are rare. Contact dermatitis from topical aminoglycosides is the most frequent clinical manifestation, as neomycin and also gentamicin and tobramycin are widely used as creams, ointments, eye drops, or topical ear drops. Concerning the evaluation of these reactions, patch testing may be useful [63].

12.5.3 NSAIDs

NSAIDs are among the most prescribed drugs in the pediatric population. Several aspects of hypersensitivity reactions to NSAIDs in the pediatric age remain to be clarified, such as their metabolism in children, the natural history of the various phenotypes of DHRs, and the importance of cofactors (e.g., infections or physical exercise). Clinical and laboratory markers that help to define endotypes are yet to be found. NSAIDs include structurally different drugs that share the capacity to inhibit cyclooxygenase isoenzymes (COX-I, COX-II, and COX-III). The rate of confirmed hypersensitivity to NSAIDs is approximately 20% of cases although these drugs (particularly ibuprofen) are known to be responsible for up to 23% of drug anaphylaxis [64]. Hypersensitivity reactions to NSAIDs can be divided into two categories: selective immune-allergic reactions (SR) and cross-intolerant reactions (CI) [54]. Patients with SR react to a single drug or NSAIDs with a shared structure. SR can have immediate onset (i.e., urticaria-angioedema and anaphylaxis) or delayed onset (i.e., fixed drug eruptions). Immediate SR is IgE-mediated, while delayed is drug-specific T-cell-mediated. In CI, clinical manifestations are triggered by more than one NSAID subclass through a combination of COX-1 inhibition and a regulatory defect in arachnoid-acid metabolism. This provokes the release of mast cell and eosinophil-derived mediators and the production of leukotrienes [64]. CI [64] can have different manifestations in children <10 years compared with those >10 years. Children with CI between 0 and 10 years present concurrently skin and respiratory reactions, while children >10 years CI are classified into three groups: the first with immediate onset of urticaria or anaphylaxis (*nonsteroidal anti-inflammatory induced urticaria angioedema anaphylaxis* (NIUAA)), the second with exacerbation of preexisting chronic urticaria (nonsteroidal *anti-inflammatory exacerbated cutaneous disease* (NECD)), and the third with exacerbations concern preexisting respiratory condition, predominantly asthma (*nonsteroidal anti-inflammatory exacerbated respiratory disease* (NERD)). Recently, a new clinical phenotype has been defined as *multiple selective immediate reactors* [65]. It includes patients who react to two or more NSAIDs while tolerating acetylsalicylic acid. In order to reach a diagnosis, medical history plays a key role in establishing the steps of diagnostic workup. Well-defined timing, clinical features, cofactors, and response to any treatment are paramount, but above all, it must be clarified whether the child presented reactions to more than one NSAID, as well as whether any NSAIDs are tolerated. Finally, personal history of atopy, allergic rhinitis, asthma, or urticaria must be investigated. Regarding diagnostic tests, they should be performed 4–6 weeks after the reaction. SPTs and IDT are not standardized and have many false negatives. Patch tests and delayed-reading IDT can be used for delayed reactions, but data on sensitivity and specificity are lacking. The DPT, therefore, remains the gold standard. The test usually starts with 1/4–1/20 of the daily dose calculated for the patient's weight and age so that the total dose is reached in 3–5 administrations, with an inter-dose interval of 1–1.5 h. A follow-up observation time of 2–6 h after the first dose is then required according to the history. DPT is not performed in cases of anaphylaxis or delayed severe drug reactions. In children, the negative predictive value of DPT is 100% for paracetamol and 94% for ibuprofen [66]. A positive challenge test for an NSAID does not discriminate between SR and CI, so a subsequent aspirin test is needed to define cross-intolerance. Some authors recommend considering testing aspirin first, as a positive DPT creates alarm in parents and makes it difficult to continue the diagnostic process. Provocation test with aspirin involves oral administration at a dose of 10 mg/kg/dose in 4–5 steps. Some pediatric studies use a higher cumulative dose of 15–20 mg/kg/dose on two consecutive days. Even in cases with confirmed CI, paracetamol is often tolerated, particularly at a dose <15 mg/kg. In the case of CI, the choice of an alternative drug is not easy in children as COX-II selective inhibitors are not approved under 12–18 years. When an NSAID induces urticaria that is prevented by the administration of anti-H1 antihistamine, the patient can tolerate a course of NSAID [54]. A preferential COX 2 inhibitor such as nimesulide can be prescribed from 12 years of age; etoricoxib (selective COX 2 inhibitor) from 16 years. Desensitization should be considered when no therapeutic alternative is available [3].

12.5.4 Perioperative Drugs

The incidence of anaphylactic reactions to perioperative drugs is lower in childhood than in adulthood, with a reported incidence among children of 1:37,000 [67]. The most frequently involved compounds are antibiotics, muscle relaxants, hypnotics, and latex. Given the number of drugs used during surgery, the diagnosis of this type of reaction often requires a long diagnostic procedure. Tests should be done 4–6 weeks after the resolution of the clinical picture and no later than 6 months after the reaction [68]. A careful history of timing, dosage, formulation, and brand of drugs that were simultaneously administered and drugs used to manage the reaction is necessary. In these settings, the discussion with the anesthesiologist may help in identifying the culprit drug [69]. Specific tests are then indicated for each type of drug [70]. In the case of a suspected hypersensitivity reaction, it is always advisable to perform the serum tryptase detection (within 30 min and 2 h after the onset of the reaction and 24 h later). Skin tests are the first step and consist of SPT and IDT with nonirritating concentrations of drugs used [3]. Specific IgE determination and BAT can be performed for some drugs. A DPT may be necessary for some drugs. We report the main categories of drugs to test.

Muscle relaxants (neuromuscular blocking agents (NMBA)): Cases of sensitization to NMBA have been reported even in patients not previously exposed, due to previous sensitization to molecules with similar structures contained in cosmetics, disinfectants, food, and drugs such as pholcodine, commonly used in cough syrup. Skin tests for NMBA have excellent sensitivity and specificity (around 100%), with persistent positivity even several years after the reaction. For some NMBA, the specific IgE assay can be performed. BAT for NMBA is potentially useful, with a sensitivity of 64–85.7% and a specificity of 93–97% [1].

Opioids: They rarely cause a true perioperative allergic reaction (2%). Adverse reactions to morphine are often PAR. Nausea and vomiting are frequent side effects that should not be confused with allergic reactions. Some opioids are semi-synthetic (e.g., fentanyl, sufentanyl, and remifentanyl) and do not cross-react with morphine [3].

Hypnotics: The most widely used is propofol, marketed as an oil-water emulsion. The presence of soya and egg lecithin in the preparation has led to the assumption that propofol is not indicated in case of allergy to these foods, but evidence is lacking [71].

Local anesthetics: True hypersensitivity reactions to these compounds are extremely rare. Most reported reactions are effectively related to side effects, overdose, injection into the circulation, and vaso-vagal crises. SPT with the commercial preparation without adrenaline should be carried out and, if negative, followed by IDT (starting with the 1/100 and 1/10 diluted solution) and eventually DPT [72].

Other allergens in perioperative settings: During an operating session, the patient may also be exposed to substances other than drugs such as disinfectants, latex, anticoagulants, antibiotics, and dextran. Such substances should be also considered the possible cause of an allergic reaction.

12.5.5 Antiepileptic

This class of drugs is often responsible for delayed skin hypersensitivity reactions such as

EMP, particularly during dose escalation, after 2–8 weeks from starting therapy. More rarely, they may cause SCAR. Reactions occur more frequently in children <12 years using aromatic antiepileptics or several drugs simultaneously. There are also significant associations with certain HLA [1]. Diagnosis is based on history, delayed reading IDT, patch test, and DTP. Delayed reading IDT and patch tests are used in case of a mild reaction and to exclude cross-reactivity, which is high (40–80% among aromatic antiepileptics). Skin tests should be carried out at least 4 weeks after the reaction. If the index reaction is severe, it is preferable to perform only patch tests. The test sensitivity depends on the drug tested, and it is higher for carbamazepine. The concentrations that must be used for IDT are not standardized. For patch tests, concentrations of 10% in vaseline are used for pure substances and 20–30% with marketed drugs (e.g., for carbamazepine). In vitro, allergy tests such as lymphocyte transformation test, cytokine determination by ELISpot or granulysin determination by cytofluorimetry can be performed. The lymphocyte transformation test appears to be more sensitive when performed in the acute phase for SJS/TEN and more sensitive when performed in the resolution phase for DRESS. In children, lymphocyte transformation tests appear to have a sensitivity of 58.4% with a specificity of 95.8% [73]. In SJS/TEN, sensitivity ranges from 37 to 86% and specificity from 86 to 100% [74]. Combining the various in vitro and in vivo methods would seem to increase the diagnostic sensitivity for reactions to antiepileptics [75].

The DPT should be performed in selected cases of mild delayed reactions. It can be administered 1/10 of the total dose and in the absence of reactions after 1–7 days, or depending on the interval of the index reaction, the remaining dose can be taken. In the case of SCARs, the DTP should not be performed [73].

12.5.6 Chemotherapeutic Agents

All chemotherapeutic agents can potentially induce hypersensitivity reactions, and they are the third leading cause of fatal drug-induced anaphylaxis in the United States [76]. Most reactions are caused by platinum compounds, taxanes, epipodophyllotoxins, and asparaginase [77].

Regarding platinum compounds, carboplatin is mainly responsible for DHRs, with an incidence of up to 46% of patients. Oxaliplatin can induce hypersensitivity reactions in about 15% of cases with severe reactions in less than 1%, whereas cisplatin is the culprit drug in about 5% of cases [76]. Taxanes can provoke DHRs in about 30% of patients, but the incidence declines to less than 5% with premedication with steroids and antihistamines [78]. Asparaginase hypersensitivity ranges from 6% to 43% of cases, with an augmented likelihood after the fourth dose [79]. Finally, the incidence of reactions to epipodophyllotoxins ranges from 6.5% to 41% [80]. Considering that in several studies with different designs and aims, variables such as atopy, previous DHRs to other drugs, age of patients, mastocytosis, and type of cancer were inconsistent risk factors, the hypersensitivity to a chemotherapeutic agent is defined as an unexpected reaction that cannot be explained by the known toxicity profile of the drug. The clinical manifestations range from cutaneous symptoms (pruritus and urticaria) to anaphylactic shock [76].

Despite their relevance in terms of frequency and entity, the ideal pathways for diagnosis, treatment, and prevention of these reactions are still unclear, and the allergy workups remain considerably heterogeneous. Platinum compounds may act as haptens to stimulate the development of specific IgE antibodies, generating a type I hypersensitivity in the following infusions. In support of IgE-mediated hypersensitivity are the rising incidence of hypersensitivity with repeated doses, the occurrence of positive skin prick tests to platinum compounds, and the presence of specific IgE [81]. Skin testing may be helpful in identifying patients with platin hypersensitivity, but their role in taxane hypersensitivity is unclear. In Table 12.5, we report the nonirritating concentrations for skin tests. Neither SPTs nor specific-IgE has been shown to have value in predicting first-time reactions, showing a high rate of false negatives. DPT is potentially indicated in patients with immediate

Table 12.5 Nonirritating concentrations of ST for chemotherapeutic agents [76]

Drug	Prick test dilutions (mg/ml)	Intradermal test dilutions (mg/ml)
Paclitaxel	<1/10 1(6)	1/1000 (0.001 [0.006]) 1/100 (0.001 [0.006]) 1/10 (0.6)
Docetaxel	1/1 4 (1)	1/100 (0.04 [0.01]) 1/10 0.4 ([0.1])
Carboplatin	1/1 (10)	1/100 (0.1) 1/10 (1)
Cisplatin	1/1 (10)	1/100 (0.01) 1/10 (0.1) 1/1 (1)
Oxaliplatin	1/1 (5)	1/100 (0.05) 1/10 (0.5) 1/1 (5)—some authors have found false positives
L-Asparaginase	A drop of reconstitute 5000 KU	0.01 ml of reconstitute 5000 KU
Methotrexate	1/1 (10)	1/100 (0.1 1/10 (1) 1/1 (10))
Procarbazine	1/1 (5)	1/100 (0.05)
Gemcitabine	1/1 (38)	1/1000 (0.0038) 1/100 (0.038) 1/10 and 1/1

reactions, including some cases of milder anaphylaxis (provided the risk assessment is favorable) and delayed reactions (provided, they are non-SCARs) [82]. However, in practice, hypersensitivity reactions (HSRs) occur during infusion, and patients should be desensitized.

Many premedication regimens, for blocking the inflammatory pathways, have been proposed for preventing DHRs. However, premedication was ineffective in preventing IgE-mediated allergic reactions to platinum salts [83]. It had no influence on the effectiveness or safety of desensitization in patients with confirmed hypersensitivity to paclitaxel [84]. The efficacy of premedication with steroids and antihistamines has been proved for preventing moderate and severe infusion reactions to taxanes, epipodophyllotoxins, asparaginase, and doxorubicin [76].

12.5.7 Immune Checkpoint Inhibitors

Immune checkpoint inhibition (CPI) with monoclonal antibodies, targeting cytotoxic T lymphocyte-associated antigen-4 (CTLA-4), programmed cell death protein 1 (PD-1), or programmed death ligand (PD-L1), has shown to be promising as an anticancer strategy. They shift the immune system toward antitumor activity by activating cytotoxic T cells. Unfortunately, this therapy is associated with different autoimmune and auto-inflammatory phenomena termed immune-related adverse events (irAEs). The irAEs are very common and affect multiple organs including skin, thyroid, lungs, GI, liver, eyes, and pancreas. Most irAEs are mild and can be reversed in a few weeks, but when severe they may require permanent discontinuation of otherwise effective therapy. Immune-related cutaneous adverse events are reported in 90% of patients treated with CTLA-4 inhibitors, 70% with PD-1/PD-L1 inhibitors, and in almost all patients receiving combined therapies. There are nonspecific maculopapular rash, vitiligo, and lichenoid dermatitis and other more severe, even if rare, effects such as bullous dermatosis, psoriasiform dermatitis, neutrophilic dermatoses, autoimmune dermato-rheumatologic diseases, and SCAR manifestations. The treatment requires prevalent topical corticosteroids, occasionally systemic corticosteroids or biologic drugs, including antitumor necrosis factor (TNF)-alpha agents. Differential diagnosis of cutaneous reactions caused by checkpoint inhibitors includes infection, systemic disease, and adverse effects of another drug [85]. There is less data regarding the incidence and clinical features of irAEs in children. Initial phase I/II clinical trials reported a lower incidence of cutaneous irAEs in children compared to adults. Phase I/II trials for pembrolizumab and nivolumab reported a 5% and 12% incidence of cutaneous eruptions, respectively. Similar to the adult population, the most common type of eruption reported in children is a "maculopapular" rash. However, other eruptions frequently reported in the adult population, such as lichenoid and bullous eruptions, have not been well-described in children, apart from a case report [86]. So far, the use of these new drugs in pediatric patients is very limited due to different immunological characteristics: pediatric tumors are usually characterized by a low tumor mutational burden, which also results in a paucity of neo-epitopes and few tumor-infiltrating T cells. The need for new strategies to improve the outcomes for pediatric patients with solid tumors induced to consider CPI for relapsing or refractory cases, for certain types of tumors, and to avoid the detrimental effects of intensive, multimodal chemotherapy. Three early trials indicated that CPIs are well tolerated in children. The most frequent irAEs were anemia, fatigue, pyrexia, and low lymphocyte counts together with pneumonitis, colitis, hepatitis, and hypophysitis [87].

12.5.8 Monoclonal Antibodies

Monoclonal antibodies (mAbs), obtained by cellular clones derived from animals that have been immunized with a specific antigen, have been used for the diagnosis and treatment of diseases since the 1970s [88]. A major concern of using rodent mAbs is the potential for triggering reactions after repeated use, with loss of efficacy due to antibodies to the species part of the therapeutic antibody, particularly if effectiveness depends on multiple uses. Biologic therapies provide the advantage of targeting specific cells or pathways, theoretically increasing efficacy and limiting complications related to the nonspecific effects of more traditional therapies [89]. The therapeutic application of mAbs in children is a developing field, and several promising results have already been obtained, such as the mAbs used in cancer therapy, in the treatment of autoimmune disorders, allergic diseases, and graft rejection in transplant-receiving patients. Hypersensitivity reactions to mAbs are increasingly frequent as this class of therapeutic agents is rapidly expanding. Despite the progressive increase of human sequences in the structure of biologicals, their immunogenicity linked to nonhuman components is not zeroed. Biologicals can induce humoral or cell-mediated hypersensitivity reactions, and reactions related to the excipients are present in the formulation. These substances are polysorbate 20 (omalizumab and benralizumab), polysorbate 80 (dupilumab, adalimumab, infliximab, canakinumab, and anakinra), mannitol (adalimumab, basiliximab, palivizumab, and etanercept), sucrose (mepolizumab, etanercept, reslizumab, and ustekinumab), and trometamol (etanercept) [90]. Immediate hypersensitivity reactions to mAbs appear until 24 h after injection, while nonimmediate reactions appear until 14 days after injection. Hypersensitivity reactions to mAbs include urticarial rash, hypotension, angioedema, hypoxia, bronchospasm, pulmonary infiltrates, and acute respiratory distress [90]. The exact mechanism of HSRs to mAbs is not fully understood. While sensitization typically occurs with repeated exposure, there are reports of reactions after the first infusion of mAbs; hence, at least some of the immediate HSRs may be caused by drug-induced cytokine release [90, 91]. In Table 12.6, the mechanisms of HSRs to mAbs described so far are illustrated.

Immediate reactions can be explained by CRR, IgE-mediated, and IgG-mediated mechanisms, but mixed reactions could occur.

The risk of developing HSR is influenced by the route of administration (higher risk with intravenous administration compared to subcutaneous administration) and the doses of immunosuppressive comedications. The following setting-specific factors have also been described:

Table 12.6 Mechanisms and clinical characterization of HSRs to mAbs

Main mechanisms	Time	Clinical	Immunology
IRR or CRR	First administration	Flushing, dyspnea, throat tightness, dizziness/hypotension, gastrointestinal symptoms, headache, increased blood pressure, chest and back pain, fever, chills, and rigors	The rapid destruction of cells targeted by the mAb through complement-mediated and or antibody-mediated cell death (ADCC) leads to the release of proinflammatory cytokines such as TNF-α and IL-6
IgE-mediated	After at least one uneventful administration with an exception: at the first infusion of cetuximab, HSRs can immediately occur	From isolated skin symptoms to anaphylactic shock and may sometimes overlap with symptoms of cytokine release (e.g., fever, rigors, chills). In 15% of infusion, patients present urticaria: 10–15% during infusion of rituximab, 2–3% during infusion of infliximab: 0.6–5% during infusion of trastuzumab; reported also for omalizumab	Activation of mast cell/ basophil
IgG-mediated	Until 6 h after infusion. After at least one uneventful infusion, sensitization would be required	Quite like those observed in IgE-mediated reactions	Activation of mast cell/ basophil
SSRL	From 5 to 7 days after infusion. Reactions may occur with the first exposure to the mAb although they most frequently develop after at least one uneventful infusion	Fever, malaise, arthralgia/arthritis, jaw pain or tightness, an erythematous (sometimes urticarial) skin eruption, purpura, and conjunctival hyperemia	Deposition of immune complexes composed of the mAb and anti-mAb IgG in small blood vessels
Nonimmediate reaction		Symmetrical drug-related intertriginous and flexural exanthema (SDRIFE) to Stevens-Johnson syndrome (SJS) and toxic epidermal necrolysis, exanthema, erythema multiform, lymphocytic infiltration of the dermal-epidermal junction with generalized erythematous squamous exanthema	Lymphocyte T activation

IRR infusion-related reactions, *CRR* cytokine release reactions, *SSLR* serum sickness-like reaction [92–101]

- The presence of anti-TNF alpha antibodies increases the risk of reactions in all autoimmune diseases.
- Reactions to infliximab are more frequent in patients suffering from rheumatoid arthritis, compared to other diseases.
- Rituximab is more immunogenic in autoimmune diseases than in cancer.
- Concomitant immunomodulatory therapy increases antibody production, especially in Crohn's disease.
- Immunogenicity can be influenced by extrinsic factors, such as contaminants or adjuvants, administration protocols, and comedication.

The following steps should be implemented for the diagnosis.

- *Skin tests:* If an immediate reaction is suspected, the first step consists of performing SPT and immediate reading IDT that should be conducted 4–6 weeks after the reaction. If a

Table 12.7 Suggested skin testing concentrations for mAbs [93]

Drug	Prick test	Intradermal test
Abciximab	0.2–2 mg/mL	0.2–2 mg/mL
Basiliximab	4 mg/mL	0.4–400 µg/mL
Cetuximab	500 µg/mL	5-50-500 µg/mL
Natalizumab	20 mg/mL	2 mg/mL
Omalizumab	12.5–125 mg/mL	1.25 µg/mL
Rituximab	10 mg/mL	0.10–1 mg/mL
Tocilizumab	20 mg/mL	0.2 mg/mL
Trastuzumab	21 mg/mL	0.21–2.1 mg/mL
Adalimumab	50 mg/mL	5–50 mg/mL
Etanercept	25 mg/mL	5 mg/mL
Infliximab	10 mg/mL	0.1–1 mg/mL
Anakinra	As is	—
Filgrastim	300 µg/mL	As is
Lenograstim	—	As is
Sagramostim	100–250 µg/mL	—

delayed reaction is suspected, the delayed reading of IDT (at 24–72 h) is used (Table 12.7). The value of skin testing is limited because they are not validated, and accuracy studies are lacking.

- DPT: The controlled administration of the mAb is not free from risks and must be executed after a careful evaluation of the risks-benefits for the patient [76]. The DPT can be considered for cases of a mild reaction or in case of an unclear history with negative skin tests. Only one study in adults has described the challenge test with mAb demonstrating that in 78% of cases, the presence of hypersensitivity was excluded and that 49% of the patients had undergone the test due to an unclear history of reaction. The DPT should be ideally performed before desensitization, to select those who effectively need this procedure. However, in practice in most cases, drug desensitization is directly performed, especially in patients with immediate reactions, including anaphylaxis. DPT can also be used to test non-cross-reactive drugs, even if cross-reactivity data is lacking in the case of biologicals.

12.6 Desensitization

Desensitization is defined as a process through which a person with a known history of hypersensitivity reaction to a given stimulus becomes progressively less responsive by exposure to increasing doses [102]. Drug desensitization is the cornerstone of the therapeutic approach to DHRs. A careful case-by-case evaluation should be done before recommending drug desensitization. It is very important to balance the risks and benefits of a given desensitization procedure for each patient, considering its effectiveness, unique mechanism of action, side effects, and possible alternatives [3]. In children, there are few conditions to prescribe a desensitization: children suffering from severe and chronic infection diseases (for example tuberculosis, HIV infection, and cystic fibrosis); children presenting a hematological or oncological conditions and a history of DHR; children suffering from chronic inflammatory diseases, requiring, for example, NSAIDs and mAbs; and children allergic to vaccines [104]. It is recommended in children with nonsevere reactions when no alternative drug is available or when the drug in question is more effective than the alternatives, and there are no risk factors for the patient [105]. Physicians and patients (and their caregivers) should be aware that desensitization may be associated with a possible risk of acute hypersensitivity reactions during the procedure. Following an attentive consultation with parents and/or tutors, informed and signed consent is required [106].

Even if this is typically used for type 1 allergic reactions with a demonstrable or presumed IgE-mediated response, other immunological reactions have been subjected to the same procedure.

This is performed by administering increasing doses of the medication over a short period of time (from several hours to a few days) until the total cumulative therapeutic dose is achieved and tolerated. The drug is given by parenteral or oral route, with the latter considered safer, easier, and less expensive when feasible [107]. A combination of two routes may also be proposed in some patients for certain drugs [7]. When the oral route is adopted, the use of suspension forms is generally preferred, since the desensitization protocol requires starting with very low doses that are easier to obtain [108]. There is no consensus on the value of premedication and co-medication during desensitization, as well as on the type and doses of drugs to be used such as antihistamines, corticosteroids, and montelukast [109]. Some protocols include intravenous administration of diphenhydramine (1 mg/kg), famotidine (20 mg in patients >12 years of age), and/or ranitidine (1.5 mg/kg) 20 min before starting desensitization. Others include a dose of dexamethasone (10 mg/m^2, maximum 20 mg) to be taken the night before the protocol and the same morning, especially when desensitizing patients to chemotherapeutic agents. In patients who previously failed a desensitization protocol or in those having experienced flushing reactions, montelukast (10 mg orally for children >14 years old, 5 mg for children 6–14 years old, 4 mg for children 2–5 years old), and/or acetylsalicylic acid (10–15 mg/kg) may be considered as additional premedication 1 h before desensitization. In patients requiring desensitization to mAb, premedication with acetaminophen (15 mg/kg) together with anti-H1 antihistamines is advised to reduce reactions due to cytokine release [110]. Nevertheless, the European Network of Drug Allergy (ENDA) and the European Academy for Allergy and Clinical Immunology (EAACI) claim that premedication with systemic corticosteroids and antihistamines is not necessary and may mask early signs of a hypersensitivity reaction [103]. Desensitization protocols have been developed and are used for patients with allergic reactions to antibiotics (mainly penicillin), insulins, sulfonamides, chemotherapeutic, biologic agents, and many others (Table 12.8).

Table 12.8 List of drugs for which desensitization protocols are reported [6]

Antimicrobial	Antifungal	Antiviral	Biologic agents	Chemotherapeutic
Ampicillin	Fluconazole	Acyclovir	Adalimumab	L-asparaginase
Aztreonam	Itraconazole	Amprenavir	Cetuximab	Carboplatin
Cefotaxime		Darunavir	Glatiramer acetate	Cisplatin
Ceftazidime		Efavirenz	Infliximab	Cytarabine
Ceftriaxone		Enfuvirtide		Docetaxel
Ciprofloxacin		Nelfinavir		Imatinib mesylate
Clarithromycin		Nevirapine		Lenalidomide
Clindamycin		Tipranavir		Mechlorethamine
Co-trimoxazole		Zidovudine		6-Mercaptopurine
Daptomycin				Oxaliplatin
Enviomycin				Paclitaxel
Ethambutol				Sunitinib
Imipenem/cilastatin				Thalidomide
Isoniazid				
Linezolid				
Meropenem				
Metronidazole				
Penicillin				
Quinidine				
Rifampicin				
Streptomycin				
Sulphadiazine				
Tobramycin				
Vancomycin				

SJS Steven-Johnson syndrome, *TEN* toxic epidermal necrolysis, *MPE* maculopapular exanthema, *DRESS* drug reaction with eosinophilia and systemic symptoms

Immunosuppressive	NAIDS	Antiepileptic	Hormonal agents	Miscellaneous
Azathioprine	Aspirin	Carbamazepine	Anastrozole	Antithymocite globulin
Cyclosporine	Flurbiprofen	Oxcarbazepine	Corticotropin	Allopurinol
Dapsone		Phenobarbital	Follicle-stimulating hormone	5-Aminosalicylic acid
Hydroxychloroquine		Phenytoin	Growth hormone	Buprenorphine
Mesalazine			Insulin	Calcitonin
Methotrexate				Calcitriol
Mycophenolate mofetil				Clopidogrel
d-Penicillamine				Colchicine
Sulfasalazine				Desferrioxamine
				Enoxaparin
				Erythropoietin
				Ferrous compounds
				Fluorescein
				Fluoxetine
				Furosemide
				Heparin
				Imiglucerase
				Interferon
				Isonicotinic acid Hydrazine
				Methylphenidate
				Neuromuscular receptor blockers
				Opioids
				Radiocontrast media
				Ubiquinone
				Warfarin

In children, NSAIDs are the most confirmed drug responsible for triggering a pediatric DHR and BLs, the most frequently suspected. However, also vaccines, chemotherapeutic agents (particularly carboplatin and L-asparaginase), mAbs, analgesics, and radiocontrast media may be associated with DHR and may be essential for the patient [111]. It is noteworthy that tolerance is temporary and can only be maintained by continuous administration of the medication. Thus, the procedure must be repeated for every new course. Standardized protocols for rapid drug desensitization to antibiotics, chemotherapeutic agents, mAb/fusion proteins, and other drugs typically last between 4 and 12 h. They usually address type 1 reactions with mast cell/basophils/IgE involvement, while slow drug desensitization protocols address delayed type IV reactions with T-cell involvement. Mixed reactions are most often seen in patients presenting urticarial rashes in a delayed fashion, in which cases rapid drug desensitization protocols obtained success [112]. Pediatricians do not have specific guidelines or recommendations on how to perform desensitization protocols for their patients. Notably, protocols in children differ from those in adults only in the cumulative dose, which should be the daily therapeutic dose [113]. Generally, it is recommended to use protocols previously tested, validated, and published on a small group of patients. Nevertheless, most often protocols must be tailored to a single patient. Caution and surveillance by well-trained specialists and nurses are mandatory in all cases, with continuous monitoring of the child. Caregivers should also be taught to recognize early signs to notify healthcare workers [106]. Before beginning the procedure, patients should be in a stable clinical condition, and any concomitant medication used for treating underlying diseases must be continued. Only beta-blockers should be discontinued as they may interfere with the treatment of a severe hypersensitivity reaction.

Despite its clinical success, little is known about the mechanisms and molecular basis of drug desensitization. Mast cells and basophils are likely to be targets of the process. For instance, mediators from these cells are released during DHRs, as well as during desensitization procedures, providing temporary tolerance. Suboptimal doses of antigen prior to the optimal dose seem to induce mast cells and basophils' unresponsiveness to the drug but not to other stimuli. Different hypotheses have been proposed to elucidate the efficacy of desensitization. Increasing subtherapeutic doses can provide sufficient antigenic determinants to bind to IgE anchored to the surface FcεRI receptors but not to cross-link such IgE. Another explanation is that the antigen may be able to induce rapid internalization of cross-linked antigen receptors, which depletes the cell surface of these receptors, thus making the cell unresponsive to the antigen [114]. Finally, the third hypothesis is that activating signal transduction components, such as SYK kinase, are depleted. In vitro tests revealed that rapid desensitization of human mast cells decreases the levels of signal-transducing molecules, such as SYK and LYN [115]. This may be due to the degradation of such molecules or to other—still unknown—mechanisms. Available data show the importance of different signal-transduction pathways for desensitization. SYK-deficient basophils do not degranulate, and STAT-6-deficient mast cells cannot be desensitized although they remain responsive to antigens and release beta-hexosaminidase [116]. In nonallergic hypersensitivity reactions, the mechanism of rapid desensitization to aspirin and other NSAIDs is believed to be based on a decreased production of leukotrienes and tryptase. Mechanisms are still unknown for non-IgE-mediated reactions. Immunocytotoxic reactions such as type II reactions or oxaliplatin immune-induced syndrome, vasculitis, serum sickness-like (type III reactions), or SCAR are contraindicated for desensitization. However, desensitization protocols for type IV DHRs are reported [117]. According to Corrado-Chagoya et al. [118], a 6-year-old boy experienced an SJS/TEN overlap syndrome to the antituberculosis drugs, and he tolerated the drugs after undergoing a desensitization protocol with premedication. Witcher et al. showed instead that a 5-year-old boy was successfully desensitized to phenobarbital after having presented a DRESS syndrome [119]. Most protocols and recommendations on desensitization focus on adults and have been transported and adapted to children.

12.7 Conclusions

In the vast realm of medical challenges, drug allergy stands as a significant one, deserving our attention. Scientific research about its pathogenetic mechanisms is still ongoing, and many of these are yet to be fully understood. However, in the last decades, we have become better equipped to predict, diagnose, and manage drug allergies by comprehending their underlying immunological processes. Moreover, by recognizing the signs, symptoms, and risk factors associated with drug allergies, we can now take proactive measures to minimize the risks and promote patient safety. We have come to realize the diversity of drug allergies, from mild skin rashes to life-threatening anaphylaxis, as well as the complex interactions between drugs, the immune system, and genetic predispositions. We know that misdiagnosis can occur for several reasons. First, adverse drug reactions can manifest with symptoms like those of a DHR, without involving the immune system. These nonimmune-mediated adverse reactions can be mistakenly identified as a true allergy, leading to a misdiagnosis and inappropriate case management. Additionally, the diagnostic tests available for drug allergies may have low diagnostic accuracy. Because of ADR frequency combined with cofactors such as common mild infections, but also due to similarities in the clinical presentation of DHR with several types of nonallergic disease, there is a consistent risk of labeling a patient as allergic even if he/she is not. This is particularly harmful to children, as they may withdraw a specific drug even when no alternatives are available. To conclude, it is paramount to stress once more how any diagnostic workup should never miss a thorough analysis of the patient's medical history and an accurate interpretation of test results. Additional tests or consultation with a specialist may be also necessary to confirm or exclude a diagnosis. Finally, drug allergy is a medical field with continuous developments that reduce the chances of misdiagnosis and improve patient care and safety.

Box 12.1 Hypersensitivity Reactions to Drugs. The Fixed Points

- Hypersensitivity reactions to drugs are the cause of 3–6% of hospital admissions and occur in 10–15% of hospitalized subjects. They can cause serious damage, such as to cause the patient's death.
- A child should not be considered allergic to drugs based on the medical history alone without having conducted the necessary allergy diagnostics. The replacement of the suspect drug with an alternative drug with a different chemical structure without clarifying the diagnosis with an allergy workup is not advisable except in an emergency as the drug alternative often has lower efficacy, higher costs, and higher side effects.
- Diagnostics of drug allergy must be conducted in allergy centers with experience and personnel trained in this area. It varies depending on the type of drug, its class, and the circumstances in which the reaction occurred (e.g., perioperative period).
- The diagnostic procedure is different in immediate and delayed reactions The pathogenetic mechanisms of drug hypersensitivity are different and not always explored with routine allergy tests (skin tests and research of specific IgE). LTT, ELISpot test, and BAT need further validation for routine use. When indicated, provocation testing should be performed under the close supervision of personnel trained in the treatment of anaphylaxis and with access to resuscitation in case of emergency.
- The provocation test is contraindicated in the event of a history of dangerous reactions for the patient (SCAR, vasculitis, and organ and hematological reactions) while, in the event of anaphylaxis, the risk/benefit ratio must be evaluated.
- Some patients show hypersensitivity to nonreplaceable drugs (e.g., insulin, biological drugs, and chemotherapy). In these cases, it is necessary to resort to desensitization procedures.

References

1. Dona I, Caubet JC, Brockow K, Doyle M, Moreno E, Terreehorst I, et al. An EAACI task force report: recognizing the potential of the primary care physician in the diagnosis and management of drug hypersensitivity. Clin Transl Allergy. 2018;8:16.
2. Park BK, Naisbitt D, Demoly P. Drug hypersensitivity. In: Allergy. 4th ed. W.B. Saunders; 2012. p. 321–30.
3. Franceschini F, Bianchi A, Bottau P, Caimmi S, Crisafulli G, Liotti L, et al. La ipersensibilità a farmaci nel bambino: come comportarsi. Riv Immunol Allergol Pediatr. 2023;37:1.
4. Pichler WJ. Drug hypersensitivity: classification and clinical features. In: Post TW, editor. UpToDate. Waltham, MA: UpToDate; 2023. (Accessed on July 5th, 2023).
5. Igea JM. The history of the idea of allergy. Allergy. 2013;68:966–73.
6. Thong B, Vervloet D. Drug allergies. Available at: https://www.worldallergy.org/education-and-programs/education/allergic-disease-resource-center/professionals/drug-allergies (Accessed on August 5th, 2023).
7. Thong B, Tan T. Epidemiology and risk factors for drug allergy. Br J Clin Pharmacol. 2010;71:684–700.
8. Schneck J, Fagot JP, Sekula P, Sassolas B, Roujeau JC, Mockenhaupt M. Effects of treatments on the mortality of Stevens-Johnson syndrome and toxic epidermal necrolysis: a retrospective study on

patients included in the prospective EuroSCAR Study. J Am Acad Dermatol. 2008;58:33–40.
9. Pichler WJ. Delayed drug hypersensitivity reactions. Ann Intern Med. 2003;139:683–93.
10. Barranco P, Lopez-Serrano MC. General and epidemiological aspects of allergic drug reactions. Clin Exp Allergy. 1998;28:61–2.
11. Ventura MT, Boni E, Cecere R, Buquicchio R, Calogiuri GF, Martignago I, et al. Importance of hypersensitivity in adverse reactions to drugs in the elderly. Clin Mol Allergy. 2018;16:7.
12. Gamboa PM. The epidemiology of drug allergy-related consultations in Spanish allergology services: alergológica-2005. J Investig Allergol Clin Immunol. 2009;19(S2):45–50.
13. Norton AE. Broyles AD, Drug allergy in children and adults: is it the double X chromosome? Ann Allergy Asthma Immunol. 2019;122:148–55.
14. Leong KP, Thong BY, Cheng YK, Tang CY, Cheng HH. Are there differences in drug allergy between the sexes? Ann Acad Med Singap. 2003;32:151.
15. Yang SC, Chen CB, Lin MY, Zhang ZY, Jia XY, Huang M, et al. Genetics of severe cutaneous adverse reactions. Front Med. 2021;8:652091.
16. Ramesh S. Antibiotic hypersensitivity in patients with CF. Clin Rev Allergy Immunol. 2002;23:123–41.
17. Caubet JC, Kaiser L, Lemaître B, Fellay B, Gervaix A, Eigenmann PA. The role of penicillin in benign skin rashes in childhood: a prospective study based on drug rechallenge. J Allergy Clin Immunol. 2011;127:218–22.
18. Shiohara T, Kano Y. A complex interaction between drug allergy and viral infection. Clin Rev Allergy Immunol. 2007;33:124–33.
19. Johansson SG, Florvaag E, Oman H, Poulsen LK, Mertes PM, Harper NJ, et al. National pholcodine consumption and prevalence of IgE-sensitization: a multicentre study. Allergy. 2010;65:498–502.
20. Landry Q, Zhang S, Ferrando L, Bourrain JL, Demoly P, Chiriac AM. Multiple drug hypersensitivity syndrome in a large database. J Allergy Clin Immunol Pract. 2020;8:258-66:e1.
21. Jagpal PK, Alshareef S, Marriott JF, Krishna MT. Characterization, epidemiology and risk factors of multiple drug allergy syndrome and multiple drug intolerance syndrome: a systematic review. Clin Transl Allergy. 2022;12:e12190.
22. Khan D. Cephalosporin allergy: current understanding and future challenges. J Allergy Clin Immunol Pract. 2019;7:2105–14.
23. Pichler WJ. Immune pathomechanism and classification of drug hypersensitivity. Allergy. 2019;74:1457–71.
24. Kloypan C, Koomdee N, Satapornpong Pempark T, Biswas M, Sukasem C. A comprehensive review of HLA and severe cutaneous adverse drug reactions: implication for clinical pharmacogenomics and precision medicine. Pharmaceuticals. 2021;14:1077.
25. Kumar M, Duraisami K, Chow B. Unlocking the non-IgE-mediated pseudo-allergic reaction. Puzzle with Mas-related G-protein coupled receptor member X2 (MRGPRX2). Cells. 2021;10:1033.
26. Grabenhenrich L, Dolle S, Moneret-Vautrin A, Köhli A, Lange L, Spindler T, et al. Anaphylaxis in children and adolescents: the European Anaphylaxis Registry. J Allergy Clin Immunol. 2016;137:1128–1137.e1.
27. Gabrielli S, Clarke A, Eismann H. Disparities in rate, triggers, and management in pediatric and adult cases of suspected drug-induced anaphylaxis in Canada. Immun Inflamm Dis. 2018;6:3–12.
28. Arnold KA, Gao J, Stein SL. A review of cutaneous hypersensitivity reactions in infants: from common to concerning. Pediatr Dermatol. 2019;36:274–82.
29. Sokumbi O, Wetter DA. Clinical features, diagnosis, and treatment of erythema multiforme: a review for the practicing dermatologist. Int J Dermatol. 2012;51:889–902.
30. Heinze A, Tollefson M, Holland KE, Chiu YE. Characteristics of pediatric recurrent erythema multiforme. Pediatr Dermatol. 2018;35:97–103.
31. Lee AY. Fixed drug eruptions. Incidence, recognition, and avoidance. Am J Clin Dermatol. 2000;1:277–85.
32. Morelli J, Tai Y, Rogers M. Fixed drug eruptions in children. J Pediatr. 1999;134:365–7.
33. Crisafulli G, Franceschini F, Caimmi S, Bottau P, Liotti L, Saretta F, et al. Mild cutaneous reactions to drugs. Acta Biomed. 2019;90:36–43.
34. Del Pozzo-Magana B, Abuzgaia A, Murray B, Rieder MJ, Lazo-Langner A. Paediatric serum sickness-like reaction: a 10-year retrospective cohort study. Paediatr Child Health. 2021;6:428–35.
35. Lee E, Koh M. Acute generalized exanthematous pustulosis in children and adolescents in Singapore: a ten-year retrospective review. Pediatr Dermatol. 2021;38:424–30.
36. Liccioli G, Marrani E, Giani T, Simonini G, Barni S, Mori F. The first pediatric case of acute generalized exanthematous pustulosis caused by hydroxychloroquine. Pharmacology. 2019;104:57–9.
37. Costa D, Seque C, Enokihara M, Porro AM. Acute generalized exanthematous pustulosis: a case series of 13 patients in Brazil. J Eur Acad Dermato Venereol. 2019;33:e52–5.
38. Szatkowski J, Schwartz R. Acute generalized exanthematous pustulosis (AGEP): a review and update. J Am Acad Dermatol. 2015;73:843–8.
39. White K, Abe R, Ardern-Jones M, Beachkofsky T, Bouchard C, Carleton B, Chodosh J, et al. SJS/TEN 2017: building multidisciplinary networks to drive science and translation. J Allergy Clin Immunol Pract. 2018;6:38–69.
40. Antoon J, Goldman J, Lee B, Schwartz A. Incidence, outcomes, and resource use in children with Stevens-Johnson syndrome and toxic epidermal necrolysis. Pediatr Dermatol. 2018;35:182–7.

41. Techasatian L, Panombualert S, Uppala R, Jetsrisuparb C. Drug-induced Stevens-Johnson syndrome and toxic epidermal necrolysis in children: 20 years study in a tertiary care hospital. World J Pediatr. 2017;13:255–60.
42. Finkelstein Y, Soon G, Acuna P, George M, Pope E, Ito S, et al. Recurrence and outcomes of Stevens-Johnson syndrome and toxic epidermal necrolysis in children. Pediatrics. 2011;128:723–8.
43. Liccioli G, Mori F, Parronchi P, Capone M, Fili L, Barni S, et al. Aetiopathogenesis of severe cutaneous adverse reactions (SCARs) in children: a 9-year experience in a tertiary care paediatric hospital setting. Clin Exp Allergy. 2020;50:61–73.
44. Liotti L, Caimmi S, Bottau P, Bernardini R, Cardinale F, Saretta F, et al. Clinical features, outcomes and treatment in children with drug induced Stevens-Johnson syndrome and toxic epidermal necrolysis. Acta Biomed. 2019;29:52–60.
45. Criado PR, Criado RF, Avancini JM, Santi CG. Drug reaction with eosinophilia and systemic symptoms (DRESS)/drug-induced hypersensitivity syndrome (DIHS): a review of current concepts. An Bras Dermatol. 2012;87:435–49.
46. Mori F, Caffarelli C, Caimmi S, Bottau P, Liotti L, Franceschini F, et al. Drug reaction with eosinophilia and systemic symptoms (DRESS) in children. Acta Biomed. 2019;29:66–7.
47. Afiouni R, Zeinaty P, Kechichian E. Pediatric drug reaction with eosinophilia and systemic symptoms: a systematic review of the literature, with a focus on relapsing cases. Pediatr Dermatol. 2021;38:125–31.
48. Cacoub P, Musette P, Descamps V. The DRESS syndrome: a literature review. Am J Med. 2011;124:588–97.
49. Kumar PA, Saroch A. Diagnostic criteria for drug rash and eosinophilia with systemic symptoms. J Family Med Prim Care. 2017;3:693–4.
50. Novembre E, Mori F, Barni S. La Drug Induced Enterocolitis Syndrome (DIES): una nuova sindrome da conoscere. RIAIP. 2020;3:2–6.
51. Di Filippo P, Venanzi A, Ciarelli F, Panetti B, Di Pillo S, Chiarelli F, et al. Drug-Induced Enterocolitis Syndrome in Children. Int J Mol Sci. 2023;24:7880.
52. Novembre E, Barni S, Saretta F, Castagnoli R, Arasi S, Mastrorilli C, et al. Rare Allergic Diseases Commission of the Italian Society of Pediatric Allergy and Immunology (SIAIP). The history of drug-induced enterocolitis syndrome. Pediatr Allergy Immunol. 2022;33(Suppl. 27):54–7.
53. García Rodríguez R, Alfaya Arias T, Borja Segade J, Méndez Díaz Y, Moreno Lozano L, Extremera Ortega A, et al. Drug-induced enterocolitis in an adult patient. J Allergy Clin Immunol Pract. 2017;5:1752–3.
54. Khan DA, Banerji A, Blumenthal KG, Phillips EJ, Solensky R, White AA, et al. Drug allergy: A 2022 practice parameter update. J Allergy Clin Immunol. 2022;150:1333–93.
55. The WHO AWaRe (Access, Watch, Reserve) antibiotic book. Geneva: World Health Organization; 2022. Available at: https://www.who.int/publications/i/item/9789240062382 (accessed on August 7th, 2023).
56. Romano A, Atanaskovic-Markovic M, Barbaud A, Bircher AJ, Brockow K, Caubet JC, et al. Towards a more precise diagnosis of hypersensitivity to beta-lactams—an EAACI position paper. Allergy. 2020;75:1300–15.
57. Blanca-Lopez N, Atanaskovic-Markovic M, Gomes E, Kidon M, Kuyucu S, Mori F, et al. An EAACI Task Force report on allergy to beta-lactams in children: Clinical entities and diagnostic procedures. Pediatr Allergy Immunol. 2021;32:1426–36.
58. Mori F, Liccioli G, Barni S, Novembre E. Management of suspected antibiotic reactions in children. Pediatr Infect Dis J. 2019;38:e149–52.
59. Grinlington L, Choo S, Cranswick N, Gwee A. Non beta-lactam antibiotic hypersensitivity reactions. Pediatrics. 2020;145:e20192256.
60. Barni S, Butti D, Mori F, Pucci N, Rossi ME, Cianferoni A, et al. Azithromycin is more allergenic than clarithromycin in children with suspected hypersensitivity reaction to macrolides. J Investig Allergol Clin Immunol. 2015;25:128–32.
61. Chow T, Khan D. Sulfonamide hypersensitivity. Clin Rev Allergy Immunol. 2022;62:400–12.
62. Zhu L, Liu A, Wong P, Arroyo AC. Road less traveled: drug hypersensitivity to fluoroquinolones, vancomycin, tetracyclines, and macrolides. Clin Rev Allergy Immunol. 2022;62:505–18.
63. Dilley M, Geng B. Immediate and delayed hypersensitivity reactions to antibiotics: aminoglycosides, clindamycin, linezolid, and metronidazole. Clin Rev Allergy Immunol. 2022;62:463–75.
64. Kidon M, Blanca-Lopez N, Gomes E, Terreehorst I, Tanno L, Ponvert C, et al. EAACI/ENDA Position Paper: Diagnosis and management of hypersensitivity reactions to non-steroidal anti-inflammatory drugs (NSAIDs) in children and adolescents. Pediatr Allergy Immunol. 2018;29:469–80.
65. Doña I, Pérez-Sánchez N, Eguiluz-Gracia I, Muñoz-Cano R, Bartra J, et al. Progress in understanding hypersensitivity reactions to nonsteroidal anti-inflammatory drugs. Allergy. 2020;75:561–75.
66. Misirlioglu ED, Toyran M, Capanoglu M, Kaya A, Civelek E, Kocabas CN. Negative predictive value of drug provocation tests in children. Pediatr Allergy Immunol. 2014;25:685–90.
67. Wakimoto M, Miller R, Kim S, Uffman JC, NafiuS OO, Tobias JD, et al. Perioperative anaphylaxis in children: a report from the Wake-Up Safe collaborative. Paediatr Anaesth. 2021;31:205–12.
68. Laguna J, Archilla J, Doña I, Corominas M, Gastaminza G, Mayorga C, et al. Practical guidelines for perioperative hypersensitivity reactions. J Investig Allergol Clin Immunol. 2018;28:216–32.

69. Garvey L, Ebo D, Mertes P, Dewachter P, Garcez T, Kopac P, et al. An EAACI position paper on the investigation of perioperative immediate hypersensitivity reactions. Allergy. 2019;74:1872–84.
70. Brockow K, Garvey L, Aberer W, Atanaskovic-Markovic M, Barbaud A, Bilo MB, et al. Skin test concentrations for systemically administered drugs, an ENDA/EAACI drug allergy interest group position paper. Allergy. 2013;68:702–12.
71. Pfützner W, Brockow K. Perioperative drug reactions—practical recommendations for allergy testing and patient management. Allergo J Int. 2018;27:126–9.
72. Malinovsky J, Chiriac A, Tacquard C, Mertes PM, Demoly P. Allergy to local anesthetics: reality or myth? Presse Med. 2016;45:753–7.
73. Mori F, Blanca-Lopez N, Caubet J-C, , Demoly P, Du Toit G, Gomes ER, et al. Delayed hypersensitivity to antiepileptic drugs in children. Pediatr Allergy Immunol. 2021;32:425–36.
74. Tang YH, Mockenhaupt M, Henry A, Bounoua M, Naldi L, Le Gouvello S et al. Poor relevance of a lymphocyte proliferation assay in lamotrigine-induced Stevens-Johnson syndrome or toxic epidermal necrolysis. Clin Exp Allergy. 2012;42:248–54.
75. Kumkamthornkul P, Udnaen S, Tansit T, Tuchinda P, Srinoulprasert Y. Evaluation of a lymphocyte transformation test and cytokine detection assay to identify phenytoin and carbamazepine provoked DRESS or SJS/TEN in epilepsy patients. Int Immunopharmacol. 2018;63:204–10.
76. Pagani M, Bavbek S, Alvarez-Cuesta E, Berna Dursun A, Bonadonna P, Castells M, et al. Hypersensitivity reactions to chemotherapy: an EAACI Position Paper. Allergy. 2022;77:388–403.
77. Pellegrino B, Boggiani D, Tommasi C, Palli D, Musolino A. Nab-paclitaxel after docetaxel hypersensitivity reaction: case report and literature review. Acta Biomed. 2017;88:329–33.
78. Kintzel PE. Prophylaxis for paclitaxel hypersensitivity reactions. Ann Pharmacother. 2001;30:367–71.
79. Narta UK, Kanwar SS, Azmi W. Pharmacological and clinical evaluation of L-asparaginase in the treatment of leukemia. Crit Rev Oncol Hematol. 2007;61:208–21.
80. Lee C, Gianos M, Klausermeyer WB. Diagnosis and management of hypersensitivity reactions related to common cancer chemotherapy agents. Ann Allergy Asthma Immunol. 2009;102:179–87.
81. Leguy-Seguin V, Jolimoy G, Coudert B, Pernot C, Dalac S, Vabres P, et al. Diagnostic and predictive value of skin testing in platinum salt hypersensitivity. J Allergy Clin Immunol. 2007;119:726–30.
82. Aberer W, Bircher A, Romano A, Blanca M, Campi P, Fernandez J, et al. Drug provocation testing in the diagnosis of drug hypersensitivity reactions: general considerations. Allergy. 2003;58:854–63.
83. Polyzos A, Tsavaris N, Kosmos C, Arnaouti T, Kalahanis N, Tsigris C, et al. Hypersensitivity reactions to carboplatin administration are common but not always severe. A 10-year experience. Oncology. 2001;61:129–33.
84. Lopez-Gonzalez P, Madrigal-Burgaleta R, Carpio-Escalona LV, Bernal-Rubio L, Guerra E, Berges-Gimeno MP, et al. Assessment of antihistamines and corticosteroids as premedication in rapid drug desensitization to paclitaxel: outcomes in 155 procedures. J Allergy Clin Immunol Pract. 2018;6:1356–62.
85. Wang E, Kraehenbuehl L, Ketosugbo K, , Kern JA, Lacouture ME, Leung DYM. Immune-related cutaneous adverse events due to checkpoint inhibitors. Ann Allergy Asthma Immunol. 2021;126:613–22.
86. Mueller KA, Cordisco MR, Scott GA, Plovanich ME. A case of severe nivolumab- induced lichen planus pemphigoides in a child with metastatic spitzoid melanoma. Pediatr Dermatol. 2023;40:154–6.
87. Nigro O, Ferrari A, Casanova M, Orbach D, Leruste A, Gatz SA, et al. Controversies on the possible role of immune checkpoint inhibitors in pediatric cancers: balancing irAEs and efficacy. Tumori. 2021;107:276–81.
88. Kohler G, Milstein C. Continuous cultures of fused cells secreting antibody of predefined specificity. Nature. 1975;256:495–7.
89. Martin-Mateos MA. Monoclonal antibodies in pediatrics: use in prevention and treatment. Allergol Immunopathol (Madr). 2007;35:145–50.
90. Brennan PJ, Rodriguez Bouza T, Hsu FI, Sloane DE, Castells MC. Hypersensitivity reactions to mAbs: 105 desensitizations in 23 patients, from evaluation to treatment. J Allergy Clin Immunol. 2009;124:1259–66.
91. Picard M, Regniér GV. Current knowledge and management of hypersensitivity reactions to monoclonal antibodies. J Allergy Clin Immunol Pract. 2017;5:600–9.
92. Maggi E, Vultaggio A, Matucci A. Acute infusion reactions induced by monoclonal antibody therapy. Expert Rev Clin Immunol. 2011;7:55–63.
93. Corominas M, Gastaminza G, Lobera T. Hypersensitivity reactions to biological drugs. J Investig Allergol Clin Immunol. 2014;24:212–25.
94. O'Meara S, Nanda KS, Moss AC. Antibodies to infliximab and risk of infusion reactions in patients with inflammatory bowel disease: a systematic review and meta-analysis. Inflamm Bowel Dis. 2014;20:1–6.
95. Maneiro JR, Salgado E, Gomez-Reino JJ. Immunogenicity of monoclonal antibodies against tumor necrosis factor used in chronic immune-mediated inflammatory conditions: systematic review and meta-analysis. JAMA Intern Med. 2013;173:1416–28.

96. Finkelman FD, Khodoun MV, Strait R. Human IgE-independent systemic anaphylaxis. J Allergy Clin Immunol. 2016;137:1674–80.
97. Van der Laken CJ, Voskuyl AE, Roos JC, Stigter van Walsum M, de Groot ER, et al. Imaging and serum analysis of immune complex formation of radiolabelled infliximab and anti-infliximab in responders and non-responders to therapy for rheumatoid arthritis. Ann Rheum Dis. 2007;66:253–6.
98. Alvarez-Cuesta E, Madrigal-Burgaleta R, Angel-Pereira D, Urena-Tavera A, Zamora- Verduga M, Lopez-Gonzalez P, et al. Delving into cornerstones of hypersensitivity to antineoplastic and biological agents: value of diagnostic tools prior to desensitization. Allergy. 2015;70:784–94.
99. Bulur I, Keseroglu HO, Saracoglu ZN, Gonul M. Symmetrical drug-related intertriginous and flexural exanthema (Baboon syndrome) associated with infliximab. J Dermatol Case Rep. 2015;9:12–4.
100. Lowndes S, Darby A, Mead G, Lister A. Stevens-Johnson syndrome after treatment with rituximab. Ann Oncol. 2002;13:1948–50.
101. Lin WL, Lin WC, Yang JY, Chang YC, Ho HC, Yang LC, et al. Fatal toxic epidermal necrolysis associated with cetuximab in a patient with colon cancer. J Clin Oncol. 2008;26:2779–80.
102. Demir S, Olgac M, Unal D, Gelincik A, Colakoglu B, Buyukozturk S. A practical and successful desensitization protocol for immediate hypersensitivity reactions to iron salts. Int Arch Allergy Immunol. 2014;165:100–3.
103. Caimmi S, Caffarelli C, Saretta F, Liotti L, Crisafulli G, Cardinale F, et al. Drug desensitization in allergic children. Acta Biomed. 2019;90:20–9.
104. Diaferio L, Giovannini M, Clark E, Castagnoli R, Caimmi D. Protocols for drug allergy desensitization in children. Expert Rev Clin Immunol. 2020;16:91–100.
105. Warrington R. Drug allergy: causes and desensitization. Hum Vaccin Immunother. 2012;8:1513–24.
106. Cernadas JR. Desensitization to antibiotics in children. Pediatr Allergy Immunol. 2013;24:3–9.
107. Cernadas JR, Brockow K, Romano A, Aberer W, Torres MJ, Bircher A, et al. General considerations on rapid desensitization for drug hypersensitivity- a consensus statement. Allergy. 2010;65:1357–66.
108. Caimmi S, Crisafulli G, Franceschini F, Liotti L, Bianchi A, Bottau P, et al. Hypersensitivity to Intravenous Iron Preparations. Children. 2022;9:1473.
109. Sherer K, Brockow K, Aberer W, Gooi JH, Demoly P, Romano A, et al. Desensitization in delayed drug hypersensitivity reactions- an EAACI position paper of the drug allergy interest group. Allergy. 2013;68:844–52.
110. Hong D, Dioun A. Indications, protocols and outcomes of drug desensitization for chemotherapy and monoclonal antibodies in adults and children. J Allergy Clin Immunol Pract. 2014;2:13–9.
111. De las Vecillas Sanches L, Alenazy LA, Garcia-Neuer M, Castells MC. Drug hypersensitivity and desensitization: mechanisms and new approaches. Int J Mol Sci. 2017;18:1316.
112. Castells MC. A new era for drug desensitization. J Allergy Clin Immunol Pract. 2015;3:639–40.
113. De Groot H, Mulder WMC. Clinical practice: drug desensitization in children. Eur J Pediatr. 2010;169:1305–9.
114. Sancho-Serra Mdel C, Simarro M. Castells.Rapid IgE desensitization is antigen specific and impairs early and late mast cell responses targeting FceRI internalization. Eur J Immunol. 2011;41:1004–13.
115. Kepley C. Antigen-induced reduction in mast cell and basophil functional responses due to reduced Syk protein levels. Int Arch Allergy Immunol. 2005;138:29–39.
116. Rodriguez Morales A, Shah N, Castells M. Antigen-IgE desensitization in signal transducer and activator of transcription 6-deficient mast cells by suboptimal doses of antigen. Ann Allergy Asthma Immunol. 2005;94:575–80.
117. Cuesta A, Madrigal-Burgaleta R, Broyles AD, Cuesta-Herranz J, Guzman-Melendez MA, Maciag MC, et al. Standards for practical intravenous rapid drug desensitization & delabelling: a WAO committee statement. World Allergy Org J. 2022;15:100640.
118. Corrado-Chagoya R, Hernandez-Romero J, Eliosa-Alvarado GA, Cruz Pantoja RA, Campos-Gutiérrez RI, Velasco-Medina AA et al. Tolerance induction to antituberculosis drugs in a patient with Stevens-Johnson syndrome/toxic epidermal necrolysis overlap. Allergy Rhinol (Providence). 2018;9:1–5.
119. Witcher RH, Ramirez MM. Successful phenobarbital desensitization after DRESS reaction in the management of refractory status epilecticus. J Pharm Pract. 2018;1:1.

IgE-Mediated Food Allergy

13

Davide Caimmi, Evangéline Clark, Giuliana Giannì, and Carlo Caffarelli

Abstract

Food allergies in children are a common concern that are defined as adverse immune responses to food proteins. Common food allergens in children include cow's milk, hen's eggs, peanuts, tree nuts, wheat, fish, and shellfish. The diagnostics of food allergies in children often involves a comprehensive evaluation of medical history, physical examination, and a specific allergy workup.

The management of food allergies in children primarily revolves around strict avoidance of allergenic foods. This includes carefully reading food labels, educating family members, teachers, and other caregivers about the child's allergy, and ensuring that the child has a safe and allergen-free environment. Moreover, professionals of healthcare should prescribe emergency medications, including epinephrine auto-injectors in children at risk of anaphylaxis. Tolerance induction protocols are currently recommended, in specific cases only, in children suffering from cow's milk, egg, or peanut allergy.

Keywords

Allergens · Anaphylaxis · Children · Cow's milk · Diagnosis · Disease management · Egg · Food allergy · IgE · Oral food challenge · Peanuts

Test your learning and check your understanding of this book's contents: use the "Springer Nature Flashcards" app to access questions using ▶ https://sn.pub/nspbjm. To use the app, please follow the instructions in Chap. 1.

Key Points

- IgE-mediated food allergy refers to immediate hypersensitivity reactions, driven by the immune system, following food consumption.
- Main food triggers of food allergy in children include cow's milk, hen's egg, and peanuts.

(continued)

D. Caimmi (✉)
Allergy Unit, University Hospital of Montpellier, Montpellier, France

IDESP, Univ Montpellier—INSERM, Montpellier, France

E. Clark
Allergy Unit, University Hospital of Montpellier, Montpellier, France

G. Giannì
UOC di Pediatria e Neonatologia, Ospedali Riuniti di Livorno, Azienda USL Toscana nord ovest, Livorno, Italy

C. Caffarelli
Clinica Pediatrica, Azienda Ospedaliero-Universitaria, Department of Medicine and Surgery, University of Parma, Parma, Italy

C. Caffarelli, G. L. Marseglia (eds.), *Textbook of Pediatric Allergy*,
https://doi.org/10.1007/978-3-031-71283-8_13

- If the clinical history is compatible with food allergy, clinicians should perform skin prick tests/serum-specific IgE (including molecular allergens, when available) to assess the sensitization profile.
- Oral food challenge remains the gold standard to diagnose food allergy.

13.1 Introduction

Food allergy (FA) has become increasingly prevalent in recent years among children and can have a significant impact on their health and daily life [1]. Understanding the triggering factors, recognizing the symptoms, and effectively managing FA are crucial for individuals and their caregivers.

The most common FA is mediated by *IgE antibodies* to a food allergen and results from a *type I hypersensitivity reaction* according to Gell and Coombs' classification. Other hypersensitivity mechanisms (types III and IV) may also be involved in FA.

We will focus on IgE-mediated FA in children. We will begin with definitions and epidemiological descriptions, and finally, we will examine the main allergens and protein families.

13.2 Epidemiology

Assessing the *prevalence* of IgE-mediated food allergy is challenging. There are large variations in study methodology, from studies relying on self-reporting questionnaires that are likely to overestimate the true prevalence to those using more rigorous double-blind placebo-controlled food challenges but including a small number of patients [1–8].

According to studies conducted between 2000 and 2012, the lifetime prevalence of self-reported food allergy (FA) ranges from 5.7% to 41.8%. Additionally, the point prevalence of self-reported FA in European children aged 6–10 years varies from 1.6% to 24.4% [1].

In childhood, food allergy seems to be increasing in prevalence in many countries, as well as in severity. Even though there are large regional differences in the prevalence of food allergy in children across Europe, cow's milk and hen's egg are the most common. Other frequent allergens include wheat, soy, peanuts, tree nuts, fish, shellfish, and various plant-source foods that are related to pollen-food allergy syndromes [8].

13.3 Mechanisms and Clinical Symptoms

Oral tolerance is the normal physiological response to the ingestion of foods. The enterocytes let through, by transcytosis, food antigens that are thus put in contact with the lymphoid tissue associated with the mucous membranes (GALT). Tolerance involves the suppression of TH_2 cells, the generation of Treg cells, with a decreased production of IgE and an increased production of IgA and IgG_4 by B cells, the suppression of T cell effector migration to tissues, the induction of IL-10-producing cells, and the suppression of tissue basophil, eosinophil, and *mast cell* activation [9]. When the tolerance response is ineffective, sensitization to certain food proteins (and thus possible occurrence of clinical manifestations of allergy) may occur. The balance between tolerance and inflammation is partly regulated by the interaction between innate and adaptive immune cells and the intestinal microbiota. Loss of tolerance can be also related to an alteration and/or inflammation of the epithelial or mucosal barrier. Sensitization to food allergens is possible not only via the digestive tract but also via the skin and less frequently via the respiratory route [10].

The immunopathological mechanisms of food allergy are mediated by IgE with the occurrence of clinical immediate hypersensitivity reactions. However, especially during the first year of life, it may coexist with immediate hypersensitivity, a form of oral tolerance deficiency, the delayed onset of which could explain the transient nature of food allergy in very young children.

Enterocytes, digestive epithelial cells, are the passageway for secretory IgA to the intestinal lumen and food macromolecules to the submucosal tissue. They express HLA class II molecules from the first week after birth, and can therefore, as such, like the M cells of Peyer's patches, play a role in the presentation of antigens to *T lymphocytes* located in the underlying lymphoid tissue. Most food antigens crossing the intestinal barrier are degraded during the trans-enterocyte passage. Some intact molecules that cross the barrier are internalized by dendritic cells and macrophages. The antigen-presenting cells process and present antigens to the T lymphocytes which will thus be activated. This activation will ultimately cause the production of antibodies by the B lymphocytes and/or a cytotoxicity reaction via the CD8+ T lymphocytes [10–12].

Specific IgE to food allergens produced by the *B lymphocytes* bind to the high-affinity receptors for IgE (FcεRI) located on mast cells and basophils. The link between allergen and the IgE-FcεRI complex determines the activation of mast cells that release preformed mediators (mainly histamine, but also tryptase for the mast cells only), then, secondarily, newly formed mediators mostly derived from the degradation of membrane phospholipids [10, 11].

This process may result in the appearance of clinical symptoms. In IgE-mediated food allergy, they occur immediately (within 1–2 h) after food intake. In certain cases, as for patients suffering from alpha-gal syndrome, symptoms may occur after a longer period (see the chapter on meat allergy).

IgE-mediated food allergy may be expressed through several different clinical symptoms [13–15]:

- Oral (tongue/lips/pharyngeal swelling with pruritus).
- Skin (urticaria, atopic eczema, angioedema, rash, and itching).
- Respiratory symptoms (nasal obstruction, rhino-conjunctivitis, wheezing, cough, and bronchospasm).
- Digestive symptoms (nausea, vomiting, abdominal pain, and diarrhea).
- Cardio-vasculaire symptoms (malaise, pallor, hypotension, and arythmies).
- Neurological symptoms (behavior change, feeling of impending illness, and loss of consciousness).
- Anaphylaxis, including anaphylactic shock, requires immediate medical attention and prompt therapy.
- Food-dependent exercise-induced anaphylaxis is a particular form of allergic reaction, often initially characterized by isolated pruritus, first at extremities, then generalized, followed by urticaria and angioedema, erythema, respiratory symptoms with profuse sweating, discomfort (syncope), headaches, and gastrointestinal disorders. The progression to laryngeal edema or cardiovascular collapse is not uncommon. Acute signs appear during physical exercise only when the children had a specific triggering food or a meal up to 4 h before exercising. Therefore, the anaphylactic reaction does not systematically occur during exercise but only if it is preceded or accompanied (and even rarely followed) by intake of the culprit food.

13.4 Diagnosis of Food Allergy

The *diagnosis of FA* begins with a thorough interrogation, followed by a dietary investigation, and, if symptoms are suggestive of an immunological mechanism possibly responsible for the reported reaction, an allergy workup. The clinical history needs to be compatible with a possible IgE-mediated food allergy. The time between food intake and the appearance of symptoms needs to follow the timing of the possible immunological mechanisms. Reactions should appear after every exposure to the food [1, 13, 16, 17]. Clinical symptoms should be those possibly elicited by an IgE-mediated reaction, after mast cells/basophils mediator release.

Skin prick tests (SPT) are the first tests to be performed. A positive result indicates the presence of specific IgE antibodies against the tested allergen. It is important to note that a positive test does not necessarily mean allergy but rather sensitization to the allergen, without obligatory clinical symptoms in case of exposure to the food in question. A correlation between the SPTs and the clinical history is suggestive of allergy, even though often not sufficient to reach a firm diagnosis [13, 16–19].

SPT to foods have a high sensitivity and negative predictive value. If the SPT results are negative, FA should be ruled out if the clinical presentation is not suggestive. However, if the clinical presentation is highly suggestive, it is necessary to re-assess the clinical history, search for hidden allergens, perform serum-specific IgE measurement, and potentially conduct an *oral food challenge* (OFC) [17–19].

If SPTs are positive, considering the low specificity and positive predictive value, further investigations should be pursued, as mentioned above, to avoid overdiagnosis.

In young children, especially with atopic eczema, a positive SPT to a food never previously ingested, such as milk, egg, or peanuts, is associated with a clinical reaction at the first exposure in about 50% of cases. It is therefore recommended that the first administration of the food has been done under medical surveillance [17–19].

Circulant-specific IgE to the whole allergen has the advantage of being widely available, not being affected by either medication intake (such as antiH_1-antihistamines) or by skin conditions (e.g., dermographism and atopic dermatitis). They are only performed as a second-line approach based on the results of skin tests and clinical correlation, or if any cutaneous or systemic condition makes it impossible to perform skin tests [13, 17, 20–22].

The presence of serum-specific IgE antibodies in food indicates a sensitization to the suspected food. Nontargeted screening for anti-food IgE antibodies is not recommended as it may lead to the discovery of asymptomatic sensitizations and unnecessary food avoidance [1, 13, 17, 21].

The measurement of IgE antibodies against each single suspected natural or recombinant molecular allergen is a valuable diagnostic tool for FA. This measurement can be performed by using single or multiplex assays. Molecular IgE testing can sometimes predict the severity of the allergy and differentiate between persistent or transient forms of food allergy [17, 20]. For example, in cow's milk allergic patients, high IgE levels to caseins may be predictive of a severe and persistent allergy [23].

The *basophil activation test* (BAT) is an in vitro test that evaluates the percentage of basophils that are activated after the bounding of IgE antibodies to their high-affinity IgE receptor through flow cytometry [17, 20]. Positivity rates depend on the allergen tested. It is not currently used in routine practice but mainly for research purposes or in specialized centers. The most common system used for the BAT requires fresh blood, which remains the main limit of such tests, and needs an equipped laboratory close to the clinic [20]. Other methods have been developed to perform the test not on fresh blood but their use is currently limited. The mast cell activation test has recently been developed to evaluate FA in vitro but still needs to be validated [20].

It is recommended to measure serum tryptase during a reaction to confirm anaphylaxis and during a nonreactive period when mast cell activation syndrome is suspected [13].

Finally, the *OFC* represents the gold standard for FA diagnosis [13, 16, 17, 24, 25]. OFC should be conducted by trained medical and nonmedical staff with equipment promptly available to manage allergic reactions, and in facilities where an intensive care unit is available, in case of a severe reaction during the test. There is no standardized protocol to perform OFC. In general, two to threefold increasing amounts of food are given at 20-min intervals starting from a low dose, i.e., 3 mg of food proteins up to a sufficient amount that should elicit a reaction in allergic patients, i.e., 1000–3000 mg of food proteins [13, 24, 25].

Proposing cutoffs for SPT and specific IgE to avoid unnecessary potentially dangerous and time-consuming OFC has been a major goal of several research in the past years. Nevertheless, it has been shown that cutoffs are only valid in a specific setting and population and cannot be generalized for the whole sensitized and/or allergic population [26, 27]. Therefore, today, these cutoffs should not be considered when approaching a child to reach a diagnosis of food allergy.

The use of *alternative tests*, such as anti-food IgG testing, lymphocyte stimulation, cytotoxicity assays, mediator release tests, provocation neutralization, applied kinesiology, or hair analysis testing, is not recommended by any scientific society.

13.5 Global Management of Food Allergy

Steps for managing FA in children are as follows [13, 14, 16]:

1. *Accurate diagnosis.*
2. *Strict avoidance*—the most effective way to manage FA is to avoid consuming allergenic foods altogether.
3. *Emergency preparedness and allergy action plan*—provide a written emergency action plan and medication. Children with allergic reactions to food should receive anti-H_1 antihistamines and corticosteroids. When children are at risk of anaphylaxis, they (as well as caregivers) should be trained on how to use epinephrine auto-injectors, which is the first drug option. Oral corticosteroids are neither effective during an acute reaction nor prevent the risk of biphasic reactions.
4. *Communication and education*—the parents can educate family, friends, and school personnel on emergency procedures. Also, it is important to educate parents and children (or guide parents to explain to their child) on the existence of a labeling *European legislation* (1169/2011—October 25th, 2011) [28]. Allergens present in a product must be listed in the ingredients (by using a different font, letter size, or background color). Such list of mandatory allergens includes cereals containing gluten, crustaceans, eggs, fish, peanuts, soybeans, cow's milk, nuts, celery, mustard sesame seeds, sulfur dioxide and sulfites at concentrations of more than 10 mg/kg or 10 mg/liter expressed as SO2, lupin, and mollusks.
5. *Nutritional balance*—removing allergenic foods from the diet may require additional attention to ensure that the patient receives all the necessary nutrients.
6. *Ongoing monitoring*—regular follow-up is essential to monitor any changes in the condition, discuss new research and treatments, and receive support and guidance.
7. *Evaluating the possibility of a tolerance induction protocol*—a possible approach to FA includes *tolerance induction* protocols. Today, sublingual immunotherapy (SLIT), epicutaneous immunotherapy (EPIT), and oral immunotherapy (OIT) are the three main approaches. OIT seems to be the preferred solution in terms of efficacy and tolerated dose. Several different OIT protocols and clinical trials have been provided, but there is no standardized procedure. The European Academy of Allergy and Clinical Immunology only advises proposing OIT to children allergic to cow's milk, egg, or peanuts. The different protocols consist of gradually increasing the administered dose of allergen, starting from a low dose. Each dose incrementation should be provided at the hospital, and the patients should continue consuming the tolerated dose at home, daily between two hospital visits. Once the patient reaches a target "maintenance" dose (which varies according to the allergen and the protocol), such dose should be continued and could be considered as a desensitization dose. Very few data are today available on the sustained unresponsiveness after this step and on the possibility of achieving an immunological tolerance, rather than just a temporary desensitization. Adverse events are common both in the build-up phase and during maintenance.

13.6 Cow's Milk Allergy

Cow's milk allergy (CMA) (Table 13.1) represents one of the most common FAs in children. It significantly impairs the quality of life of patients and families, and it has considerable healthcare costs [1]. CMA has an estimated prevalence of

Table 13.1 Essential information on cow's milk allergy

Skin prick test	Extract or fresh cow's milk (or even infant formula, if necessary)	
Main molecular allergens	Alpha-lactalbumin (Bos d 4)	Denaturation by heat
	Beta-lactoglobulin (Bos d 5)	
	Caseins (Bos d 8)	Resistant to heat
Diagnosis	Combination of medical history evaluation, allergy tests (such as skin prick tests or blood tests), and possibly OFC under medical supervision	
Management	Elimination diet Education Epinephrine auto-injector if necessary In persistent forms, patients may benefit from tolerance induction protocols	
Cross-reactivity	Especially with other mammalian milks (mostly, goat and sheep's milk) Possible with meat	
Natural history	Toward natural tolerance acquisition	

0.54–3% around the world [29]. A positive SPT and specific IgE to CMA have a prevalence ranging between 1.8 and 7.5% in the first years of life [30]. The development of tolerance to CMA occurs gradually during childhood and adolescence, influenced by various factors. Over 50% of children with CMA also experience reactions to other foods [31]. The presence of a family history of atopy is a significant risk factor, whether or not familiar atopy manifests as a food allergy.

13.6.1 Allergens and Cross-Reactive Reactions

Cow's milk contains between 30 and 35 g/L of proteins. Cow's milk allergens are denominated as Bos d from *Bos domesticus*. More than 50% of the individuals with CMA are sensitized to caseins and whey proteins (alpha-lactalbumin or Bos d 4 and beta-lactoglobulin or Bos d 5). The allergenicity of cow's milk proteins is modified by extensive heating. Caseins (Bos d 8) are more resistant to heating compared to whey proteins, which have reduced allergenicity after heating [23]. Milk baked with a flour-based compound (matrix effect) is often tolerated by children with CMA.

Cross-reactivity between cow's milk, goat's milk, and sheep's milk has been demonstrated. These cross-reactions appear to be common (for example, up to 92% cross-reactivity between cow's milk and goat's milk). Various combinations of different milks are possible, and some patients may also be allergic to caseins from sheep and goat's milk, but not to those in cow's milk [32]. Furthermore, induction of tolerance to cow's milk does not necessarily imply tolerance to cross-reacting mammalian milk. In case of allergy to sheep and/or goat's milk, patients should be aware that it is not mandatory to highlight these products on food labels, following the European legislation, which could lead to possible inadvertent exposure.

Cross-reactivity between cow's milk and beef or veal meat is rare (10–20%), and such cross-reactivity primarily mainly indicates a cross-sensitization rather than the risk of a clinical reaction [32]. Therefore, cow's milk allergy should not necessarily lead to the avoidance of animal meat.

13.6.2 Clinical Aspects

Typically, the diagnosis is suggested in a breastfed infant who shortly after formula intake develops acute urticaria. The clinical signs may vary from digestive symptoms (50–60% of cases) to cutaneous symptoms (10–39% of cases) or respiratory symptoms (20–30% of cases). Anaphylactic shock (9% of cases) may be the first manifestation. The severity of the allergic reaction does not predict the long-term prognosis [33].

Severe allergic reactions, often including bronchospasm and/or anaphylactic shock, have been reported following the injection of methylprednisolone containing bovine lactose (typically contaminated with cow's milk proteins) as an emergency treatment for an acute allergy. Therefore, clinicians should be aware of this possible contraindication in patients allergic to cow's milk proteins [34].

13.6.3 Diagnosis

The diagnostic workup for CMA follows what was previously mentioned for all FA. SPTs should be performed either with standardized extracts or fresh milk or the particular infant formula using the *prick-by-prick* technique. SPTs are also valuable for investigating potential cross-reactivity with other mammalian milk, such as goat's milk and sheep's milk. Both SPT and specific serum IgE for cow's milk and its various proteins (mainly α-lactalbumin, β-lactoglobulin, and casein) are commercialized [23, 27, 33].

OFC represents the gold standard for the diagnosis. Gradually increasing amounts of milk are given under strict medical supervision, until reaching the typical consumption dose, i.e., at a 20–30-min interval 0.1 – 0.3 – 0.9 – 3 – 9.1 – 30.3 – 90.9 ml of milk [25]. The OFC either confirms the presence of an allergy to cow's milk proteins and allows for assessment of the dose and the cumulated dose eliciting the allergic reaction or demonstrates tolerance to them.

13.6.4 Treatment

The fundamental principle of treating CMA is complete avoidance of milk proteins. It is crucial to introduce suitable substitute products to prevent nutritional deficiencies during the period of milk avoidance. In infants, exclusive breastfeeding is recommended, and the mother should adhere to a dairy-free diet to prevent rare reactions caused by cow's milk proteins contained in breast milk. A written emergency action plan should be provided, along with the conditions that need the administration of epinephrine auto-injectors.

Children can gradually develop tolerance to milk proteins. When CMA occurs in the first few weeks of life, half of the cases reach tolerance by 3 years of age and more than 90% by 15 years of age [35]. In children with persistent CMA, a tolerance induction protocol could be helpful to reduce the risk of an allergic reaction upon accidental exposure or even to provide a desensitization to this food [36–38].

13.7 Hen's Egg Allergy

Hen's egg allergy is documented to be one of the most prevalent FA among children (Table 13.2). The prevalence of hen's egg allergy in children varies in Europe between 1.6% and 2.8% [39].

Table 13.2 Essential information on hen's egg allergy

Skin prick test	Extract, raw, and cooked white and yolk	
Main molecular allergens	Ovalbumin (gal d 2)	Denaturation by heat
	Ovomucoid (gal d 1)	Resistant to heat
Diagnosis	Combination of medical history evaluation, allergy tests (such as skin prick tests or blood tests), and possibly OFC under medical supervision (first cooked, then raw)	
Management	Elimination diet Education Epinephrine auto-injector if necessary In persistent forms, patients may benefit from tolerance induction protocols	
Cross-reactivity	Low risk Beware of possible role of gal d 5 in the bird-egg syndrome	
Natural history	Toward natural tolerance acquisition	

Widely consumed in various forms, hen's egg, a source of proteins and lipids, is introduced into the diet around the age of 9 months and is the cause of numerous reactions. Egg allergy is usually diagnosed in childhood. Table 13.2 summarizes the main aspects of this allergy.

13.7.1 Allergens and Cross-Reactive Reactions

One medium-sized egg has a weight of about 60 g and contains about 6.5 g of protein. The albumen weighs 30 g, with 3 g of protein. The yolk weighs 20 g, with 3.5 g of protein. Hen's egg allergens are denominated as Gal d for *Gallus domesticus*. Gal d 1 (ovomucoid), Gal d 2 (ovalbumin), Gal d 3 (transferrin/conalbumin), and Gal d 4 (lysozyme) are in the egg albumen. In the yolk, the main allergen is Gal d 5 (α-livetin). Ovomucoid is resistant to heat and digestion, while ovalbumin, the most abundant protein (54% of the total egg white proteins), is sensitive to heat. Alpha-livetin or serum albumin is responsible for a possible cross-reaction between eggs and bird proteins.

Cross-reactivity of eggs mainly occurs among species of Galliformes (such as chicken, quail, turkey, guinea fowl, and pheasant), with cross-sensitization rates reaching up to 69%. Cross-reactivity is less common between Galliformes and Columbiformes (pigeons, doves, and related species), with cross-sensitization rates of up to 44%. It is also less frequent between Galliformes and Anseriformes (ducks, geese, teal, etc.) or between Galliformes and Charadriiformes (woodcocks, snipes, gulls, and terns). Some individuals may experience allergic reactions when consuming duck or goose eggs, but they can safely ingest hen's eggs without presenting any hypersensitivity reaction [40].

13.7.2 Clinical Aspects

The clinical manifestations of egg allergy are similar to those of FA in general. They most commonly occur upon ingestion of eggs or products containing eggs, but other routes of exposure are possible, such as direct skin contact or contact with egg proteins on mucous membranes [40]. It should be noted that contact with urticaria to eggs does not necessarily correlate with a reaction to eating eggs. Fatal anaphylaxis following the ingestion of egg proteins in children and adolescents has been exceptionally reported [41].

The tolerance of baked eggs can be observed in more than half of children allergic to cooked eggs [42]. Some children who tolerate cooked eggs react to raw eggs. In general, egg allergy has a favorable prognosis, with 50% of allergic individuals outgrowing the allergy by the age of 6 years [39]. Prognostic markers for tolerance have been identified, such as low levels of specific egg IgE antibodies (ovomucoid and ovalbumin), a rapid decline over time in wheal size in prick tests or specific egg IgE levels, early age at diagnosis, mild initial symptoms, and tolerance to cooked and/or baked eggs.

13.7.3 Diagnosis

As with other manifestations of FA, the allergy workup includes a detailed clinical history, SPT with extracts or fresh egg, and detection of specific IgE levels. The gold standard remains the OFC. During the challenge, one egg should be given, with a first dose of about 3 mg of egg proteins and the last up to 3000 mg [25]. The acquisition of tolerance to egg is determined by the OFC, first with cooked egg and then, if necessary, with raw egg.

13.7.4 Treatment

The treatment is based on avoiding products containing eggs. Patient education, sometimes with the assistance of a dietitian, is essential to learn how to read labels, create suitable menus, adapt recipes, recognize early signs of an allergic reaction, and administer initial treatments.

The diet is tailored to children's tolerance levels. Children who tolerate baked eggs or cooked eggs are allowed to consume them, even if they react to cooked or raw egg ingestion, respectively. Children with persistent egg allergy may, on a case-by-case basis, benefit from tolerance induction protocols [36–38].

13.8 Peanut Allergy

The peanut (*Arachis hypogaea*) is an annual herbaceous plant belonging to the Fabaceae family (legume or bean) grown in tropical and warm-temperate regions for its seeds and oil. Peanuts, also known as groundnuts, earthnuts, goober peas, monkey nuts, pygmy nuts, and pig nuts, are not classified as tree nuts.

Peanut allergy (PA) (Table 13.3) is a prevalent FA among children and adolescents in Anglo-Saxon countries, and its frequency and severity are on the rise [43]. The United States, United Kingdom, Canada, and Australia have the highest prevalence rates, ranging from 1% to 2%. The increasing prevalence of PA is worrisome due to its significant impact on public health, as it is the primary cause not only of severe anaphylactic reactions but also of fatalities.

The causes for this increase are not fully understood. Several factors have been suggested. These include the widespread consumption of peanuts, the persistence of peanut allergens in the environment after consumption, and the enhanced absorption of peanut allergens through an impaired skin barrier in children with atopic dermatitis.

Studies conducted over the last 10 years (such as the LEAP, LEAP-on, and EAT studies) found that introducing peanuts into the diet of infants aged 4–8 months may provide protection against the development of PA in countries with high levels of consumption [44].

PA is considered a persistent allergy, being only 15–20% of allergic children able to recover. PA significantly impacts the quality of life. In comparison to individuals with insulin-dependent diabetes, severe asthma, or chronic rheumatoid disease, the quality of life is more affected in individuals with PA [45, 46].

13.8.1 Allergens and Cross-Reactive Reactions

The allergenicity of peanuts depends on different cooking methods. Raw or roasted peanuts are more allergenic than fried or boiled peanuts. A total of 16 peanut allergens have been sequenced: from *Arachis hypogaea* 1 (Ara h 1) to Ara h 17, excluding only Ara h 4. Among peanut components, there are two cupins (Ara h 1 and Ara h 3), three albumins (Ara h 2, Ara h 6, and Ara h 7), one profilin (Ara h 5), a protein-related-10 protein (PR-10) (Ara h 8), four oleosins (Ara h 10, Ara h 11, Ara h 14, and Ara h 15), three nonspe-

Table 13.3 Essential information on peanut allergy

Skin prick test	Extract, or prick by prick	
Main molecular allergens	Ara h 1 (cupin) Ara h 2 (albumin) Ara h 3 (cupin) Ara h 6 (conglutin)	Main markers of true peanut allergy (especially, Ara h 2 and Ara h 6)
	Ara h 8 (PR-10)	Usually, oral syndrome only
	Ara h 9 (LTP)	From minor to severe symptoms, depending on the population
Diagnosis	Combination of medical history evaluation, allergy tests (such as skin prick tests or blood tests), and possibly OFC under medical supervision	
Management	Elimination diet Education Epinephrine auto-injector if necessary In persistent forms, patients may benefit from tolerance induction protocols	
Cross-reactivity	Especially with legumes and tree nuts	
Natural history	Toward the persistence of the allergy	

cific lipid transfer proteins (LTP) (Ara h 9, Ara h 16, and Ara h 17), and two defensins (Ara h 12 and Ara h 13).

The four major peanut components, whose positivity is associated with clinically possibly severe reactions, are Ara h 1, Ara h 2, Ara h 3, and Ara h 6 [47]. Of these four, the 2-S albumin Ara h 2 is the most specific marker for severe reactions. Reactivity to some peanut components may result from cross-reactivity to respiratory allergens, and it is associated with mild allergic reactions or even with tolerance to peanuts. Cross-sensitizations mainly to tree nuts and legumes (especially lupine, soybeans, and peas) are possible.

13.8.2 Clinical Aspects

Symptoms of PA are likely to be severe. Fatal anaphylaxis can occur, as confirmed by various epidemiological studies [41, 48, 49].

Atopy is often present in individuals with PA. Studies showed that 60–75% of patients with PA had asthma and/or atopic dermatitis, and 55–60% had allergic rhinitis. The coexistence of asthma further increases the risk of severe anaphylactic reactions to peanuts [50, 51].

Deaths have been reported due to PA. Among the 31 deaths from FA reported between 2001 and 2006 in the United States, 17 (54.8%) were attributed to PA which was the leading cause of food allergy-related deaths [48]. In the United Kingdom, an analysis of hospitalizations for overall anaphylaxis over two decades revealed that peanuts remain the leading cause of fatal food-related allergic reactions [41].

In addition to ingestion, PA symptoms can also occur after inhalation or contact. This event may especially take place during air travel, when in contact with peanut consumers or through kissing someone who has previously consumed peanuts.

13.8.3 Diagnosis

The diagnosis of PA relies on the patient's medical history, SPT, and measurement of specific IgE levels [52, 53]. It may be followed by an OFC that is the gold standard and the only means to achieve a definite diagnosis. Many recombinant peanut allergens are currently commercially available: rAra h 1, rAra h 2, rAra h 3, rAra h 6, rAra h 8, and rAra h 9. The recombinant rAra h 2 may help to confirm the diagnosis of PA (in conjunction with the positive results of specific IgE testing for whole peanut and skin tests).

13.8.4 Treatment

The treatment of PA involves avoiding peanuts. However, peanut avoidance may be challenging because peanuts are a ubiquitous allergen that is often "hidden" in various products. It is therefore important for patients and caregivers to pay attention to food labeling. Peanuts can be found in a wide range of food items, including breakfast cereals, breads, snacks, dairy products, ice cream, beverages, soups, meat substitutes, and processed meats.

The avoidance of other legumes and tree nuts is based on the patient's medical history and allergy workup.

Symptomatic treatment of an allergic reaction depends on its severity and may involve anti-H_1 antihistamines and corticosteroids. The treatment of choice for any anaphylactic reaction is intramuscular adrenaline.

Oral, sublingual, and epicutaneous peanut *tolerance protocols* are currently being developed. These different therapeutic approaches involve administering increasing amounts of the allergen, followed by a maintenance dose that the patient regularly consumes, and may help patients to increase the eliciting dose and therefore reactive threshold [36–38].

13.9 Other Food Allergies

Some other food groups can trigger allergic reactions in children (Table 13.4).

13.9.1 Tree Nut Allergy

Allergy to tree nuts affects 0.5–1.2% of the population [54]. It is a leading cause of mortality due to food-induced anaphylaxis, along with peanuts and milk [41, 48, 49].

Table 13.4 Other main foods responsible for food allergy in children

Food	Main allergens	Specificity
Tree nuts	Almond Hazelnut Walnut Cashew Pistachio Pecan nut Macadamia nut Brazil nut	Cross-reactions are possible between tree nuts, especially between walnut and pecan nuts and between cashew and pistachio
Wheat	Tri a 12 (profilin) Tri a 15 (α-amylase inhibitor) Tri a 14 (LTP) Tri a 19 (omega-5-gliadin)	Role of tri a 15 in baker's asthma Role of tri a 19 in exercise-induced anaphylaxis
Seafood	Beta-parvalbumins Tropomyosins	Differentiate between allergies to fishes, crustaceans, and mollusks
Meat	Albumins Alpha-gal	Possible delayed anaphylaxis in patients suffering from alpha-gal syndrome

Tree nuts include a variety of nuts, such as almonds, hazelnuts, walnuts, cashews, pistachios, Brazil nuts, pecan nuts, and macadamia nuts, which belong to different families and botanical groups. Some of the main families of tree nuts are as follows:

- *Rosaceae* family: almond (*Prunus dulcis*).
- *Anacardiaceae* family: cashew (*Anacardium occidentale*) and pistachio (*Pistacia vera*).
- *Betulaceae* family: hazelnut (*Corylus avellana*).
- *Proteaceae* family: macadamia nut (*Macadamia integrifolia*).
- *Lecythidaceae* family: Brazil nut (*Bertholletia excelsa*).

Of note, certain foods are related to tree nuts but are not classified as such:

- Peanuts and chestnut legumes or members of the *Fabaceae* family.
- Coconut belongs to the *Arecaceae* family or palm tree.
- Nutmeg is a spice and seed from the *Myristicaceae* family.
- Pine nuts are seeds belonging to the *Pinaceae* family.

Vicilins, 2S-albumins, profilins, heveins, and LTP are the major allergens of tree nuts. There is no evidence that the detection of IgE to molecular allergens is superior to SPT or serum-specific IgE to extracts to identify allergic patients.

Cross-reactivity can occur among different tree nut varieties and with other allergens such as pollen proteins. Main cross-reactions, within the same tree nut family, may especially occur between walnut and pecan and between cashew nut and pistachio [55].

13.9.2 Wheat Allergy

Wheat (*Triticum aestivum*) is a widely consumed food grain that grows in different climatic areas. Wheat allergy is the most common of all cereal allergies. It often develops during infancy or early childhood. In the general population, resolution occurs in most patients by the age of 5 years. In the atopic population, resolution occurs later, often during adolescence. In the European general population, the prevalence of wheat allergy in children varies from 0.2% to 1.3%, with higher prevalence rates in Northern European countries [56]. In the United States, it is 0.4%. In the pediatric population, wheat allergy is reported in 18% of children with FA, ranking after milk, peanut, and tree nut allergies [57].

Wheat belongs to the grass family *Poaceae* and contains many allergenic proteins, divided into four groups or fractions: albumins (soluble in water), globulins (soluble in dilute saline), gliadins (soluble in alcohol/water mixtures), and glutenins (extracted in dilute acid). The latter two classes account for 85% of wheat proteins and are known as gluten.

The major allergens of wheat are Tri a 12 (profilin) involved in cross-sensitization between pollen and food; Tri a 15 (α-amylase inhibitor) implicated in baker's asthma; Tri a 14 (LTP) involved in severe allergic reactions in the Mediterranean region; Tri a 37 (α-purothionine) associated with severe reactions; and Tri a 19 (omega-5-gliadin) implicated in *food-dependent exercise-induced anaphylaxis* in adults and older children, while in young children, this allergen is associated with immediate allergic reactions [58].

Wheat allergy may present with various symptoms, ranging from simple urticaria to anaphylaxis and baker's asthma. It is frequently reported to elicit food-dependent exercise-induced anaphylaxis [58].

Tolerance induction to wheat has been performed in children and adults with similar efficacy to that of milk and egg [38].

13.9.3 Seafood Allergy

Allergy to seafood (fishes and shellfish that are mollusks and crustaceans) is one of the major FA in children [56, 59, 60]. The prevalence of seafood allergy varies between regions due to differences in the consumption of these foods. The highest prevalence was found in the Asia-Pacific region.

Muscular β-parvalbumins are the major allergens in IgE-mediated allergic reactions to fish (70–95% of patients). They are widely present in the white muscle of bony fish and exhibit variable structural homology between species, even among closely related ones. Alpha-parvalbumins are primarily found in cartilaginous fish such as rays and sharks. They have moderate homology with the beta-parvalbumins of certain species. The IgE reactivity of parvalbumins is generally not affected by cooking or digestion although some preservation and processing methods can alter the fish's protein profile in vitro. There is generally no cross-reactivity with crustaceans or mollusks. Furthermore, fish-allergic individuals generally do not react to fish eggs [59].

Shrimp is the most consumed seafood worldwide. Muscular tropomyosins are the major allergens in crustaceans. Cross-reactivity between different crustacean species is common. Tropomyosins are heat-stable and resistant to digestion. However, cooking may increase their reactivity. Mollusks can be divided into gastropods (abalone, whelks, and snails), cephalopods (squid, octopuses, and cuttlefish), and bivalves (mussels, oysters, and clams). About 40% of individuals allergic to one type of crustacean may experience reactions when exposed to another crustacean, while 17–40% of those allergic to one type of mollusk may react to a different type of mollusk. It is worth noting that 45% of individuals allergic to crustaceans react to mollusks, and conversely, 81% of those allergic to mollusks react to crustaceans [60, 61].

The only effective and recommended prophylaxis for allergic reactions to seafood is avoidance.

13.9.4 Meat Allergy

Meat can be classified into different categories: red meat (beef, veal—bovine under 6 months of age, horse, pork, lamb, goat, etc.), white meat (poultry and rabbit), and game meat. Allergies to meat, particularly red meat, are considered rare (affecting 1–2% of food-allergic individuals for pork and beef). It is mainly associated with bovine albumin allergies in some atopic children. Primary beef allergy affects young atopic children (atopic dermatitis). It is typically caused by Bos d 6 (bovine albumin), although other allergens have been implicated (such as Bos d 7 immunoglobulin). It is often (>90%) associated with CMA and other sensitizations (atopic background). Sensitization occurs through intestinal or cutaneous routes, and symptoms range from exacerbation of atopic dermatitis to anaphylactic shock. Tolerance over time is common (90% at 3 years). Although the cross-reactivity rate with other meats rich in albumin is unknown, the theoretical risk is high [62].

Alpha-gal syndrome affects individuals of all ages, including nonatopic patients (50% of cases). It developed in 95% of mammalian meat-allergic individuals in an American series. Alpha-gal is not a protein, but a carbohydrate. Sensitization mainly occurs through tick bites [63]. Patients present with urticaria, gastrointestinal symptoms, and anaphylactic reactions, appearing generally 3–6 h after meat ingestion. This allergy tends to diminish or disappear after a few years. Alpha-gal is resistant to cooking and digestion [62].

Primary poultry allergy affects adolescents and young adults with atopic conditions. It is mainly caused by Gal d 7 from chicken (myosin light chain 1), although other allergens such as Gal d 8 have been implicated. It is not associated with egg allergy, whereas less than 5% of individuals allergic to chicken eggs are allergic to chicken meat. However, it is associated with sensitization to fish and/or crustaceans in one-third of cases. The allergen is resistant to cooking and digestion [64].

The primary management approach is strict avoidance of meats implicated in the reactions.

13.10 Protein Families

Special attention should be given to patients presenting with a *pollen-food allergy syndrome* (PFAS). Allergic reactions are mainly triggered by pan-allergens that are present both in pollens and in fruits and vegetables and induce symptoms ranging from an oral allergy syndrome to anaphylactic reactions [65–67]. The main pan-allergens are profilins, PR-10, LTPs, thaumatin-like proteins (TLPs), and gibberellin-regulated proteins (GRPs) (Table 13.5).

13.10.1 Profilins

Profilin is a small, actin-binding protein found in both plant and animal cells. It plays a crucial role in cytoskeletal dynamics and cell motility. Profilin acts as an allergen by sensitizing individuals primarily through inhalation or ingestion. Profilin allergy is commonly associated with pollen allergies such as birch or grass pollen. This can lead to cross-reactivity with various fruits, vegetables, and other plant-derived foods. Examples of fruits include banana, pineapple, melon, tomato, apple, pear, cherry, lychee, and peach, among others. Some vegetables that can cause cross-reactivity are celery, zucchini, and paprika. Legumes, such as peanuts and soybeans, as well as nuts such as hazelnuts (Cor a 2), can also be involved [65].

In addition to birch pollen, symptoms associated with profilins may also involve pollens from timothy grass (Phl p 12), mugwort (Art v 4), ragweed (Amb a 8), or plane (Pla a 3).

Profilin is present in both the pulp and peel of fruits, and it is sensitive to heat denaturation and digestion by pepsin. However, celery profilin

Table 13.5 Main protein families, responsible for pollen-food allergy syndrome

Family	Main allergen	Main respiratory allergens	Main food allergens
Profilins	Bet v 2	Birch and other *Fagaceae*, grass, mugwort, ragweed, pellitory, olive, ash, cypress, palm	Apple, peach, pear, melon, kiwi, celery, carrot, orange, peanut, soy, tomato, pineapple, hazelnut, mustard, sunflower, fig
PR-10	Bet v 1	Birch (but also other *Betullaceae* and *Fagaceae*)	Apple, peach, pear, strawberry, apricot, cherry, raspberry, kiwi, celery, carrot, peanut, soy, hazelnut, tomato, walnut
LTP	Pru p 3	Olive tree, artemisia, ambrosia, pellitory, plane tree, hemp	Apple, peach, cherry, grape, orange, tomato, hazelnut, walnut, peanut, lettuce, corn, wheat
TLP	Mal d 2	*Cupressaceae*, plane tree, birch, olive tree, mugwort	Peach, apple, pear, plum, cherry, banana, kiwi, grape, melon, almond
GRP	Pru p 7	*Cupressaceae*	Peach, apple, apricot, cherry, orange, lemon, grenade, pepper, potato, carrot, sesame

seems to be heat-resistant. Profilin is unable to trigger sensitization through the gastrointestinal tract [65]. When individuals sensitized to profilin consume raw fruits, reactions typically occur in the oral cavity (pollen food allergy syndrome (PFAS)). However, it is important to note that serious systemic symptoms have also been reported in some cases [68].

13.10.2 PR-10

PR-10 proteins are a family of allergenic proteins that are structurally conserved across different plants, including pollen, fruits, and vegetables. They are involved in plant defense mechanisms and are recognized as major allergens in respiratory allergy and FA. Bet v 1 from birch pollen and Mal d 1 from apples are major allergens of the PR-10 family [65].

Allergens of the PR-10 family are contained in numerous fruits, such as Pru p 1 in peaches, Pru ar 1 in apricots, Pru av. 1 in cherries, Fra a 1 in strawberries, Pyr c 1 in pears, and Act d 8 in kiwi fruit. They are also present in vegetables, including Api g 1 in celeriac and Dau c 1 in carrots, as well as in legumes such as soybean (Gly m 4), mungo bean (Vig r 1), and peanut (Ara h 8). These proteins often exhibit cross-reactivity, leading to similar allergic reactions when exposed to related allergens. Most reactions are limited to the oral cavity. However, systemic reactions have been reported, particularly in the presence of cofactors [68]. Therefore, the prescription of adrenaline should be considered in specific cases.

13.10.3 LTP

LTPs are a group of proteins found in various plants, including fruits, vegetables, nuts, and seeds. They play a role in plant defense for their antifungal and antibacterial activities. They are heat-stable and resistant to digestion due to the presence of four disulfide bridges. LTP sensitization is more prevalent in Mediterranean countries, where it is thought to be associated with systemic allergic reactions [65]. LTPs are present, with varying degrees of homology, in numerous plants: *Rosaceae* family: peach (Pru p 3); apple (Mal d 3); plum (Pru d 3); pear (Pyr c 3); cherry (Pru av. 3); apricot (Pru ar 3); strawberry (Fra a 3); raspberry (Rub i 3); rose (Ros r 3); nuts: hazelnut (Cor a 8); chestnut (Cas s 8); walnut (Jug r 3); almond (Pru du 3); seeds: peanut (Ara h 9); broad bean (Pha v 3); sunflower (Hel a 3); mustard (Sin a 3); sesame (Ses i LTP); wheat (Tri a 14); rice (Ory s 14); corn (Zea m 14); barley (Hor v 14); other foods: kiwi (Act c 10, Act d 10); pomegranate (Pun g 3); lemon (Cit l 3); orange (Cit s 3); tomato (Luc e 3); grape (Vit v 1); lettuce (Lac s 1); onion (All lc 3); celery (Api g 2); carrot (Dau c 3); parsley (Pet c 3); and cauliflower (Bra o 3). LTP is contained in latex (Hev b 12) and in aeroallergens: mugwort (Art v 3); pellitory (Par j 2); plane tree (Pla a 3); olive tree (Ole e 7); ragweed (Amb a 6); and cannabis (Can s 3).

LTP is 30 times more abundant in the peel than in the pulp of peaches but present in similar concentrations in the peel/pulp of other fruits such as plums and apricots. Sensitization to LTP occurs through dietary exposure, although cutaneous (harvesters and market gardeners) and respiratory routes are also possible. The role of sensitization to cannabis LTP (Can s 3) is somewhat surprising, preceding sensitization to other food-related LTPs [69].

A commercial extract of peach contains LTP (Pru p 3) and gibberellin. Even if Pru p 3 differs from other LTPs, it is often used to determine whether an individual is sensitized to LTPs. Management involves avoiding both raw and cooked offending foods and continuing to consume tolerated foods, even in the presence of cross-sensitization to LTP. The patient should be aware of possible reactions with cofactors and have an emergency kit with adrenaline available when at risk for anaphylaxis. Tolerance induction techniques remain experimental, but studies focusing on immunotherapy with Pru p 3 allergen extract have shown positive results [70].

13.10.4 TLP

TLPs are a class of plant proteins that are widely distributed in various plant species. They are named after the first identified member of this protein family, thaumatin, which was originally discovered in the tropical fruit *Thaumatococcus daniellii*. TLPs are characterized by their ability to impart a sweet taste and contribute to the defense mechanisms of plants against pathogen-attacks, especially fungal ones. This family of proteins is widely recognized as a pan-allergen family responsible for the occurrence of cross-reactivity between pollen and various fruits [65].

TLPs act as allergens and can be found in different types of pollen, including *Cupressaceae* pollen allergens, pollen from plane trees, birch, mugwort, and nettle. These TLPs are associated with FA, specifically involving peach (Pru p 2), apple (Mal d 2), pear (Pyr pv 2), plum (Pru d 2), cherry (Pru av. 2), banana (Mus a 4), kiwi (Act d 2), grape (Vit v TLP), melon (Cuc TLP), and almond (Pru du 2).

13.10.5 GRPs

GRPs are allergens responsible for plant-based food allergies. These proteins have mainly been identified in peach (Pru p 7), apricot (Pru m 7), orange (Cit s 7), and pomegranate (Pun g 7) [65, 71–73]. GRPs exhibit stability against heat and digestion. They can induce systemic and often severe reactions, even in children. Allergic individuals to GRPs may react not only to fruits from the *Rosaceae* family, such as peaches, apricots, apples, strawberries, and cherries but also to fruits from the *Rutaceae* family, such as lemons and oranges. When diagnosing systemic reactions to fruits, particularly in cases where Pru p 3-specific IgE is negative, allergy to GRPs should be considered.

13.11 Summary

Food allergies seem to have an increase in prevalence and incidence, especially in children. Most frequent clinical symptoms are related to IgE-mediated reactions that occur immediately after food intake (even though rarely up to 4 h).

The main symptoms include skin signs (hives and itching) but also gastrointestinal ones (nausea, vomiting, and diarrhea), or even respiratory and cardiovascular ones. Anaphylaxis can occur.

Diagnosis begins with a thorough history, followed by a dietary investigation, SPT (with extracts or with the *prick-by-prick* technique), and specific IgE determination. OFC is the gold standard for diagnosing food allergy. It is also helpful to determine the reactive dose or demonstrate the tolerance to a specific allergen.

In patients with a diagnosis of food allergy, an elimination diet of the culprit food remains the main therapy. Patients and caregivers should be educated to avoid accidental exposure and to treat reactions. Allergen immunotherapy protocol may be proposed in specific cases when the allergy seems to be persistent. CMA, hen's egg allergy, and PA are the worldwide main food allergies in children. Knowing the allergens to be tested for each one of these foods is important to set up the correct management of the disease and to propose possible targeted therapies, such as oral immunotherapy. Other common food allergies in children include tree nuts, wheat, seafood (fishes, mollusks, and crustaceans), and meat. Some children may present reactions to molecular allergens that act as pan-allergens because they are present in different foods. Main family proteins potentially responsible for these cross-reactivities include profilins, PR-10, LTP, TLP, and GRP.

References

1. Caimmi D, Caffarelli C, Licari A, Miraglia del Giudice M, Calvani M, Marseglia GL, et al. Food allergy in primary care. Acta Biomed. 2021;92(S7):e2021521.
2. Ballmer-Weber B, Lidholm J, Fernandez-Rivas M, Seneviratne S, Hanschmann KM, Vogel L, et al. IgE recognition patterns in peanut allergy are age dependent: perspectives of the EuroPrevall study. Allergy. 2015;70:391–407.
3. Eigenmann PA, Sicherer SH, Borkowski TA, Cohen BA, Sampson HA. Prevalence of IgE-mediated food allergy among children with atopic dermatitis. Pediatrics. 1998;101:E8.
4. Gupta RS, Springston EE, Warrier MR, Smith B, Kumar R, Pongracic J, et al. The prevalence, severity, and distribution of childhood food allergy in the United States. Pediatrics. 2011;128:e9–e17.
5. Lyons SA, Clausen M, Knulst AC, Ballmer-Weber BK, Fernandez-Riva M, Barreales L, et al. Prevalence of food sensitization and food allergy in children

across Europe. J Allergy Clin Immunol Pract. 2020;8:2736–46.
6. Osterballe M, Mortz CG, Hansen TK, Andersen KE, Bindslev-Jensen C. The prevalence of food hypersensitivity in an unselected population of children and adults. Pediatr Allergy Immunol. 2005;16:567–73.
7. Rona RJ, Keil T, Summers C, Gislason D, Madsen C, Summers C, et al. The prevalence of food allergy: a meta-analysis. J Allergy Clin Immunol. 2007;120:638–46.
8. Sicherer SH, Munoz-Furlong A, Godbold JH, Sampson HA. US prevalence of self-reported peanut, tree nut, and sesame allergy: 11-year follow-up. J Allergy Clin Immunol. 2010;125:1322–6.
9. Spolidoro GCI, Ali MM, Amera YT, Nyassi S, Lisik D, Ionnidou A, et al. Prevalence estimates of eight big food allergies in Europe: updated systematic review and meta-analysis. Allergy. 2023;8:351–68.
10. Sampson HA, O'Mahony L, Burks AW, Plaut M, Lack G, Akdis CA. Mechanisms of food allergy. J Allergy Clin Immunol. 2018;141:11–9.
11. Eigenman PA. Mechanisms of food allergy. Pediatr Allergy Immunol. 2009;20:5–11.
12. Tsuji NM, Kosaka A. Oral tolerance: intestinal homeostasis and antigen-specific regulatory T cells. Trends Immunol. 2008;29:532–40.
13. Muraro A, Werfel T, Hoffmann-Sommergruber K, Roberts G, Beyer K, Bindslev-Jenses C, et al. EAACI food allergy and anaphylaxis guidelines: diagnosis and management of food allergy. Allergy. 2014;69:1008–25.
14. Sampson HA, Muñoz-Furlong A, Campbell RL, Adkinson NF Jr, Bock SA, Branum A, et al. Second symposium on the definition and management of anaphylaxis: summary report—second National Institute of allergy and infectious disease/Food Allergy and Anaphylaxis Network symposium. J Allergy Clin Immunol. 2006;117:391–7.
15. Sharma HP, Bansil S, Uygungil B. Signs and symptoms of food allergy and food-induced anaphylaxis. Pediatr Clin N Am. 2015;62:1377–92.
16. Boyce JA, Assa'ad A, Burks AW, Jones SM, Sampson HA, Wood RA, et al. Guidelines for the diagnosis and management of food allergy in the United States: summary of the NIAID-sponsored expert panel report. J Allergy Clin Immunol. 2010;126:1105–18.
17. Foong RX, Dantzer JA, Wood RA, Santos AF. Improving diagnostic accuracy in food allergy. J Allergy Clin Immunol Pract. 2021;9:71–80.
18. Peters RL, Allen KJ, Dharmage SC, Tang MLK, Koplin JJ, Ponsonby AL, et al. Skin prick test responses and allergen-specific IgE levels as predictors of peanut, egg, and sesame allergy in infants. J Allergy Clin Immunol. 2013;132:874–80.
19. Peters RL, Gurrin LC, Allen KJ. The predictive value of skin prick testing for challenge-proven food allergy: a systematic review. Pediatr Allergy Immunol. 2012;23:347–52.
20. Arasi S, Barni S, Matrorilli C, Comberiati P, Chiera F, Pelosi U, et al. Role of *in vitro* testing in food allergy. Pediatr Allergy Immunol. 2020;31(S26):36–8.
21. Bernstein IL, Li JT, Bernstein DI, Hamilton R, Spector SL, Tan R, et al. Allergy diagnostic testing: an updated practice parameter. Ann Allergy Asthma Immunol. 2008;100(S3):1–148.
22. Sampson HA. Predictive values of food-specific IgE in food allergy. Rev Fr Allergol. 1998;38:914–20.
23. Restani P, Ballabio C, Di Lorenzo C, Tripodi S, Fiocchi A. Molecular aspects of milk allergens and their role in clinical events. Anal Bioanal Chem. 2009;395:47–56.
24. Ballmer-Weber B, Beyer K. Food challenges. J Allergy Clin Immunol. 2018;141:69–71.
25. Sampson HA, Gerth van Wijk R, Bindslev-Jensen C, Sicherer S, Teuber SS, Burks AW, et al. Standardizing double-blind, placebo-controlled oral food challenges: American Academy of Allergy, Asthma & Immunology-European academy of allergy and clinical immunology PRACTALL consensus report. J Allergy Clin Immunol. 2012;130:1260–74.
26. Calvani M, Arasi S, Bianchi A, Caimmi D, Cuomo B, Dondi A, et al. Is it possible to make a diagnosis of raw, heated, and baked egg allergy in children using cutoffs? A systematic review. Pediatr Allergy Immunol. 2015;26(6):509–21.
27. Cuomo B, Indirli GC, Bianchi A, Arasi S, Caimmi D, Dondi A, et al. Specific IgE and skin prick tests to diagnose allergy to fresh and baked cow's milk according to age: a systematic review. Ital J Pediatr. 2017;43:93.
28. Regulation (EU) No 1169/2011 of the European Parliament and of the Council of 25 October 2011 on the provision of food information to consumers. http://eur-lex.europa.eu. Last access on August 29th 2023.
29. Rona RJ, Keil T, Summers C, Gislason D, Zuidmeer L, Sodergren E, et al. The prevalence of food allergy: a meta-analysis. J Allergy Clin Immunol. 2007;120:638–46.
30. Giannetti A, Toschi Vespasiani G, Ricci G, Miniaci A, di Palmo E, Pession A. Cow's milk protein allergy as a model for food allergies. Nutrients. 2021;13:1525.
31. Groetch M, Sampson HA. Chapter 52: management of food allergy. In: From: Pediatric allergy: principles and practice. 2nd ed. Elsevier; 2010.
32. Garcia BE, Lizaso MT. Cross-reactivity syndromes in food allergy. J Investig Allergol Clin Immunol. 2011;21:162–70.
33. Rancé F, Dutau G. Actualités sur la prise en charge de l'allergie aux protéines du lait de vache (APLV). Rev Fr Allergol. 2009;49:S28–33.
34. Medicinal products containing lactose of bovine origin for IV/IM use in acute allergic reactions. http://eur-lex.europa.eu. Last access on August 29th, 2023.
35. Skripak JM, Matsui EC, Mudd K, Wood RA. The natural history of IgE-mediated cow's milk allergy. J Allergy Clin Immunol. 2007;120:1172–7.

36. Mori F, Giovannini M, Barni S, Jilenez-Saiz R, Munblit D, Biagioni B, et al. Oral immunotherapy for food-allergic children: a pro-con debate. Front Immunol. 2021;12:636612.
37. Pajno GB, Fernandez-Rivas M, Arasi S, Roberts G, Akdis CA, Alvaro-Lozano M, et al. EAACI guidelines on allergen immunotherapy: IgE-mediated food allergy. Allergy. 2018;73:799–815.
38. Rodriguez del Rio P, Alvarez-Perea A, Blumchen K, Caimmi D, Caubet JC, Kostantinopoulos AP, et al. Food immunotherapy practice: nation differences across Europe, the FIND project. Allergy. 2022;77:920–32.
39. Benhamou AH, Caubet JC, Eigenmann PA, Nowak-Wegrzyn A, Marcos CP, Reche M, et al. State of the art and new horizons in the diagnosis and management of egg allergy. Allergy. 2010;65:283–9.
40. Añíbarro B, Seoane FJ, Vila C, Lombardero M. Allergy to eggs from duck and goose without sensitization to hen egg proteins. J Allergy Clin Immunol. 2000;105:834–6.
41. Pumphrey RSH, Gowland MH. Further fatal allergic reactions to food in the United Kingdom, 1999-2006. J Allergy Clin Immunol. 2007;119:1018–9.
42. Des Roches A, Nguyen M, Paradis L, Primeau MN, Singer S. Tolerance to cooked egg in an egg allergic population. Allergy. 2006;61:900–1.
43. Teufel M, Biedermann T, Rapps N, Hausteiner C, Henningsen P, Enck P, et al. Psychological burden of food allergy. World J Gastroenterol. 2007;13:3456–65.
44. Fisher HR, Du Toit G, Bahnson HT, Lack G. The challenges of preventing food allergy: lessons learned from LEAP and EAT. Ann Allergy Asthma Immunol. 2018;121:313–9.
45. Sicherer SH, Sampson HA. Food allergy. J Allergy Clin Immunol. 2006;117(2S):S470–5.
46. Avery NJ, King RM, Knight S, Hourihane JO. Assessment of quality of life in children with peanut allergy. Pediatr Allergy Immunol. 2003;14:378–82.
47. Lange L, Beyer K, Kleine-Tebbe J. Benefits and limitations of molecular diagnostics in peanut allergy. Allergo J Int. 2014;23:158–63.
48. Bock SA, Muñoz-Furlong A, Sampson HA. Further fatalities caused by anaphylactic reactions to food, 2001–2006. J Allergy Clin Immunol. 2007;119:1016–8.
49. Sampson HA. Peanut anaphylaxis. J Allergy Clin Immunol. 1990;86:1–3.
50. Lagreula M, Chiriac AM, Leoni MC, Demoly P, Caimmi D. Risk factors for developing food-induced bronchospasm during oral food challenge. Pediatr Allergy Immunol. 2017;28:598–602.
51. Caffarelli C, Garrubba M, Greco C, Mastrorilli C, Povesi DC. Asthma and food allergy in children: is there a connection or interaction? Front Pediatr. 2016;4:34.
52. Astier C, Morisset M, Roitel O, Codreanu F, Jacquenet S, Franck P, et al. Predictive value of skin prick tests using recombinant allergens for diagnosis of peanut allergy. J Allergy Clin Immunol. 2006;118:250–6.
53. Roberts G, Lack G. Diagnosing peanut allergy with skin prick and specific IgE testing. J Allergy Clin Immunol. 2005;115:1291–6.
54. Cox AL, Eigenmann PA, Sicherer SH. Clinical relevance of cross-reactivity in food allergy. J Allergy Clin Immunol Pract. 2021;9:82–99.
55. Stiefel G, Anagnostou K, Boyle RJ, Brathwaite N, Ewan P, Fox AT, et al. BSACI guideline for the diagnosis and management of peanut and tree nut allergy. Clin Exp Allergy. 2017;47:719–39.
56. Gupta RS, Springston EE, Warrier MR, Smith B, Kumar R, Pongracic J, et al. The prevalence, severity, and distribution of childhood food allergy in the United States. Pediatrics. 2011;128:e9–17.
57. Järvinen KM, Sicherer SH, Sampson HA, Nowak-Wegrzyn A. Use of multiple doses of epinephrine in food-induced anaphylaxis in children. J Allergy Clin Immunol. 2008;122:133–8.
58. Ricci G, Andreozzi L, Cipriani F, Giannetti A, Gallucci M, Caffarelli C. Wheat allergy in children: a comprehensive update. Medicina (Kaunas). 2019;55:400.
59. Buyuktiryaki B, Masini M, Mori F, Barni S, Liccioli G, Sarti L, at al. IgE-mediated fish allergy in children. Medicina (Kaunas). 2021;57:76.
60. Giovannini M, Beken B, Buyuktiryaki B, Barni S, Liccioli G, Sarti L, et al. IgE-mediated shellfish allergy in children. Nutrients. 2023;15:2714.
61. Pascal M, Grishina G, Yang AC, Sanchez-Garcia S, Lin J, Towle D, et al. Molecular diagnosis of shrimp allergy: efficiency of several allergens to predict clinical reactivity. J Allergy Clin Immunol Pract. 2015;3:521–9.
62. Wilson JM, Platt-Mills TA-E. Red meat allergy in children and adults. Curr Opin Allergy Clin Immunol. 2019;19:229–35.
63. Commins SP, James HR, Kelly LA, Pochan SL, Workman LJ, Perzanowski MS, et al. The relevance of tick bites to the production of IgE antibodies to the mammalian oligosaccharide galactose-α-1,3-galactose. J Allergy Clin Immunol. 2011;127:1286–93.
64. Hemmer W, Klug C, Swoboda I. Update on the bird-egg syndrome and genuine poultry meat allergy. Allergo J Int. 2016;25:68–75.
65. Poncet P, Sénechal H, Charpin D. Update on pollen-food allergy syndrome. Expert Rev Clin Immunol. 2020;16:561–78.
66. Mastrorilli C, Cardinale F, Giannetti A, Caffarelli C. Pollen-food allergy syndrome: a not so rare disease in childhood. Medicina (Kaunas). 2019;55:641.
67. Dramburg S, Hilger C, Santos AF, de Las VL, Aalberse RC, Aceved N, et al. EAACI molecular allergology user's guide 2.0. Pediatr Allergy Immunol. 2023;34(S28):e13854.

68. Asero R, Ariano R, Aruanno A, Barzaghi C, Borrelli P, Busa M, et al. Systemic allergic reactions induced by labile plant-food allergens: seeking potential cofactors. A multicenter study. Allergy. 2021;76:1473–9.
69. Decuyper II, Rihs HP, van Gasse AL, Elst J, de Puysseleyr L, Faber MA, et al. Cannabis allergy: what the clinician needs to know in 2019. Expert Rev Clin Immunol. 2019;15:599–606.
70. Martin Iglesias MA, Garcia Rodriguez R, Palacios Cañas A, Meneses Sotomayor JV, Clar Castello M, Feo Brito F. Combined LTP sublingual and oral immunotherapy in LTP syndrome: efficacy and safety. J Clin Med. 2023, 1823;12:1823.
71. Ando Y, Miyamoto M, Kato M, Nakayama M, Fukuda H, Yoshihara S. Pru P 7 predicts severe reactions after ingestion of peach in Japanese children and adolescents. Int Arch Allergy Immunol. 2019;181:183–90.
72. Barni S, Caimmi D, Chiera F, Comberiati P, Mastrorilli C, Pelosi U, et al. Phenotypes and endotypes of peach allergy: what is new? Nutrients. 2022;14:998.
73. Klingebiel C, Chantran Y, Arif-Lusson R, Ehrenberg AE, Östling J, Poisson A, et al. Pru p 7 sensitization is a predominant cause of severe, cypress pollen-associated peach allergy. Clin Exp Allergy. 2019;49:526–36.

14 Non-IgE-Mediated Gastrointestinal Food Allergies in Children

Enza D'Auria and Giovanna Monti

Abstract

Non-IgE-mediated gastrointestinal food allergies (non-IgE-GI-FAs) encompass a spectrum of disorders, including food protein-induced allergic proctocolitis (FPIAP), acute and chronic food protein-induced enterocolitis syndrome (FPIES), food protein-induced enteropathy (FPE), and food protein-induced motility disorders (FPIMDs). Cow's milk, soy, and wheat are the three most common trigger foods. The pathogenesis of these disorders remains poorly understood, and diagnostic markers are still lacking. The results of the skin prick test or measurement of the food-specific serum IgE level is generally negative although positive results may occur in some form, e.g., "atypical" FPIES. Therefore, the diagnosis relies on the demonstration of clear clinical improvement after food allergen elimination and the reemergence of symptoms upon challenge. Non-IgE-GI-FAs may overlap in terms of clinical and histologic features among themselves and with eosinophilic gastroenteropathies, which makes diagnosis challenging in clinical practice.

The treatment requires the elimination of offending food allergens until tolerance has developed. In breastfed infants, a maternal avoidance diet is sufficient to control symptoms in most cases.

In formula-fed infants, treatment usually involves the use of an extensively hydrolyzed or amino acid-based formula in more severe cases.

Generally, non-IgE-GI-FAs have a favorable prognosis; the majority resolve by 1 year in patients with FPIAP, 1–3 years in patients with FPE, and 1–5 years in patients with FPIES, with significant differences regarding specific foods. There is an urgent need to better define the prevalence and natural history of FPIES and the pathogenesis of non-IgE-GI-FAs in order to identify useful diagnostic markers.

Keywords

Non-IgE-mediated gastrointestinal food allergies · Food protein-induced allergic proctocolitis · Food protein-induced enterocolitis syndrome · Food protein-induced enteropathy · Food protein-induced motility disorders Atypical FPIES · Trigger foods · Vomiting Diarrhea · Enteropathy · Failure to thrive Avoidance diets · Extensively hydrolyzed formulas · Elemental formulas · Tolerance

E. D'Auria (✉)
Department of Biomedical and Clinical Science, Allergy Unit, Buzzi Children's Hospital, University of Milan, Milan, Italy
e-mail: enza.dauria@unimi.it

G. Monti
Department of Child Pathology and Care, Allergy Unit, Regina Margherita Children's Hospital, Turin, Italy

C. Caffarelli, G. L. Marseglia (eds.), *Textbook of Pediatric Allergy*,
https://doi.org/10.1007/978-3-031-71283-8_14

Test your learning and check your understanding of this book's contents: use the "Springer Nature Flashcards" app to access questions using ▶ https://sn.pub/nspbjm. To use the app, please follow the instructions in Chap. 1.

Key Points

- FPIAP is one of the most common causes of rectal bleeding in infants, otherwise healthy.
- Acute form of FPIES may be severe, leading to dehydration and shock.
- Clinical presentation of acute FPIES may mimic different medical and surgical conditions during infancy.
- The cardinal symptom of FPE is non-bloody chronic diarrhea, which is associated with malabsorption and enteropathy with failure to thrive in most cases.
- Specific IgE to foods is absent in most cases, and the diagnosis is mainly clinical.
- FPIMD should be suspected in cases of persisting GI symptoms, e.g., regurgitation, vomiting, colic, and constipation, which do not respond to conventional treatment.
- The diagnosis of non-IgE-GI-FAs mostly relies on the demonstration of clinical improvement after food allergen elimination and the reemergence of symptoms upon reintroduction.

14.1 Introduction

The term "food allergy" (FA) refers to an immunological adverse reaction to one or more specific foods that can be triggered and reproduced repeatedly. It can be differentiated by its pathogenetic mechanism into immunoglobulin-E-mediated, non-IgE-mediated, or mixed IgE/non-IgE-mediated allergies [1].

Non-IgE-mediated gastrointestinal food allergies (non-IgE-GI-FAs) encompass a spectrum of disorders, which have in common primary involvement of the gastrointestinal system (Fig. 14.1).

They are characterized by an inflammatory process of the gut—either subacute or chronic [2]; unlike IgE-mediated allergies, signs of non-IgE-mediated reactions typically occur from hours to days after exposure as a consequence of several hits of food exposure to the gut.

Non-IgE-mediated gastrointestinal food allergic disorders include food protein-induced allergic proctocolitis (FPIAP), food protein-induced enterocolitis syndrome (FPIES), food protein-induced allergic enteropathy (FPE), and food protein-induced motility disorders (FPIMD), meaning that disorders presenting with GI symptoms, not included in the above mentioned "classical" non-IgE-mediated gastrointestinal food allergy, improve after dietary elimination of specific food proteins [3, 4].

This chapter focuses on the clinical manifestations, epidemiology, pathogenesis, diagnosis, and management strategies of non-IgE-GI-FAs.

Fig. 14.1 Classification of non-IgE-mediated gastrointestinal food allergies

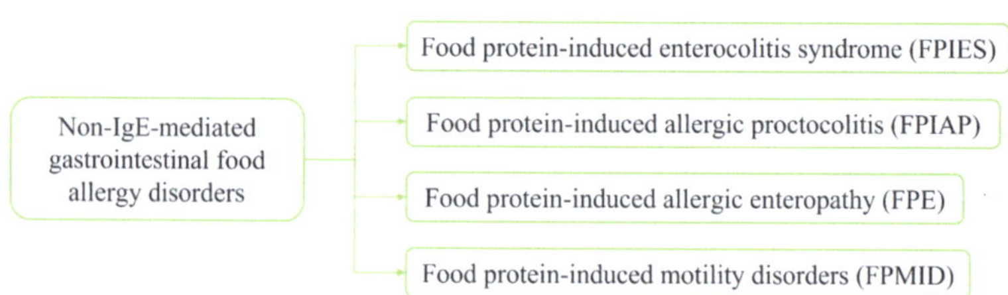

14.2 Epidemiology

The exact prevalence of non-IgE-mediated gastrointestinal food allergies is not well established, as studies on this topic are few, and the data are not definitive. Moreover, since symptoms are often aspecific, these disorders are frequently misdiagnosed, and the true prevalence is difficult to estimate.

FPIAP is the most represented entity within non-IgE-mediated gastrointestinal food allergies. It is among the most common causes of rectal bleeding in infants, accounting for up to 60% rectal bleeding in otherwise healthy infants [5]. The reported prevalence of this disease varies widely, ranging from 0.16% to 17% [6, 7]. The discrepancy in prevalence rates in different studies may be accounted for by the differences in screening and diagnosis of disease.

The age of onset of FPIAP is generally within the first 6 months of life (typically in the first 1–4 weeks postdelivery). It is estimated that the majority of infants develop tolerance by the first year of life, with 99% within 3 years [4, 8, 9]. With respect to FPE, the age of onset is highly dependent on the time of first exposure to the antigen, specifically cow's milk. Typically, symptoms begin between 2 and 9 months of age, within weeks after the introduction of the food.

FPE is quite uncommon, and its prevalence is considered to be in decline compared with the last decade [10]. The occurrence in breastfed infants is controversial, as few data are available, and they are prominently from case reports. In the majority of cases, the disease was clinically presumed and not confirmed through endoscopy [4].

Epidemiological data regarding FPIES are limited, and the actual prevalence of this condition is not well known. The lack of accurate epidemiological data may also be the result of different clinical phenotypes, absence of specific diagnostic markers, frequent misdiagnosis, lack of diagnostic criteria until 2017 [11], and a code for the disease (K52.21) that was only established in 2015 by the International Statistical Classification of Diseases and Related Health Problems [12].

Assessing the data from large case series of patients and prospective birth cohorts, the acute pediatric FPIES cumulative incidence seems to range between 0.015% (Australia) and 0.7% (Spain) [13–16]. The prevalence of acute FPIES reported in the adult population was 0.22% [17]. Overall, the results of these studies suggest that FPIES is not as uncommon a condition as initially hypothesized. There are few reports on the evolution of FPIES incidence over time, although the perception is that it is increasing [15, 18–21]. The prevalence of chronic FPIES is mostly unknown. The case studies described in the scientific literature mostly consisted of a limited number of patients [22–26]; two studies date back to the 1960s and the 1970s [22, 23], and in some studies, the diagnosis of chronic FPIES remained presumptive in some children [27, 28].

The prevalence of FPIMD is even more difficult to establish since symptoms, such as regurgitation, vomiting, and colic, are very common in infants and children and overlap with gastrointestinal functional disorders [29, 30].

According to epidemiological data, the expected coexistence of cow's milk allergy and gastroesophageal reflux disease (GERD) would occur, by far, in <1% of the breastfed or formula-fed infants [4].

The association of cow's milk allergy (CMA)-GERD has been reported in 16–56% of cases with persistent gastrointestinal symptoms and suspicion of GERD, irrespective of breast or formula feeding [29].

Recently, the incidence of food allergies in infants and children with constipation was reported to be 15% in a large case series [31].

14.3 Trigger Foods

Cow's milk (CM) is one of the foods most commonly associated with food allergies. The estimated prevalence of CM allergy ranges widely, from 3% for food-challenged allergies to 6% for self-reported overall lifetime allergies [9].

As far as non-IgE-GI-FAs is concerned, CM is the major causative agent, followed by soy, wheat, eggs, and corn.

Table 14.1 Cow's milk- and soy-induced FPIES

Author	Country	Percent (n) Cow's milk	Percent (n) Soy	Subject number
Caubet et al. (2014) [43]	USA	44 (70)	41 (66)	160
Ruffner et al. (2013) [42]	USA	67 (309)	41 (190)	462
Blackman et al. (2019) [34]	USA	49 (36)	31 (23)	74
Lee et al. (2021) [46]	Australia	30 (50)	13 (22)	168
Mehr et al. (2009) [19]	Australia	20 (7)	7 (16)	230
Mehr et al. (2017) [16]	Australia	33 (76)	34 (12)	35
Ludman et al. (2014) [40]	UK	46 (25)	11 (6)	54
Stiefel et al. (2022) [41]	UK	34 (33)	5.2 (7)	98
Barni et al. (2019) [44]	Italy	43 (21)	0 (0)	48
Miceli Sopo et al. (2014) [25]	Italy	67 (44)	4 (3)	66
Argiz et al. (2021) [45]	Italy/Spain	15 (28)	0.6 (1)	179
Diaz et al. (2019) [36]	Spain	40 (48)	0.8 (1)	120
Lange et al. (2022) [27]	Germany	28 (40)	1.16 (1)	142
Lemoine et al. (2022) [28]	France	60 (108)	0.5 (1)	179
Douros et al. (2019) [21]	Greece	35 (27)	0 (0)	78
Xepapadaki et al. (2019) [120]	Greece	45.5 (33)	0 (0)	72
Ullberg et al. (2021) [47]	Sweden	26 (30)	6 (7)	113
Nishimura et al. (2022) [39]	Japan	13 (3)	8 (24.7)	23

FPIAP can affect both breastfed and formula-fed children, and in 50–65% of cases, the culprit antigen is CM. The maternal consumption of CM proteins (in particular β-lactoglobulin) leads to their excretion in breast milk (BM), inducing FA in the breastfed infant [5]. Other dietary triggers of FPIAP that may be present in the maternal diet are soy, wheat, egg, and goat or sheep's milk proteins [4]. After weaning, the same food proteins are able to trigger the disease directly through the infant's diet. In formula-fed infants, the agents that are most commonly related to FPIAP are CM and soy [5].

Almost any food can be a trigger for FPIES. However, depending on different geographical areas and different eating habits, trigger foods may vary in type and frequency; moreover, in some countries, some foods considered in previous years as rare triggers of FPIES have been reported with increasing frequency [20, 32–34]. The clinical form (acute or chronic) of FPIES also holds different triggers: the chronic form is caused mainly by CM, followed by soy, and rarely by other foods [22–26, 35–37]. FPIES can be caused by liquid food or solid food. Liquid food-induced FPIES accounts for about 65% of cases [38], and CM is the leading liquid food cause of FPIES worldwide [14, 16, 18, 19, 21, 27, 28, 36, 39–47] (see Table 14.1). Soy-FPIES is most reported in the USA [34, 42, 43] and Japan [39], while in Europe, it is very underrepresented [40, 44], presumably due to the decreased use of soy either as a soy formula or as a complementary food (e.g., yogurt or cheese) during weaning. Solid foods commonly implicated in large case series are reported in Table 14.2. The majority of children with FPIES react to a single food, but multiple forms have been reported (6%–69% depending on the case series) [16, 18, 19, 21, 27, 28, 34, 36, 41–47].

Table 14.2 Solid foods commonly implicated in large case series

Author	Country	Rice	Oat	Corn	Wheat	Egg	Fish	Poultry	Beef	Lamb	Pork	Banana	Potato	Sweet potato
		n (%)	*n* (%)	*n* (%)	*n* (%)	*n* (%)	*n* (%)	*n* (%)	*n* (%)	*n* (%)	*n* (%)	*n* (%)	*n* (%)	*n* (%)
Caubet et al. (2014) [43]	USA	36 (22.5)	26 (16.2)	1 (0.6)	2 (1.2)	4 (2.4)	10 (6.2)	5 (3.1)	5 (3.1)	1 (0.6)	NR	NR	NR	4 (2.4)
Ruffner et al. (2013) [42]	USA	88 (19)	74 (16)	37 (8)	46 (10)	51 (11)	14 (3)	40 (8.6)	101 (22)	2 (0.5)	74 (16)	16 (3.5)	8 (2)	19 (4.1)
Blackman et al. (2019) [34]	USA	39 (53)	26 (35)	5 (7)	4 (5)	NR	1 (1)	7 (9.4)	1 (1)	NR	NR	18 (24)	6 (8)	16 (22)
Lee et al. (2021) [46]	Australia	75 (45)	18 (11)	NR	NR	20 (12)	19 (11)	11 (7)	NR	NR	NR	16 (8)	NR	NR
Mehr et al. (2009) [19]	Australia	14 (40)	2 (6)	NR	NR	NR	1 (3)	1 (3)	NR	1 (3)	NR	1 (3)	NR	2 (6)
Mehr et al. (2017) [16]	Australia	102 (45)	21 (9)	2 (1)	8 (3.5)	27 (12)	12 (5)	19 (8)	6 (3)	3 (1)	NR	9 (4)	5 (2)	7 (3)
Ludman et al. (2014) [40]	UK	2 (4)	3 (6)	1 (2)	6 (11)	7 (13)	8 (12)	4 (7)	2 (4)	NR	NR	3 (6)	1 (2)	NR
Stiefel et al. (2022) [41]	UK	6 (4.4)	7 (5)	NR	3 (2.2)	22 (16.3)	19 (14)	6 (4.4)	2 (1.5)	1 (0.7)	1 (0.7)	8 (6)	2 (1.5)	5 (3.7)
Ullberg et al. (2021) [47]	Sweden	9 (8)	25 (22)	4 (3.5)	1 (0.8)	7 (6)	28 (25)	7 (6)	1 (0.8)	NR	1 (0.8)	1 (0.8)	3 (2.6)	3 (2.6)
Barni et al. (2019) [44]	Italy	6 (1.2)	NR	1 (2)	2 (4)	7 (14.5)	10 (21)	NR	2 (4)	NR	NR	NR	NR	NR
M Sopo et al. (2014) [25]	Italy	NR	3 (4)	1 (2)	NR	4 (6)	8 (12)	2 (3)	NR	NR	NR	NR	NR	NR
Argiz et al. (2021) [45]	Italy/Spain	4 (2.2)	NR	NR	3 (1.7)	35 (19.5)	102 (57)	NR	NR	NR	NR	NR	NR	NR
Diaz et al. (2019) [36]	Spain	12 (10)	NR	NR	1 (0.8)	13 (10.8)	39 (32.5)	2 (1.7)	1 (0.8)	NR	NR	1 (0.8)	1 (0.8)	NR
Lange et al. (2022) [27]	Germany	6 (4.6)	3 (2.3)	NR	5 (3.8)	6 (4.6)	27 (20.7)	7 (5.4)	12 (9.2)	1 (0.6)	3 (2.3)	2 (1.2)	6 (4.6)	2 (1.2)
Lemoine et al. (2022) [28]	France	NR	NR	NR	NR	29 (16.2)	21 (11.7)	NR	NR	NR	NR	NR	NR	NR
Douros et al. (2019) [21]	Greece	7 (8.9)	NR	NR	NR	4 (5.1)	42 (54)	4 (5.1)	2 (2.5)	NR	NR	NR	NR	NR
Xepapadaki et al. (2019) [120]	Greece	7 (9.7)	NR	NR	NR	5 (7)	25 (34.7)	2 (2.8)	NR	NR	NR	NR	NR	NR
Nishimura et al. (2022) [39]	Japan	1 (4.3)	NR	NR	3 (13)	7 3 (0)	1 (4.3)	NR	NR	NR	NR	NR	NR	NR

NR not reported

14.4 Pathogenesis

Non-IgE-mediated gastrointestinal food allergies are characterized by an inflammatory response against food, which is not associated with the production of circulating IgEs and the following activation of mast cells and basophils. This entails that a variety of pathogenetic mechanisms may play a role in the development of these allergic disorders [48].

In FPIAP, the antigen of the offending food determines cell-mediated inflammation of the gut mucosa, particularly in the sigmoid colon and rectum. This causes edema and erosion of the epithelium, with the consequence of bloody stools [4].

Upon biopsy, allergic proctocolitis was found to be associated with a significant focal increase in the number of eosinophils in the colonic mucosa. Specifically, a finding of 60 eosinophils/10 high-power fields in the lamina propria strongly suggests the diagnosis of FPIAP even though these histopathological features are not pathognomonic of the disease.

Due to the zonal distribution of eosinophils in FPIAP, multiple mucosal biopsy specimens are needed in order to confirm the diagnosis [49].

The malabsorption that characterizes FPE instead is the result of structural damage to the mucosa of the jejunum. Specifically, villous atrophy with crypt hyperplasia and inflammation have been reported to be associated with thickening of the basement membrane and increased mitotic activity in the jejunal crypts. This mechanism is thought to be mediated mostly by T cells, particularly CD3+ alpha/beta T-cell-receptor-bearing cells, together with suppressor-cytotoxic CD8+ cells, which infiltrate the epithelial membrane with a patchy distribution.

Furthermore, TIA1, a cytotoxic granule-associated protein that is specific to T lymphocytes and natural killer (NK) cells, is found to be increased in patients with FPE and decreased upon elimination diet [10].

From an immunological point of view, the immunological response to antigens is mediated by the proliferation and differentiation of Th2 lymphocytes, which leads to the production of cytokines. Recent evidence has found increased levels of IL-4 and IL-13 in infants with non-IgE-mediated FAs even after a few days after the introduction of a special diet [50].

A profound activation of the innate immune system (with the involvement of monocytes, neutrophils [PMNs], eosinophils [EOS], and NK cells) has been demonstrated [51] in patients with active FPIES. As for PMNs, in addition to their activation, there was also a significant increase in circulating levels [51]. In other studies, in patients with active FPIES, the recruitment of PMNs and increased levels of IL-8, a chemoattractant for PMNs, as well as increased expression of genes involved in granulocyte adhesion and diapedesis and of those involved in innate immunity signals during positive oral food challenge (OFC), were observed [52–55]. The role sustained by PMN in the immunopathogenesis of FPIES is also demonstrated by the fact that increased circulating PMNs are often detected during acute FPIES reactions [51] and that an increase in these cells, peaking at 6 h after the onset of OFC (≥1500 cells/mL above the baseline count), is part of the diagnostic criteria for defining positive evidence [56].

No significant change [57] or decrease [52] in absolute EOS counts was observed in patients with positive OFCs, in whom increased fecal EOS-derived neurotoxin [57] and major basic protein [58] were instead observed [57].

Studies aimed at investigating the involvement of the T-cell-mediated response in FPIES have shown conflicting results. An in vitro enhanced antigen-specific T lymphocyte proliferative response was reported [59, 60] in active FPIES. This activation is followed by the release of high levels of the proinflammatory cytokines TNF-α and TH-2 (IL-10 and IL-4). However, more recent studies have not confirmed these observations [54]. Goswami et al. [51] demonstrated pan-T-cell activation and redistribution from the circulation in patients with active FPIES.

Lower baseline serum levels of IL-10 in patients with active CM-FPIES [54] and an increase in IL-10 expressed by CD3+ cells after the acquisition of tolerance [61] was reported, suggesting a key role of IL-10 in the acquisition of tolerance in patients with CM-FPIES.

Chung et al. [62] observed increased TNF-α expression and concurrently reduced expression of TGF-β1 receptors in duodenal biopsies from infants with FPIES compared with those from the control group. TGF-β, which plays a key role in ensuring the integrity of the intestinal barrier, is reduced in the stimulated supernatants of children with CM-FPIES in the active phase compared with those who have outgrown it [63]. In addition, TNF-α increases gastrointestinal permeability, leading to third spacing fluid loss with subsequent dehydration, and potentiates the synthesis of prostaglandins, eliciting the relaxation of vascular smooth muscle tone [64] as well as hypotension, contributing to the pathogenesis of shock in the most severe cases of FPIES.

Recently, Berin et al. [53], in symptomatic FPIES OFCs, observed a proinflammatory cytokine release with an IL-17 inflammatory signature (mainly IL-17, IL-22, and IL-2), in addition to the REG1A protein, which is expressed in the intestine and regulates mucosal barrier function downstream of the Th17 cytokine IL-22.

An important role in the onset of the typical symptoms of FPIES, primarily vomiting, may be held by serotonin (5-HT), as suggested by the prompt response of the acute picture to the use of ondansetron, a central selective serotonin receptor antagonist [65].

5-HT causes increases in both intestinal motility and fluid secretion, in addition to nausea and vomiting, through stimulation of smooth muscle and sensory nerves in the stomach, including the vagus nerve. The question is raised as to what stimulus induces the secretion of 5-HT since enterochromaffin cells play a chemosensory role and are not immunocompetent. Recent studies have shown that 5-HT is also produced by T lymphocytes [66] and this could hint at immune-neuroendocrine communication at the level of the intestinal tract, one of whose ultimate effectors could be enterochromaffin cell, leading to 5HT secretion.

Lozano-Ojalvo et al. [67] demonstrated that the levels of a total of 34 metabolites, including inosine and urate of the purine signaling pathway, were increased during OFCs performed on patients with symptomatic FPIES. The level of the serotonin metabolite 5-hydroxyindole acetate was significantly elevated after the reaction. The activation of the purinergic pathway during FPIES reactions shown in this study provides a possible mechanism connecting inflammation and vomiting by triggering serotonin release from the gastric and duodenal mucosa.

Although the exact pathogenesis remains still understood, motility alterations due to neuroimmune interactions seem to play an important role in the development of FPIMD [68, 69].

14.5 Clinical Manifestations

Non-IgE-GI-FAs are a heterogeneous group of food allergies and, as previously explained, can involve a variety of organ systems. The differentiating factors between the entities analyzed in this chapter are gastrointestinal symptoms. The onset may be in the first weeks of life, normally with a delay period from the first exposure to the allergen, and is usually subacute or chronic. The spectrum of clinical manifestation is wide and can range from mild hematochezia to severe vomiting and diarrhea and from subacute symptoms (some hours after food ingestion) to progressive and chronic presentations (i.e., anemia or faltering growth). There are a range of nonspecific symptoms that span all of the entities under the non-IgE-GI-FAs umbrella. These are regurgitation, vomiting, crying, abdominal gas, and distention, constipation, or diarrhea.

14.6 Food Protein-Induced Allergic Proctocolitis (FPIAP)

FPIAP affects both formula-fed and BM-fed infants. Children who are fed solely formula are more likely to develop this pathology compared with children who are fed a combination of BM and cow's milk-based formula or BM exclusively [7]. This could be due to the protective effect of immunomodulatory substances present in mothers' milk or of the different intestinal microbiomes of the breastfed infant, together with exposure to lower levels of CM proteins in human milk. The exact prevalence of this disease among exclusively breastfed infants remains unknown [5].

FPIAP is considered to be at the milder end of the severity spectrum of non-IgE-GI-FAs [70]. Infants develop symptoms within the first months of life; they typically present with intermittent, moderately bloody, loose stools in otherwise seemingly well infant. Other causes of bleeding (constipation and/or anal fissures, infections, and inflammatory intestinal diseases) should be excluded [4, 5]. In some cases, occasional vomiting may occur, but it is not the main symptom; minor symptoms such as gas colic and increased bowel movement can also be present [5]. In a small percentage of cases, the onset can be acute within 12 h after ingestion of the offending food [5].

14.7 Food Protein-Induced Allergic Enteropathy (FPE)

Also known as CM-sensitive enteropathy, FPE becomes clinically apparent soon after the integration of CM into the infant's diet, most frequently in the first 2 months of life. The cardinal symptom of FPE is nonbloody chronic diarrhea, associated with malabsorption. It is usually caused by CM but may be due to soy or egg. The latter can lead to a range of consequences, from steatorrhea to protein-losing enteropathy with hypoalbuminemia and hypoproteinemia [71]. The disease is associated with failure to thrive (FTT) in more than half of the cases. Other symptoms that have been described in children with FPE are vomiting, abdominal distension, lack of appetite, and carbohydrate intolerance [5]; the latter is likely due to the celiac-like effects of CM protein on the mucosa of the small intestine [1]. Elimination of the trigger food leads to the regression of symptoms within 1–4 weeks, while patchy villous atrophy normalizes several months after apparent clinical healing [10].

14.8 Food Protein-Induced Enterocolitis Syndrome (FPIES)

FPIES may occur in both acute and chronic manifestations [72, 73]. The acute form is characterized by the manifestation of repeated projectile vomiting after 1–4 h from the isolated consumption of the trigger food, often associated with persistent and intense pallor, floppiness, and less frequently hypothermia and lethargy, which feature the most severe forms. In 5–20% of cases, it also appears a progression toward dehydration, hypotension, and shock. Diarrhea, which is discontinuous, has a late onset (5–8 h) [72, 73]. Laboratory findings may show leukocytosis with a predominance of neutrophils, thrombocytosis, and metabolic acidosis; transient methemoglobinemia has also been reported in severe cases [74, 75]. In some subjects, mild elevations in C-reactive protein values and the occurrence of fever, both during acute emergency department (ED) episodes and positive OFC, have been reported [75, 76].

The reaction may require emergency treatment in a medical setting, but usually resolves after a few hours, after the offending food's exclusion.

In acute FPIES, the reaction appears mostly coinciding with the first or second direct contact with the culprit food or during its reintroduction after a suspension timeframe, or again if the food is not assumed daily [16, 72, 73].

The chronic FPIES onset may be subtle due to repeated exposure to the culprit food (CMF or soy-based infant formula [SF]) in newborns and young infants) [22–26, 36]. There was recently a report of two cases of chronic FPIES by fish [37] in infancy and a case of late onset of chronic FPIES induced by eggs, beef, and salmon in a young adult [35].

The described clinical presentation is characterized by intermittent but progressive emesis and/or watery diarrhea, at times with mucus and/or blood in the stool, failure to thrive or progressive weight loss, and possible evolution into the most severe forms, such as dehydration to hypovolemic shock. Laboratory data reveal leukocytosis with neutrophilia and metabolic acidosis and less commonly anemia and hypoalbuminemia [22–26, 36]. It has also been reported in some cases of particular severity methemoglobinemia (Table 14.1) [77, 78].

The symptoms disappear from a few days up to 2 weeks after the elimination of the trigger food, whose subsequent ingestions following a

Table 14.3 Comparison of FPIAP, chronic FPIES, and FPE

	FPIAP	Chronic FPIES	FPE
Age at onset	Within the first 6 months of life	Weeks or months after the first introduction of the trigger food; CM and soy up to 2 years	Between 2 and 9 months of age
Food protein implicated	CM, soy, wheat, egg, goat, and sheep's milk	CM, soy, and egg	CM, soy, wheat, and eggs
Main symptoms	Bloody and loose stool	severe diarrhea, intermittent but progressive emesis, and dehydration up to hypovolemic shock in more severe cases	Nonbloody diarrhea, malabsorption, and FTT
Additional symptoms	Gas colic, increased bowel movement, gagging, food refusal, and irritability	Edema, failure to thrive, and bloody stools	Vomiting, abdominal distention, fussiness, carbohydrate intolerance
Laboratory findings	Peripheral eosinophilia, and mild anemia	Leukocytosis with neutrophilia and metabolic acidosis and less commonly anemia and hypoalbuminemia and methemoglobinemia in more severe cases	Iron deficiency anemia, positive FOB test, hypoalbuminemia, and eosinophilia
GI tract affected	Sigmoid colon and rectum	Small intestine, colon, and rectum	Jejunum
Biopsy macroscopic findings	Focal erythema, ulceration, diffuse nodularity, and loss of vascular pattern	Variable patchy, villous atrophy, occasional mucosal erosions, and prominent rectal ulceration	Villous atrophy
Microscopic findings	Focal increase in eosinophils (60 eosinophils/10 high-power field) in the lamina propria of the colonic mucosa	Cryptal eosinophilic abscesses	Crypt hyperplasia, thickening of the basement membrane, increased mitotic activity in the jejunal crypts, and T-cell infiltration of the epithelial membrane
Treatment	Exclusion of culprit food from the maternal or infant's diet	Avoidance of the offending foods, symptoms clear in 3–10 days, 80% respond to hydrolysate and 20% require an elemental formula	Avoidance of the offending food
Prognosis	Resolves within 1 year	CM tends to resolve by age 3–5 years, rice-induced FPIES: 50% outgrow by age 5 years	Resolves in 1–3 years

period of avoidance cause the outbreak of a typical acute episode (acute-on chronic form). This is the most important criterion for a chronic FPIES diagnosis; hence, for an infant presenting a clinical picture compatible with a suspected chronic FPIES, a trial of food elimination followed by supervised OFCs to potential food triggers might be necessary for a conclusive diagnosis. Without a confirmatory challenge, the diagnosis of chronic FPIES remains presumptive [11].

Table 14.3 shows the characteristics of the major non-IgE-GI-FAs.

14.9 Food Protein-Induced Gastrointestinal Motility Disorders

Regurgitation, vomiting, and colic are among the most common disorders that occur during infancy and early childhood. Infant regurgitation and colic are defined by the Rome IV criteria as functional gastrointestinal disorders (FGIDs) of infancy [79]. In at least a subset of infants with these functional disorders, improvement after the dietary elimination of specific food proteins has been demonstrated.

In some children with gastroesophageal reflux (GER) due to CMA, a particular pH-metric esophageal pattern with a gradual drop in pH after a meal has been noted [80]. However, this finding is not present in all infants who respond to the diet and has not been confirmed by other authors [81]. pH-impedance analysis showed that patients with CMA have predominantly a non-acid GER component [82] that can be even more painful than acid GER [83], but do not benefit from therapy with acid inhibitors.

FPIMD should be particularly suspected in the presence of regurgitation associated with chronic diarrhea or blood in the stool, other atopic manifestations (eczema) or a positive family history of allergy.

The involvement of symptoms in different organ systems in association with regurgitation increases the likelihood of CMA [84].

Food protein-induced constipation is a poorly defined clinical entity, and only a small proportion of constipation in children <2 years of age is due to food allergies [85].

14.10 Diagnosis and Differential Diagnosis

The diagnosis of non-IgE-GI-FAs is challenging as it is based on the recognition of a pattern of symptoms that are often nonspecific and may overlap from one disorder to another. Furthermore, there are no pathognomonic diagnostic markers.

A careful allergy-focused history is the starting point for the diagnosis of non-IgE-GI-FAs. In particular, the characterization of the clinical picture, the temporal relationship between the ingestion of the trigger food and the onset of symptoms, the quantity of food causing the reaction, and most importantly, the reproducibility of the symptoms upon food ingestion are key points when obtaining the medical history. A family history of atopy is often present.

The cornerstone for the diagnosis remains the avoidance diet, either for the weaned child or for the nursing mother in the case of non-IgE-GI-FAs in breast-fed infants, which is usually the case with FPIAP [4]. After symptom resolution under dietary elimination, it is possible to perform an OFC, which is the gold standard for diagnosing non-IgE-GI-FAs. If symptoms reappear upon reintroduction of the offending food, the diagnosis is confirmed [73].

After excluding other diseases in differential diagnosis, a convincing history of typical characteristic signs and symptoms, which rapidly resolve after withdrawal of the suspected trigger food and that in case of multiple episodes recur at repeated exposures to the suspect food or foods, is in most cases sufficient to confirm the diagnostic suspicion of acute FPIES [11].

Diagnostic clinical criteria for acute FPIES according to international guidelines were published in 2017 [11]. While most cases of acute FPIES fall under these diagnostic criteria, they nevertheless fail to capture all the clinical phenotypes of acute FPIES, particularly the milder ones. Even in the case of multiple episodes after intake of the same food but a consistently mild clinical picture, it would not be feasible to place the diagnosis of acute FPIES according to the 2017 criteria and the child should undergo diagnostic OFC [86]. It can be challenging to establish whether there is hypotension, hypothermia, or lethargy; however, parents may report the presence of "cold skin," floppiness, decreased activity level, or poor responsiveness to vocal recall.

It is not an easy task to place the diagnostic suspicion of acute FPIES. A pathognomonic clinical picture, as well as specific hematochemical, fecal, and instrumental markers, is missing. Without a thorough understanding of the disease, it is very difficult to associate an acute reaction with solid foods that are commonly considered nonallergenic (e.g., rice or potato). Acute FPIES also presents issues of differential diagnosis with different conditions of an allergic nature or otherwise [87] (Table 14.4).

The diagnosis of FPIES in the neonatal period, even more so in preterm newborns, is even more challenging, and FPIES should be especially carefully differentiated from necrotizing enterocolitis (NEC), as its management, morbidity and mortality are remarkably different [88]. For both pathological conditions, the symp-

Table 14.4 Acute FPIES: clinical phenotypes and differential diagnosis

	Mild	Moderate	Severe
	1–2 vomiting ± Diarrhea	>3 vomiting ± Diarrhea	>3 vomiting ± Diarrhea ± Mucus/blood
		Pallor	Intense pallor ± Hypotermia
		Decreased activity level ± Mild floppiness	Lethargy Floppiness ± Hypotension to shock
	↓	↓	↓
	Maldigestive symptoms		
Infectious	Gastroenteritis	Gastroenteritis	Sepsis
Allergic	Immediate gastrointestinal hypersensitivity	Anaphylaxis	Anaphylaxis
Surgical			Necrotizing enterocolitis Hypertrophic pyloric stenosis Intussusception Volvolus Hirschprung disease

Children with sepsis were likely to present with fever, tachycardia, tachypnea, and hypotension; those with GE presented mainly with diarrhea, sometimes bloody, and fever; high CRP values were also present in both infectious forms. In comparison, children with FPIES were characterized by lethargy, floppiness, pallor without fever, hypothermia, and normal CRP. Leukocytosis, lymphocytosis, and thrombocytosis were more commonly seen in FPIES than in sepsis or GE. Patients with acute FPIES presented a greater rapidity of response to oral rehydration therapy and especially to elimination of the trigger food

IGH and anaphylaxis are characterized by very short latency (from a few minutes to 30′) between the intake of the trigger food and the onset of symptoms, the presence of abdominal crampy pain and possible psychomotor agitation (anaphylaxis), in addition to the positivity of sIgE for the trigger food, although it can also be found in so-called atypical FPIES [72]

toms, laboratory measures, and radiographic findings are nonspecific, and an overlap in clinical presentation can make a differential diagnosis between NEC and FPIES difficult. Cases of term [89] and preterm, low-weight for age newborns [90] were described as affected by CM-FPIES initially diagnosed as NEC, characterized by eosinophilia, leukocytosis with neutrophilia and thrombocytosis, other than the occurrence of multiple episodes and correlation of symptom onset and resolution with feed changes (modification of diet to an extensively hydrolyzed formula [eHF] or an amino acid-based formula [AAF]) [89, 90]. In the early stage, abdominal ultrasound (AU) can be useful for differentiating NEC and FPIES [91]. Laboratory abnormalities are associated with non-IgE-GI-FAs (Table 14.3).

Skin prick test (SPT) and sIgE are usually negative. However, some infants with FPIAP [92] and approximately 25–30% of patients with FPIES might develop IgE to the food trigger, the so-called atypical FPIES [2, 93].

Other diagnostic tests for non-IgE-GI-FAs are under investigation, but their role is far to be defined [94]. Invasive confirmatory tests, such as endoscopy, are necessary to confirm the diagnosis of FPE. Histology findings include jejunal villous atrophy, crypt hyperplasia, and inflammation, similar to those found in celiac disease although less severe [95, 96]. Otherwise, biopsy is not recommended in FPIAP unless there is uncertainty in the diagnosis or when symptoms persist despite the elimination diet. It has been demonstrated that clinical signs and symptoms such as diarrhea, rectal bleeding, irritability, and urticaria are associated in more than 70% of cases to abnormal biopsies, while <50% of children with pathological biopsies present with faltering growth or reflux/vomiting [97].

The differential diagnosis of FPIAP includes all of the conditions that may be associated with hematochezia in young infants, such as anal fissures, NEC, Meckel's diverticulum and intussusception, very early onset IBD (although it is quite rare), vascular malformations, coagulation defects, and thrombocytopenia.

FPE should be differentiated from chronic FPIES, coeliac disease, secondary lactose intolerance, cystic fibrosis, autoimmune enteropathies, metabolic disorders, congenital disaccharide malabsorption, chronic kidney disease, sepsis and immunodeficiencies, and/or chronic infection.

Infectious gastroenteritis (viral, bacterial or parasitic) is frequent in this age group and may present with similar features to non-IgE-GI-FAs and should therefore be excluded in the diagnostic workup of these pathologies [98].

Also, chronic FPIES can present different phenotypes, characterized by different clinical pictures and laboratory and instrumental data, which make it difficult to raise the diagnostic suspicion, possibly even more than for the acute form. Chronic FPIES can mimic a wide spectrum of other medical and surgical conditions, peculiar to newborns and young infants (Table 14.5). If diagnostic doubts are not raised, the risk will be, on the one hand, the implementation of unnecessary and invasive investigations and treatments and, on the other hand, the evolution into clinical pictures of a particular severity.

Indications for the OFC in FPIES are listed in Table 14.6.

Since OFC in these patients has a risk of severe reactions or that otherwise requires intervention with intravenous fluids, steroids, or both, it should always be carried out under medical supervision by a trained team with emergency drugs available, and it is also recommended for a venous access to be placed before the trial begins [11].

Diagnostic criteria for the interpretation of OFCs according to international guidelines were published in 2017 [11].

Over the last few years, several protocols for performing OFCs in patients with FPIES have been published [13, 39, 43, 44, 99–103], some of which, after 2017 [39, 44, 99–101], vary substantially regarding the doses of the food at each feeding, the total dose and the timing between one dose and the next, as well as the total observation period (Table 14.7). The important differences among all the protocols that have been proposed suggest the need for international standardization of the approach to OFCs in FPIES and for studies to further investigate the characteristics of patients who need to test the food in a hospital setting and those who might be partially or exclusively introduced at home.

In general, the diagnosis of FPIMD as well as the majority of non-IgE-GI-FAs is clinical and should be suspected in cases of persisting GI symptoms, e.g., regurgitation, vomiting, colic, and constipation, which do not respond to conventional treatment.

Treatment with acid inhibitors is not significantly effective in infants with regurgitation or vomiting and/or protracted crying without instrumental evidence of GERD [104]. However, proton pump inhibitors are often empirically prescribed [105] but should be reserved for infants with pathological acid exposure time or a significant temporal association between symptoms and acid GER during pH impedance or with evidence of esophagitis [84] or with evidence of esophagitis.

Endoscopic examination of the upper gastrointestinal tract should be considered in some patients in case of more severe symptoms with frequent regurgitation or vomiting. Esophageal biopsies allow for the differentiation between GERD and eosinophilic esophagitis [106].

Table 14.5 Differential diagnosis of chronic FPIES

Medical conditions	
Gastrointestinal reflux disease	No diarrhea, no dehydration, vomiting usually minimal
Infectious gastroenteritis	Viral: fever present, slower course over days, no specific food trigger
	Bacterial: watery or bloody diarrhea, fever, positive stool culture, response to antibiotics
Sepsis	Fever present, treatment with fluid resuscitation alone does not improve
Inborn errors of metabolism	Inability to process sugars, amino acids, and organic acids; many patients may self-avoid food that cannot be metabolized (avoidance of fruit in fructose intolerance and dairy in galactosemia)
Intractable diarrhoea of infancy (IDI)	Permanent intestinal failure associated with a high rate of digestive loss, no specific food trigger, villous atrophy at histopathological analysis
Severe lactase deficiency	Low prevalence under 5–6 years of age; frequently positive family history of lactose intolerance; the symptoms disappear taking milk and lactose-free dairy products
Inadequate energy production:	Failure to thrive, heart and muscle involvement, splenomegaly, hypoglycemia, no diarrhea or
Mitochondrial, fatty acid	Food avoidance oxidation disorders, glycogen storage disorder
Lysosomal storage disorders	Hepatosplenomegaly, developmental delay, short stature, chronic pain
Congenital disorder of glycosylation	Low tone, seizures, dysmorphic features
Congenital methemoglobinemia (type I)	Mostly asymptomatic, no vomiting or diarrhea, general fatigue, dyspnea
Primary immunodeficiency	Not specific to food, abnormality in lymphocyte counts, immunoglobulins, etc.
Surgical conditions	
Hypertrophic pyloric stenosis	No diarrhea, diagnosis with ultrasound
Intussusception	Severe cramping abdominal pain—intermittent, not associated with specific food, abdominal mass on examination, detectable on ultrasound
Malrotation/volvulus	Not associated with a specific food; sepsis from necrotic bowel, fluid resuscitation alone does not improve symptoms
Necrotizing enterocolitis	In FPIES: eosinophilia, leukocytosis with neutrophilia and thrombocytosis, other than the occurrence of multiple episodes and correlation of symptom onset and resolution with feed changes [75, 76]; pneumatosis intestinalis and portal venous gas may be present in the early stage but decreased significantly at the second hour from the onset [79]. Bowel wall thickening was absent in the nonaffected part of all infants with FPIES, but diffused in infants with NEC; positive rate of reduced intestinal motility outside the lesion area: 100% in NEC and 0% in FPIES [79]
Hirschsprung's disease	Abdominal distension, constipation, delayed passage of meconium, bilious emesis
Allergic disorders	
Food protein-induced allergic proctocolitis (FPIAP)	Well-appearing, thriving infant; no vomiting, resolution sooner (approximately 1 y of age)
Food protein-induced enteropathy (FPE)	Small bowel injury and malabsorption. No lethargy, pallor, or dehydration, and no metabolic derangements. Diagnosis confirmed with endoscopy and biopsy

Adapted with permission from Nowak-Wegrzyn et al. [17]

Table 14.6 Indication to perform oral food challenge (OFC) in FPIES

1. Diagnosis of acute FPIES (for cases in which the history is unclear, the time course of symptoms is atypical, symptoms persist despite removing the suspected trigger food or foods from the diet)
2. Etiologic diagnosis (food trigger not identified, for example, if the infant presented with an acute episode after eating a mix of foods. In this case, multiple separate OFCs for foods contained in the meal and no longer taken after the episode would be appropriate)
3. Diagnosis of chronic FPIES
4. Assessment of the tolerance achievement to the trigger food
5. Introduction into a medical setting of foods that are potentially cross-reactive with the trigger food or for which a high level of co-reactivity was reported
6. First introduction of foods at high risk of reaction (infants with multiple forms of FPIES or with previous severe acute reactions)

Table 14.7 Different protocols for performing OFCs in FPIES published since 2017

Author	Dose and dose interval	Post-OFC observation	Positive OFC	Reaction time	Severe reactions
Nishimura et al. (2022) [39]	One food challenge dose (1/50, 1/10, 1/2, and full dose) per day for 4 days	4 h	$N = 8/23$ (34.8%)	1/50 full doses on the first day (75% of positive patients) 7/8 positive OFCs: within 4 h 1/8: after over 8 h	None
Guenther et al. (2020) [101]	0.03–0.6 g food protein/kg body, divided in 3 equal doses, over 30 min. An age-appropriate serving could be given 3 h later at the discretion of the provider (51% of OFCs)		$N = 10/88$ (11%)	Symptoms developed after a median cumulative dose of 0.35 g/kg (range 0.2–0.6 g/kg, serving size 50–100% based on age-appropriate serving size estimates), within 2–3 h after completion of the initial divided dose. No subject had a reaction after administration of an age-appropriate serving following the initial divided dose	None
Infante et al. (2019) [99]	Method 1: 12.5%, 25%, 50%, remaining dose every 30′, during the same day Method 2: 25%, 50%, and 100% of a standard serving size per age in 2/3 nonconsecutive days	Method 1: 2 h Method 2: 4 h	$N = 43/75$ (57.3%) $N = 32/75$ (42.7%)	Method 1:95.3% of children reacted when they had eaten the whole meal Method 2: 81.25% developed the symptoms at the first day with a lower dose of the food	Method 1: admission to ED, 39.5% Hospitalization in ICU: 42% Method 2: Admission to ED, 12.5% Hospitalization in ICU: 25%
Wang et al. (2019) [100]	Protocol 2024–2016: 2-dose challenge, receiving a cumulative of 1/4–1/3 serving size for age Protocol 2016–2017: 1-dose protocol: administration of 1/3 of serving size for age	4 h Upon discharge, families were generally instructed to increase the dose every 3 days over 9 to 12 days	$N = 30/169$ (18%)	17 (10%) during initial challenge Symptoms occurred at least 85 min after dosing 13 (7.7%) during home introduction	Admission to ED: 4 (2.4%) Hospitalization in ICU: 1 (0.6)%
Barni et al. (2019) [44]	25% of the total dose (0.3 g food protein/kg body weight) followed by a full dose 4 h later if no reaction was observed		$N = 19/54$ (35.2%)	100% of positive OFCs after 25% of the full dose mean time latency: 136 min	$N = 9$ (47%) Hospitalization in ICU: none

14.11 Treatment and Management

Treatment of non-IgE-mediated-GI-FAs is based on the strict maternal dietary exclusion of the offending food in breastfed infants, otherwise on an elimination diet for non-breastfed infants. The maternal elimination diet should be maintained for 2–4 weeks with the support of a dietician in order to avoid deficiencies or nutritional imbalances. After that period, when symptom resolution takes place, CM proteins—or the suspected offending food—could be reintroduced into the mothers' diet in order to verify the recurrence of allergies in the baby.

Recently, international guidelines suggested that in the case of exclusively breastfed infants, CM could be reintroduced into the mother's diet at home in previously consumed amounts [107]. Instead, when home reintroduction is done in weaned infants, the British guidelines (iMAP—Milk Allergy in Primary Care) suggest following a consensus-based milk ladder in order to give the infant food, which is increasingly allergenic [107]. It should be underlined that this management could be applied until now only to infants affected by mild-moderate non-IgE-mediated gastrointestinal allergy to CM. Moreover, before home-based reintroduction, possible IgE-mediated mechanisms should be ruled out [4]. No data are available for home reintroduction of other allergens in breastfed infants before or after weaning. In this case, each case should be studied to determine if reintroduction is appropriate based on the severity of the presentation and the risk profile [4].

Age-appropriate allergy-focused diet history tools should be taken by healthcare providers in order to determine the need for allergy testing and therefore guide the elimination diet [4, 108]. FPIAP is a benign condition with rapid resolution and an excellent prognosis.

A recent study by Jang et al. [109] aiming to clarify the etiology of small rectal bleeding in not-sick newborns showed that FPIAP is a rare cause of small rectal bleeding while idiopathic neonatal transient colitis (INTC) is far more prevalent.

Hence, in infants who are otherwise healthy, it is possible to adopt a wait-and-see approach, postponing the start of an elimination diet for 1 month, in order to assess whether the disease regresses spontaneously [92].

This option should be discussed with parents, and their distress toward the condition should be taken into account to decide on the possibility of holding off treatment.

If symptoms continue after 1 month or if the parents opt for the immediate initiation of treatment, an elimination diet is started. When the symptoms, specifically hematochezia, stop, the next step is the assessment of IgE positivity via SPT or specific IgE testing: if these are negative, the food may be gradually reintroduced at home; if positive, the allergy must be treated as an IgE-mediated reaction, requiring OFC for the reintroduction of the suspected food in the diet. However, in the event that symptoms persist after the elimination of the culprit food, it is necessary to exclude other conditions characterized by hematochezia [94].

The avoidance diet—either of the mother if the child is breastfed or the infant—usually first excludes CM since, as mentioned, it is the antigen most commonly implicated in the development of non-IgE-mediated-GI-FAs. Other foods that can be eliminated if the sole exclusion of CM is not enough are eggs, nuts, or whichever food the parents suspect. Once the allergen is detected, it should be excluded from the diet for the first year of life. Symptoms should resolve rapidly after the start of the elimination diet, within 3 days and up to a few weeks [5]. In the majority of cases, CM is the causative agent of FPE, hence the name CM-sensitive enteropathy, and the exclusion of this food from the diet leads to symptom resolution within 1–4 weeks.

eHF is considered the first-line treatment for cow's milk or soy enteropathy in infants. In more severe cases, AAF is indicated [70].

When symptoms do not resolve, other foods that may be eliminated from the diet are soy, wheat, and eggs, which can also induce FPE. While clinically the condition regresses rapidly after the onset of a diet, histological remission may take up to several months [94].

Reintroduction in breastfed infants is not recommended in case of suspected FPIES or in the presence of severe associated symptoms. In case the elimination-reintroduction challenge gives ambiguous results in the breastfed infant, experts suggest reintroducing the food in the child after weaning [4].

In FPIAP and FPE, the reintroduction of trigger food can safely be performed at home. In the case of FPIAP, the onset of rectal bleeding 6–72 h after food ingestion confirms the diagnosis. For FPE, the reappearance of symptoms usually takes longer; the affected infant experiences vomiting and diarrhea within 40–72 h following food administration. Management of acute and chronic FPIES is based on eliminating diet of the triggering food and all of its known and hidden sources. The eventuality of a reaction to a low threshold is indeed quite rare [110]; thus generally potential traces of trigger food indicated on the label of packaged foods can be allowed.

During weaning, the exclusion of FPIES trigger food from the maternal diet is not usually requested unless chronic or acute symptoms or FPIES appears, which is rare but still possible [25, 26, 111–113]. In CM-FPIES, if the BM is unavailable or insufficient, the use of eHF is recommended [11]. The use of an AAF is indicated in case of nonresponse to eHF in chronic-FPIES or acute reactions after taking eHF, which have been reported in some cases [114, 115], as well as in severe FPIES [56].

Parents and caregivers need to be educated about intervention in cases of acute reactions resulting from the accidental intake of the trigger food and provided with an action plan that also carries directions for primary care physicians (ambulance and ED personnel), who may not always be able to recognize an already known FPIES and promptly institute the correct treatment.

Perhaps one of the most difficult aspects in the management of the disease is the decision regarding the first introduction of "high-risk" FPIES foods not yet included in the child's diet, which concerns the choice of these foods, the appropriate time for introduction (before or after 1 year of age), and the location of the introduction (at home or in a protected environment), as well as the possible availability of venous access whenever the introduction takes place in the hospital. Specific allergy tests have no utility in guiding all these choices, as their negativity does not exclude the possibility that the patient may have a reaction to their first introduction. It has been suggested that in countries where acute FPIES in children is vastly caused by a single food, unrestricted weaning advice seems appropriate in most patients [45].

Tolerance to one food from the food group is considered a favorable prognostic indicator for tolerance to other foods from the same group [11]; vice versa, patients with FPIES have an increased risk of reacting to foods from the same category (e.g., rice and oats, chicken meat and turkey meat), which should therefore be introduced with caution in case of FPIES caused by one of them. Coassociations between foods not belonging to the same group should also be taken into account. Empirical guidelines for selecting weaning foods for infants with FPIES are reported in the 2017 International guidelines [11].

If an acute reaction occurs at home, the level of intervention may vary depending upon the severity of presenting symptoms. For mild symptoms (1–2 vomiting episodes and no associated lethargy), oral rehydration, ondansetron (for ages 6 months and older, no known cardiac problems, no family history of syncope suggestive of prolonged QT syndrome), and close monitoring at home for 4–6 h from the onset of symptoms are suggested [65].

For moderate or severe symptoms (>3 episodes of emesis with associated moderate to severe lethargy), emergency care and/or hospitalization may be required [65].

In an emergency setting, fluid rehydration with a normal saline bolus (10–20 mL/kg repeated as needed), a single dose of methylprednisolone (1 mg/kg, maximum 60–80 mg), and ondansetron (0.15 mg/kg, with a maximum dose of 8 mg) may be considered. In severe cases, close attention to electrolyte abnormalities such as acidemia, correction of anemia, and intensive cardiorespiratory support may be indicated [65].

In acute management of FPIES, the first priority should be hemodynamic support, given the risk for dehydration or shock with progressive FPIES symptoms [65]. Vasopressors may be needed for hypotension not immediately responsive to fluid resuscitation [115].

Ondansetron is a serotonin 5-HT3 receptor antagonist reported to improve emesis, which may occur in the FPIES OFC [116–118]. It is available in oral form as a tablet, rapidly disintegrating tablet, oral film, and liquid for IM or IV use. The dose of ondansetron is 0.15 mg/kg, with a maximum dose of 8 mg. The dose may be repeated once if the patient vomits within 10 min after the first.

The treatment of FPIMD relies on a trial of an avoidance diet for 2–4 weeks. If a patient ameliorates after an avoidance diet, the diagnosis needs to be confirmed by subsequent cow's milk challenge to avoid unnecessary dietary restrictions for the mother or infant [3].

14.12 Natural History

The majority of infants with FPIAP develop tolerance by the first year of life, with 99% within 3 years [4, 8, 9].

Most children with FPIES acquire spontaneous tolerance for the culprit food by school age [56], but the age of resolution varies depending on the type of food and country of origin of the patients and on the timing of rechallenge of the trigger food, which differs between studies and never proceeds at regular intervals due to a variety of causes, including parents' reluctance to rechallenge or the limited availability of OFC appointments. Although the timing of an OFC has no definitive standard, in the United States, diagnostic OFCs are usually attempted within 12–18 months after the most recent reaction [11].

Tolerance to CM has been reported in 88–100% of cases by 3 years of age in Israel [13], Korea [119], Australia [103], Italy [18], and France [28]. However, the passing of CM- or soy-FPIES in the USA has been reported in only 52–70% of cases by 3 years of age, with 15–28% of children still presenting CM- or soy-related allergies at 5 years of age [42, 100].

Tolerance to solid foods is also reported in varying percentages depending on the case series and the type of food reevaluated.

By 3 years of age, 20–90% of children with rice-FPIES are tolerant [18, 43, 100, 103, 120, 121], with the highest percentages reported in Australian children [103].

Grain-FPIES was overcome in 53–75% of cases by 3 years of age [43, 100, 103].

Egg tolerance was achieved in 100% of the reevaluated Italian and Greek children [18, 120] but in only 12.5% of the Australian patients [103]. In Japan, yolk-FPIES was overcome by the age of 2 years in 64.3% of patients [122]. Egg white OFCs were performed before tolerance acquisition of egg yolk, and in no event did the patients manifest an egg white-FPIES.

Fish tolerance was achieved in 25–100% of cases by 8 years of age [102, 103, 120, 123].

FPE generally resolves by 1–3 years of life.

The natural history of FPIMD is poorly understood.

14.13 Conclusions

Gastrointestinal symptoms are a common clinical problem in infants and young children. The spectrum of clinical manifestations of non-IgE-GI-FAs is wide and ranges from mild hematochezia to severe vomiting and diarrhea, which can lead to shock in the acute form of FPIES to FTT in the chronic form of FPIES and in children with FPE.

Although non-IgE-GI-FAs are increasingly recognized in children, the diagnosis may be challenging due to a lack of diagnostic markers and clinical overlaps among themselves, with eosinophilic gastroenteropathies and other pediatric gastroenterological conditions that occur during infancy and childhood.

The diagnosis of non-IgE-mediated food allergies requires a high degree of clinical suspicion and careful dietary assessment. A multidisciplinary team involving allergists, gastroenterologists, dieticians, and speech pathologists is recommended when managing complex cases.

The prognosis for most non-IgE-mediated conditions is favorable.

The exact prevalence of these entities, especially FPIES, remains largely unknown and needs to be determined. In addition, there is an urgent need to better characterize the pathogenesis of these disorders in order to identify diagnostic biomarkers and develop new treatment strategies.

Take-Home Messages

- Non-IgE-GI-FAs may overlap among themselves, with eosinophilic gastroenteropathies and with other nonallergic gastroenterological conditions.
- Clinical manifestations may be severe and lead to shock in acute FPIES and enteropathy with failure to thrive in a chronic form of FPIES and in children with FPE.
- In most cases, diagnosis relies on the demonstration of clear clinical improvement after food allergen elimination and the reemergence of symptoms upon challenge.
- Biopsy is necessary to confirm the diagnosis of FPE.
- Prognosis of non-IgE-GI-FAs is favorable.

Glossary

AAF	Amino acid-based formula
BM	Breast milk
CMA	Cow's milk allergy
CM	Cow's milk
EOS	Eosinophils
ED	Emergency department
eHF	Extensively hydrolyzed formula
FA	Food allergy
FTT	Failure to thrive
FPIAP	Food protein-induced allergic proctocolitis
FPIES	Food protein-induced enterocolitis syndrome
FPE	Food protein-induced allergic enteropathy
FPIMD	Food protein-induced motility disorders
FGIDs	Functional gastrointestinal disorders
GER	Gastroesophageal reflux
GERD	Gastroesophageal reflux disease
INTC	Idiopathic neonatal transient colitis
NK	Natural killer
NEC	Necrotizing enterocolitis
Non-IgE-GI-FAs	Non-IgE-mediated gastrointestinal food allergies
OFC	Oral food challenge
PMN	Neutrophil
5-HT	Serotonin
SF	Soy-based infant formula
eHF	Extensively hydrolyzed formula
SPT	Skin prick test

References

1. Johansson SGO, Bieber T, Dahl R, Friedmann PS, Lanier BQ, Lockey RF, et al. Revised nomenclature for allergy for global use: report of the Nomenclature Review Committee of the World Allergy Organization, October 2003. J Allergy Clin Immunol. 2004;113:832–6.
2. Zhang S, Sicherer S, Berin MC, Agyemang A. Pathophysiology of non-IgE-mediated food allergy. Immunotargets Ther. 2021;10:431–46.
3. Berni Canani R, Caffarelli C, Calvani M, Martelli A, Carucci L, Cozzolino T, et al. Diagnostic therapeutic care pathway for pediatric food allergies and intolerances in Italy: a joint position paper by the Italian Society for Pediatric Gastroenterology Hepatology and Nutrition (SIGENP) and the Italian Society for Pediatric Allergy and Immunology (SIAIP). Ital J Pediatr. 2022;48:87.
4. Meyer R, Chebar Lozinsky A, Fleischer DM, Vieira MC, Du Toit G, Vandenplas Y, et al. Diagnosis and management of Non-IgE gastrointestinal allergies in breastfed infants—an EAACI position paper. Allergy. 2020;75:14–32.
5. Nowak-Węgrzyn A, Katz Y, Mehr SS, Koletzko S. Non-IgE-mediated gastrointestinal food allergy. J Allergy Clin Immunol. 2015;135:1114–24.
6. Elizur A, Cohen M, Goldberg MR, et al. Cow's milk associated rectal bleeding: a population based prospective study. Pediatr Allergy Immunol. 2012;23:766–70.
7. Martin VM, Virkud YV, Seay H, Hickey A, Ndahayo R, Rosow R, et al. Prospective assessment of pediatrician-diagnosed food protein-induced allergic proctocolitis by gross or occult blood. J Allergy Clin Immunol Pract. 2020;8:1692–9.
8. Buyuktiryaki B, Kulhas Celik I, Erdem SB, Capanoglu M, Civelek E, Guc BU, et al. Risk factors influencing tolerance and clinical features of

food protein-induced allergic proctocolitis. J Pediatr Gastroenterol Nutr. 2020;70:574–9.
9. Lozinsky AC, de Morais MB. Eosinophilic colitis in infants. J Pediatr (Rio J). 2014;90:16–21.
10. Savilahti E. Food-induced malabsorption syndromes. J Pediatr Gastroenterol Nutr. 2000;30:S61–6.
11. Nowak-Węgrzyn A, Chehade M, Groetch ME, Spergel JM, Wood RA, Allen K, et al. International consensus guidelines for the diagnosis and management of food protein-induced enterocolitis syndrome: Executive summary-Workgroup Report of the Adverse Reactions to Foods Committee, American Academy of Allergy, Asthma & Immunology. J Allergy Clin Immunol. 2017;139:1111–1126.e4.
12. Cianferoni A. Food protein-induced enterocolitis syndrome epidemiology. Ann Allergy Asthma Immunol. 2021;126:469–77.
13. Katz Y, Goldberg MR, Rajuan N, Cohen A, Leshno M. The prevalence and natural course of food protein-induced enterocolitis syndrome to cow's milk: a large-scale, prospective population-based study. J Allergy Clin Immunol. 2011;127(3):647–53.
14. Alonso SB, Ezquiaga JG, Berzal PT, Tardón SD, San José MM, López PA, et al. Food protein-induced enterocolitis syndrome: Increased prevalence of this great unknown-results of the PREVALE study. J Allergy Clin Immunol. 2019;143:430–3.
15. Ruffner MA, Wang KY, Dudley JW, Cianferoni A, Grundmeier RW, Spergel JM, et al. Elevated atopic comorbidity in patients with food protein-induced enterocolitis. J Allergy Clin Immunol Pract. 2020;8:1039–46.
16. Mehr S, Frith K, Barnes EH, Campbell DE, FPIES Study Group. Food protein-induced enterocolitis syndrome in Australia: a population-based study, 2012–2014. J Allergy Clin Immunol. 2017;140:1323–30.
17. Nowak-Wegrzyn A, Warren CM, Brown-Whitehorn T, Cianferoni A, Schultz-Matney F, Gupta RS. Food protein-induced enterocolitis syndrome in the US population-based study. J Allergy Clin Immunol. 2019;144:1128–30.
18. Sopo SM, Giorgio V, Dello Iacono I, Novembre E, Mori F, Onesimo R. A multicentre retrospective study of 66 Italian children with food protein-induced enterocolitis syndrome: different management for different phenotypes. Clin Exp Allergy. 2012;42:1257–65.
19. Mehr S, Kakakios A, Frith K, Kemp AS. Food protein-induced enterocolitis syndrome: 16-year experience. Pediatrics. 2009;123:e459–64.
20. Akashi M, Hayashi D, Kajita N, Kinoshita M, Ishii T, Tsumura Y, et al. Recent dramatic increase in patients with food protein-induced enterocolitis syndrome (FPIES) provoked by hen's egg in Japan. J Allergy Clin Immunol Pract. 2022;10:1110–2.
21. Douros K, Tsabouri S, Feketea G, Grammeniatis V, Koliofoti EG, Papadopoulos M, et al. Retrospective study identified fish and milk as the main culprits in cases of food protein-induced enterocolitis syndrome. Acta Paediatr. 2019;108:1901–4.
22. Gryboski JD. Gastrointestinal milk allergy in infants. Pediatrics. 1967;40:354–62.
23. Powell GK. Milk- and soy-induced enterocolitis of infancy. Clinical features and standardization of challenge. J Pediatr. 1978;93:553–60.
24. Hwang JB, Lee SH, Kang YN, Kim SP, Suh SI, Kam S. Indexes of suspicion of typical cow's milk protein-induced enterocolitis. J Korean Med Sci. 2007;22:993–7.
25. Miceli Sopo S, Monaco S, Greco M, Scala G. Chronic food protein-induced enterocolitis syndrome caused by cow's milk proteins passed through breast milk. Int Arch Allergy Immunol. 2014;164:207–9.
26. Weinberger T, Feuille E, Thompson C, Nowak-Węgrzyn A. Chronic food protein-induced enterocolitis syndrome: characterization of clinical phenotype and literature review. Ann Allergy Asthma Immunol. 2016;117:227–33.
27. Lange L, Gernert S, Berger M, Arens A, Rache L, Delissen J, et al. Different patterns of foods triggering FPIES in Germany. J Allergy Clin Immunol Pract. 2022;10:1063–9.
28. Lemoine A, Colas A-S, Le S, Delacourt C, Tounian P, Lezmi G. Food protein-induced enterocolitis syndrome: a large French multicentric experience. Clin Transl Allergy. 2022;12:e12112.
29. Salvatore S, Agosti M, Baldassarre ME, D'Auria E, Pensabene L, Nosetti L, et al. Cow's milk allergy or gastroesophageal reflux disease-can we solve the dilemma in infants? Nutrients. 2021;13:297.
30. Meyer R, Vandenplas Y, Lozinsky AC, Vieira MC, Canani RB, Dupont C, et al. Diagnosis and management of food allergy-associated gastroesophageal reflux disease in young children-EAACI position paper. Pediatr Allergy Immunol. 2022;33:e13856.
31. Sissoko NDN, Chen W, Wang C, Wu Y, Zheng X, Dong X, et al. Associations between functional constipation and non-IgE-mediated food allergy in infants and children. Allergol Immunopathol (Madr). 2023;51:163–73.
32. Goodman M, Feuille E. Is avocado an emerging culprit in food protein-induced enterocolitis syndrome? Ann Allergy Asthma Immunol. 2019;122:218–20.
33. Cherian S, Neupert K, Varshney P. Avocado as an emerging trigger for food protein-induced enterocolitis syndrome. Ann Allergy Asthma Immunol. 2018;121:369–71.
34. Blackman AC, Anvari S, Davis CM, Anagnostou A. Emerging triggers of food protein-induced enterocolitis syndrome: lessons from a pediatric cohort of 74 children in the United States. Ann Allergy Asthma Immunol. 2019;122:407–11.
35. Gonzalez-Delgado P, Ruano-Zaragoza M, Gutierrez A, Lopez F, Fernandez J. Chronic adult food protein-induced enterocolitis syndrome. Ann Allergy Asthma Immunol. 2020;125:716–7.

36. Díaz JJ, Espín B, Segarra O, Domínguez-Ortega G, Blasco-Alonso J, Cano B, et al. Gastrointestinal Allergy Working Group of the Spanish Society of Pediatric Gastroenterology, Hepatology and Nutrition (SEGHNP). Food protein-induced enterocolitis syndrome: data from a multicenter retrospective study in Spain. J Pediatr Gastroenterol Nutr. 2019;68:232–6.
37. Infante S, Albéndiz-Gutiérrez VJ, Alvarez-Perea A, Cabrera-Freitag P, Morales-Cabeza C, Fuentes-Aparicio V, et al. Chronic food protein-induced enterocolitis syndrome due to solid food. J Allergy Clin Immunol Pract. 2020;8:2077–8.
38. Agyemang A, Nowak-Wegrzyn A. Food protein-induced enterocolitis syndrome: a comprehensive review. Clin Rev Allergy Immunol. 2019;57:261–71.
39. Nishimura K, Yamamoto-Hanada K, Sato M, Toyokuni K, Ogita H, Kiguchi T, et al. Remission of acute food protein-induced enterocolitis syndrome confirmed by oral food challenges in Japan. Nutrients. 2022;14:4158.
40. Ludman S, Harmon M, Whiting D, du Toit G. Clinical presentation and referral characteristics of food protein-induced enterocolitis syndrome in the United Kingdom. Ann Allergy Asthma Immunol. 2014;113:290–4.
41. Stiefel G, Alviani C, Afzal NA, Byrne A, du Toit G, DunnGalvin A, et al. Food protein-induced enterocolitis syndrome in the British Isles. Arch Dis Child. 2022;107:123–7.
42. Ruffner MA, Ruymann K, Barni S, Cianferoni A, Brown-Whitehorn T, Spergel JM. Food protein-induced enterocolitis syndrome: insights from review of a large referral population. J Allergy Clin Immunol Pract. 2013;1:343–9.
43. Caubet JC, Ford LS, Sickles L, Järvinen KM, Sicherer SH, Sampson HA, et al. Clinical features and resolution of food protein-induced enterocolitis syndrome: 10-year experience. J Allergy Clin Immunol. 2014;134:382–9.
44. Barni S, Sarti L, Mori F, Liotti L, Pucci N, Novembre E. A modified oral food challenge in children with food protein-induced enterocolitis syndrome. Clin Exp Allergy. 2019;49:1633–6.
45. Argiz L, Infante S, Machinena A, Bracamonte T, Echeverria L, Prieto A, et al. Children with acute food protein-induced enterocolitis syndrome from Spain and Italy usually tolerate all other food groups. Clin Exp Allergy. 2021;51:1238–41.
46. Lee E, Barnes EH, Mehr S, Campbell DE. An exploration of factors associated with food protein-induced enterocolitis syndrome: birth, infant feeding and food triggers. Pediatr Allergy Immunol. 2021;32:742–9.
47. Ullberg J, Fech-Bormann M, Fagerberg UL. Clinical presentation and management of food protein-induced enterocolitis syndrome in 113 Swedish children. Allergy. 2021;76:2115–22.
48. Cianferoni A. Non-IgE mediated food allergy. Curr Pediatr Rev. 2020;16:95–105.
49. Odze RD, Bines J, Leichtner AM, Goldman H, Antonioli DA. Allergic proctocolitis in infants: a prospective clinicopathologic biopsy study. Hum Pathol. 1993;24:668–74.
50. Savino F, Giuliani F, Giraudi S, Savino F, Giuliani F, Giraudi S, et al. Analysis of serum Th2 cytokines in infants with non-IgE mediated food allergy compared to healthy infants. Nutrients. 2022;14:1565. et al. Analysis of serum Th2 cytokines in infants with non-IgE mediated food allergy compared to healthy infants. Nutrients. 2022;14:1565.
51. Goswami R, Blazquez AB, Kosoy R, Rahman A, Nowak-Węgrzyn A, Berin MC. Systemic innate immune activation in food protein-induced enterocolitis syndrome. J Allergy Clin Immunol. 2017;139:1885–1896.e9.
52. Kimura M, Ito Y, Shimomura M, Morishita H, Meguro T, Adachi Y, et al. Cytokine profile after oral food challenge in infants with food protein-induced enterocolitis syndrome. Allergol Int. 2017;66:452–7.
53. Berin MC, Lozano-Ojalvo D, Agashe C, Baker MG, Bird JA, Nowak-Wegrzyn A. Acute FPIES reactions are associated with an IL-17 inflammatory signature. J Allergy Clin Immunol. 2021;148:895–901.
54. Caubet JC, Bencharitiwong R, Ross A, Sampson HA, Berin MC, Nowak-Węgrzyn A. Humoral and cellular responses to casein in patients with food protein-induced enterocolitis to cow's milk. J Allergy Clin Immunol. 2017;139:572–83.
55. Mehr S, Lee E, Hsu P, Anderson D, de Jong E, Bosco A,et al. Innate immune activation occurs in acute food protein-induced enterocolitis syndrome reactions. J Allergy Clin Immunol. 2019;144:600–2.
56. Mathew M, Leeds S, Nowak-Węgrzyn A. Recent update in food protein-induced enterocolitis syndrome: pathophysiology, diagnosis, and management. Allergy Asthma Immunol Res. 2022;14:587–603.
57. Wada T, Matsuda Y, Toma T, Koizumi E, Okamoto H, Yachie A. Increased CD69 expression on peripheral eosinophils from patients with food protein-induced enterocolitis syndrome. Int Arch Allergy Immunol. 2016;170:201–5.
58. Baker MG, Cecilia Berin M, Sicherer S. Update on Food Protein-Induced Enterocolitis Syndrome (FPIES). Curr Allergy Asthma Rep. 2022;22:113–22.
59. Van Sickle GJ, Powell GK, McDonald PJ, Goldblum RM. Milk- and soy protein-induced enterocolitis: evidence for lymphocyte sensitization to specific food proteins. Gastroenterology. 1985;88:1915–21.
60. Hoffman KM, Ho DG, Sampson HA. Evaluation of the usefulness of lymphocyte proliferation assays in the diagnosis of allergy to cow's milk. J Allergy Clin Immunol. 1997;99:360–6.
61. Mori F, Barni S, Cianferoni A, Pucci N, de Martino M, Novembre E. Cytokine expression in CD3+ cells in an infant with food protein-induced enterocolitis syndrome (FPIES): case report. Clin Dev Immunol. 2009;2009(1):679381.

62. Chung HL, Hwang JB, Park JJ, Kim SG. Expression of transforming growth factor beta1, transforming growth factor type I and II receptors, and TNF-alpha in the mucosa of the small intestine in infants with food protein-induced enterocolitis syndrome. J Allergy Clin Immunol. 2002;109:150–4.
63. Konstantinou GN, Bencharitiwong R, Grishin A, Caubet JC, Bardina L, Sicherer SH,et al. The role of casein-specific IgA and TGF-β in children with food protein-induced enterocolitis syndrome to milk. Pediatr Allergy Immunol. 2014;25:651–6.
64. Askari B, Ferreri NR. Regulation of prostacyclin synthesis by angiotensin II and TNF-alpha in vascular smooth muscle. Prostaglandins Other Lipid Mediat. 2001;63:175–87.
65. Leonard SA, Miceli Sopo S, Baker MG, Fiocchi A, Wood RA, Nowak-Węgrzyn A. Management of acute food protein-induced enterocolitis syndrome emergencies at home and in a medical facility. Ann Allergy Asthma Immunol. 2021;126:482–488.e1.
66. Ahern GP. 5-HT and the immune system. Curr Opin Pharmacol. 2011;11:29–33.
67. Lozano-Ojalvo D, Chen X, Dunkin D, Agashe C, Baker MG, Bird JA, et al. Untargeted serum metabolomic analysis reveals a role for purinergic signaling in FPIES. J Allergy Clin Immunol. 2023;151:797–802.
68. Schäppi MG, Borrelli O, Knafelz D, Williams S, Smith VV, Milla PJ, et al. Mast cell-nerve interactions in children with functional dyspepsia. J Pediatr Gastroenterol Nutr. 2008;47:472–80.
69. Borrelli O, Barbara G, Di Nardo G, Cremon C, Lucarelli S, Frediani T, et al. Neuroimmune interaction and anorectal motility in children with food allergy-related chronic constipation. Am J Gastroenterol. 2009;104:454–63.
70. Caubet J-C, Szajewska H, Shamir R, Nowak-Węgrzyn A. Non-IgE-mediated gastrointestinal food allergies in children. Pediatr Allergy Immunol. 2017;28:6–17.
71. Tracy MS, Yasuda JL, Rufo PA. Protein-losing enteropathy in the setting of iron deficiency anemia: a case series. JPGN Rep. 2020;1:e009.
72. Nowak-Wegrzyn A, Berin MC, Mehr S. Food protein-induced enterocolitis syndrome. J Allergy Clin Immunol Pract. 2020;8:24–35.
73. Labrosse R, Graham F, Caubet J-C. Non-IgE-mediated gastrointestinal food allergies in children: an update. Nutrients. 2020;12:2086.
74. Sicherer SH. Food protein-induced enterocolitis syndrome: case presentations and management lessons. J Allergy Clin Immunol. 2005;115:149 56.
75. Pecora V, Prencipe G, Valluzzi R, Dahdah L, Insalaco A, Cianferoni A, et al. Inflammatory events during food protein-induced enterocolitis syndrome reactions. Pediatr Allergy Immunol. 2017;28:464–70.
76. Kimura M, Ito Y, Tokunaga F, Meguro T, Shimomura M, Morishita H, et al. Increased C-reactive protein and fever in Japanese infants with food protein-induced enterocolitis syndrome. Pediatr Int. 2016;58:826–30.
77. Yogo N, Fujito S. Methaemoglobinaemia due to food protein-induced enterocolitis syndrome. Arch Dis Child. 2021;106:1117.
78. Geljic A, Hojsak I. Methaemoglobinaemia in two exclusively breastfed infants with food protein-induced enterocolitis syndrome. J Paediatr Child Health. 2021;57:941–2.
79. Benninga MA, Faure C, Hyman PE, St James Roberts I, Schechter NL, Nurko S. Childhood functional gastrointestinal disorders: neonate/toddler. Gastroenterology. 2016;150(6):1443–55.
80. Cavataio F, Iacono G, Montalto G, Soresi M, Tumminello M, Carroccio A. Clinical and pH-metric characteristics of gastro-oesophageal reflux secondary to cows' milk protein allergy. Arch Dis Child. 1996;75:51–6.
81. Milocco C, Torre G, Ventura A. Gastro-oesophageal reflux and cows' milk protein allergy. Arch Dis Child. 1997;77:183–4.
82. Borrelli O, Mancini V, Thapar N, Giorgio V, Elawad M, Hill S, et al. Cow's milk challenge increases weakly acidic reflux in children with cow's milk allergy and gastroesophageal reflux disease. J Pediatr. 2012;161:476–481.e1.
83. Salvatore S, Pagliarin F, Huysentruyt K, Bosco A, Fumagalli L, Van De Maele K, et al. Distress in infants and young children: don't blame acid reflux. J Pediatr Gastroenterol Nutr. 2020;71:465–9.
84. Rosen R, Vandenplas Y, Singendonk M, Cabana M, DiLorenzo C, Gottrand F, et al. Pediatric Gastroesophageal Reflux Clinical Practice Guidelines: Joint Recommendations of the North American Society for Pediatric Gastroenterology, Hepatology, and Nutrition and the European Society for Pediatric Gastroenterology, Hepatology, and Nutrition. J Pediatr Gastroenterol Nutr. 2018;66:516 54.
85. Iacono G, Cavataio F, Montalto G, Florena A, Tumminello M, Soresi M, et al. Intolerance of cow's milk and chronic constipation in children. N Engl J Med. 1998;339:1100–4.
86. Miceli Sopo S, Gelsomino M, Rivetti S, Del Vescovo E. Food protein-induced enterocolitis syndrome: proposals for new definitions. Medicina (Kaunas). 2019;55:216.
87. Lee E, Barnes EH, Mehr S, Campbell DE. Differentiating acute food protein-induced enterocolitis syndrome from its mimics: a comparison of clinical features and routine laboratory biomarkers. J Allergy Clin Immunol Pract. 2019;7:471–8.
88. Srinivasan P, Brandler M, D'Souza A, Millman P, Moreau H. Allergic enterocolitis presenting as recurrent necrotizing enterocolitis in preterm neonates. J Perinatol. 2010;30:431–3.

89. Lenfestey MW, de la Cruz D, Neu J. Food protein-induced enterocolitis instead of necrotizing enterocolitis? A neonatal intensive care unit case series. J Pediatr. 2018;200:270–3.
90. D'Auria E, Cocchi I, Monti G, Sartorio MUA, Daniele I, Lista G, et al. Food protein-induced enterocolitis syndrome in preterm newborns. Pediatr Allergy Immunol. 2022;33:e13676.
91. Guo Y, Si S, Jia Z, Lv X, Wu H. Differentiation of food protein-induced enterocolitis syndrome and necrotizing enterocolitis in neonates by abdominal sonography. J Pediatr. 2021;97:219–24.
92. Cetinkaya PG, Ocak M, Sahiner UM, Sekerel BE, Soyer O. Food protein-induced allergic proctocolitis may have distinct phenotypes. Ann Allergy Asthma Immunol. 2021;126:75–82.
93. Connors L, O'Keefe A, Rosenfield L, Kim H. Non-IgE-mediated food hypersensitivity. Allergy Asthma Clin Immunol. 2018;14:56.
94. Calvani M, Anania C, Cuomo B, D'Auria E, Decimo F, Indirli GC, et al. Non-IgE- or mixed IgE/non-IgE-mediated gastrointestinal food allergies in the first years of life: old and new tools for diagnosis. Nutrients. 2021;13:226.
95. Variend S, Placzek M, Raafat F, Walker-Smith JA. Small intestinal mucosal fat in childhood enteropathies. J Clin Pathol. 1984;37:373–7.
96. Iyngkaran N, Abdin Z, Davis K, Boey CG, Prathap K, Yadav M, et al. Acquired carbohydrate intolerance and cow milk protein-sensitive enteropathy in young infants. J Pediatr. 1979;95:373–8.
97. Shah N, Foong R-XM, Borrelli O, Volonaki E, Dziubak R, Meyer R, et al. Histological findings in infants with Gastrointestinal food allergy are associated with specific gastrointestinal symptoms; retrospective review from a tertiary centre. BMC Clin Pathol. 2015;15:12.
98. Al-Iede M, Sarhan L, Alshrouf MA, Said Y. Perspectives on non-IgE-mediated gastrointestinal food allergy in pediatrics: a review of current evidence and guidelines. J Asthma Allergy. 2023;16:279–91.
99. Infante S, Marco-Martín G, Zubeldia JM, Fuentes-Aparicio V, Alvarez-Perea A,et al. Oral food challenge in food protein-induced enterocolitis syndrome by fish: is there any room for improvement? Int Arch Allergy Immunol. 2019;179:215–20.
100. Wang KY, Lee J, Cianferoni A, Ruffner MA, Dean A, Molleston JM, et al. Food protein-induced enterocolitis syndrome food challenges: experience from a large referral center. J Allergy Clin Immunol Pract. 2019;7:444–50.
101. Guenther MW, Crain M, Parrish CP, Bird JA. An observed serving dose may not be necessary following a standard divided-dose FPIES oral food challenge. J Allergy Clin Immunol Pract. 2020;8:1462–4.
102. Vazquez-Ortiz M, Machinena A, Dominguez O, Alvaro M, Calvo-Campoverde K, Giner MT, et al. Food protein-induced enterocolitis syndrome to fish and egg usually resolves by age 5 years in Spanish children. J Allergy Clin Immunol Pract. 2017;5:512–515.e1.
103. Lee E, Campbell DE, Barnes EH, Mehr SS. Resolution of acute food protein-induced enterocolitis syndrome in children. J Allergy Clin Immunol Pract. 2017;5:486–8.
104. Gieruszczak-Białek D, Konarska Z, Skórka A, Vandenplas Y, Szajewska H. No effect of proton pump inhibitors on crying and irritability in infants: systematic review of randomized controlled trials. J Pediatr. 2015;166:767–70.
105. Levy EI, Salvatore S, Vandenplas Y, de Winter JP. Prescription of acid inhibitors in infants: an addiction hard to break. Eur J Pediatr. 2020;179:1957–61.
106. Koletzko S, Niggemann B, Arato A, Dias JA, Heuschkel R, Husby S, et al. Diagnostic approach and management of cow's-milk protein allergy in infants and children: ESPGHAN GI Committee practical guidelines. J Pediatr Gastroenterol Nutr. 2012;55:221–9.
107. Venter C, Brown T, Meyer R, Walsh J, Shah N, Nowak-Węgrzyn A, et al. Better recognition, diagnosis and management of non-IgE-mediated cow's milk allergy in infancy: iMAP—an international interpretation of the MAP (Milk Allergy in Primary Care) guideline. Clin Transl Allergy. 2017;7:26.
108. Skypala IJ, Venter C, Meyer R, deJong NW, Fox AT, Groetch M, et al. The development of a standardised diet history tool to support the diagnosis of food allergy. Clin Transl Allergy. 2015;5:7.
109. Jang H-J, Kim AS, Hwang J-B. The etiology of small and fresh rectal bleeding in not-sick neonates: should we initially suspect food protein-induced proctocolitis? Eur J Pediatr. 2012;171:1845–9.
110. Mane SK, Hollister ME, Bahna SL. Food protein-induced enterocolitis syndrome to trivial oral mucosal contact. Eur J Pediatr. 2014;173:1545–7.
111. Monti G, Castagno E, Liguori SA, Lupica MM, Tarasco V, Viola S, et al. Food protein-induced enterocolitis syndrome by cow's milk proteins passed through breast milk. J Allergy Clin Immunol. 2011;127:679–80.
112. Tan J, Campbell D, Mehr S. Food protein-induced enterocolitis syndrome in an exclusively breast-fed infant-an uncommon entity. J Allergy Clin Immunol. 2012;129:873–4.
113. Baldo F, Bevacqua M, Corrado C, Nisticò D, Cesca L, Declich V, et al. FPIES in exclusively breastfed infants: two case reports and review of the literature. Ital J Pediatr. 2020;46:144.
114. Joshi SR, Bird JA. Cow's milk-associated chronic food protein-induced enterocolitis syndrome exacerbated by extensively hydrolyzed formula. Ann Allergy Asthma Immunol. 2018;120:532–3.
115. Kabuki T, Joh K. Extensively hydrolyzed formula (MA-mi) induced exacerbation of food protein-induced enterocolitis syndrome (FPIES) in a male infant. Allergol Int. 2007;56:473–6.
116. Miceli Sopo S, Bersani G, Monaco S, Cerchiara G, Lee E, Campbell D, Mehr S. Ondansetron

in acute food protein-induced enterocolitis syndrome, a retrospective case-control study. Allergy. 2017;72:545–51.

117. Holbrook T, Keet CA, Frischmeyer-Guerrerio PA, Wood RA. Use of ondansetron for food protein-induced enterocolitis syndrome. J Allergy Clin Immunol. 2013;132:1219–20.
118. Watts SW, Morrison SF, Davis RP, Barman SM. Serotonin and blood pressure regulation. Pharmacol Rev. 2012;64:359–88.
119. Hwang J-B, Sohn SM, Kim AS. Prospective follow-up oral food challenge in food protein-induced enterocolitis syndrome. Arch Dis Child. 2009;94:425–8.
120. Xepapadaki P, Kitsioulis NA, Manousakis E, Manolaraki I, Douladiris N, Papadopoulos NG. Remission patterns of food protein-induced enterocolitis syndrome in a Greek pediatric population. Int Arch Allergy Immunol. 2019;180:113–9.
121. Nowak-Wegrzyn A, Sampson HA, Wood RA, Sicherer SH. Food protein-induced enterocolitis syndrome caused by solid food proteins. Pediatrics. 2003;111:829–35.
122. Watanabe Y, Sakai H, Nihei M, Miura K, Kumaki S. Early tolerance acquisition in hen's egg yolk-associated food protein-induced enterocolitis syndrome. J Allergy Clin Immunol Pract. 2021;9:2120–2122.e2.
123. Miceli Sopo S, Monaco S, Badina L, Barni S, Longo G, Novembre E, et al. Food protein-induced enterocolitis syndrome caused by fish and/or shellfish in Italy. Pediatr Allergy Immunol. 2015;26:731–6.

Eosinophilic Esophagitis in Children

15

Martina Votto, Ilaria Brambilla, Silvia Maria Elena Caimmi, Riccardo Castagnoli, Maria De Filippo, Alessandro Raffaele, Gian Luigi Marseglia, and Amelia Licari

Abstract

Eosinophilic esophagitis (EoE) is an emerging antigen-mediated disease of unknown etiology limited to the esophagus. EoE is a multifactorial disease typically characterized by T helper 2 inflammation. Pathogenesis is not entirely understood and is likely non-IgE mediated. Food allergens trigger EoE, stimulating the dysregulated immune cells through an impaired esophageal epithelial barrier. Clinical presentation of EoE depends on age and mainly includes food refusal, vomiting, abdominal or chest pain, dysphagia, and food impaction. Upper gastrointestinal endoscopy is the gold standard to diagnose and monitor EoE. The goal of treatment is to achieve clinical, endoscopic, and histological ("deep") remission to prevent esophageal fibrosis and improve the quality of life. In children, cornerstones of therapy are proton pump inhibitors, topical steroids (swallowed fluticasone and viscous budesonide), and food elimination diets. Over recent decades, much progress has been made toward a greater understanding of the EoE pathogenesis and new therapeutic approaches. Dupilumab is the first biological therapy recently approved in the US for adolescents (≥12 years) and adults with active EoE. Due to its chronic nature, EoE management requires long-term therapy and regular follow-up.

Keywords

Adolescents · Allergy · Children · Comorbidities · Dupilumab · Eosinophilic esophagitis · Eosinophils · Esophagus · Foods Food elimination diet · Long-term follow-up Proton pump inhibitor · Quality of life T-Helper 2 (Th2) inflammation · Topical steroids

Test your learning and check your understanding of this book's contents: use the "Springer Nature Flashcards" app to access questions using ▶ https://sn.pub/nspbjm. To use the app, please follow the instructions in Chap. 1.

M. Votto (✉) · R. Castagnoli · M. De Filippo
G. L. Marseglia · A. Licari
Pediatric Unit, Department of Clinical, Surgical, Diagnostic and Pediatric Sciences, University of Pavia, Pavia, Italy

Pediatric Clinic, Fondazione IRCCS Policlinico San Matteo, Pavia, Italy
e-mail: martina.votto@unipv.it

I. Brambilla · S. M. E. Caimmi
Pediatric Clinic, Fondazione IRCCS Policlinico San Matteo, Pavia, Italy

A. Raffaele
Pediatric Surgery Unit, Department of Maternal and Child Health, Fondazione IRCCS-Policlinico San Matteo, Pavia, Italy

C. Caffarelli, G. L. Marseglia (eds.), *Textbook of Pediatric Allergy*,
https://doi.org/10.1007/978-3-031-71283-8_15

Key Points

- Eosinophilic esophagitis (EoE) is a T helper 2 (Th2)-mediated disease exclusively involving the esophagus with a multifactorial mechanism.
- EoE diagnosis requires a combination of clinical symptoms (which are heterogeneous and vary with age), endoscopic, and histological findings (≥15 eosinophils/high power field).
- Treatment of EoE is based on three "D": (1) Drugs (topical corticosteroids, proton pump inhibitors, and biologics); (2) Diets (exclusive elemental diet and empirical food elimination diet); and (3) Dilation in case of esophageal stenosis.
- EoE is a chronic disease requiring long-term treatment and follow-up, especially in children.

Eosinophilic esophagitis (EoE) is a chronic, antigen-mediated disease that explicitly involves the esophagus [1]. The first case of EoE was reported in 1978 and was misinterpreted as an esophageal motility disorder [2]. Subsequently, esophageal eosinophilia was considered a feature of gastroesophageal reflux disease (GERD) [3]. EoE was characterized as a distinct clinical entity by Attwood and Straumann only in the early 1990s [4, 5]. Since then, several efforts have been made to understand the pathophysiology and natural history of this proteiform disease.

15.1 Epidemiology

EoE has evolved from a rare condition to a commonly encountered disease in pediatric clinical practice and a significant cause of upper gastrointestinal morbidity [6]. The global prevalence of EoE is 0.5–1 cases/1000 persons [6]. In children, the pooled incidence of EoE is 6.6 cases/100,000 persons-year, whereas the overall prevalence is 34 cases/100,000 children [6]. In the Netherlands, the incidence rates increased from 0.01/100,000 (95% CI: 0.0–0.04) in 1995 to 3.16/100,000 (95% CI: 2.90–3.44) in 2019 [7]. The prevalence of pediatric EoE varies from 2.3/100,000 in Denmark to 90.7/100,000 in Ohio [6]. During the last years, several studies reported a dramatic increase in EoE epidemiology, especially in children in Western Countries [8–14]. This increase in EoE epidemiology was, at least partially, an actual increase and not an artificial effect due to raised awareness. This phenomenon occurred parallelly with the dramatic increase in the global prevalence of allergic diseases observed during the past few decades and might be in part explained by the hygiene hypothesis [15, 16]. Despite some genetic factors associated with an increased risk of developing EoE, environmental factors are probably the most relevant players in disease occurrence [6]. In children living in Westernized Countries, one of the most impressive changes in environmental factors exposure observed in the last decades is related to dietary habits with increased consumption of modified and enriched foods [17].

Although EoE mainly affects adults between 20 and 40 years, all age groups can be affected, with a particular prevalence in the male sex (M:F = 3:1) [18].

15.2 Pathogenesis

The pathogenesis of EoE is still largely undefined. It is commonly considered a multifactorial disease in which genetic and environmental factors may play a role [17]. These factors are responsible for altering the esophageal barrier through intricate interactions, with loss of cell-to-cell adhesion mechanisms and consequent increased permeability, allowing abnormal exposure to allergens and other luminal components [19, 20]. Alteration of the esophageal barrier leads to the epithelial release of alarmins, like thymic stromal lymphopoietin (TSLP) and interleukin (IL)-33. These mediators drive the differentiation of T helper 2 (Th2) effector cells, with the consequent production of several Th2 cytokines (IL-4, IL-5, IL-9, and IL-13) and massive recruitment of eosinophils [21]. Simultaneously, luminal antigens, encountering antigen-presenting cells, activate specific antigen Th2 differentiation, with additional releasing of inflammatory cytokines, eosinophils recruitment, and plasma cell activation with specific IgE production [21]. Therefore, IgEs, that are pivotal in several atopic diseases, do not have a primary role in EoE pathogenesis [17].

The role of genetic factors in EoE pathogenesis was postulated starting from clinical evidence, showing that EoE prevalence varies among sex and ethnicity. Epidemiological studies showed that EoE is more common in White than Black or Hispanic children [22, 23]. Besides, having a first-degree family member affected by EoE increases the risk for disease occurrence (OR, 16.3; 95% CI, 9.4–28.3) [24]. This risk is markedly higher in monozygotic twins than in dizygotic (41% vs. 22%) [25]. Despite this evidence, twin studies report a low disease concordance, pointing to the crucial role of environmental risk factors. The effect of genetics seems to unfold in conjunction with environmental factors, including early-life exposures [17]. Early life is a critical period during which the immune system and gut microbiota mature and become susceptible to early environmental exposures [17]. A few studies focused on the role of early life exposures [26–30]. Formula feeding, neonatal intensive care admission, prematurity, maternal fever, antibiotic and acid suppressants use in infancy, and cesarean delivery were all considered potential early risk factors of EoE [17].

The role of genetics has been supported by the results of candidate-gene and genome-wide association studies, highlighting the role of different *loci* involved in the Th2 inflammatory response and the regulation of epithelial barrier structure and function in EoE patients [31–34]. The esophageal epithelial barrier integrity is ensured by desmosomes, tight and adherence junctions, and several genes involved in epithelial cell differentiation, including filaggrin and desmoglein-1. A genetic variation in these genes was detected in EoE patients [35]. The most potent association concerned the dysregulated calpain 14 (CAPN14) expression, an enzyme involved in esophageal barrier regulation via the IL-13 pathway [31–33].

EoE is characterized by a typical Th2 inflammatory response and a high prevalence of other atopic comorbidities [36, 37]. Different genetic alterations were detected in EoE patients, mainly related to the Th2 response, resulting in the upregulation of eotaxin-3, transforming growth factor β (TGF-β), and periostin, respectively involved in eosinophil chemotaxis and adhesion, with the consequent production of TSLP [31, 38]. TSLP is considered a crucial mediator involved in the EoE inflammatory cascade. Although TSLP is also expressed in other atopic disorders, its production is unrelated to other concomitant allergic diseases [32, 33].

EoE is also associated with different monogenic inherited diseases. Connective tissue disorders, such as Marfan and Ehlers Danlos Syndromes, share a common pathogenic mechanism through the dysregulation of the TGF-β signaling. Children with autosomal dominant Hyper-IgE Syndrome (HIES) and Netherton Syndrome have also significantly increased the incidence of EoE [39, 40].

15.3 Diagnosis

EoE is characterized clinically by symptoms of esophageal dysfunction and histologically by ≥15 eosinophils per high power field (eos/HPF) [41]. Other causes of esophageal eosinophilia should always be ruled out, particularly GERD, coeliac disease, Crohn's disease, achalasia, HIES, and drug hypersensitivity. Pediatricians should diagnose EoE based on a combination of symptoms, and histological and endoscopic findings, as no single feature is sufficient to establish a definitive diagnosis. Therefore, essential diagnostic instruments are: (1) medical history, (2) endoscopic features, and (3) histological examination. Upper gastrointestinal (GI) endoscopy is currently the gold standard for the diagnosis and follow-up of EoE [41]. Therefore, there is a critical need for non-invasive tools and biomarkers to replace such invasive monitoring. Despite several efforts to identify potential non-invasive biomarkers, none have been incorporated into guideline recommendations [42].

15.3.1 Clinical Features and Heterogeneity of EoE

EoE symptoms vary with age [1, 43]. Toddlers and young children generally experience food refusal, feeding difficulties, recurrent vomiting and/or regurgitation, and failure to thrive. School-aged children often reported abdominal/epigastric pain, and refractory gastroesophageal reflux, whereas adolescents and adults present dysphagia and food impaction [43]. Children can also develop compensative feeding habits (drinking during meals, eating slowly, chewing carefully, cutting food into small pieces, lubricating foods with sauces or liquids) or avoiding some foods (meat, crusty bread, and pills) [44].

Notably, clinical, endoscopic, and histological features reflect the evolution of EoE inflammation through time, as reported in Fig. 15.1. Different clinical patterns or phenotypes have been identified [45]. The "inflammatory" pattern is generally observed in children and is defined by the endoscopic evidence of edema, erythema, linear furrowing, and the prevalent eosinophilic infiltration at the biopsy [45–47]. Instead, the "fibro-stenotic" phenotype affects adults who typically experience dysphagia and food impaction episodes [44–47]. This phenotype is endoscopically characterized by fixed esophageal rings and/or strictures resulting from tissue remodeling and esophageal fibrosis [44–47]. The clinical and histological heterogeneity might reflect and partially explain the heterogeneous response to currently available therapies [45]. While diet and medical therapies may reduce tissue fibrosis in childhood, this remodeling process may persist despite the resolution of inflammation in adulthood [48]. Recently, Shoda et al. identified three potential endotypes of EoE, using a machine learning approach to analyze the histological, endoscopic, and molecular features of patients with EoE. The first endotype (EoEe1) was recognized in 35% of the cohort and was mainly characterized by minimal eosinophilic inflammation and steroid responsiveness. The EoEe2 endotype affected 29% of patients, showing a prevalent Th2 inflammation, pediatric-onset, and low steroid response. Finally, 36% of

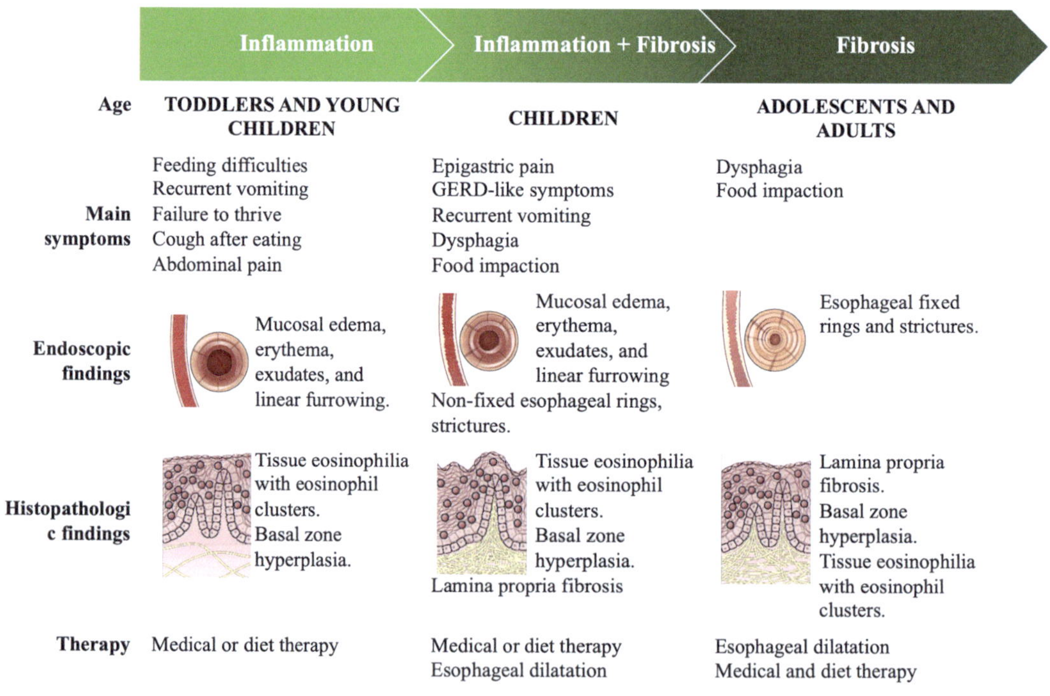

Fig. 15.1 Natural history and clinical heterogeneity of eosinophilic esophagitis (Modified from Votto et al., 2022 [113])

the EoE cohort (EoEe3) presented an adult-onset and structuring disease [49]. Therefore, according to this endotype classification, patients with the EoEe1 endotype might successfully be treated with diet and steroid therapy, and children with the EoEe2 endotype might benefit from the anti-Th2 immune agents (i.e., dupilumab) [50]. Finally, adult patients with the EoEe3 endotype are more challenging to treat with available therapies; thus, esophageal dilatations are the only current solution to esophageal stenosis [50].

Several studies have shown that patients with EoE have concomitant allergic comorbidities, such as allergic rhinitis, asthma, atopic dermatitis, and IgE-mediated food allergy [36]. The prevalence of asthma reaches 60% in pediatric series [51]. The prevalence of IgE-mediated food allergy varies between 25% and nearly 70% [52, 53]. Eczema was also significantly more frequent in EoE patients than in controls [52, 53]. These findings have led many researchers to consider EoE the final step of the atopic march [54].

Several non-atopic diseases are associated with EoE, such as inflammatory bowel disease, connective tissue disorders, autism and attention deficit hyperactivity disorders, esophageal atresia, celiac disease, as well as the monogenic disorders previously reported [51, 55–58].

Recently, Biedermann et al. identified a new clinically defined syndrome in adults with EoE called the food-induced immediate response of the esophagus (FIRE) [59]. FIRE syndrome encompasses esophageal symptoms occurring rapidly after contact with the esophageal surface with a specific food. This syndrome is mainly triggered by fruits, vegetables, and drinks, just like the pollen food allergy syndrome (PFAS). Therefore, FIRE symptoms originate in the esophagus instead of the oropharyngeal cavity. Prominent symptoms are highly pronounced unpleasant and even painful retrosternal symptoms strictly linked to the ingestion of a specific food trigger, usually appearing shortly after the exposure with a latency of fewer than 5 min with limited duration, as most patients perceive symptoms for <30 min. These symptoms are also distinguished and unrelated to dysphagia and GERD [59, 60]. FIRE has been described in only one pediatric case [61]. The pathogenesis of this novel syndrome is still unclear; a local immunologic factor causing an immediate mucosa response has been postulated. However, FIRE may be underestimated in children because symptoms could be attributed to EoE, and patients are too young to distinguish between typical EoE, PFAS, and FIRE symptoms [61].

15.3.2 Endoscopic and Histological Features

Upper GI endoscopy is the first step in the diagnostic work-up of EoE. Several characteristic endoscopic findings can also be recognized in children. A graded endoscopic score system has been developed to standardize endoscopic findings [62]. The EREFS is a summation and scoring of the five most prominent endoscopic signs of EoE observed during the endoscopy:

- **Edema (E)** is the loss of vascular markings (present 1, absent 0);
- **Rings (R)** or esophageal trachealization (none 0, mild 1, moderate 2, severe 3);
- **Exudates (E)** or white plaques (none 0, mild 1, severe 2);
- **Furrows (F)** or vertical lines (none 0, mild 1, severe 2);
- **Strictures (S)** (present 1, absent 0).

Edema, exudates, and furrows are considered inflammatory components, whereas the rings and strictures reflect fibrotic components. An EREFS score < 2 corresponds to endoscopic remission.

Unlike other GI tracts, the normal esophagus is entirely devoid of eosinophils, where a small number of tissue eosinophils are physiologically present. Histologically, ≥15 eosinophils in one HPF are necessary for defining EoE and monitoring disease activity [63]. Other histological findings have been observed in eosinophilic esophagitis, such as spongiosis (dilation of intercellular spaces), increased mast cell and lymphocyte numbers, basal zone hyperplasia, and papillary elongation [64]. Recently, Collins et al. developed a histological scoring system [64].

The eosinophilic esophagitis histological scoring system (EoE-HSS) evaluates eight features: eosinophil density, basal zone hyperplasia, eosinophil abscesses, eosinophil surface layering, dilated intercellular spaces, surface epithelial alteration, dyskeratotic epithelial cells, and lamina propria fibrosis [64].

15.4 Therapy

EoE treatment aims to control symptoms and esophageal inflammation and prevent complications. The therapeutic options are divided into three categories: Drugs (medical therapy), Diet (elimination of culprit foods), and Dilation (mechanical therapy) [1, 43]. The only currently approved treatment options for EoE are budesonide effervescent tablets for adults in most European Countries and dupilumab, approved by FDA for patients ≥12 years [65]. Therefore, treatments routinely used in pediatric clinical practice, like proton pump inhibitors (PPIs) or topical corticosteroids, are not approved for EoE, so they are prescribed off-label.

15.4.1 Pharmacological Therapy (Table 15.1)

15.4.1.1 Swallowed Topical Corticosteroids

Topical corticosteroids are effective in inducing EoE remission. Oral steroids can clinically and histologically treat the disease; however, they carry significant known side effects if used long-term. Given the chronicity and life-long duration of EoE, long-term treatment with oral or systemic steroids is not recommended [63]. Meta-analyses of topical corticosteroids in the form of swallowed fluticasone or viscous budesonide demonstrate the superiority of these medications to placebo for esophageal eosinophilia, endoscopic findings, and GI symptoms [66]. A further meta-analysis confirmed the efficacy of swallowed budesonide compared to placebo [67]. A recent randomized trial to compare fluticasone and viscous budesonide for EoE treatments showed that viscous budesonide provided a significantly higher level of esophageal exposure to the therapeutic agent with lower eosinophil counts [68]. Moreover, some evidence shows that oral

Table 15.1 Pharmacological therapy of EoE in children and adolescents

	Proton pump inhibitors (PPIs)	Slurry budesonide	Swallowed fluticasone
Dosage	Children: 1 mg/kg/day Adolescents: 20–40 mg/day	<10 years: 1 mg/day >10 years: 2 mg/day	<10 years: 440 mcg twice daily >10 years: 880 mcg twice daily
Special instruction	• Twice daily • 30 min before meals	• Mixed with sucralose (5 g of sucralose), honey, or 2.5 mL aminoacidic formula per mg of budesonide to make a total volume of 8–12 mL	• Do not use the spacer • Do not inhale
General considerations	• Initial treatment 8–12 weeks • Effective in 54% of children	• Administering the second dose at bedtime • Avoid eating/drinking 30 min after use • Safe and well tolerated	
Long-term maintenance	• PPIs are safe • The response is more sustained in inflammatory phenotype (70%)	• Esophageal candidiasis 4–5% • Consider periodic monitoring for adrenal insufficiency, bone metabolism, and growth • The strategy is to decrease the dose to the lowest effective level • Limited data on optimal dosage and side effects of long-term use	

budesonide can reverse esophageal fibrosis [69]. Despite regular therapy, the increase in esophageal eosinophil counts is also described [70, 71].

There are many unresolved questions about the chronic use of topical steroids. There is no consensus regarding dosage, formulation, frequency, and how to obtain remission using minimal steroid dosage. Long-term side effects are a significant concern, and no studies have been conducted regarding bone health in patients for longer than 1 year [72]. The most common side-effect of topical steroids is oral and esophageal candidiasis [73]. Topical corticosteroids are typically administered once or twice daily, and dosing depends on age and disease severity. Patients should spray fluticasone without a spacer in the back of their mouth and swallow at the dose. No food or drink is allowed 30 min after administering the medication [72].

15.4.1.2 Proton Pump Inhibitors

The response rates to PPI therapy in the EoE population can vary widely from 30% to 70% [41]. In a meta-analysis of 32 studies on PPI treatment in EoE, 50.5% of patients achieved histologic remission [74]. The dosage effective in EoE treatment is 1–2 mg/kg in children and 40 mg of omeprazole (or equivalent dosages for other PPIs) once or twice daily. The mechanism of action of PPIs in EoE is still unclear. PPIs are well-established inhibitors of gastric parietal H+/K + -ATPase, and this effect may reduce acidic injury to the esophagus and cause epithelial healing. Also, PPIs show anti-cytokine properties, directly inhibiting epithelial STAT6, a key transcription factor for the secretion of pro-inflammatory chemokines and cytokines [75, 76]. No clinical features or biomarkers discern a patient who will respond to PPI monotherapy from resistance. Differences in the pathophysiology between PPI-responsive and PPI-resistant EoE remain determined and might be related to different genetic polymorphisms or molecular transcripts.

15.4.1.3 Biological Therapies

The increasing knowledge of EoE pathogenesis has allowed several therapeutic targets to be identified and tested. The humanized antibodies against IL-5, such as mepolizumab and reslizumab, were tested in three controlled trials in children and adults with active EoE, demonstrating reduced tissue eosinophilia and a favorable safety profile. Unfortunately, clinical improvement was minimal [77–79]. A phase III trial using benralizumab, a monoclonal antibody against the IL-5 receptor, is active [79, 80].

Two RCTs with the anti-IL-13 agent and one with the anti-IL-4 receptor antagonist dupilumab showed promising results [81, 82]. In a phase II study, a monoclonal antibody against IL-13 improved endoscopic and histological disease activity in the short and long term146, 147. Dupilumab is currently the most advanced biologic therapy in EoE treatment. Dupilumab is a human monoclonal antibody targeting the α-chain subunit of the IL-4 receptor, which is shared between IL-4 and IL-13 [83]. The phase III study of dupilumab demonstrated significant beneficial treatment effects on clinical symptoms, eosinophil counts, and esophageal distension [79].

Therefore, FDA first, then EMA, recently approved dupilumab for treating adolescents (≥12 years) and adults with active EoE. Trials in children younger than 12 years are active but preliminary results showed promising effects.

15.4.2 Diet Therapies (Table 15.2)

15.4.2.1 Diet Therapy

In 1995, Kelly et al. successfully demonstrated the efficacy of the exclusive aminoacidic-based formula diet in children with EoE [84]. The elemental diet (ED) consists of removing all foods. Thus, patients are exclusively fed with an aminoacidic-based formula for at least 6 weeks [41, 85, 86]. The ED is the most effective treatment, and several studies reported high complete remission rates in children with active EoE [87]. EoE patients treated with the ED experienced a significant reduction in their symptoms and achieved complete histologic remission in 90% and 94% of pediatric and adult cases, respectively. Moreover, the highest efficacy rates are primarily observed in patients with a non-stenotic phenotype [88–92]. In toddlers or young

Table 15.2 Diet treatments of EoE in children and adolescents

Diet therapy	Rationale	Indications	Advantages	Disadvantages
Elemental diet	Exclusive administration of aminoacidic-based formula. Possibility to introduce one or two less allergenic foods (generally vegetables or fruits) in addition to the aminoacidic-based formula	• Toddlers or young children with severe active EoE • Severe cases • Rescue therapy or temporary solution in refractory cases	• Rapid and complete remission in 2 weeks • Better acceptance in young children and toddlers • Rescue therapy or temporary solution in adults with non-stricturing EoE • Pediatric formulas are almost nutritionally complete • Nutritional supplement	• Poor palatability and low patient's compliance • The administration through NG or G-tube may induce feeding skills regression • High cost and insurance Coverage • Less effective in stricturing EoE
Empiric food elimination diet (FED)	**Step-up approach** (from 1–2 FED to 6 FED)	• Pediatric patients • Moderate symptoms • A diet rich in milk and wheat	• Early identification of trigger food • Short diagnostic process • Avoid unnecessary diet restrictions	• Less effective
	Top-down approach (from 6 FED to 1–2 FED)	• Adults and adolescents with normal or high BMI • Severe symptoms • Baseline diet rich in fruits and vegetables • Much time to prepare alternative meals and high financial resources	• More effective	• Up to 7 endoscopies, one after every single food reintroduction. • Several diet restrictions. • Low compliance. • Risk of nutritional deficiencies

children with active EoE complicated by failure to thrive, the ED has generally been considered a valid and valuable therapeutic option with the highest patient compliance [93]. In children with multiple food triggers and subsequent high diet restrictions, ED can also be used as a supplement of protein and energy necessary for adequate growth and puberty spurt [93]. Although the ED can induce rapid disease remission in only 2 weeks, several disadvantages limit its adherence [94]. The poor palatability, highly restrictive nature, costs, and psychosocial isolation are the main reasons for treatment discontinuation and low compliance [88, 93, 95]. To remedy these issues, the ED is often modified, introducing one or two less allergenic foods (generally vegetables or fruits) in addition to the aminoacidic-based formula [88, 93]. For these reasons, ED is often not considered a first-line approach because of its limitations [93]. Therefore, it is a therapeutic option in severe EoE cases, or it is often proposed as rescue therapy or a temporary solution in adults and adolescents with refractory EoE [88, 93].

15.4.2.2 Empirical Food Elimination Diet (FED)

FED is the most widely used diet treatment for EoE. The first proposed FED was founded on avoiding the six (6-FED) most common food triggers of EoE in the Western diet: milk, wheat/gluten, egg, soy/legumes, peanut/tree nuts, and seafood/fish [96]. The efficacy (histologic remission) of 6-FED is about 74% in children [97]. In children, the most common food trigger is cow's milk (up to 85% of cases), followed by wheat/gluten (up to 60% of cases), egg, and soy/legumes, with geographic variations [87]. Consequently, nuts and fish/seafood rarely trigger EoE. Most children who histologically recover with 6-FED are allergic to only 1–3 foods [47]. Although 6-FED is less restrictive than the elemental diet, avoiding all six food groups can still be challenging. Several drawbacks limit the adherence to 6-FED due to the high level of dietary restriction and the need for frequent upper GI endoscopies to identify the culprit food(s) [93]. For these reasons, 6-FED is generally not considered the ideal therapeutic approach in children. Subsequent studies proposed and assessed less restrictive FEDs that avoided the most common EoE food triggers. The 4-FED (milk, wheat, egg, and soy/legumes-free diet) induced histologic remission in 54%of children [98, 99]. In studies evaluating the efficacy of 4-FED, milk and wheat were the most common triggers of EoE [93]. Children avoiding these two foods (2-FED) achieved complete remission in 40% of cases. The elimination of cow's milk (1-FED) demonstrated disease-remission rates of 44–51% in pediatric patients [88]. In a recent systematic review with meta-analysis, the overall efficacy of a milk-free diet was about 70% [97].

Recently, Molina-Infante et al. proposed a step-up approach that consists of the initial elimination of one (1-FED) or two (2-FED) more common allergenic foods (milk and wheat) [100]. If complete remission is not achieved, the diet is further restricted to a 4 and eventually to 6 foods [100].

The step-up approach is generally preferred in children because it leads to faster and earlier identification of food triggers, avoids unnecessary diet restrictions, and reduces the number of endoscopies.

15.4.2.3 Allergy-Test Directed Elimination Diet

Studies found that atopy patch tests, skin prick tests, and food-specific serum IgEs did not reliably predict food triggers and did not have a clear role in evaluating patients with EoE [41, 101]. A meta-analysis revealed that this approach induces histologic remission in about 46% of patients, and efficacy rates were significantly lower in adults than children [97]. According to this evidence, current American and European guidelines do not recommend an allergy-test-directed elimination diet [41, 101].

15.4.3 Esophageal Dilation

Esophageal strictures might occur despite the therapy, especially in adults requiring esophageal dilatation to treat structural alterations. Patients tolerating esophageal dilations show long-lasting symptomatic relief but do not present improved histologic features [102].

15.5 Monitoring of EoE

EoE is a chronic disease that requires lifelong therapy [41, 101]. Neither guidelines nor consensus recommendations on the long-term management of EoE have been published so far. A diagnostic work-up includes the assessment of symptoms and growth, endoscopic alterations, and histological abnormalities. The diagnostic work-up should be performed around 3–4 months after initiating a novel treatment or after each relevant therapeutical change [103]. Under stable conditions and solid adherence to treatment, a diagnostic work-up once per year is adequate for most patients.

Patients following a dietary regimen should be widely informed of the need for repeated follow-up endoscopies. Food reintroduction in patients on a 6-FED requires at least six endoscopies and several months to identify the culprit food(s). In children exclusively fed with the aminoacidic-based formula, the food-reintroduction process is even longer and loaded by several endoscopies.

Once the culprit food(s) is identified, the long-term diet therapy is only based on exclusively avoiding the food(s) responsible for esophageal inflammation [104].

Recent evidence suggests that children treated with topic steroids can undergo a progressive dose reduction after a successful induction therapy until the lowest effective dose. This approach was effective in about 50% of children treated with viscous budesonide and was safe [105].

15.5.1 Nutritional Issues and Assessment

Several factors may negatively influence the nutritional status of patients with EoE. Children with EoE generally present GI symptoms, like vomiting or food refusal, that may limit adequate nutritional intake [106]. Patients with previous food impaction episodes may risk developing anxiety and eating disorders, compromising adequate nutrient intake [95, 107].

Another critical point is that EoE is often delayed or misdiagnosed, especially in the first two decades of life [108, 109]. A longer diagnostic time significantly impairs a child's growth and is associated with tissue remodeling complications, such as esophageal rings and strictures [108, 109].

The coexistence of multiple food allergies might be a further reason for failure to thrive and undernutrition. On the other hand, long-term restrictive FEDs may compromise adequate micronutrient intake, although they do not appear to worsen child growth or body mass index (BMI) [106, 110]. Nutritionists have a crucial role in pediatric EoE. A nutritionist should meticulously evaluate the diet of patients to determine the degree of exposure to high-risk groups of foods and the potential nutritional and psychological effects of their elimination [111, 112]. Before beginning diet therapy and during the follow-up period, pediatricians should periodically assess the nutritional status of children and rule out potential nutritional deficiencies. Then, clinical (symptoms, comorbidities, feeding habits/disorders) and anthropometric data should be collected and carefully evaluated to address the best therapeutic choice.

Another critical point concerns the patient's education. Pediatricians should carefully inform patients and their families regarding what they can eat and provide the appropriate resources for additional information [93]. Patients should also be advised on the risk of potential allergen contamination. According to specific local legislation, clinicians should educate patients and families to read and correctly interpret the labels of food products [93]. The precautionary allergen labeling ("may contain") is not mandatory in some countries [93]. However, the risk of allergen cross-contamination and trace exposure for foods reporting this warning is variable and still not established in EoE patients [93].

15.5.2 Multidisciplinary Assessment

The multidisciplinary approach (allergist, gastroenterologist, endoscopist, nutritionist, psychologist) is crucial to pediatric EoE management [106]. In highly specialized centers, all these specialists should be present during the entire course of the disease and guarantee the transition from the pediatric to the adult setting. Allergists should identify other coexisting atopic comorbidities (eczema, allergic rhinitis, asthma, food/drug allergy, and anaphylaxis) and adequately treat uncontrolled symptoms. Allergy assessment is also fundamental to prevent potential IgE-mediated reactions when foods (especially milk) are reintroduced. Strict clinical and endoscopic follow-up is required to evaluate patient compliance, long-term treatment side effects, and assess disease remission.

The chronic nature of EoE, comorbidities, long-term restrictive therapies, and strict endoscopic follow-up are the main stressful factors for patients and their families [95]. It is evident that EoE significantly impacts the QoL of patients [95]. Therefore, psychological support should be provided when behavioral, mood diseases, or eating disorders are suspected [95].

Take-Home Messages

- EoE is a chronic inflammatory disease limited to the esophagus, affecting children and adults equally.
- To date, upper gastrointestinal endoscopy is the gold standard for diagnosing and monitoring EoE.
- Therapy aims to achieve a "deep remission" (symptom control and normalizing endoscopic and histologic features) and prevent esophageal fibrosis.
- Due to its chronic natural history, the need for several endoscopies, and long-term therapies, EoE has a relevant burden on children and their families, significantly affecting patients' quality of life.

References

1. Licari A, Votto M, D'Auria E, Castagnoli R, Caimmi SME, Marseglia GL. Eosinophilic gastrointestinal diseases in children: a practical review. Curr Pediatr Rev. 2020;16:106–14.
2. Landres RT, Kuster GG, Strum WB. Eosinophilic esophagitis in a patient with vigorous achalasia. Gastroenterology. 1978;74:1298–301.
3. Winter HS, Madara JL, Stafford RJ, Grand RJ, Quinlan JE, Goldman H. Intraepithelial eosinophils: a new diagnostic criterion for reflux esophagitis. Gastroenterology. 1982;83:818–23.
4. Attwood SE, Smyrk TC, Demeester TR, Jones JB. Esophageal eosinophilia with dysphagia. A distinct clinicopathologic syndrome. Dig Dis Sci. 1993;38:109–16.
5. Straumann A, Spichtin HP, Bernoulli R, Loosli J, Vögtlin J. Idiopathic eosinophilic esophagitis: a frequently overlooked disease with typical clinical aspects and discrete endoscopic findings. Schweiz Med Wochenschr. 1994;124:1419–29.
6. Dellon ES, Hirano I. Epidemiology and natural history of eosinophilic esophagitis. Gastroenterology. 2018;154:319–32.
7. de Rooij WE, Barendsen ME, Warners MJ, van Rhijn BD, Verheij J, Bruggink AH, et al. Emerging incidence trends of eosinophilic esophagitis over 25 years: results of a nationwide register-based pathology cohort. Neurogastroenterol Motil. 2021;33:e14072.
8. Votto M, Raffaele A, De Filippo M, Caimmi S, Brunero M, Riccipetitoni G, et al. Eosinophilic gastrointestinal disorders in children and adolescents: a single-center experience. Dig Liver Dis. 2022;54:214–20.
9. Navarro P, Arias Á, Arias-González L, Laserna-Mendieta EJ, Ruiz-Ponce M, Lucendo AJ. Systematic review with meta-analysis: the growing incidence and prevalence of eosinophilic oesophagitis in children and adults in population-based studies. Aliment Pharmacol Ther. 2019;49:1116–25.
10. Allin KH, Poulsen G, Melgaard D, Frandsen LT, Jess T, Krarup AL. Eosinophilic oesophagitis in Denmark: population-based incidence and prevalence in a nationwide study from 2008 to 2018. United European Gastroenterol J. 2022;10:640–50.
11. Arias Á, Lucendo AJ. Incidence and prevalence of eosinophilic oesophagitis increase continiously in adults and children in Central Spain: a 12-year population-based study. Dig Liver Dis. 2019;51:55–62.
12. Prasad GA, Alexander JA, Schleck CD, Zinsmeister AR, Smyrk TC, Elias RM, et al. Epidemiology of eosinophilic esophagitis over three decades in Olmsted County, Minnesota. Clin Gastroenterol Hepatol. 2009;7:1055–61.
13. Hruz P, Straumann A, Bussmann C, Heer P, Simon HU, Zwahlen M, et al. Escalating incidence of eosinophilic esophagitis: a 20-year prospective, population-based study in Olten County, Switzerland. J Allergy Clin Immunol. 2011;128:1349–50.
14. van Rhijn BD, Verheij J, Smout AJ, Bredenoord AJ. Rapidly increasing incidence of eosinophilic esophagitis in a large cohort. Neurogastroenterol Motil. 2013;25:47–52.
15. Thomsen SF. Epidemiology and natural history of atopic diseases. Eur Clin Respir J. 2015;2:24642.
16. Brooks C, Pearce N, Douwes J. The hygiene hypothesis in allergy and asthma: an update. Curr Opin Allergy Clin Immunol. 2013;13:70–7.
17. Votto M, Marseglia GL, De Filippo M, Brambilla I, Caimmi SME, Licari A. Early life risk factors in pediatric EoE: could we prevent this modern disease? Front Pediatr. 2020;8:263.
18. Kapel RC, Miller JK, Torres C, Aksoy S, Lash R, Katzka DA. Eosinophilic esophagitis: a prevalent disease in the United States that affects all age groups. Gastroenterology. 2008;134:1316–21.
19. Celebi Sozener Z, Ozdel Ozturk B, Cerci P, Turk M, Gorgulu Akin B, Akdis M, et al. Epithelial barrier hypothesis: effect of the external exposome on the microbiome and epithelial barriers in allergic disease. Allergy. 2022;77:1418–49.
20. Cianferoni A, Jensen E, Davis CM. The role of the environment in Eosinophilic Esophagitis. J Allergy Clin Immunol Pract. 2021;9:3268–74.
21. Ruffner MA, Kennedy K, Cianferoni A. Pathophysiology of eosinophilic esophagitis: recent advances and their clinical implications. Expert Rev Clin Immunol. 2019;15:83–95.

22. Liacouras CA, Spergel JM, Ruchelli E, Verma R, Mascarenhas M, Semeao E, et al. Eosinophilic esophagitis: a 10-year experience in 381 children. Clin Gastroenterol Hepatol. 2005;3:1198–206.
23. Mansoor E, Cooper GS. The 2010–2015 prevalence of eosinophilic esophagitis in the USA: a population-based study. Dig Dis Sci. 2016;61:2928–34.
24. Allen-Brady K, Firszt R, Fang JC, Wong J, Smith KR, Peterson KA. Population-based familial aggregation of eosinophilic esophagitis suggests a genetic contribution. J Allergy Clin Immunol. 2017;140:1138–43.
25. Alexander ES, Martin LJ, Collins MH, Kottyan LC, Sucharew H, He H, et al. Twin and family studies reveal strong environmental and weaker genetic cues explaining heritability of eosinophilic esophagitis. J Allergy Clin Immunol. 2014;134:1084–92.
26. Jensen ET, Kappelman MD, Kim HP, Ringel-Kulka T, Dellon ES. Early life exposures as risk factors for pediatric eosinophilic esophagitis. J Pediatr Gastroenterol Nutr. 2013;57:67–71.
27. Radano MC, Yuan Q, Katz A, Fleming JT, Kubala S, Shreffler W, et al. Cesarean section and antibiotic use found to be associated with eosinophilic esophagitis. J Allergy Clin Immunol Pract. 2014;2:475–7.
28. Jensen ET, Kuhl JT, Martin LJ, Rothenberg ME, Dellon ES. Prenatal, intrapartum, and postnatal factors are associated with pediatric eosinophilic esophagitis. J Allergy Clin Immunol. 2018;141:214–22.
29. Jensen ET, Gupta SK. Early life factors and Eosinophilic Esophagitis: building the evidence. J Pediatr Gastroenterol Nutr. 2018;67:549–50.
30. Witmer CP, Susi A, Min SB, Nylund CM. Early infant risk factors for pediatric eosinophilic esophagitis. J Pediatr Gastroenterol Nutr. 2018;67:610–5.
31. O'Shea KM, Aceves SS, Dellon ES, Gupta SK, Spergel JM, Furuta GT, et al. Pathophysiology of eosinophilic esophagitis. Gastroenterology. 2018;154:333–45.
32. Kottyan LC, Rothenberg ME. Genetics of eosinophilic esophagitis. Mucosal Immunol. 2017;10:580–8.
33. Chang X, March M, Mentch F, Nguyen K, Glessner J, Qu H, et al. A genome-wide association meta-analysis identifies new eosinophilic esophagitis loci. J Allergy Clin Immunol. 2022;149:988–98.
34. Sleiman PM, Wang ML, Cianferoni A, Aceves S, Gonsalves N, Nadeau K, et al. GWAS identifies four novel eosinophilic esophagitis loci. Nat Commun. 2014;5:5593.
35. Chang JW, Jensen ET, Dellon ES. Nature with nurture: the role of intrinsic genetic and extrinsic environmental factors on Eosinophilic Esophagitis. Curr Allergy Asthma Rep. 2022;22:163–70.
36. Rossi CM, Lenti MV, Merli S, Licari A, Votto M, Marseglia GL, et al. Primary eosinophilic gastrointestinal disorders and allergy: clinical and therapeutic implications. Clin Transl Allergy. 2022;12:e12146.
37. Capucilli P, Hill DA. Allergic comorbidity in eosinophilic esophagitis: mechanistic relevance and clinical implications. Clin Rev Allergy Immunol. 2019;57:111–27.
38. Blanchard C, Mingler MK, McBride M, Putnam PE, Collins MH, Chang G, et al. Periostin facilitates eosinophil tissue infiltration in allergic lung and esophageal responses. Mucosal Immunol. 2008;1:289–96.
39. Arora M, Bagi P, Strongin A, Heimall J, Zhao X, Lawrence MG, et al. Gastrointestinal manifestations of STAT3-deficient hyper-IgE syndrome. J Clin Immunol. 2017;37:695–700.
40. Paluel-Marmont C, Bellon N, Barbet P, Leclerc-Mercier S, Hadj-Rabia S, Dupont C, et al. Eosinophilic esophagitis and colonic mucosal eosinophilia in Netherton syndrome. J Allergy Clin Immunol. 2017;139:2003–5.
41. Dellon ES, Liacouras CA, Molina-Infante J, Furuta GT, Spergel JM, Zevit N, et al. Updated international consensus diagnostic criteria for eosinophilic esophagitis: proceedings of the AGREE conference. Gastroenterology. 2018;155:1022–33.
42. Votto M, De Filippo M, Castagnoli R, Delle Cave F, Giffoni F, Santi V, et al. Non-invasive biomarkers of eosinophilic esophagitis. Acta Biomed. 2021;92:e2021530.
43. Cianferoni A, Spergel JM. Eosinophilic esophagitis and gastroenteritis. Curr Allergy Asthma Rep. 2015;15:58.
44. Muir AB, Brown-Whitehorn T, Godwin B, Cianferoni A. Eosinophilic esophagitis: early diagnosis is the key. Clin Exp Gastroenterol. 2019;12:391–9.
45. Ruffner MA, Cianferoni A. Phenotypes and endotypes in eosinophilic esophagitis. Ann Allergy Asthma Immunol. 2020;124:233–9.
46. Hirano I, Sharaf R, Stollman N, Wang K, Falck-Ytter Y, Chan E, et al. Spotlight: treatment of eosinophilic esophagitis (EoE). Gastroenterology. 2020;158:1788.
47. Steinbach EC, Hernandez M, Dellon ES. Eosinophilic Esophagitis and the Eosinophilic gastrointestinal diseases: approach to diagnosis and management. J Allergy Clin Immunol Pract. 2018;6:1483–5.
48. Shaheen NJ, Mukkada V, Eichinger CS, Schofield H, Todorova L, Falk GW. Natural history of eosinophilic esophagitis: a systematic review of epidemiology and disease course. Dis Esophagus. 2018;31:doy015.
49. Shoda T, Wen T, Aceves SS, Abonia JP, Atkins D, Bonis PA, et al. Eosinophilic oesophagitis endotype classification by molecular, clinical, and histopathological analyses: a cross-sectional study. Lancet Gastroenterol Hepatol. 2018;3:477–88.
50. Keely S, Talley NJ. Endophenotyping eosinophilic oesophagitis: a new era for management? Lancet Gastroenterol Hepatol. 2018;3:449–50.
51. Capucilli P, Cianferoni A, Grundmeier RW, Spergel JM. Comparison of comorbid diagnoses in children with and without eosinophilic esophagitis in a large population. Ann Allergy Asthma Immunol. 2018;121:711–6.

52. González-Cervera J, Arias Á, Redondo-González O, Cano-Mollinedo MM, Terreehorst I, Lucendo AJ. Association between atopic manifestations and eosinophilic esophagitis: a systematic review and meta-analysis. Ann Allergy Asthma Immunol. 2017;118:582–90.
53. Hill DA, Dudley JW, Spergel JM. The prevalence of eosinophilic esophagitis in pediatric patients with IgE-mediated food allergy. J Allergy Clin Immunol Pract. 2017;5:369–75.
54. Hill DA, Grundmeier RW, Ramos M, Spergel JM. Eosinophilic esophagitis is a late manifestation of the allergic march. J Allergy Clin Immunol Pract. 2018;6:1528–33.
55. Talathi S, Knight T, Dimmitt R, Mestre J, Jester T. Concurrent eosinophilic esophagitis in pediatric patients with inflammatory bowel disease: a case series. Ann Allergy Asthma Immunol. 2019;123:313–6.
56. Abonia JP, Wen T, Stucke EM, Grotjan T, Griffith MS, Kemme KA, et al. High prevalence of eosinophilic esophagitis in patients with inherited connective tissue disorders. J Allergy Clin Immunol. 2013;132:378–86.
57. Peterson K, Firszt R, Fang J, Wong J, Smith KR, Brady KA. Risk of autoimmunity in EoE and families: a population-based cohort study. Am J Gastroenterol. 2016;111:926–32.
58. Kottyan L, Spergel JM, Cianferoni A. Immunology of the ancestral differences in eosinophilic esophagitis. Ann Allergy Asthma Immunol. 2019;122:443–4.
59. Biedermann L, Holbreich M, Atkins D, Chehade M, Dellon ES, Furuta GT, et al. Food-induced immediate response of the esophagus-a newly identified syndrome in patients with eosinophilic esophagitis. Allergy. 2021;76:339–47.
60. Holbreich M, Straumann A. Features of food-induced immediate response in the esophagus (FIRE) in a series of adult patients with eosinophilic esophagitis. Allergy. 2021;76:2893–5.
61. Votto M, Naso M, De Filippo M, Marseglia A, Raffaele A, Marseglia GL, et al. Food-induced immediate response of the esophagus: a first report in the pediatric age. Allergy. 2022;77:711–2.
62. Hirano I, Moy N, Heckman MG, Thomas CS, Gonsalves N, Achem SR. Endoscopic assessment of the oesophageal features of eosinophilic oesophagitis: validation of a novel classification and grading system. Gut. 2013;62:489–95.
63. Liacouras CA, Furuta GT, Hirano I, Atkins D, Attwood SE, Bonis PA, et al. Eosinophilic esophagitis: updated consensus recommendations for children and adults. J Allergy Clin Immunol. 2011;128:3–20.
64. Collins MH, Martin LJ, Alexander ES, Boyd JT, Sheridan R, He H, et al. Newly developed and validated eosinophilic esophagitis histology scoring system and evidence that it outperforms peak eosinophil count for disease diagnosis and monitoring. Dis Esophagus. 2017;30:1–8.
65. Biedermann L, Straumann A, Greuter T, Schreiner P. Eosinophilic esophagitis-established facts and new horizons. Semin Immunopathol. 2021;43:319–35.
66. Murali AR, Gupta A, Attar BM, Ravi V, Koduru P. Topical steroids in eosinophilic esophagitis: systematic review and meta-analysis of placebo-controlled randomized clinical trials. J Gastroenterol Hepatol. 2016;31:1111–9.
67. Rawla P, Sunkara T, Thandra KC, Gaduputi V. Efficacy and safety of budesonide in the treatment of Eosinophilic Esophagitis: updated systematic review and meta-analysis of randomized and non-randomized studies. Drugs R D. 2018;18:259–69.
68. Dellon ES, Sheikh A, Speck O, Woodward K, Whitlow AB, Hores JM, et al. Viscous topical is more effective than nebulized steroid therapy for patients with eosinophilic esophagitis. Gastroenterology. 2012;143:321–4.
69. Aceves SS, Newbury RO, Chen D, Mueller J, Dohil R, Hoffman H, et al. Resolution of remodeling in eosinophilic esophagitis correlates with epithelial response to topical corticosteroids. Allergy. 2010;65:109–16.
70. Eluri S, Runge TM, Hansen J, Kochar B, Reed CC, Robey BS, et al. Diminishing effectiveness of long-term maintenance topical steroid therapy in PPI non-responsive eosinophilic esophagitis. Clin Transl Gastroenterol. 2017;8:e97.
71. Collins CA, Palmquist J, Proudfoot JA, Qian A, Wangberg H, Khosh-Hemmat E, et al. Evaluation of long-term course in children with eosinophilic esophagitis reveals distinct histologic patterns and clinical characteristics. J Allergy Clin Immunol. 2019;144:1050–7.
72. Cianferoni A. Eosinophilic esophagitis and other eosinophilic disorders of the gastrointestinal tract. Pediatr Allergy Immunol. 2020;31(Suppl 24):25–7.
73. Jensen ET, Huang KZ, Chen HX, Landes LE, McConnell KA, Almond MA, et al. Longitudinal growth outcomes following first-line treatment for pediatric patients with eosinophilic esophagitis. J Pediatr Gastroenterol Nutr. 2019;68:50–5.
74. Lucendo AJ, Arias Á, Molina-Infante J. Efficacy of proton pump inhibitor drugs for inducing clinical and histologic remission in patients with symptomatic esophageal eosinophilia: a systematic review and meta-analysis. Clin Gastroenterol Hepatol. 2016;14:13–22.
75. Wen T, Dellon ES, Moawad FJ, Furuta GT, Aceves SS, Rothenberg ME. Transcriptome analysis of proton pump inhibitor-responsive esophageal eosinophilia reveals proton pump inhibitor-reversible allergic inflammation. J Allergy Clin Immunol. 2015;135:187–97.
76. Zhang X, Cheng E, Huo X, Yu C, Zhang Q, Pham TH, et al. Omeprazole blocks STAT6 binding to the eotaxin-3 promoter in eosinophilic esophagitis cells. PLoS One. 2012;7:e50037.

77. Straumann A, Conus S, Grzonka P, Kita H, Kephart G, Bussmann C, et al. Anti-interleukin-5 antibody treatment (mepolizumab) in active eosinophilic oesophagitis: a randomised, placebo-controlled, double-blind trial. Gut. 2010;59:21–30.
78. Spergel JM, Rothenberg ME, Collins MH, Furuta GT, Markowitz JE, Fuchs G 3rd, et al. Reslizumab in children and adolescents with eosinophilic esophagitis: results of a double-blind, randomized, placebo-controlled trial. J Allergy Clin Immunol. 2012;129:456–63.
79. Biedermann L, Straumann A. Mechanisms and clinical management of eosinophilic oesophagitis: an overview. Nat Rev Gastroenterol Hepatol. 2023;20:101–19.
80. Hassani M, Koenderman L. Immunological and hematological effects of IL-5(Rα)-targeted therapy: an overview. Allergy. 2018;73:1979–88.
81. Rothenberg ME, Wen T, Greenberg A, Alpan O, Enav B, Hirano I, et al. Intravenous anti-IL-13 mAb QAX576 for the treatment of eosinophilic esophagitis. J Allergy Clin Immunol. 2015;135:500–7.
82. Hirano I, Collins MH, Assouline-Dayan Y, Larry E, Gupta SK, et al. A randomized, double-blind, placebo-controlled trial of a novel recombinant, humanized, anti-interleukin-13 monoclonal antibody (RPC4046) in patients with active eosinophilic esophagitis: results of the HEROES study. United European Gastroenterol J. 2016;4:A1–156.
83. Licari A, Castagnoli R, Marseglia A, Olivero F, Votto M, Ciprandi G, et al. Dupilumab to treat type 2 inflammatory diseases in children and adolescents. Paediatr Drugs. 2020;22:295–310.
84. Kelly KJ, Lazenby AJ, Rowe PC, Yardley JH, Perman JA, Sampson HA. Eosinophilic esophagitis attributed to gastroesophageal reflux: improvement with an amino acid-based formula. Gastroenterology. 1995;109:1503–12.
85. Lucendo AJ, Molina-Infante J, Arias Á, von Arnim U, Bredenoord AJ, Bussmann C, et al. Guidelines on eosinophilic esophagitis: evidence-based statements and recommendations for diagnosis and management in children and adults. United European Gastroenterol J. 2017;5:335–58.
86. De Bortoli N, Penagini R, Savarino E, Marchi S. Eosinophilic esophagitis: update in diagnosis and management. Position paper by the Italian Society of Gastroenterology and Gastrointestinal Endoscopy (SIGE). Dig Liver Dis. 2017;49:254–60.
87. Molina-Infante J, Lucendo AJ. Dietary therapy for eosinophilic esophagitis. J Allergy Clin Immunol. 2018;142:41–7.
88. Chehade M, Aceves SS. Treatment of Eosinophilic Esophagitis: diet or medication? J Allergy Clin Immunol Pract. 2021;9:3249–56.
89. Henderson CJ, Abonia JP, King EC, Putnam PE, Collins MH, Franciosi JP, et al. Comparative dietary therapy effectiveness in remission of pediatric eosinophilic esophagitis. J Allergy Clin Immunol. 2012;129:1570–8.
90. Markowitz JE, Spergel JM, Ruchelli E, Liacouras CA. Elemental diet is an effective treatment for eosinophilic esophagitis in children and adolescents. Am J Gastroenterol. 2003;98:777–82.
91. Warners MJ, Vlieg-Boerstra BJ, Verheij J, van Rhijn BD, Van Ampting MT, Harthoorn LF, et al. Elemental diet decreases inflammation and improves symptoms in adult eosinophilic oesophagitis patients. Aliment Pharmacol Ther. 2017;45:777–87.
92. Peterson KA, Byrne KR, Vinson LA, Ying J, Boynton KK, Fang JC, et al. Elemental diet induces histologic response in adult eosinophilic esophagitis. Am J Gastroenterol. 2013;108:759–66.
93. Cianferoni A, Shuker M, Brown-Whitehorn T, Hunter H, Venter C, Spergel JM. Food avoidance strategies in eosinophilic oesophagitis. Clin Exp Allergy. 2019;49:269–84.
94. Visaggi P, Mariani L, Pardi V, Rosi EM, Pugno C, Bellini M, et al. Dietary management of eosinophilic esophagitis: tailoring the approach. Nutrients. 2021;13:1630.
95. Votto M, Castagnoli R, De Filippo M, Brambilla I, Cuppari C, Marseglia GL, et al. Behavioral issues and quality of life in children with eosinophilic esophagitis. Minerva Pediatr. 2020;72:424–32.
96. Kagalwalla AF, Sentongo TA, Ritz S, Hess T, Nelson SP, Emerick KM, et al. Effect of six-food elimination diet on clinical and histologic outcomes in eosinophilic esophagitis. Clin Gastroenterol Hepatol. 2006;4:1097–102.
97. Arias A, González-Cervera J, Tenias JM, Lucendo AJ. Efficacy of dietary interventions for inducing histologic remission in patients with eosinophilic esophagitis: a systematic review and meta-analysis. Gastroenterology. 2014;146:1639–48.
98. Kagalwalla AF, Wechsler JB, Amsden K, Schwartz S, Makhija M, Olive A, et al. Efficacy of a 4-food elimination diet for children with eosinophilic esophagitis. Clin Gastroenterol Hepatol. 2017;15:1698–707.
99. Molina-Infante J, Arias A, Barrio J, Rodríguez-Sánchez J, Sanchez-Cazalilla M, Lucendo AJ. Four-food group elimination diet for adult eosinophilic esophagitis: a prospective multicenter study. J Allergy Clin Immunol. 2014;134:1093–9.
100. Molina-Infante J, Arias Á, Alcedo J, Garcia-Romero R, Casabona-Frances S, Prieto-Garcia A, et al. Step-up empiric elimination diet for pediatric and adult eosinophilic esophagitis: the 2-4-6 study. J Allergy Clin Immunol. 2018;141:1365–72.
101. Hirano I, Chan ES, Rank MA, Sharaf RN, Stollman NH, Stukus DR, et al. AGA Institute and the joint task force on allergy-immunology practice parameters clinical guidelines for the management of eosinophilic esophagitis. Gastroenterology. 2020;158:1776–86.
102. Schoepfer AM, Gonsalves N, Bussmann C, Conus S, Simon HU, Straumann A, et al. Esophageal dilation in eosinophilic esophagitis: effectiveness, safety, and impact on the underlying inflammation. Am J Gastroenterol. 2010;105:1062–70.

103. Greuter T, Alexander JA, Straumann A, Katzka DA. Diagnostic and therapeutic long-term management of eosinophilic esophagitis—current concepts and perspectives for steroid use. Clin Transl Gastroenterol. 2018;9:e212.
104. Lucendo AJ. Meta-analysis-based guidance for dietary management in eosinophilic esophagitis. Curr Gastroenterol Rep. 2015;17:464.
105. Oliva S, Volpe D, Russo G, Veraldi S, Papoff P, Giordano C, et al. Maintenance therapy with the lowest effective dose of oral viscous budesonide in children with eosinophilic esophagitis. Clin Gastroenterol Hepatol. 2022;20:2905–7.
106. Votto M, De Filippo M, Olivero F, Raffaele A, Cereda E, De Amici M, et al. Malnutrition in eosinophilic gastrointestinal disorders. Nutrients. 2020;13:128.
107. Mehta H, Groetch M, Wang J. Growth and nutritional concerns in children with food allergy. Curr Opin Allergy Clin Immunol. 2013;13:275–9.
108. Schoepfer AM, Safroneeva E, Bussmann C, Kuchen T, Portmann S, Simon HU, et al. Delay in diagnosis of eosinophilic esophagitis increases risk for stricture formation in a time-dependent manner. Gastroenterology. 2013;145:1230–6.
109. Lenti MV, Savarino E, Mauro A, Penagini R, Racca F, Ghisa M, et al. Diagnostic delay and misdiagnosis in eosinophilic oesophagitis. Dig Liver Dis. 2021;53:1632–9.
110. Colson D, Kalach N, Soulaines P, Vannerom Y, Campeotto F, Talbotec C, et al. The impact of dietary therapy on clinical and biologic parameters of pediatric patients with eosinophilic esophagitis. J Allergy Clin Immunol Pract. 2014;2:587–93.
111. Mehta P, Furuta GT, Brennan T, Henry ML, Maune NC, Sundaram SS, et al. Nutritional state and feeding behaviors of children with Eosinophilic Esophagitis and gastroesophageal reflux disease. J Pediatr Gastroenterol Nutr. 2018;66:603–8.
112. Groetch M, Venter C, Skypala I, Vlieg-Boerstra B, Grimshaw K, Durban R, et al. Dietary therapy and nutrition management of eosinophilic esophagitis: a work group report of the American Academy of allergy, asthma, and immunology. J Allergy Clin Immunol Pract. 2017;5:312–24.
113. Votto M, De Filippo M, Lenti MV, Rossi CM, Di Sabatino A, Marseglia GL, et al. Diet therapy in eosinophilic esophagitis. Focus on a personalized approach. Front Pediatr. 2022;9:820192.

16 Urticaria in the Allergic Child

Domenico Minasi, Amelia Licari, and Sara Manti

Abstract

Urticaria is common in children, and it causes frequent medical visits, emergency room accesses, and diagnostic tests. Based on the duration of the illness, urticaria is classified as acute urticaria (AU) (≤ 6 weeks), prevalent in the child, or chronic urticaria (CU) (> 6 weeks). This distinction also reflects the impact of urticaria on the patient's life. The exact pathogenesis of urticaria is still poorly understood, but there is broad consensus in considering urticaria a mast cell-driven disease. In allergic children with food allergy, asthma, or allergic rhinitis, urticaria can occur occasionally or recurrently; it can also be a symptom of an existing clinical condition (e.g., food allergy) or arise independently. A summary of current knowledge of urticaria in allergic children and its management is presented.

Keywords

Urticaria · Children · Comorbidities · Diagnosis · Management · Treatment

Test your learning and check your understanding of this book's contents: use the "Springer Nature Flashcards" app to access questions using ▶ https://sn.pub/nspbjm. To use the app, please follow the instructions in Chap. 1.

16.1 Introduction

Urticaria is common in children, and it causes frequent medical visits, emergency room accesses, and diagnostic tests. Urticaria is characterized by the development of wheals (hives), angioedema, or both. Based on the duration of illness, it is classified as acute urticaria (AU) (≤ 6 weeks), prevalent in children, or chronic (CU) (> 6 weeks). It is further classified as spontaneous or common (up to 70–80% of cases) or inducible when exposure to a specific causal agent induces symptoms onset [1].

Epidemiological data on the prevalence and incidence of urticaria in children are sparse; however, some studies report a prevalence of AU

D. Minasi (✉)
Pediatric Unit, Great Metropolitan Hospital Reggio Calabria, Reggio Calabria, Italy

A. Licari
Pediatric Clinic, Fondazione IRCCS Policlinico San Matteo, University of Pavia, Pavia, Italy

S. Manti
Pediatric Unit, Department of Human Pathology of Adult and Evolutive Age "Gaetano Barresi", University of Messina, Messina, Italy

C. Caffarelli, G. L. Marseglia (eds.), *Textbook of Pediatric Allergy*,
https://doi.org/10.1007/978-3-031-71283-8_16

ranging from 1% to 16.2%, with the highest incidence in infants and preschoolers, while CU presents both the prevalence and the incidence below 1% in children [2, 3]. In allergic children with food allergy, asthma, or allergic rhinitis, urticaria can occur occasionally or recurrently; it can be a symptom of an existing clinical condition (e.g., food allergy) or arise independently.

16.2 Clinical Presentation

Urticaria is a skin eruption characterized by wheals that have a central swelling due to dermal edema, surrounded by erythema, a fleeting nature (each wheal resolves within 24 h, but new lesions may appear) and cause itching or burning sensation. The skin lesions have defined or serpiginous borders, variable distribution, size, and shape (rounded, annular, polycyclic, or geographic). In infants and early childhood, urticaria is typically generalized and presented with annular or geographic plaques in most cases due to the structure of the baby's skin. The infant's skin shows a higher rate of water absorption and desorption than adults; a microvasculature network poorly developed in the first months of life; a decreased cohesion between **the** epidermis and dermis; and a low collagen and elastic fibers content. All these factors may contribute to edema formation in the dermal layer [4].

In AU, the morphology and distribution of the lesions can help define the cause. Linear lesions are typical of dermographism, and small wheals with a large erythematous halo are typical of cholinergic and aquagenic urticarial. In contrast, wheals are more frequently large, round, or multiform in post-infectious urticaria. Angioedema is associated with urticaria in up to 50% of cases [5].

Angioedema is defined as a sudden, pronounced swelling of the submucosal or subcutaneous tissue involving areas like the lips, eyelids, auricles, scrotum, throat, back of the hands, and feet. It is sometimes painful but not itching, and its resolution is slower than for wheals (up to 72 h). Urticaria/angioedema in childhood is not life-threatening, and the prognosis is generally good, but it can significantly impair the quality of life for patients and their families [3].

16.3 Pathophysiology

The exact pathogenesis of urticaria is still poorly understood, but there is broad consensus in considering urticaria a mast cell-driven disease. The activation and degranulation of mast cells, which remains central in the pathophysiological process of urticaria and consequent to the dysregulation of mast cells and basophils, causes the release of inflammatory mediators responsible for the formation of wheals and angioedema [6].

Mast cell activation is a complex process that can be started on an immunological pathway (hypersensitivity (HS) reaction mediated by antibodies and/or cells such as IgE-mediated type I HS reaction but also type II, III, and IV HS reaction) or non-immunological basis, through the interaction between ligand and membrane receptors involved in innate immunity (e.g. complement, toll-like, cytokines, chemokines, opioids) or directly by xenobiotics (haptens, drugs) [7]. Mast cell activation results in the release of histamine and other inflammatory mediators, thus inducing sensory nerve stimulation (pruritus), vasodilatation (erythema), extravasation (edema), and the recruitment of other immune cells (infiltrate). Urticaria without angioedema or pruritus may be caused by non-histaminergic autoinflammatory mechanisms involving the cryopyrin and interleukin (IL)-1 pathway, while non-histaminergic angioedema can be related to bradykinin and fibrinolytic dysregulation, as well as primary defects in vascular integrity [8]. These pathophysiological aspects should be considered to assess and manage the child with urticaria adequately.

16.4 Urticaria and Allergic Rhinitis

In children with pollen-allergic rhinitis, urticaria can occur as part of the Pollen Food Allergy Syndrome (PFAS), an immunoglobulin

E (IgE)-mediated allergic disease caused by a cross-reaction among pollens and vegetable foods [9]. In these children, exposure to raw foods of plant origin that contain cross-antigens for inhaled allergens induces an immune response with activation and degranulation of mast cells, the release of preformed inflammatory mediators, and consequent onset of symptoms. However, clinical manifestations occur only in a subset of pollen-sensitized children. Some patients react to a specific food, while others to multiple foods [10, 11]. Symptoms of PFAS are usually limited to the oropharyngeal mucosa (oral allergy syndrome—OAS), occur immediately, within 5 to 10 min, after consuming fresh fruits, vegetables, nuts, legumes, and seeds, and typically last from a few minutes to half an hour. Symptoms include lip and oropharyngeal pruritus, paresthesia, angioedema of the oral mucosa, lips, tongue, palate, and pharynx, ear pruritus, and laryngeal constriction [12, 13].

Urticaria, associated or not with angioedema or other systemic symptoms, such as nausea, abdominal pain, diarrhea, and hypotension, was highlighted in about 2–10 cases of PFAS, and anaphylaxis in 1–2% [14].

However, it should be noted that since there are no diagnostic tests capable of distinguishing which children may develop a systemic reaction, each oral allergy syndrome must be carefully evaluated because it could be the first symptom of a more severe reaction [15].

A careful evaluation of the clinical history is crucial in diagnosing urticaria related to PFAS. However, the oral food challenge (OFC) is considered the gold standard diagnostic tool in children with suspected food allergies (FAs).

Component-resolved diagnostics (CRD) represents another reliable instrument for diagnosis, as it allows the establishment and comparison of individual sensitization profiles based on cross-reactive proteins.

16.5 Urticaria and Asthma

Asthma and urticaria are partially mediated by increased histamine release from highly activated mast cells; however, they are pathophysiologically different because mast cell degranulation in these two conditions results from different mechanisms. Data on the prevalence of urticaria in allergic asthmatic children are limited. In two pediatric populations studied for the association of asthma with extra-respiratory symptoms, asthma was significantly associated with urticarial in 25.2% of cases [16].

In a recent study conducted to evaluate the incidence and characteristics of urticaria in patients with allergic asthma, urticaria occurred in 23.6% of the enrolled subjects. Particularly, urticaria was significantly more frequent in asthmatic patients with positive skin prick tests for inhalant allergens (mainly seasonal pollens), and it occurred mainly during seasonal asthma exacerbation. The study also found that asthmatics with more severe symptoms were more likely to experience hives. Seasonal allergies could therefore be a link between asthma and hives [17].

16.6 Urticaria and Food Allergy (FA)

FA is an adverse and reproducible immunological response following exposure to a specific food that must be distinct from food intolerance, a non-immune reaction related to metabolic, toxic, pharmacological, or undefined mechanisms. Any food can potentially trigger an allergic reaction [18].

The prevalence of FAs has increased in the last two to three decades and represents a public health problem, especially in industrialized countries. In Europe [19] and the United States [20], 6–8% of children suffer from FAs, respectively.

FAs can be determined by different IgE-mediated, non-IgE-mediated or mixed, IgE- and non-IgE-mediated, immunological reactions.

In IgE-mediated FA, the clinical manifestations appear rapidly after contact with food and result from the release of mediators caused by the activation of dermal mast cells. Mast cells have the high-affinity receptor for IgE on the surface, which can be activated by crosslinking with IgE [18]. Non-IgE-mediated FA is due to T-cell-driven inflammatory responses.

FA symptoms can occur after direct contact with the skin, after inhalation, or, more frequently, after ingesting the allergen. They can lead to a wide range of cutaneous, gastrointestinal, respiratory, cardiovascular, or neurological clinical manifestations. Symptoms can occur singly or concurrently, simultaneously or at different times, ranging from mild local to fatal or near-fatal anaphylaxis [21].

AU is a frequent symptom in children with IgE-mediated FA; however, food allergens have been documented as the cause in less than 7% of all urticaria cases in several studies [22].

When urticaria is triggered by food, it is detectable for a close cause-effect relationship. Characteristically, it occurs within a few hours (max 2 h) from contact/ingestion with the allergen, always occurs every time the child comes into contact/ingestion with the allergen and does not last long. The reactions to alpha-gal content in non-primate mammals meat occur instead after 2–6 h from exposure.

If food allergens cause hives, the most common eliciting foods are milk, eggs, fish, and nuts, but additives, such as Na benzoate, can also be a trigger [23, 24].

Foods such as fish (tuna, sardines), cheeses (emmental), fruits (strawberry), and vegetables (especially tomatoes) can be possible triggers of recurrent urticaria, especially in patients intolerant to histamine or with deficiency of the enzyme diamine oxidase, responsible for histamine degradation [25, 26]. Food allergy is a rare cause of childhood chronic urticarial (CU). In a case series of children with CU, the prevalence of FAvaried from 0% to 8.6% [3].

In the child with FA, a diagnostic workup appears indicated when the clinical history suggests a close relationship with a specific trigger to which the patient was exposed shortly before the onset of urticaria symptoms.

16.7 Treatment

Primarily, treatment for AU should aim to eliminate the triggering agent from the child's body.

The 2nd-generation antihistamines are the first-line treatment of AU, also thanks to their good safety profile [1].

Except for astemizole and terfenadine, 2nd-generation antihistamines, such as cetirizine, desloratadine, fexofenadine, levocetirizine, loratadine, ebastine, rupatadine, and bilastine, are minimally or non-sedating and free of anticholinergic effects. It is suggested regular use of 2nd-generation antihistamines for the treatment of patients with urticaria; conversely, the use of different 2nd-generation antihistamines at the same time should be discouraged [1]. In case of an unsatisfactory response to standard treatment doses, patients with urticaria will benefit from up-dosing of antihistamines up to fourfold.

Systemic corticosteroids are recommended in case of antihistamines ineffectiveness. In the onset of AU, mast cell-released mediators (such as leukotrienes, cytokines, and platelet-activating factor), basophils, lymphocytes, and eosinophils can also be involved. The latter may be relatively refractory to the treatment with antihistamines and require a brief burst of systemic corticosteroid; thus, prednisone or prednisolone may be added for a few days to control symptoms.

In patients unresponsive to high doses of H1-antihistamines, omalizumab, a monoclonal anti-IgE antibody, must be considered a helpful add-on treatment. Dosing is independent of total serum IgE levels; the recommended dose is 300 mg every 4 weeks. It prevents angioedema development, improves quality of life, and is suitable for long-term treatment [1]. Omalizumab is efficacy also in treating cholinergic urticaria, cold or solar urticaria, heat urticaria, dermographism, and delayed pressure urticaria. In light of its lower safety profile and the evidence that it is off-label for urticaria, ciclosporin A should be considered only in patients with severe urticaria refractory to a high dose of antihistamine and omalizumab in combination [1].

The recommended treatment algorithm for urticaria is reported in Fig. 16.1.

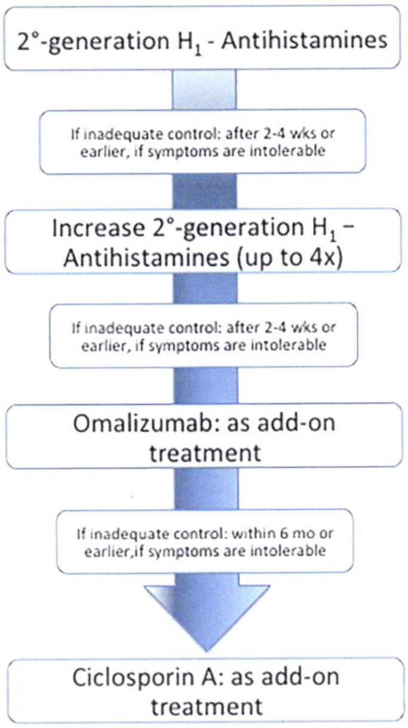

Fig. 16.1 Recommended treatment algorithm for urticaria

References

1. Zuberbier T, Abdul Latiff AH, Abuzakouk M, Aquilina S, Asero R, Baker D, et al. The international EAACI/GA²LEN/EuroGuiDerm/APAAACI guideline for the definition, classification, diagnosis, and management of urticaria. Allergy. 2022;77:734–66.
2. Brüske I, Standl M, Weidinger S, Klümper C, Hoffmann B, Schaaf B, et al. Epidemiology of urticaria in infants and young children in Germany – results from the German LISAplus and GINIplus Birth Cohort Studies. Pediatr Allergy Immunol. 2014;25:36–42.
3. Caffarelli C, Paravati F, El Hachem M, Duse M, Bergamini M, Simeone G, et al. Management of chronic urticaria in children: a clinical guideline. Ital J Pediatr. 2019;45:101.
4. Minasi D, Manti S, Chiera F, Marseglia GL. Marseglia acute urticaria in the infant. Pediatr Allergy Immunol. 2020;31:49–51.
5. Mortureux P, Léauté-Labrèze C, Legrain-Lifermann V, Lamireau T, Sarlangue J, Taïeb A. Acute urticaria in infancy and early childhood: a prospective study. Arch Dermatol. 1998;134:319–23.
6. Saini S, Shams M, Bernstein JA, Maurer M. Urticaria and angioedema across the ages. J Allergy Clin Immunol Pract. 2020;8:1866–74.
7. Hennino A, Bérard F, Guillot I, Saad N, Rozières A, Nicolas JF. Pathophysiology of urticaria. Clin Rev Allergy Immunol. 2006;30:3–11.
8. Huston DP, Sabato V. Decoding the enigma of Urticaria and angioedema. J Allergy Clin Immunol Pract. 2018;6:1171–5.
9. Werfel T, Asero R, Ballmer-Weber BK, Beyer K, Enrique E, Knulst AC, et al. Position paper of the EAACI: food allergy due to immunological cross-reactions with common inhalant allergens. Allergy. 2015;70:1079–90.
10. Kelava N, Lugović-Mihić L, Duvancić T, Romić R, Situm M. Oral allergy syndrome—the need of a multidisciplinary approach. Acta Clin Croat. 2014;53:210–9.
11. Aalberse RC. Structural biology of allergens. J Allergy Clin Immunol. 2000;106:228–38.
12. Mastrorilli C, Cardinale F, Giannetti A, Caffarelli C. Pollen-food allergy syndrome: a not so rare disease in childhood. Medicina (Kaunas). 2019;55:641.
13. Caffarelli C, Coscia A, Baldi F, Borghi A, Capra L, Cazzato S, et al. Characterization of irritable bowel syndrome and constipation in children with allergic diseases. Eur J Pediatr. 2007;166:1245–52.
14. Bedolla-Barajas M, Kestler-Gramajo A, Alcalá-Padilla G, Morales-Romero J. Prevalence of oral allergy syndrome in children with allergic diseases. Allergol Immunopathol (Madr). 2017;45:127–33.
15. Kleine-Tebbe J, Vogel L, Crowell DN, Haustein UF, Vieths S. Severe oral allergy syndrome and anaphylactic reactions caused by a Bet v 1- related PR-10 protein in soybean, SAM22. J Allergy Clin Immunol. 2002;110:797–804.
16. Ronchetti R, Villa MP, Matricardi PM, La Grutta S, Barreto M, Pagani J, et al. Association of asthma with extra-respiratory symptoms in schoolchildren: two cross-sectional studies 6 years apart. Pediatr Allergy Immunol. 2002;13:113–8.
17. Vadasz Z, Kessel A, Hershko AY, Maurer M, Toubi E. Seasonal exacerbation of asthma is frequently associated with recurrent episodes of acute Urticaria. Int Arch Allergy Immunol. 2016;169:263–6.
18. Calvani M, Anania C, Caffarelli C, Martelli A, Miraglia Del Giudice M, Cravidi C, et al. Food allergy: an updated review on pathogenesis, diagnosis, prevention and management. Acta Biomed. 2020;91:e2020012.
19. Nwaru BI, Hickstein L, Panesar SS, Roberts G, Muraro A. Sheikh A, et al. Prevalence of common food allergies in Europe: a systematic review and meta-analysis. Allergy. 2014;69:992–1007.
20. Gupta RS, Springston EE, Warrier MR, Smith B, Kumar R, Pongracic J, et al. The prevalence, severity, and distribution of childhood food allergy in the United States. Pediatrics. 2011;128:e9–17.
21. Cafarotti A, Giovannini M, Begìn P, Brough HA, Arasi S. Management of IgE-mediated food allergy in the 21st century. Clin Exp Allergy. 2023;53:25–38.
22. Ricci G, Giannetti A, Belotti T, Dondi A, Bendandi B, Cipriani F, et al. Allergy is not the main trigger of urticarial in children referred to the emergency room. J Eur Acad Dermatol Venereol. 2010;24:1347–8.

23. Mastrorilli C, Caffarelli C, Hoffmann-Sommergruber K. Food allergy and atopic dermatitis: prediction, progression, and prevention. Pediatr Allergy Immunol. 2017;28:831–40.
24. Tosca MA, Castagnoli R, Brambilla I, Santoro A, Procaccianti M, Giannetti A, et al. Urticaria in childhood. Acta Biomed. 2020;91:e2020013.
25. Kudryavtseva AV, Neskorodova KA, Staubach P. Urticaria in children andadolescents: an updated review of the pathogenesis and management. Pediatr Allergy Immunol. 2019;30:17–24.
26. Ensina LF, Min TK, Félix MMR, de Alcântara CT, Costa C. Acute Urticaria and anaphylaxis: differences and similarities in clinical management. Front Allergy. 2022;3:840999.

17 Angioedema in the Pediatric Population: A Practical Approach

Mauro Cancian and Riccardo Senter

Abstract

Angioedema is characterized by subcutaneous and submucosal accumulation of fluids caused by increased permeability of vascular endothelium.

In most cases, especially in pediatric age, the swelling is caused by the release of histamine and other vasoactive molecules by mast cells, both when it is associated with urticaria and when isolated.

However, there are also forms mediated by bradykinin, including hereditary angioedema (HAE) due to C1-INH deficiency. This is a rare genetic disease that typically begins in childhood and is not always promptly identified. New variants of HAE with normal levels of C1INH have been discovered in recent years, whilst other mutations still remain unknown.

This chapter aims to provide a practical approach to the differential diagnosis of angioedema without wheals, with particular regard to the pediatric population and to the main therapeutic indications in these forms.

Keywords

Angioedema · Hereditary angioedema · Mast cell · Pediatric · Contact system · C1 Inhibitor · Bradykinin · ITACA · Berotralstat · Icatibant · Lanadelumab · pdC1INH · hrC1INH

Test your learning and check your understanding of this book's contents: use the "Springer Nature Flashcards" app to access questions using ▶ https://sn.pub/nspbjm. To use the app, please follow the instructions in Chap. 1.

17.1 Angioedema Classification

Edema is defined as swelling due to the abnormal presence of fluid in the tissues of the body, which may be associated to various conditions including renal, cardiac, vascular, hepatic, endocrine, or lymphatic diseases [1].

The word ***angioedema*** (AE) derives from the combination of two terms from ancient Greek, αγγείον (vessel) and οίδημα (edema). This immediately indicates that it is an endothelial disorder, different from edema of other origins where the leakage of plasma into the interstitial space is primarily governed by oncotic pressures

M. Cancian (✉) · R. Senter
Department of Systems Medicine, Azienda Ospedale Università di Padova, Padua, Italy
e-mail: mcancian@unipd.it

C. Caffarelli, G. L. Marseglia (eds.), *Textbook of Pediatric Allergy*,
https://doi.org/10.1007/978-3-031-71283-8_17

and Starling's laws. In these cases, fluid accumulation has a territorial distribution and can occur, for example, in the distal parts of the lower limbs or intraperitoneally, depending on the causes. In angioedema, first described in 1586 by Marcello Donati in De medica historia mirabili, the subcutaneous tissue of any district (limbs, face, genitals, etc.) and the mucosa/submucosa of the gastrointestinal, urogenital, and respiratory systems can be affected. In rare cases, involvement of the brain can also occur (Fig. 17.1) [1–3].

The classification of angioedema can be approached from various perspectives, all of which are useful in understanding a condition that can be isolated or associated and overlap with other diseases. The term angioedema, indeed, simply identifies a condition in which increased endothelial permeability leads to the leakage of plasma from the microcirculation. It is therefore necessary to differentiate the mechanisms of endothelial activation in order to identify the different mediators and prescribe specific therapies (Fig. 17.2).

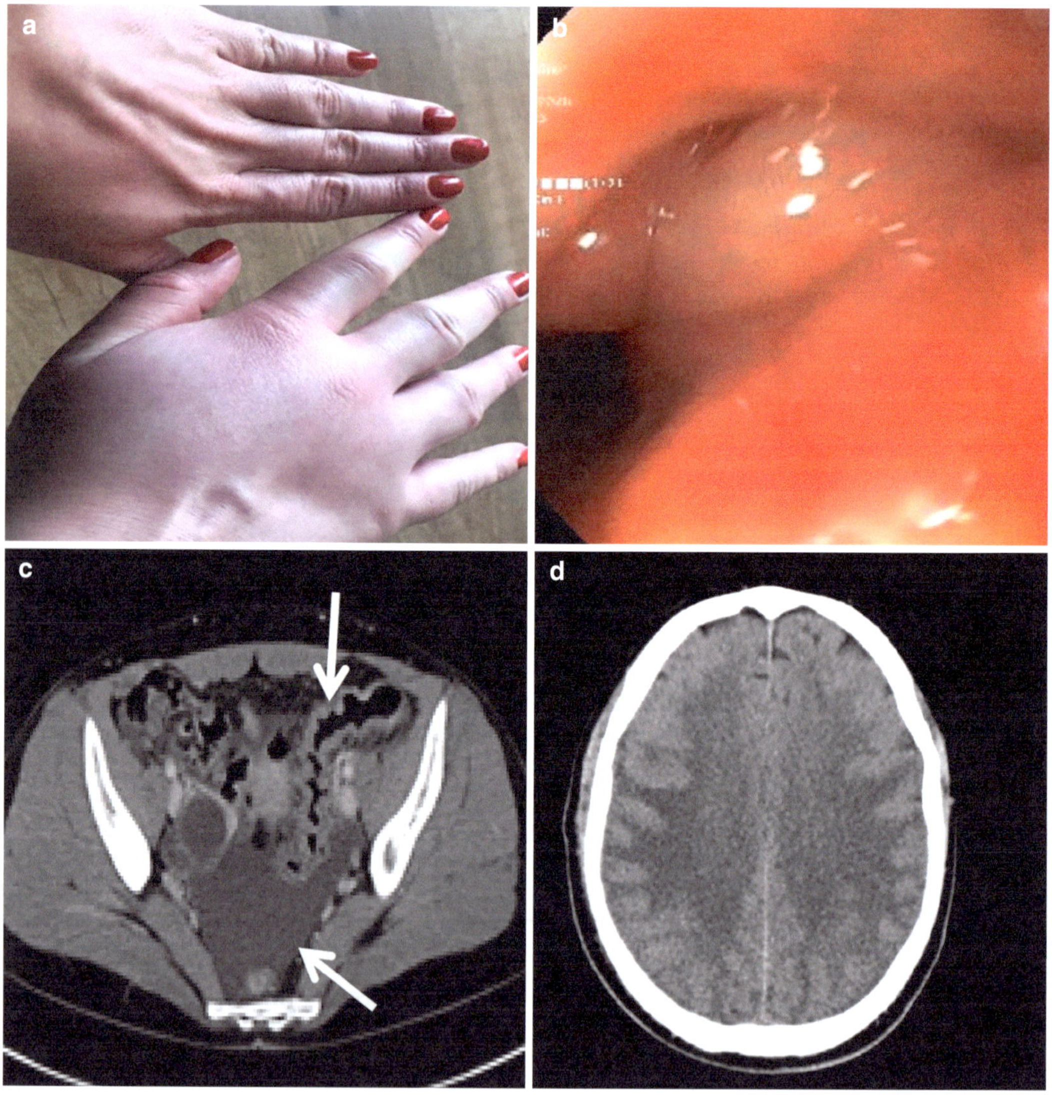

Fig. 17.1 Subcutaneous (**a**), Laryngeal (**b**), Abdominal (**c**) and Cerebral (**d**) Angioedema. Personal cases series

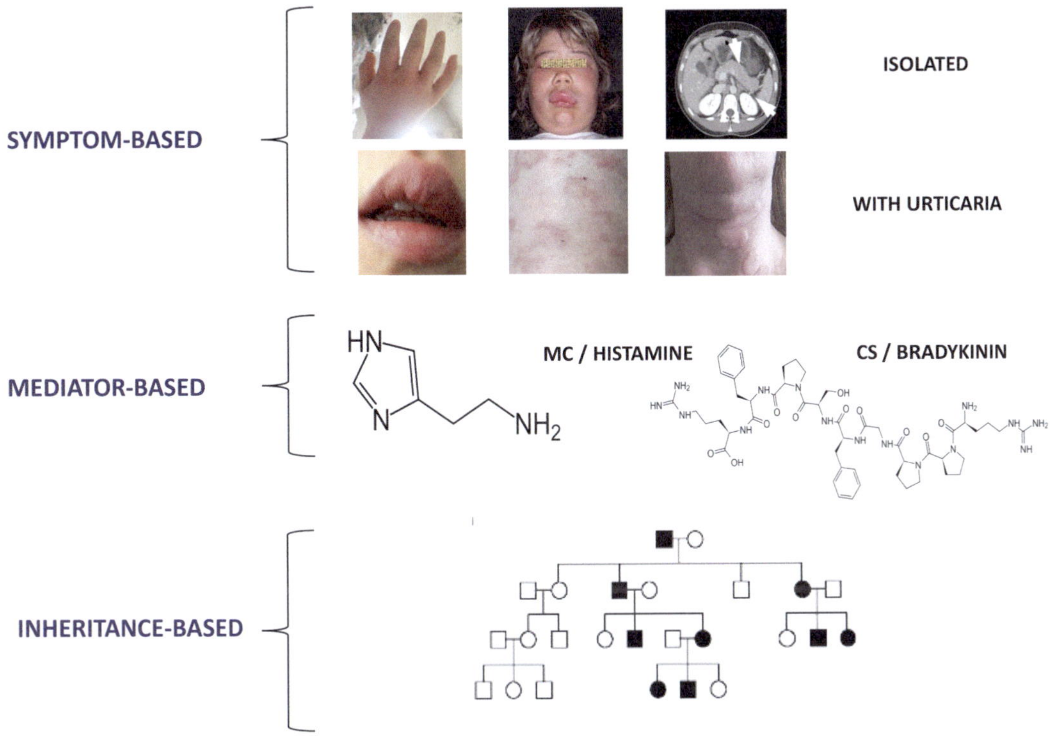

Fig. 17.2 Practical approach to discriminate among different forms of angioedema. *MC* Mast cell, *CS* Contact system. Personal cases series

The first approach is based on symptoms, determining whether angioedema occurs in an isolated manner, "primary angioedema," or if it is associated or alternates with wheals [4–8]. This distinction is very useful from a practical point of view, because:

- In the majority of cases, angioedema is associated with urticaria [9, 10].
- When urticaria is present, whether acute or chronic, and whether allergic, inducible or spontaneous, the final event is always mast cell (MC) activation leading to release of histamine and other mediators [11, 12].

Urticaria, which involves the epidermis and superficial layers of the dermis, is pruritic and tends to regress rapidly with the use of antihistamines and corticosteroids. In angioedema, which affects deeper layers, itching is absent, and there is a sensation of tension and pain. Although mediated by mast cells, angioedema regresses more slowly with antiallergic medications compared to urticaria, as the amount of fluid present is much larger and reabsorption occurs through the lymphatic vessels [4, 6, 8–10].

Angioedema associated or alternating with urticaria, which represents the most common variant of AE in adults and even more in the pediatric population, is always a variant of urticaria and should be diagnosed and treated according to international guidelines, as explained in detail in the chapter dedicated to urticaria in this book [13, 14].

The second approach aims to identify the final mediator of AE. In angioedema associated with urticaria, this is not challenging because, as emphasized, MC are always the effector cells. In isolated AE, on the other hand, in addition to histamine and other preformed or newly formed mast cell mediators, such as Platelet Activating Factors, leukotrienes, and cytokines, ***bradykinin*** (BK) may be involved. Bradykinin is a small vasoactive peptide identified while studying

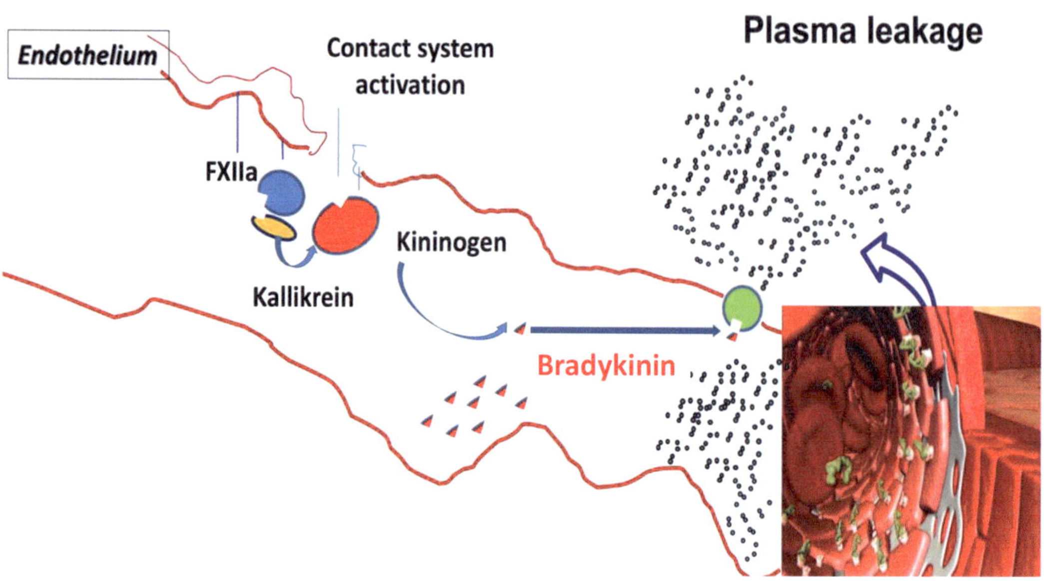

Fig. 17.3 Bradykinin-mediated angioedema. *FXIIa* Factor XII activated

snake venom and initially called a slow-reacting substance of anaphylaxis. Circulating BK, produced by activation of the contact system, causes plasma leakage from blood vessels by activating the endothelial BKβ2 receptor (Fig. 17.3) [15, 16]. Acute episodes of bradykinin-mediated angioedema, which are much less common than histamine-mediated ones, are refractory to antiallergic therapy (antihistamines, steroids, epinephrine) and should be treated with drugs that antagonize bradykinin production (plasma-derived or recombinant C1-inhibitor concentrates, kallikrein antagonists) or block its receptor (icatibant) [17–19].

Unfortunately, we do not have clinically useful biomarkers that can help in distinguishing between MC-mediated and BK-mediated angioedema on acute attacks: serum tryptase, which represents a specific marker of MC degranulation, is typically not increased in histaminergic angioedema probably because of the relatively small number of cells involved. On the opposite versant, the short half-life and very low plasma concentrations of bradykinin do not allow to demonstrate contact system activation [12, 16].

Therefore, as the reabsorption of fluids in angioedema of any origin can take several hours even with appropriate therapy, in cases of recurrent, primary idiopathic angioedema the only strategy to identify the type of angioedema with reasonable accuracy is the response to continuative prophylaxis. If angioedema responds to continuous administration of antihistamines or, if uneffective, to omalizumab, it can be classified as MC-mediated. Otherwise, it can be presumed to be BK-induced [13, 14, 18, 19].

The third classification criterion is based on the hereditary nature of angioedema. If there is a hereditary pattern, which in the case of angioedema is autosomal dominant with variable penetrance, a MC-mediated form can be excluded and any efforts should be addressed to differentiate between hereditary angioedema (HAE) caused by C1INH deficiency (C1INH-HAE) and HAE with normal C1-INH [19–22].

This approach, which reflects the Hereditary Angioedema Working Group's classification of angioedema, still represents the most practical, comprehensive, and educational way to deal with AE (Fig. 17.4) [23].

However, a new classification has recently been proposed, the DANCE project promoted by the international AE network ACARE, which divides angioedema into five categories: (1) MC-mediated, (2) BK-mediated, (3) caused by vascular endothelium dysfunction, (4) drug-

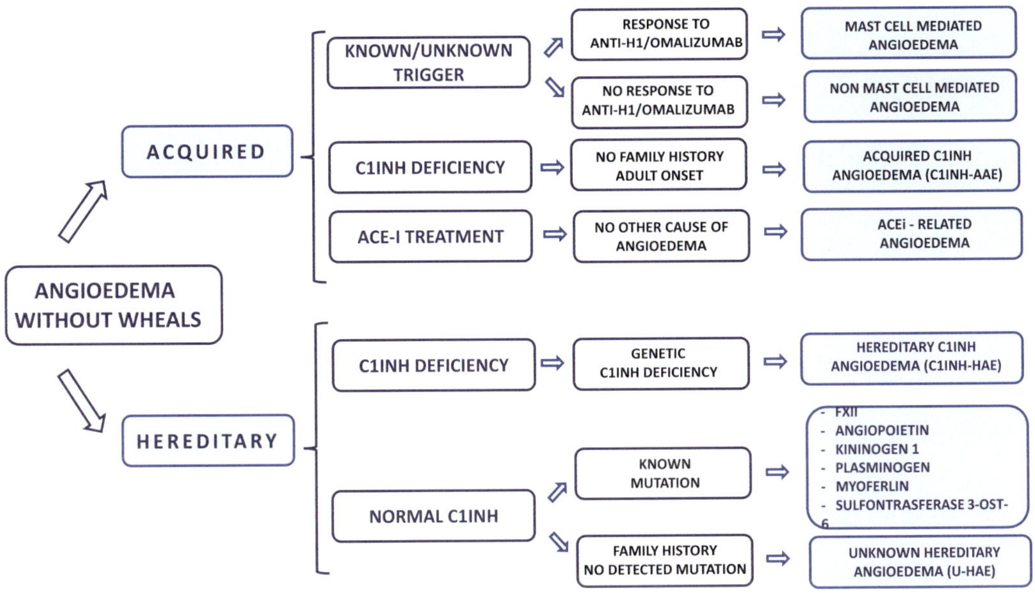

Fig. 17.4 Angioedema classification (Modified from Ref. [23]). *FXII* Factor XII, *C1INH* C1 Inhibitor, *HAE* Hereditary angioedema, *AAE* Acquired angioedema, *ACEi* Angiotensin converting enzyme inhibitor, *H1* Histamine H1 receptor

induced, and (5) unknown origin/mechanism. Although this classification is less intuitive and presents overlaps mixing endotypes (types 1–3) with triggers (type 4, where the pathogenic mechanisms vary depending on the drugs involved), it will likely become the future reference for the nomenclature of angioedema [24].

17.2 Mast Cell-Mediated, Pediatric Angioedema Without Wheals

Although in childhood angioedema associated with urticaria is much more common than primary angioedema, the latter can still occur in the pediatric population with an incidence that is not well known [5].

In most cases, it is an IgE-mediated, type 1 hypersensitivity reaction. The most common allergens in children are foods, followed by medications and, to a lesser extent, insect stings. Usually, the temporal relationship between exposure to the stimulus and the onset of symptoms guides the diagnosis, which can be further investigated by classic diagnostic methods: prick tests; prick-by-prick tests with fresh foods; intradermal tests for medications; specific IgE testing (ImmunoCAP®, ISAC Panel®, ALEX Test®); basophil activation test; provocation tests, etc. [25, 26]

The mast cell and basophil, whose contribution is likely more significant in other forms of allergy than in AE, can also be activated by other immunological mechanisms (autoimmunity, immune complexes) or in a non-immune-mediated manner (physical stimuli; direct degranulation by contrast media, muscle relaxants, or other medications; spontaneous activation) (Fig. 17.5): this complicates the differential diagnosis, as except for physical forms diagnostic methods are more limited and less standardized.

A further possibility to be considered is angioedema induced by nonsteroidal anti-inflammatory drugs (NSAIDs), which is a common symptom of adverse drug reaction to this therapeutic class in children. ***NSAID hypersensitivity*** is likely correlated with a defect in the cyclooxygenase metabolic pathway, which probably causes an increase in proinflammatory cysteinyl leukotrienes. The diagnosis is exclusively clinical, and potential cross-reactivity among different NSAIDs should always be taken into account [27–29].

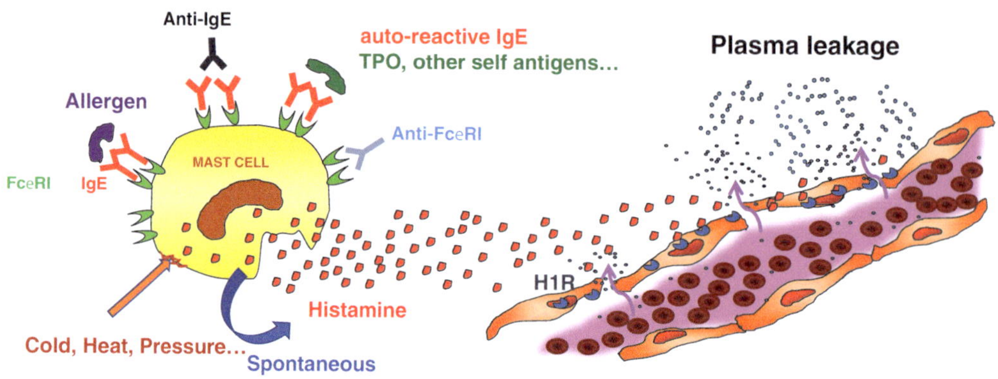

Fig. 17.5 Mast cell-mediated angioedema. *FcεRI* high affinity receptor for IgE, *H1* Histamine H1 receptor, *TPO* Thyroperoxidase

In pediatric age, more frequently than in adults, angioedema may also be caused by ***viral or bacterial infections*** and the suspicion arises from the presence of systemic symptoms (fever, arthralgia, myalgia, headache, general malaise, etc.). Mast cells are likely involved to a lesser extent, for example, by anaphylatoxins C3a and C5a activated by circulating immune complexes, while cytokines and other proinflammatory mediators often play a role [5, 10, 19, 30].

In any case, regardless of the stimuli and individual pathogenetic mechanisms, MC-mediated angioedema tends to persist less than those of other origins and respond, especially in children, to symptomatic therapy. AE is rarely part of an anaphylactic reaction, but if the upper airways are involved, maintaining their patency should always be the main goal [31]. In recurrent idiopathic forms, where specific biomarkers do not exist, the response to antihistamine prophylaxis or omalizumab represents the most valid diagnostic criterion to assess if mast cells are involved [18].

17.3 Hereditary Angioedema Due to C1-Inhibitor Deficiency in the Pediatric Population

The first cases of angioedema in the modern era of medicine had been reported by Henrick Quincke, who identified family clusters with this complaint in 1892 [32]. As reviewed by Reshef et al. [3], in the following years Sir William Osler defined this disease as angioneurotic edema, thus underlining the origin of swelling from blood vessel but without any evidence of organic causes.

After that, Crowder and Crowder demonstrated the autosomal dominant transmission, and it took about a century before Virginia Donaldson identified ***C1INH deficiency*** as the cause of the disease in 1964, and Erich Nussberger bradykinin as the final mediator in 1998.

Finally, in the last two decades, six new variants of angioedema with normal C1INH have been discovered, and hereditary forms of angioedema of unknown origin still exist [21, 22].

C1INH is a protease inhibitor belonging to the serpin family, which blocks the activation of the complement cascade and also exerts many actions on the contact system (Fig. 17.6): in particular, it inhibits the enzymatic activity of kallikrein and thus the generation of bradykinin from high molecular weight kininogen [33–35]. Reduced or absent C1INH activity results therefore in increased BK production, predisposing to plasma leakage from the microcirculation [36, 37]. When an additional stimulus locally activates the contact system, plasma leaks from the capillary and elicits angioedema.

Painful swelling and functional limitation are observed when subcutaneous tissue is affected; gastrointestinal and urogenital angioedema elicits abdominal colic, which may mimic an acute abdomen and lead to inappropriate surgery;

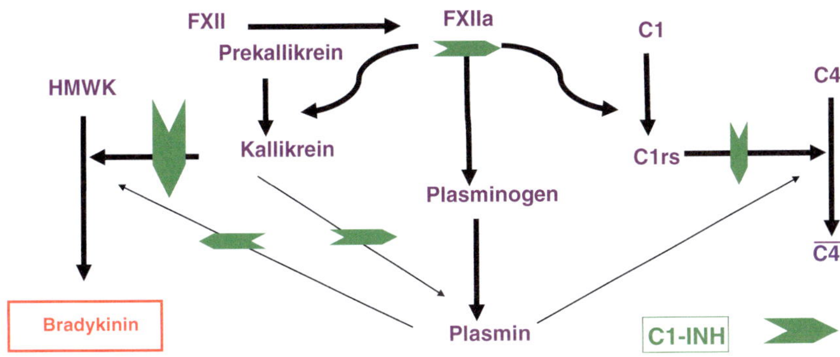

Fig. 17.6 C1-Inhibitor activity. *FXII* Factor XII, *FXIIa* Factor XII activated, *C1INH* C1 Inhibitor, *C* Complement, *HMWK* High molecular weight kininogen

Table 17.1 Complement assessment in hereditary angioedema due to C1-inhibitor deficiency

C1INH-HAE	C1INH	C1INH	C4	C3	C1q
Type	Quantitative	Functional	Quantitative	Quantitative	Quantitative
Type I HAE	<50%	<50%	Reduced	Normal	Normal
Type II HAE	>50%	<50%	Reduced	Normal	Normal

C1INH C1 Inhibitor, *C* Complement, *HAE* Hereditary angioedema

laryngeal attacks are dramatic, life-threatening events [38–41].

Although trauma, surgery, airway endoscopy, dental procedures, and stressful conditions may favor angioedema onset, in most cases, acute attacks occur spontaneously due to local activation of the contact system by unknown triggers.

Patients sometimes experience prodromes as nonitching ***erythema marginatum***, irritability, sense of hunger, asthenia, or other symptoms, but in many cases, there are no presaging signs [42–44].

Hereditary angioedema caused by a deficiency of C1-inhibitor is a ***rare disease*** with an estimated prevalence of 1 in 50,000 [45–51]. It can be presented in two different forms:

1. C1INH-HAE Type 1, which accounts for 85% of cases, is characterized by absent or reduced production of C1-inhibitor (lacking protein).
2. C1INH-HAE Type 2, less common (15%), is characterized by normal or even increased synthesis of C1-inhibitor, which lacks inhibitory activity (dysfunctional protein) [17, 38].

The pattern of autosomal dominant inheritance and the clinical characteristics are identical in both types, whilst the diagnostic approach differs: while in type 1, it is sufficient to demonstrate a quantitative deficit of C1INH, in type 2, it is necessary to verify its functional activity by enzyme-linked immunosorbent or chromogenic assays, with the last one showing higher sensitivity and specificity [17, 19, 38, 52–54]. As a first-level screening test, or when C1INH assessment is not available, measuring the concentration of plasma C4 is very useful as its levels are reduced in around 95% of patients with C1INH deficiency (Table 17.1) [19, 49, 54, 55].

Special attention should be given to interpreting assays in the first year of life, when the complement system is still immature and an excessively early assay could lead to false positives [56, 57]. Thus in infancy, as well as in rare case of doubt and for prenatal (chorionic villous sampling or amniocentesis) or preimplantation diagnosis of HAE, mutational analysis of Serping1—the gene on chromosome 11 that encodes for C1INH—may be considered [19, 21, 55–59].

Finally, it should always be considered that the term 'hereditary' means that the disease can be transmitted to offspring, but not necessarily that a parent of a patient is affected. De novo mutations,

Table 17.2 ITACA Survey on pediatric population with hereditary angioedema

Study population and findings	Male	Female
Numerosity: 76 subjects from 66 independent families	44 (57.9%)	32 (42.1%)
Age: mean, years (SD): 11.7 (4.88), range 2–21	12.5 (4.8)	10.6 (4.61)
Age of onset: median, years (IQR): 4 (2–7.5)	3 (2–7.5)	4 (2.25–6.75)
Age at diagnosis (n = 64): median, years (IQR): 4(2–8)	4 (2.5–8)	3.5 (2–6.25)
Diagnosis delay among the already symptomatic (n = 35): median, years (IQR): 1 (1–3)	1 (1–3)	1 (1–2.75)
Plasma C1INH function (n = 55): median, % (SD) = 23.63 ± 16.56%, range 0–57.3%	24.6 (18)	24.7 (15.3)
Plasma C4 level (n = 49) mean±SD = 0.06±0.02, range 0.01–0.13	0.056 (0.02)	0.064 (0.02)
At least one attack during life (%): 59/76 (77.6)	36/44 (81.8)	23/32 (71.9)
At least one treated attack during life (n = 62; %): 48/62 (77.4)	28/37 (75.8)	20/25 (80)
Long-term prophylaxis (%): 6 (7.9)	5 (11.4)	1 (3.2)
Probands (%): 3(3.9)	3 (6.81)	0 (0)
Number of attacks in the reference period: median (IQR): 2.5 (0–8)	4 (0–8)	1 (0–7.75)

C1INH C1 inhibitor, *SD* Standard deviation, *IQR* interquartile range

in fact, represent 20% of C1-INH-HAE cases, and whilst a positive family history strengthens the diagnostic suspicion, a negative familial anamnesis does not exclude it [19, 20, 55].

Although the diagnosis of C1-INH-HAE is not particularly complex, and new tools and networks may now support centers lacking the proper facilities, the diagnostic delay is still significant, especially in individuals with type 2 C1INH-HAE and/or no family history. The negative consequences of this delay are particularly relevant, considering the severity of symptoms and the fact that hereditary angioedema has pediatric onset, as typical of most congenital diseases [49, 56, 57, 60–64].

Onset of swelling has been indeed reported to present mostly in childhood, with median age of first episode ranging from 5 to 11 years and mean diagnostic age of diagnosis and diagnostic delay highly variable in different surveys [65–69].

A recent survey by the ***Italian Network for Hereditary and Acquired Angioedema*** (ITACA, www.angioedemaitaca.org) evaluated 76 HAE patients from 66 independent families, ranging in age from 2 to 21 years and referring to the Centers of Reference of Civitanova Marche, Genoa, Milan, Padua, Palermo, Pescara, Naples, and Rome.

Retrospective data on family history, disease onset, symptom localization, number of attacks within a homogeneous one-year period, and other characteristics were collected through interviews with patients or their parents and by aggregating data entered into the ***ITACA disease registry***, approved by local ethics committees.

The demographic characteristics of the cohort and the main findings are reported in Table 17.2: it is noteworthy that 78% of the young patients had experienced and treated at least one attack in their lifetime, with some of them having suffered from several acute episodes during the observation period. The diagnostic delay was less significant compared to previous reports, but it was confirmed to be higher in de novo mutations compared to children of parents with diagnosed disease (unpublished data).

Interestingly, adolescents or parents of younger patients mostly reported subcutaneous localization as the site of angioedema onset, while abdominal attacks were by far the most frequent during the 12-month observation period (Fig. 17.7). This is likely due to the fact that abdominal discomfort is very common in the pediatric population, and it is usually interpreted as a form of infectious or functional gastrointestinal disorder.

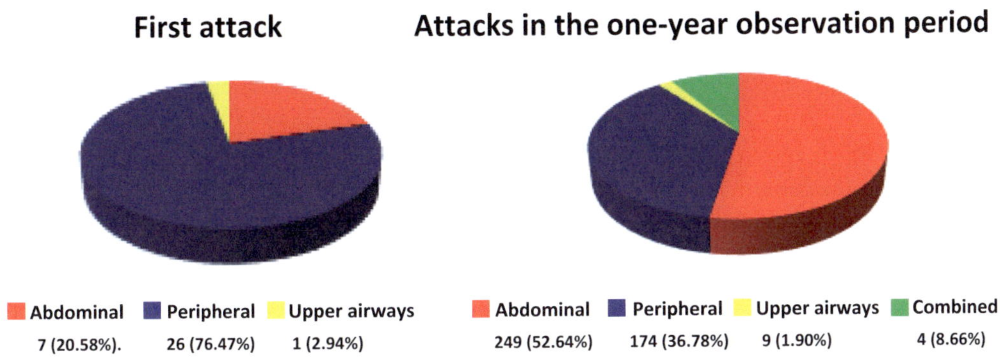

Fig. 17.7 ITACA survey: attacks location in a pediatric population with Hereditary angioedema. The proportion of abdominal and subcutaneous attacks were different between the first attack reported and the attacks recorded in the one-year observation period ($p < 0{,}001$)

Puberty appears to represent a turning point in the course of the disease, as shown by a multicenter study conducted by ITACA reporting that the proportion of symptomatic patients increased significantly after puberty in both males and females. Moreover, the numbers of acute attacks were significantly higher after ***puberty*** when comparing both one-year and three-year periods pre/after menarche/semenarche. Symptom worsening after puberty occurred to a greater extent in female subjects than in males: this is related to hormonal factors, and it is well known that estrogens can trigger or worsen angioedema unlike progestins, which can be used in women with C1-INH-HAE and which according to some authors might even exert a protective effect [19, 20, 55]. On the contrary, there was no significant variation in the location of the attacks, which were reported mostly as abdominal and subcutaneous, both before and after puberty by both genders [70].

All these data highlight the importance of early diagnosis of pediatric C1INH-HAE, allowing patients to be treated as soon as possible with the specific drugs that are now numerous and suitable for every condition and age group, as resumed in Table 17.3. The main goal remains to prevent mortality caused by laryngeal attacks and reduce the subcutaneous, gastrointestinal, and urogenital symptoms of acute episodes through on-demand treatment (ODT) with bradykinin receptor antagonists (icatibant) and plasma-derived or human-recombinant C1-inhibitor concentrates (pdC1INH and hrC1INH, respectively). Additionally, short-term prophylaxis (STP) with pdC1INH shortly before events predisposing to angioedema, such as surgery, airway endoscopy, and invasive dental procedures, can also be planned [19, 71, 72].

Nevertheless, the unpredictable nature of acute episodes and their negative consequences on normal daily, school, and social activities contribute to a significant disease burden and reduced Quality of Life (QoL) for both the young patients and their parents, relatives, and care-givers [73–75].

Thus, the most recent guidelines recommend, when appropriate, the use of long-term prophylaxis (LTP) with subcutaneous or intravenous pdC1INH concentrates, as well as of subcutaneous (lanadelumab) or oral (berotralstat) kallikrein antagonists, to prevent angioedema attacks and ideally eliminate the overall impact of the disease (before the advent of specific medications, tranexamic acid was frequently used in children, while attenuated androgens have always been contraindicate) [19, 71, 72].

In parallel, many other innovative drugs are at present on pipeline, targeted to every level of the contact system pathway up to Factor XII. Genetic therapy is also being considered [76].

Table 17.3 Therapy of hereditary angioedema in Europe

Marketed Brand	Drug	Posology	Route/Interval of administration	Therapeutic Indications*	Age Restrictions**
Berinert	pd-C1INH	20 IU/kg 60 IU/Kg	i.v./on occasion s.c./twice a week	OD/STP LTP	None ≧12 years
Cinryze	pd-C1INH	1000 IU	i.v./on occasion i.v./twice a week	OD/STP LTP	≧2 years
Rhucin	Conestat alfa hr-C1INH	50 IU/kg 4200 IU if BW > 84 kg	i.v./on occasion	OD	≧2 years
Firazyr generics	Icatibant	10–30 mg/1–3 ml weight based	s.c./on occasion	OD	≧2 years
Takhzyro	Lanadelumab	300 mg/2 ml	s.c./every 2–4 weeks	LTP	≧12 years
Orladeyo	Berotralstat	150 mg per day	oral/daily	LTP	≧12 years
various generics	Tranexamic acid	Approximately 20 mg per kg per day	oral/daily	LTP	≧1 years***
Danazol generics	Danazolol	<200 mg per day	oral/daily	LTP	≧16 years***

C1INH C1 inhibitor, *pd* plasma derived, *hr* human recombinant, *BW* body weight, *s.c.* subcutaneous, *i.v.* intravenous, *OD* on demand, *STP* short-term prophylaxis, *LTP* long-term prophylaxis, *IU* international unit
*special limitations for pregnancy and lactation
**age restrictions may vary among different countries
***off-label in some countries

17.4 Hereditary Angioedema With Normal C1INH

In recent years, at least six additional forms of hereditary angioedema (HAE) not caused by antigenic or functional deficiency of C1-INH have been identified, starting with the mutation of ***Factor XII*** which is the most common one [21, 22].

There are no specific biomarkers for these variants, which can only be diagnosed by demonstrating the genetic defect. Penetrance is lower compared to C1INH-HAE and particularly in Factor XII mutations, of which we have greater experience and a substantial case series available; symptoms seem to be hormone-dependent presenting mostly in women, especially after puberty and/or after the introduction of estrogen-containing contraceptive pill [22, 77].

Although we have no method available to measure BK plasma levels, bradykinin is hypothesized to be the final mediator in the majority of these variants, while in others, an endothelial defect might be underlying the disease [22, 24].

In any case, since specific therapies are not yet available, patients are treated with the same therapies and strategies used for C1INH-HAE [19, 22].

17.5 Acquired Angioedema Due to C1INH Deficiency

Much rarer than hereditary angioedema, with a prevalence of approximately 1 in 500,000, acquired C1-INH deficiency (C1INH-AAE) can also be observed. There are no genetic deficiencies, and the disease is not hereditary. In addition to a reduction in C4 and C1INH antigen and functional levels, there is often a decrease in circulating C1q. In some cases, anti-C1INH antibodies may also be found [78].

These forms are associated with autoimmune disorders, particularly systemic lupus erythematosus, or proliferative diseases (monoclonal gammopathies, marginal zone lymphomas) that may precede or follow the detection of C1INH deficiency. Onset occurs in adulthood, and therefore they are not of primary interest in pediatrics [78].

C1INH-AAE is treated similarly to hereditary forms of C1INH deficiency, and after addressing the underlying pathology, the angioedema typically regresses [19, 78].

17.6 Drug-Induced, Bradykinin-Mediated Angioedema

The half-life of bradykinin is very short, as it is rapidly degraded by specific proteases among which ***angiotensin-converting enzyme*** (ACE) is the main one. This explains why ACE inhibitors (ACEi) can induce or predispose to angioedema even years after their introduction in therapy, and why along with estrogens ACEi are absolutely contraindicated in hereditary angioedema, in acquired C1INH deficiency and in patients with recurrent angioedema of unknown origin [79].

The diagnosis is based on clinical evaluation since there are no specific diagnostic tests. Other drugs such as angiotensin receptor blockers (sartans), dipeptidyl peptidase-4 inhibitors (gliptins), and neprilysin inhibitors are suspected of causing angioedema through bradykinin. However, as their therapeutic indications primarily concern adults, analysis of adverse effects induced by these drugs is beyond the scope of this chapter [79, 80].

17.7 Idiopathic Angioedema (Angioedema of Unknown Origin)

Even after a careful assessment, some patients with angioedema can still not be included in any of the above-described categories. This applies especially to adults and children with recurrent angioedema and no family history, who do not show alterations in C1 inhibitor functional activity, in whom genetic mutations potentially related to angioedema are absent and who do not respond to either antihistamines or omalizumab.

Current research on angioedema is particularly focused on this class of patients, aiming to identify new AE variants and therapies more effective than the anecdotal ones, including tranexamic acid or anti-leukotrienes, usually prescribed in these cases.

Key Points

- Angioedema is defined as subcutaneous or submucosal swelling resulting from increased endothelium permeability, which in most cases—especially in pediatric age—is elicited by histamine and other mediators released by mast cells.
- Less frequently, angioedema is caused by a vasoactive peptide, bradykinin, produced through activation of the contact system.
- Bradykinin-mediated angioedema include hereditary angioedema caused by C1 inhibitor deficiency, a disease that typically begins in childhood and can affect the subcutaneous tissue and mucous membranes of the upper airways, gastrointestinal tract, and genitourinary system.
- This is an autosomal dominant-inherited disease, easily diagnosable by assessing plasma levels of C4 and functional and antigenic C1 inhibitor. Specific therapies are available for on-demand use and short- and long-term prophylaxis.

Take-Home Messages

- Primary angioedema, in which no wheal occurs, is usually elicited by histamine and other mediators released by mast cell upon allergic or non-allergic activation.
- When angioedema in childhood is refractory to antihistamines and steroids, bradykinin-mediated, hereditary angioedema should be suspected even if family history is negative.
- The first diagnostic step in hereditary angioedema is to assess complement levels (C4, antigen and functional C1 inhibitor). Serping1 gene-analysis may

(continued)

be helpful in case of doubts or in infancy, when the complement system is still immature. In subjects with a positive familial anamnesis and normal levels of circulating C4 and C1INH, genetic assessment of the known mutations is mandatory.

- Diagnostic accuracy is essential to enable patients to receive specific therapy currently available: plasma-derived or human recombinant C1INH concentrates; BK2-receptor antagonist icatibant; kallikrein antagonists (berotralstat and lanadelumab).

References

1. Leung AK, Robson WL. Oedema in children. J R Soc Promot Heal. 2000;120:212–9.
2. Mansi M, Zanichelli A, Coerezza A, Suffritti C, Wu MA, Vacchini R, et al. Presentation, diagnosis and treatment of angioedema without wheals: a retrospective analysis of a cohort of 1058 patients. J Intern Med. 2015;277:585–93.
3. Reshef A, Kidon M, Leibovich I. The story of angioedema: from Quincke to bradykinin. Clin Rev Allerg Immunol. 2016;51:121–39.
4. Kesh S, Bernstein J. Isolated angioedema: a review of classification and update on management. Ann Allergy Asthma Immunol. 2022;129:692–702.
5. Liotti L, Pecoraro L, Mastrorilli C, Castagnoli R, Saretta F, Mori F, et al. Pediatric angioedema without wheals: how to guide the diagnosis. E Life. 2023;13:1021.
6. Kudryavtseva AV, Neskorodova KA, Staubach P. Urticaria in children and adolescents: an updated review of the pathogenesis and management. Pediatr Allergy Immunol. 2019;30:17–24.
7. Riedl M, Maurer M. The road to better urticaria and angioedema management. J Allergy Clin Immunol Pract. 2021;9:2243–4.
8. Guo C, Saltoun C. Urticaria and angioedema. Allergy Asthma Proc. 2019;40:437–40.
9. Pier J, Bingemann TA. Urticaria, angioedema, and anaphylaxis. Pediatr Rev. 2020;41:283–92.
10. Pattanaik D, Lieberman JA. Pediatric angioedema. Curr Allergy Asthma Rep. 2017;17:60.
11. Kolkhir P, Giménez-Arnau AM, Kulthanan K, Peter J, Metz M, Maurer M. Urticaria. Nat Rev Dis Primers. 2022;8:61.
12. Elieh Ali Komi D, Wöhrl S, Bielory L. Mast cell biology at molecular level: a comprehensive review. Clin Rev Allergy Immunol. 2020;58:342–65.
13. Zuberbier T, Latiff AHM, Abuzakouk M, Aquilina S, Asero R, Baker D, et al. The international EAACI/GA²LEN/EuroGuiDerm/APAAACI guideline for the definition, classification, diagnosis, and management of urticaria. Allergy. 2022;77:734–66.
14. Tsabouri S, Arasi S, Beken B, Church MK, Alvaro-Lozano M, Caffarelli C et al. A European survey of management approaches in chronic urticaria in children: EAACI pediatric urticaria taskforce. Pediatr Allergy Immunol. 2022;33:e13674.
15. Long AT, Kenne E, Jung R, Fuchs TA, Renné T. Contact system revised: an interface between inflammation, coagulation, and innate immunity. J Thromb Haemost. 2016;14:427–37.
16. Hofman Z, de Maat S, Hack CE, Maas C. Bradykinin: inflammatory product of the coagulation system. Clin Rev Allergy Immunol. 2016;51:152–61.
17. Cicardi M, Zuraw BL. Angioedema due to bradikynin dysregulation. J Allergy Clin Immunol Pract. 2018;6:1132–41.
18. Maurer M, Magerl M. Differences and similarities in the mechanisms and clinical expression of bradykinin-mediated vs. Mast cell-mediated angioedema. Clin Rev Allergy Immunol. 2021;61:40–9.
19. Maurer M, Magerl M, Betschel S, Aberer W, Ansotegui IJ, Aygören-Pürsün E et al. The international WAO/EAACI guideline for the management of hereditary angioedema-the 2021 revision and update. Allergy. 2022;77:1961–90.
20. Busse PJ, Christiansen SC. Hereditary angioedema. N Engl J Med. 2020;382:1136–48.
21. Germenis AE, Margaglione M, Pesquero JB, Farkas H, Cichon S, Csuka D, et al. International consensus on the use of genetics in the management of hereditary angioedema. J Allergy Clin Immunol Pract. 2020;8:901–11.
22. Shamanaev A, Dickeson SK, Ivanov I, Litvak M, Sun MF, Kumar S et al. Mechanisms involved in hereditary angioedema with normal C1-inhibitor activity. Front Physiol. 2023;14:1146834.
23. Cicardi M, Aberer W, Benerji A, Bas M, Bernstein JA, Bork K, et al. Classification, diagnosis, and approach to treatment for angioedema: consensus report from the hereditary angioedema international working group. Allergy. 2014;69:602–16.
24. Reshef A. A global consensus on the definition, acronyms, nomenclature, and classification of angioedema (the DANCE initiative). Flash communication, EAACI Annual Congress, Hamburg 2023.

25. Hamilton RG, Hemmer W, Nopp A, Kleine-Tebbe J. Advances in IgE testing for diagnosis of allergic disease. J Allergy Clin Immunol Pract. 2020;8:2495–504.
26. Bezirganoglu H, Arik Yilmaz E, Sahiner UM, Soyer O, Sekerel BE, Teksam O et al. The common triggers of urticaria in children admitted to the pediatric emergency room. Pediatr Dermatol. 2022;39:695–701.
27. Stevens W, Buchheit K, Cahill KN. Aspirin-exacerbated diseases: advances in asthma with nasal polyposis, urticaria, angioedema, and anaphylaxis. Curr Allergy Asthma Rep. 2015;15:69.
28. Capriles-Behren E, Caplin J, Sanchez-Borges M. NSAID facial angioedema in a selected pediatric atopic population. J Investig Allergol Clin Immunol. 2000;10:277–9.
29. Sanchez-Borges M, Capriles-Behrens E, Caballero-Fonseca F. Hypersensitivity to non-steroidal anti-inflammatory drugs in childhood. Pediat Allergy Immunol. 2004;15:376–80.
30. Ensina LF, Brandão LS, Neto HC, Ben-Shoshan M. Urticaria and angioedema in children and adolescents: diagnostic challenge. Allergol Immunopathol. 2022;50:17–29.
31. Tanverdi MS, Wiersma A, Kim KM, Hicks AG, Mistry RD. Anaphylaxis in children. Pediatr Emerg Care. 2022;38:456–61.
32. Quincke H. Uber akutes umschriebenes Hautoedem. Mschr Prakt Dermatol. 1882;1:160–9.
33. Davis AE, Mejia P, Lu F. Biological activities of C1 inhibitor. Mol Immunol. 2008;45:4057–63.
34. Schoenfeld AK, Lahrsen E, Alban S. Regulation of complement and contact system activation via C1 inhibitor potentiation and factor XIIa activity modulation by sulfated glycans–structure-activity relationships. PLoS One. 2016;11:e0165493.
35. Karknaukhova E. C1-inhibitor: structure, functional diversity and therapeutic development. Curr Med Chem. 2022;29:467–88.
36. Davis AE. The pathophysiology of hereditary angioedema. Clin Immunol. 2005;114:3–9.
37. Cugno M, Zanichelli A, Foieni F, Caccia S, Cicardi M. C1-inhibitor deficiency and angioedema: molecular mechanisms and clinical progress. Trends Mol Med. 2009;15:69–78.
38. Zuraw BL. Clinical practice. Hereditary angioedema. N Engl J Med. 2008;359:1027–36.
39. Rubinstein E, Stolz LE, Sheffer AL, Stevens C, Bousvaros A. Abdominal attacks and treatment in hereditary angioedema with C1-inhibitor deficiency. BMC Gastroenterol. 2014;14:71.
40. Bork K, Siedlecki K, Bosch S, Schopf RE, Kreuz W. Asphyxiation by laryngeal edema in patients with hereditary angioedema. Mayo Clin Proc. 2000;75:349–54.
41. Bork K. Recurrent angioedema and the threat of asphyxation. Dtsch Arztebl Int. 2010;107:408–14.
42. Craig T. Triggers and short-term prophylaxis in patients with hereditary angioedema. Allergy Asthma Proc. 2020;41:S30–4.
43. Kemp JG, Craig TJ. Variability of prodromal signs and symptoms associated with hereditary angioedema attacks: a literature review. Allergy Asthma Proc. 2009;30:493–9.
44. Leibovich-Nassi I, Golander H, Somech R, Har-Even D, Reshef A. New instruments for the evaluation of prodromes and attacks of hereditary angioedema (HAE-EPA). Clin Rev Allergy Immunol. 2021;61:29–39.
45. Aygören-Pürsün E, Magerl M, Maetzel A, Maurer M. Epidemiology of Bradykinin-mediated angioedema: a systematic investigation of epidemiological studies. Orphanet J Rare Dis. 2018;3:73.
46. Stray-Pedersen A, Abrahamsen TG, Frøland SS. Primary immunodeficiency diseases in Norway. J Clin Immunol. 2000;20:477–85.
47. Roche O, Blanch A, Caballero T, Sastre N, Callejo D, López-Trascasa M. Hereditary angioedema due to C1 inhibitor deficiency: patient registry and approach to the prevalence in Spain. Ann Allergy Asthma Immunol. 2005;94:498–503.
48. Bygum A. Hereditary angio-oedema in Denmark: a nationwide survey. Br J Dermatol. 2009;161:1153–8.
49. Zanichelli A, Arcoleo F, Barca MP, Borrelli P, Bova M, Cancian M, et al. A nationwide survey of hereditary angioedema due to C1 inhibitor deficiency in Italy. Orphanet J Rare Dis. 2015;6:11.
50. Schöffl C, Wiednig M, Koch L, Blagojevic D, Duschet P, Hawranek T, et al. Hereditary angioedema in Austria: prevalence and regional peculiarities. Dtsch Dermatol Ges. 2019;17:416–23.
51. Lumry WR, Settipane RA. Hereditary angioedema: epidemiology and burden of disease. Allergy Asthma Proc. 2020;41:S08–13.
52. Gompels MM, Lock RJ, Morgan JE, Osborne J, Brown A, Virgo PF. A multicentre evaluation of the diagnostic efficiency of serological investigation for C1 inhibitor deficiency. Clin Pathol. 2002;55:145–7.
53. Wagenaar-Bos IG, Drouet C, Aygören-Pursun E, Bork K, Bucher C, Bygum A et al. Functional C1-inhibitor diagnostics in hereditary angioedema: assay evaluation and recommendations. J Immunol Methods. 2008;338:14–20.
54. Porebski G, Kwitniewski M, Reshef A. Biomarkers in Hereditary Angioedema. Clin Rev Allergy Immunol. 2021;60:404–15.
55. Cancian M, ITACA. Diagnostic and therapeutic management of hereditary angioedema due to C1-inhibitor deficiency: the Italian experience. Curr Opin Allergy Clin Immunol. 2015;15:383–91.
56. Farkas H, Martinez-Saguer I, Bork K, Bowen T, Craig T, Frank M, et al. International consensus on the diagnosis and management of pediatric patients with hereditary angioedema with C1 inhibitor deficiency. Allergy. 2017;72:300–13.
57. Pedrosa M, Phillips-Angels E, López-Lera A, López-Trascasa M, Caballero T. Complement study versus C1INH gene testing for the diagnosis of Type I Hereditary angioedema in children. J Clin Immunol. 2016;36:16–8.

58. Loules G, Zamanakou M, Parsopoulou F, Vatsiou S, Psarros F, Csuka D et al. Targeted next-generation sequencing for the molecular diagnosis of hereditary angioedema due to C1-inhibitor deficiency. Gene. 2018;667:76–82.
59. Drouet C, López-Lera A, Ghannam A, López-Trascasa M, Cichon S, Ponard D, et al. SERPING1 Variants and C1-INH biological function: a close relationship with C1-INH-HAE. Front Allergy. 2022;3:835503.
60. Cancian M, Perego F, Senter R, Arcoleo F, De Pasquale T, Zoli A, et al. Pediatric angioedema: essential features and preliminary results from the Hereditary Angioedema Global Registry in Italy. Pediatr Allergy Immunol. 2020;31:22–4.
61. Lai Y, Zhang G, Inhaber N, Bernstein JA, Cwik M, Zhou Z, et al. A robust multiplexed assay to quantify C1-inhibitor, C1q, and C4 proteins for in vitro diagnosis of hereditary angioedema from dried blood spot. J Pharm Biomed Anal. 2021;95:113844.
62. Förster TM, Magerl M, Maurer M, Zülbahar S, Zielke S, Inhaber N, et al. HAE patient self-sampling for biomarker establishment. Orphanet J Rare Dis. 2021;28:399.
63. Isono M, Kokado M, Kato K. Why does it take so long for rare disease patients to get an accurate diagnosis? A qualitative investigation of patient experiences of hereditary angioedema. PLoS One. 2022;17:e0265847.
64. Zanichelli A, Magerl M, Longhurst H, Fabien V, Maurer M. Hereditary angioedema with C1 inhibitor deficiency: delay in diagnosis in Europe. Allergy Asthma Clin Immunol. 2013;9:29.
65. Farkas H. Pediatric hereditary angioedema due to C1-inhibitor deficiency. Allergy Asthma Clin Immunol. 2010;6:18.
66. Nanda MK, Elenburg S, Bernstein J, Assa'ad AH. Clinical features of pediatric angioerdema. J Allergy Clin Immunol Pract. 2015;3:392–5.
67. Christiansen SC, Davis DK, Castaldo AJ, Zuraw BL. Pediatric hereditary angioedema: onset, diagnostic delay, and disease severity. Clin Pediatr. 2016;55:935–42.
68. Karadža-Lapić L, Barešić M, Vrsalović R, Ivković-Jureković I, Sršen S, Prkačin I, et al. Hereditary angioedema due to C1-inhibitor deficiency in pediatric patients in Croatia – first national study, diagnostic and prophylactic challenges. Acta Clin Croat. 2019;58:139–46.
69. Andrási N, Balla Z, Visy B, Szilágyi Á, Csuka D, Varga L, et al. Diagnosing pediatric patients with hereditary C1-inhibitor deficiency—experience from the Hungarian Center of Reference and Excellence. Front Allergy. 2022;3:860355.
70. Cancian M, Triggianese P, Modica S, Arcoleo F, Bignardi D, Brussino L et al. The impact of puberty on the onset, frequency, location, and severity of attacks in hereditary angioedema due to C1-inhibitor deficiency: a survey from the Italian Network for Hereditary and Acquired Angioedema (ITACA). Front Pediatr. 2023;11:1141073.
71. Tachdjian R, Kaplan AP. A comprehensive manangement approach in pediatric and adolescent patents with hereditary angioedema. Clin Pediatr. 2023;12:99228231155703.
72. Krack AT, Bernstein JA, Ruddy RM. Recognition, evaluation and management of pediatric hereditary angioedema. Pediatr Emer Care. 2012;37:218–25.
73. Bork K, Anderson JT, Caballero T, Craig T, Johnston DT, Li HH, et al. Assessment and management of disease burden and quality of life in patients with hereditary angioedema: a consensus report. Allergy Asthma Clin Immunol. 2021;17:40.
74. Savarese L, Bova M, De Falco C, Guarino MD, De Luca Picione R, Petraroli A et al. Emotional processes and stress in children affected by hereditary angioedema with C1-inhibitor deficiency: a multicenter, prospective study. Orphanet J Rare Dis. 2018;13:115.
75. Savarese L, Freda MF, De Luca Picione R, Dolce P, De Falco R, Alessio M et al. The experience of living with a chronic disease in pediatrics from the mothers' narrative: the clinical interview on parental sense of grip on the disease. Health Psychol Open. 2020;7:2055102920971496.
76. Zanichelli A, Montinaro V, Triggiani M, Arcoleo F, Visigalli D, Cancian M. Emerging drugs for the treatment of hereditary angioedema due to C1-inhibitor deficiency. Expert Op Emerging Drugs. 2023;27:103–10.
77. Bork K, Barnstedt SE, Koch P, Traupe H. Hereditary angioedema with normal C1-inhibitor activity in women. Lancet. 2000;356:213–7.
78. Cugno M, Castelli R, Cicardi M. Angioedema due to acquired C1-inhibitor deficiency: a bridging condition between autoimmunity and lymphoproliferation. Autoimmun Rev. 2008;8:156–9.
79. Montinaro V, Cicardi M. ACE inhibitor-mediated angioedema. Int Immunopharmacol. 2020;78:106081.
80. Stone C, Brown NJ. Angiotensin-converting enzyme inhibitor and other drug-associated angioedema. Immunol Allergy Clin N Am. 2017;37:483–95.

18 Allergy-Related Eosinophilia in Children

Francesca Bravin, Giulia Stiaccini, Diego Peroni, and Pasquale Comberiati

Abstract

Eosinophilia (an increased eosinophil count) can be found both in the peripheral blood and in tissues in several medical conditions. The most frequent causes of blood and tissue eosinophilia include atopic diseases, parasitic infections, malignancies, immunodeficiency, and vasculitis. A careful history and physical examination along with directed clinical evaluation may help determine the cause. Allergic diseases are characterized by type-2 eosinophilic inflammation and are usually associated with mild eosinophilia in the bloodstream (<1500 cells/microliter).

This chapter focuses on allergy-related eosinophilia and highlights how eosinophilic inflammation contributes to the pathogenesis of allergic rhinitis, asthma, atopic dermatitis, and eosinophilic gastrointestinal disorders.

Keywords

Allergy · Atopy · Asthma · Children · Eosinophils · Eosinophilia · Eosinophilic esophagitis · Immunity · Allergic rhinitis · Atopic dermatitis

Abbreviations

AEC	Absolute eosinophil count
HE	Hypereosinophilia
HES	Hypereosinophilic syndrome
EGPA	Eosinophilic granulomatosis with polyangiitis
GPA	granulomatosis with polyangiitis
MBP	Major basic protein
EPO	eosinophil peroxidase
EDN	eosinophil-derived neurotoxin
ECP	Eosinophilic cationic protein
AD	Atopic dermatitis
FeNO	fraction of exhaled nitric oxide
EGID	Eosinophil-associated gastrointestinal disorder
EoE	Eosinophilic esophagitis
EGE	Eosinophilic gastroenteritis
EC	Eosinophilic colitis
HPF	High power field

Authors Francesca Bravin and Giulia Stiaccini equally contributed as the first author.

F. Bravin · G. Stiaccini · D. Peroni (✉)
P. Comberiati (✉)
Department of Clinical and Experimental Medicine, Section of Paediatrics, University of Pisa, Pisa, Italy
e-mail: diego.peroni@unipi.it; pasquale.comberiati@unipi.it

C. Caffarelli, G. L. Marseglia (eds.), *Textbook of Pediatric Allergy*,
https://doi.org/10.1007/978-3-031-71283-8_18

Test your learning and check your understanding of this book's contents: use the "Springer Nature Flashcards" app to access questions using ▶ https://sn.pub/nspbjm. To use the app, please follow the instructions in Chap. 1.

Key Points

- The most frequent causes of blood and tissue eosinophilia include atopic diseases, parasitic infections, malignancies, immunodeficiency, and vasculitis.
- Allergic diseases are usually associated with mild eosinophilia (<1500 cells/microliter). However, atopic dermatitis can be associated with moderate eosinophilia (1500–5000 cells/microliter) during acute phases.
- Measurement of tissue eosinophilia is recommended for the diagnosis of eosinophil-associated gastrointestinal disorders and some forms of cellular nonallergic chronic rhinitis.
- Noninvasive useful tools for evaluating eosinophilic inflammation of the airways include the induced sputum test and the fraction of exhaled nitric oxide (FeNO).
- Blood eosinophilia is not necessarily a reliable marker for tissue eosinophilia. Thus, measurement of blood eosinophilia is not recommended either for the diagnosis or the management of allergic diseases but can help in choosing a biological therapy for severe asthma.

18.1 Introduction

Eosinophilia (an increased eosinophil count) can be found both in the peripheral blood and in tissues in several medical conditions. Peripheral blood eosinophil levels vary by age, with upper reference limits being higher in younger children. Based on peripheral blood eosinophil count, eosinophilia can be classified as mild, moderate, or severe. Eosinophilia can also be classified into primary, secondary, and idiopathic based on its etiology. The causes of eosinophilia in children can be grouped into five categories, which include allergic disorders, parasitic infections, leukemia/lymphomas, vasculitis, and immunodeficiencies. Tissue eosinophilia usually results from increased recruitment of activated eosinophils from the bloodstream. Once recruited into tissues, activated eosinophils in high concentrations can cause tissue damage and dysfunction [1–3].

This chapter focuses on allergy-related eosinophilia and highlights how eosinophilic inflammation contributes to the pathogenesis of allergic rhinitis, asthma, atopic dermatitis, and eosinophilic gastrointestinal disorders.

18.2 Eosinophils

Eosinophils are bonemarrow–derived cells of the granulocyte lineage whose development and terminal differentiation are under the control of several cytokines (interleukin [IL]-3, granulocyte-macrophage colony-stimulating factor [GM-CSF], and IL-5), with IL-5 being the cytokine primarily responsible for eosinophilopoiesis.

The level of eosinophils in the blood is highest in the morning and lowest in the afternoon. The nucleus is composed of two connected lobes, and the cytoplasm is filled with granules that stain red on hematoxylin and eosin staining.

They have an approximate half-life of 8–18 h in the bloodstream. Under normal homeostatic conditions, most eosinophils leave the circulation and migrate into specific tissues where they can reside for several weeks. The gastrointestinal tract serves as the largest tissue reservoir for eosinophils, where these cells are normally present in the mucosal tissue from the stomach to the large intestine.

Moreover, they also reside in diverse tissues such as the female genital tract, mammary glands, and thymus. Recently, immunomodulatory functions of eosinophils have increasingly come into focus, with murine models demonstrating a role for eosinophils in plasma cell homeostasis in bone marrow and regulation of glucose metabolism in adipose tissue.

Their functional roles are multifaceted and include antigen presentation; the release of lipid-derived, peptide, and cytokine mediators for acute and chronic inflammation; responses to helminth and parasite clearance through degranulation; and ongoing homeostatic immune responses.

Eosinophil granules contain a wide array of preformed cytokines, chemokines, enzymes, and growth factors, leading to diverse biological functions of eosinophils in infection and inflammation. They can release eosinophil-derived neurotoxin (EDN) and eosinophil cationic protein, which are members of the RNase A family of granule proteins that exhibit ribonuclease activity. These proteins, involved in host defense against viruses, may play a role in tissue remodeling. and connective tissue disorders. In addition to the preformed mediators stored in the granules, eosinophils can also release newly synthesized mediators, including IL-4, which possesses the ability to stimulate adaptive immunity. Moreover, major basic proteins 1 and 2, eosinophil peroxidase (EPO), EDN, eosinophil cationic protein and cytokines like TGF-β that may lead to thrombosis and tissue fibrosis and injury [4 9].

18.3 Eosinophilia

Eosinophilia is defined as an increase in the number of eosinophils in the peripheral blood, observed in absolute eosinophil count (AEC) above the upper limit of normal. The AEC represents the frequency of circulating eosinophils in the peripheral blood (in cells per microliter), which is calculated by multiplying the percentage of eosinophils by the total white blood cell count.

AEC in the peripheral blood varies by age, with higher upper threshold limits seen in infants and toddlers compared to adolescents and adults.

Eosinophilia is defined as an AEC greater than 450 cells/microL or 500 cells/microL in some studies. Traditionally, eosinophilia severity has been classified into mild (AEC from the upper limit of normal to 1.500 cells/microL), moderate (AEC 1.500–5.000 cells/microL), and severe (AEC greater than 5.000 cells/microL) [1, 10].

Hypereosinophilia is defined by an AEC greater than >1500 cells/microL, obtained on at least two separate occasions (interval ≥1 month) with or without organ damage. The threshold of 1500/μl has been identified in literature because, above this count, it significantly increases the chance of organ damage. Tissue hypereosinophilia, on the other hand, can be defined as a percentage of eosinophils that exceeds 20% of all nucleated cells in the bone marrow or tissue infiltration that is deemed extensive by a pathologist. Tissue eosinophilia can occur either with or without concurrent eosinophilia in the peripheral blood [1].

Unfortunately, the severity of eosinophilia is rarely helpful for identifying the cause, except at extremes. Among a recent cohort of pediatric patients with hypereosinophilia, the extremes were represented by *eosinophilic* gastrointestinal diseases and other atopic disorders (mild hypereosinophilia) versus immune deficiencies and neoplasms (severe hypereosinophilia) [10].

18.4 Causes of Eosinophilia

Eosinophils are multifunctional leukocytes implicated in the pathogenesis of numerous inflammatory conditions. Peripheral eosinophilia can be primary, secondary, and idiopathic. Primary eosinophilia is usually seen in the context of hematologic malignancies, such as acute and chronic myeloid leukemia, and myeloproliferative disorders. In those conditions, eosinophil counts are usually greater than 5000/microL, and values >20,000 cells/microL are highly suggestive for myeloproliferative disorders. Secondary eosinophilia is associated with many other conditions [1–3].

The commonest causes of eosinophilia are summarized in Table 1. Parasitic infections, neo-

Table 18.1 Causes of eosinophilia

Allergic Disorders	Parasites	Lymphocytic/Hematologic-Neoplastic disorders	Vasculitis and immune rheumatologic diseases
Allergic rhinitis Asthma Eosinophilic Gastrointestinal disorders Atopic dermatitis Drug allergy	Helminths Ectoparasites Isospora Sarcocystis Scabies	Hematologic malignancy (LH, CML, CEL) Sezary syndrome Solid tumors	Eosinophilic granulomatosis with polyangiitis (EGPA) Sarcoidosis Alps HyperIgE syndrome
Mild to moderate eosinophilia	Mild to moderate eosinophilia	Moderate to severe eosinophilia	Moderate to severe eosinophilia

plastic disorders, vasculitis, and immunodeficiencies are out of the scope of this chapter and will only be briefly described.

A variety of infections may be associated with eosinophilia; these include helminths (worms), fungi, protozoa, bacteria, the retroviruses HIV and human T cell lymphotropic virus type 1 (HTLV-1), and scabies (a mite infestation). Most acute bacterial infections and viral infections are not associated with eosinophilia. A wide variety of parasites can elicit eosinophilia. The pattern and degree of eosinophilia in parasitic infections result from the development, migration, and distribution of the parasite within the host, as well as from the host's immune response. Parasites tend to elicit marked eosinophilia when they or their products come into contact with immune effector cells in tissues, particularly during migration. When mechanical barriers separate the parasite from the host, or when parasites no longer invade tissues, the stimulus to eosinophilia is usually low. Therefore, eosinophilia is highest in infections with a phase of parasite development that involves migration through tissues, such as trichinosis, ascariasis, gnathostomiasis, strongyloidiasis, schistosomiasis, and filariasis [11, 12].

Besides conditions where eosinophils or their precursor cells undergo malignant transformation, eosinophilia can arise due to the production of eosinophilopoietic cytokines. Eosinopoietin production has been attributed to both CD4+ and CD8+ T cells. Hodgkin's disease is commonly linked to eosinophilia, with the production of IL-5 by Reed-Sternberg cells being well-documented. Primary cutaneous T-cell lymphoma and Sezary syndrome frequently exhibit both blood and dermal eosinophilia. In addition to lymphomas, certain other malignancies can occasionally be associated with elevated eosinophil levels in the bloodstream. Tumor-associated eosinophilia is observed in nonkeratinizing cervical tumors of large-cell type, undifferentiated lung carcinomas of large-cell nature, squamous cell carcinomas affecting the lungs, vagina, penis, skin, and nasopharynx. It is also seen in adenocarcinomas of the stomach, large bowel, and uterine body, as well as transitional cell carcinoma of the bladder [13, 14].

Eosinophilic granulomatosis with polyangiitis (EGPA, previously known as Churg-Strauss syndrome) is the major vasculitis syndrome associated with eosinophilia. EGPA is one of the ANCA-associated vasculitides (AAV), a group of multisystemic diseases that also include microscopic polyangiitis and granulomatosis with polyangiitis (GPA, formerly Wegener's granulomatosis). The pediatric form of EGPA usually presents with asthma, eosinophilia, sinusitis, nasal polyps, and lung infiltrates.

Finally, several immunodeficiency syndromes should be considered in the evaluation of pediatric patients who present with hypereosinophilia and atopy [15, 16] (Table 2).

Table 18.2 Main immunodeficiency syndrome associated with eosinophilia

STAT3 Deficiency	DOCK8 Deficiency	GIOBBE Syndrome	WISKOTT-ALDRICH Syndrome	IPEX Syndrome	OMENN Syndrome
Immune dysregulation Atopic manifestations and eosinophilia	Recurrent infections Atopic dermatitis Elevated IgE levels and eosinophilia	Eczema Abscesses Recurrent pneumonia Candidiasis Characteristic facies Dentition abnormalities Scoliosis IgE > 2000 IU/mL Eosinophilia	Eczema Recurrent infections Thrombocytopenia Elevated IgE levels	Autoimmune manifestations (including enteropathy, endocrinopathy, dermatitis) Eosinophilia	Erythrodermia Failure to thrive Dhiarrea intractable diarrhea Hypoprotidemia Serious early infections Lymphadenopathy and hepatosplenomegaly Eosinophilia Lymphocytosis

18.5 Allergy-Related Eosinophilia in Children

Allergic diseases are characterized by type-2 eosinophilic inflammation. Allergic diseases encompass a diverse range of conditions affecting various organ systems, such as the skin, the respiratory system, and the gastrointestinal tract. In allergic inflammatory reactions, eosinophils have been considered terminal effector cells, but recent studies have shown that they are also involved in the early stages of the development of allergic diseases. Blood eosinophilia is usually mild in allergic diseases but can be moderate in atopic dermatitis during an acute phase. Blood eosinophilia is not necessarily a reliable marker for tissue eosinophilia. Thus, the measurement of blood eosinophilia is not recommended either for the diagnosis or the management of allergic diseases, but can help in choosing a biological therapy for severe asthma [17].

18.5.1 Allergic Rhinitis and Cellular Nonallergic Rhinitis

Allergic rhinitis is a common allergic disease characterized by chronic nasal symptoms, such as nasal obstruction, rhinorrhea, itching, and sneezing, that can be associated with ocular symptoms such as redness, itching, and watery eyes.

Previously, allergic rhinitis was classified as either seasonal or perennial based on the timing of symptoms. However, the current classification system, as outlined by the Allergic Rhinitis and its Impact on Asthma (ARIA) guidelines, categorizes it as intermittent and persistent, and each form can either be mild or moderate-severe.

Inhaled allergens are the primary triggers of allergic rhinitis. Perennial allergic rhinitis is characterized by a sustained immunoglobulin E (IgE)-mediated inflammatory response to year-round environmental aeroallergens. These allergens can include dust mites, mold spores, animal dander (such as from cats or dogs), and certain occupational allergens present in workplaces like laboratories or factories. Allergic rhinitis can also be triggered by seasonal allergens, such as tree pollen, grass, and weed pollen leading to intermittent symptoms. The diagnosis of allergic rhinitis is based on characteristic symptoms and the evidence of allergic sensitization to aeroallergens, measured either by skin prick tests (SPT) or the presence of allergen-specific IgE (sIgE) in serum.

Eosinophils strongly contribute to the pathophysiology of allergic rhinitis. Eosinophils are recruited to the nasal tissue during the late phase of the allergic reaction and release various mediators and cytokines, which contribute to chronic inflammation and nasal obstruction that characterize allergic rhinitis. Although blood eosinophilia is not always present in allergic rhinitis, when it does occur, it is typically mild. The measurement of nasal eosinophils is not recommended as a diagnostic tool in patients with allergic rhinitis. The nasal eosinophil count can vary depending on the experience and skills of the investigator, as well as other factors such as sampling technique and sample processing. Several factors (like normal physiological variability, age-related differences, sampling difficulties, and interpretation challenges) contribute to the limitations of measuring nasal eosinophils in clinical practice for the diagnosis of allergic rhinitis. However, nasal cytology is deemed helpful for the diagnosis of the different forms of cellular nonallergic rhinitis, which include nonallergic rhinitis with neutrophils (NARNE), nonallergic rhinitis with eosinophils (NARES), nonallergic rhinitis with mast cells (NARMA), nonallergic rhinitis with eosinophils and mast cells (NARESMA).

Because most patients with allergic rhinitis showed extensive eosinophilic degranulation in the nasal mucosa, researchers have tried to identify eosinophilic inflammation by measuring the eosinophil-specific cationic proteins contained in their granules (i.e. major basic protein (MBP), EDN, eosinophil cationic protein (ECP), and EPO). However, the analysis of the eosinophil-specific cationic proteins is not recommended due to inconsistent results and technical limitations [18–20].

18.5.2 Asthma

Asthma is a chronic inflammatory disorder of the lower airways, that is associated with airway hyperresponsiveness and variable airflow obstruction, which leads to episodic symptoms of shortness of breath, wheezing, and cough. Currently, two main inflammatory phenotypes of asthma are recognized, namely the "type 2 high" and "type 2-low/non-type 2" asthma.

Type 2-high asthma is characterized by lymphocyte T helper 2 and innate lymphoid cell 2 (ILC2) -driven immune-inflammatory responses and represents the phenotype affecting almost all children and half of adults with asthma. Characteristic inflammatory and immune biomarkers of type 2-high asthma are high levels of blood and sputum eosinophils, increased fractional exhaled nitric oxide (FeNO), and high levels of serum total IgE.

Type 2-high asthma includes both allergic asthma and eosinophilic asthma. Allergic asthma tends to begin during childhood and is associated with a personal and often a family history of atopy and markers of type 2 inflammation including elevated total and specific IgE levels, FeNO, and blood eosinophil count. Eosinophilic asthma tends to develop in adulthood, has a female predominance, and is associated with elevated blood eosinophil count (usually >300 cells/mm^3, or at least>150 cells/mm^3), a low rate of atopy, high or normal FeNO, reduced pulmonary function from the beginning, comorbidities, such as obesity and nasal polyposis, and high rates of exacerbations and medical resources use.

Eosinophilia in type 2-high asthma is usually <1500/microL and correlates with disease severity. An eosinophilia ≥1500/microL in patients with asthma symptoms should prompt consideration of other eosinophilic pulmonary conditions (such as allergic bronchopulmonary aspergillosis, EGPA, or nasal polyposis).

In allergic asthma, type 2 helper T lymphocytes are believed to drive the disease pathobiology. In genetically susceptible individuals, inhalation of aeroallergens activates specialized antigen-presenting cells that steer the differentiation of naive T lymphocytes toward TH2 cells, which produce cytokines such as interleukin-4 (IL-4), IL-5, IL-9 and IL-13 and lead to IgE switching in B cells, airway eosinophilia and mucous hypersecretion. In nonallergic eosinophilic asthma, air pollutants, microbes and glycolipids induce the release of epithelium-derived cytokines, including IL-33, IL-25 and TSLP, which activate ILC2s in an antigen-independent manner via their respective receptors (IL-17RB, ST2 and TSLPR). Activated ILC2s produce high amounts of IL-4, IL-5 and IL-13, leading to eosinophilia, mucous hypersecretion, and airway hyperreactivity.

A diagnosis should be made based on the symptom patterns (e.g., wheeze, shortness of breath, and dry cough), evidence of variability in airflow limitation in the presence of airway inflammation, likelihood of alternative diagnoses, and response to treatment. Lung function tests can be used to aid the diagnosis of asthma in children over the age of 5 years. Spirometry testing is commonly used to assess airflow obstruction and reversibility.

Methods for directly evaluating eosinophilic inflammation of the airways include bronchial biopsy, bronchoalveolar lavage, the induced sputum test, and the FeNO. Bronchial biopsy and bronchoalveolar lavage have been considered the gold standards for evaluating eosinophilic inflammation of the airways. However, because these tests are very invasive, the induced sputum test and FeNO are the most widely used. Sputum eosinophil counts decrease with corticosteroid treatment and are increased by allergen challenge. Targeting the reduction in sputum eosinophil counts with therapy showed reduced exacerbation numbers and symptom severity in adults with asthma. However, data on sputum eosinophil counts are lacking in children due to the technical difficulty in obtaining sputum samples. Fleming et al. reported that monitoring induced sputum in children did not significantly reduce overall exacerbations or improve asthma control. In this study, follow-up every 3 months revealed that exacerbations were reduced in the short term, suggesting that more frequent measurements would be needed to confirm a clinically useful effect. There are some technical difficulties in obtaining a sputum sample in school-aged children, which makes it not feasible in preschool-age children. In addition, the hypertonic saline used to induce sputum can cause asthma exacerbations. Also, the results of the sputum test are not immediately available after the sampling because skilled inspectors are required to examine the samples.

Measuring FeNO is a noninvasive method for evaluating type-2 inflammation in the airway. The test is relatively simple, and its results are immediately available. Many studies have shown a positive relationship between FeNO and sputum eosinophil count. Nitric oxide is produced by the nitric oxide synthase (NOS), which exists in five isoforms: three constitutive and two inducible. In the airways, iNOS, one of the inducible isoforms, produces nitric oxide upon stimulation by certain cytokines, mainly IL-4 and IL-13. Such cytokines are crucial in the pathogenesis of type-2 high asthma. FeNO is considered normal if <20 parts per billion (ppb) in children and <25 ppb in adults.

Lastly, serum periostin is a recently introduced test that is used to indirectly evaluate eosinophilic airway inflammation in patients with asthma. In several reports, serum periostin levels were significantly correlated with sputum eosinophil counts. However, a recent study by Wagener et al. showed that serum periostin had lower accuracy than blood eosinophils and FeNO for evaluating eosinophilic inflammation in asthmatic patients [21–29].

18.5.3 Atopic Dermatitis

Atopic dermatitis (AD), also referred to as atopic eczema, is a multifactorial skin condition that arises from a combination of genetic susceptibility and environmental factors. This complex interplay contributes to the development of a diverse array of clinical manifestations associated with the disease. AD affects a significant portion of children and is particularly prevalent in infants, with approximately 20% of those under the age of two being affected by the condition.

Atopic dermatitis frequently correlates with increased levels of serum IgE and a personal or family history of type I allergies, allergic rhinitis, and asthma. The presence of eosinophils within the inflammatory infiltrate of AD has been well-established. Most AD patients exhibit elevated eosinophil numbers and levels of eosinophil granule proteins in their peripheral blood, which correlate with disease activity. Furthermore, eosinophil granule proteins, known for their cytotoxic activity, are highly deposited in the skin lesions of AD patients.

Although significant advancements have been made in understanding the immunological aspects associated with AD, the underlying pathogenesis of this condition remains unclear. Skin barrier abnormalities and immune dysregulation play significant roles in the development of AD. Disruptions in the skin barrier allow for increased penetration of allergens and irritants, triggering an immune response. This immune response is characterized by excessive activity of T helper 2 and T helper 22 cells, leading to increased production of IgE through the activation of interleukins.

In infants, the skin lesions often first appear at 2–6 months of age and show an age-related distribution. Prominent clinical observations encompass redness, swelling, dryness, open sores, weeping and scabbing, and thickened skin, although these manifestations differ depending on the patient's age and the duration of the lesions. In children, skin lesions typically affect the face, hands, flexural areas (the antecubital and popliteal fossae, wrists, and ankles), and trunk.

The evaluation relies on the patient's symptoms and overall condition, as there are no distinctive indicators or definitive biomarkers to conclusively determine the evolution of AD. Most children overcome AD by school age.

The Scoring Atopic Dermatitis (SCORAD) index is the most widely used tool for assessing the severity of AD in children. Other validated tools for AD severity assessment include the Eczema Area and Severity Index (EASI), and the Investigator Global Assessment (IGA) scale [30–33].

18.5.4 Gastrointestinal Disorders

Primary eosinophilic gastrointestinal disorders (EGIDs) are a range of conditions characterized by significant eosinophilic inflammation affecting various segments of the gastrointestinal (GI) tract. These disorders manifest in the absence of secondary causes such as infections or drug reactions. Eosinophils are normal constituents of the GI tract, except in the esophagus. Depending on the localization of the pathological eosinophilic inflammation, the EGIDs are classified as eosinophilic esophagitis (EoE), eosinophilic gastritis (EG), eosinophilic gastroenteritis (EGE) and eosinophilic colitis (EC). The clinical presentation of EGIDs varies depending on the age of onset and the specific layer of the GI tract affected, including the mucosa, muscular layer, or serosa. Eosinophils typically exhibit an activated phenotype and their infiltration results in symptoms associated with organ dysfunction.

Although EGIDs are not considered allergic diseases per se, these patients, and in particular those affected with EoE, often report a concomitant history of atopic conditions. EoE is the most studied EGID and is a chronic immune-mediated, antigen-driven disease, that is influenced by a complex interplay of genetic and environmental factors, including early life exposures to allergens. These factors contribute to epithelial barrier dysfunction, allergic sensitization, and prominent Type 2 inflammation. Food allergens are the major trigger of inflammation in EoE, although selected diets based on positive food allergy tests have been shown to be less effective than empirical diets that remove six major allergenic foods irrespective of allergy testing. EoE can manifest with a diverse range of symptoms, which vary with age. In young children and toddlers, common symptoms include vomiting, recurrent abdominal pain, feeding refusal, and failure to thrive, whereas adolescents and adults frequently report dysphagia and food impaction, which can indicate more advanced tissue remodeling in the esophagus (Table 3).

The diagnosis of EoE is often delayed due to the nonspecific nature of symptoms and the copying mechanism that patients can unconsciously develop (e.g., eating slowly, extensive chewing of foods and prolongation of mealtimes, cutting down in small pieces or pureed meat and high textured foods, lubricating foods with sauces, drinking more liquids to wash down meal and high texture foods, avoiding pills and foods likely to cause dysphagia, such as meats and breads).

EGIDs can be suspected at endoscopy, and imaging can help judge the extent of the disease; however, a biopsy is needed to confirm the diagnosis. Standard guidelines for non-EoE EGIDs are currently lacking, but it is agreed that a definitive diagnosis requires recurrent GI symptoms, increased eosinophils for high power field (HPF) in biopsy specimens, and the absence of secondary causes of GI eosinophilia. The gold standard for EoE diagnosis is biopsy findings that demonstrate increased intraepithelial esophageal eosinophil counts without concomitant eosinophilic infiltration in the stomach or duodenum.

The diagnostic threshold in EoE is >15 eosinophils/HPF (standard size of around 0.3 mm^2).

On the other hand, without diagnostic guidelines, there is uncertainty about the number and location of biopsies required for optimal non-EoE EGIDs diagnosis. In addition, there is a physiological number of eosinophils, which increases from the duodenum to the caecum and decreases from the right colon to the rectum. Experts and the Food and Drug Administration

Table 18.3 Eosinophilic esophagitis age-related clinical manifestations

Infants	Children	Adolescents
Failure to thrive. Food refusal. Regurgitation. Vomiting. Irritability.	Vomiting. Abdominal pain. Difficulty of swallowing. Reflux-like symptoms. Selective/abnormal diet. Failure to thrive.	Dysphagia (22%). Reflux-like symptoms (1–8%). Food impaction (50%).

now accept ≥30 eosinophils per HPF in ≥5 HPFs in gastric biopsies and/or in ≥3 HPFs in duodenum biopsies as the diagnostic criteria for EG and EGE. The number of eosinophils currently needed per HPF for diagnosis in EC are only suggestions derived from case series and have not yet been validated in different populations. Various studies used different pathological cut-offs, suggesting values ranging from >50 eosinophils/HPF in the right colon, >42 in the transverse colon, and >32 in the descending colon, to >100, >84, and >64, respectively, for an accurate diagnosis.

Currently, no noninvasive biomarkers are available for the diagnosis and monitoring of EGIDs. Blood eosinophils can be normal, but most patients with EGE and EC have at least mild peripheral eosinophilia. Severe eosinophilia (>1.500/mm^3) was observed in patients with predominantly serosal forms of EGE, but in these cases, it is necessary to rule out any form of hypereosinophilic syndromes [34–41].

18.5.5 Emerging Therapies

Glucocorticoids offer by far the most effective treatment for controlling allergic diseases such as allergic rhinitis, asthma, and AD. They act on various cells and pathways involved in the allergic inflammatory response. They primarily work by suppressing the production and release of pro-eosinophil cytokines (IL-5, IL-3, and GM-CSF) by T cells and structural cells such as fibroblasts and epithelial cells. Glucocorticoids amplify the rate of spontaneous cell death of eosinophils by having direct effects on pro-apoptotic signaling pathways and through the increased generation of cell-damaging molecules such as reactive oxygen species (ROS) by eosinophils. Glucocorticoids also promote the clearance of apoptotic eosinophils from tissues by enhancing the phagocytic capacity of macrophages. Traditionally, therapy for eosinophilic disorders has primarily focused on glucocorticoids. However, long-term or high-dose use of glucocorticoids can lead to significant side effects, and drug resistance can develop in some individuals, reducing their effectiveness. Therefore, there has been a growing focus on developing alternative treatments that target different aspects of eosinophilic disorders.

The introduction of biologic therapy (monoclonal antibodies) has revolutionized the management of refractory allergic diseases such as asthma, AD, and other eosinophilic conditions such as EoE. Some of these biological therapies target the eosinophilic inflammation blocking either IL-5 or IL-5 receptor (i.e. mepolizumab, and benralizumab), whereas other biologicals target broader type-2 inflammation (dupilumab) and IgE-mediated allergic inflammation (omalizumab) [42–44].

18.6 Chapter-End Summary

The causes of peripheral blood eosinophilia range from benign eosinophilia to malignancy; a careful history and physical examination along with directed clinical evaluation may help determine the cause. Allergic diseases are characterized by type-2 eosinophilic inflammation. Allergic diseases are usually associated with mild eosinophilia (<1500 cells/microliter). Atopic Dermatitis can be associated with moderate eosinophilia (1500–5000 cells/microliter) during acute phases. Blood eosinophilia is not necessarily a reliable marker for tissue eosinophilia. Thus, the measurement of blood eosinophilia is not recommended either for the diagnosis or the management of allergic diseases, but it can help in choosing a biological therapy for severe asthma.

References

1. Valent P, Klion AD, Roufosse F, Simon D, Metzgeroth G, Leiferman KM, et al. Proposed refined diagnostic criteria and classification of eosinophil disorders and related syndromes. Allergy. 2023;78:47–59.
2. Gotlib J. World Health Organization-defined eosinophilic disorders: 2017 update on diagnosis, risk stratification, and management. Am J Hematol. 2017;92:1243–59.

3. Costagliola G, Marco SD, Comberiati P, D'Elios S, Petashvili N, Di Cicco ME, et al. Practical approach to children presenting with eosinophila and hypereosinophilia. Curr Pediatr Rev. 2020;16:81–8.
4. Abdala-Valencia H, Coden ME, Chiarella SE, Jacobsen EA, Bochner BS, Lee JJ, et al. Shaping eosinophil identity in the tissue contexts of development, homeostasis, and disease. J Leukoc Biol. 2018;104:95–108.
5. Jacobsen EA, Helmers RA, Lee JJ, Lee NA. The expanding role(s) of eosinophils in health and disease. Blood. 2012;120:3882–90.
6. Chu VT, Fröhlich A, Steinhauser G, Scheel T, Roch T, Fillatreau S, et al. Eosinophils are required for the maintenance of plasma cells in the bone marrow. Nat Immunol. 2011;12:151–9.
7. Wu D, Molofsky AB, Liang HE, Ricardo-Gonzalez RR, Jouihan HA, Bando JK, et al. Eosinophils sustain adipose alternatively activated macrophages associated with glucose homeostasis. Science. 2011;332:243–7.
8. Acharya KR, Ackerman SJ. Eosinophil granule proteins: form and function. J Biol Chem. 2014;289:17406–15.
9. Wang SA. The diagnostic work-up of hypereosinophilia. Pathobiology. 2019;86:39–52.
10. Burris D, Rosenberg CE, Schwartz JT, Zhang Y, Eby MD, Abonia JP, et al. Pediatric hypereosinophilia: characteristics, clinical manifestations, and diagnoses. J Allergy Clin Immunol Pract. 2019;7:2750–2758.e2.
11. O'Connell EM, Nutman TB. Eosinophilia in infectious diseases. Immunol Allergy Clin N Am. 2015;35:493–522.
12. Antonucci R, Vacca N, Boz G, Locci C, Mannazzu R, Cherchi C, et al. Parasitic Hypereosinophilia in childhood: a diagnostic challenge. Mediterr J Hematol Infect Dis. 2018;10:e2018034.
13. Grisaru-Tal S, Itan M, Klion AD, Munitz A. A new dawn for eosinophils in the tumour microenvironment. Nat Rev Cancer. 2020;20:594–607.
14. Lam BD, Hale AJ, Bullis SM, He Y, Khan S, Freed JA. A retrospective review of 193 cases of severe eosinophilia in the Northeast United States. Am J Med. 2021;134:e374–7.
15. Fijolek J, Radzikowska E. Eosinophilic granulomatosis with polyangiitis – advances in pathogenesis, diagnosis, and treatment. Front Med. 2023;3:1145257.
16. Groh M, Pagnoux C, Baldini C, Bel E, Bottero P, Cottin V, et al. Eosinophilic granulomatosis with polyangiitis (Churg-Strauss) (EGPA) Consensus Task Force recommendations for evaluation and management. Eur J Intern Med. 2015;26:545–53.
17. Jesenak M, Diamant Z, Simon D, Tufvesson E, Seys SF, Mukherjee M, et al. Eosinophils-from cradle to grave: an EAACI task force paper on new molecular insights and clinical functions of eosinophils and the clinical effects of targeted eosinophil depletion. Allergy. 2023;78:3077–102.
18. Wise SK, Damask C, Roland LT, Ebert C, Levy JM, Lin S, et al. International consensus statement on allergy and rhinology: allergic rhinitis – 2023. Int Forum Allergy Rhinol. 2023;13:293–859.
19. Bousquet J, Schünemann HJ, Samolinski B, Demoly P, Baena-Cagnani CE, Bachert C, et al. World Health Organization Collaborating Center for Asthma and Rhinitis. Allergic Rhinitis and its Impact on Asthma (ARIA): achievements in 10 years and future needs. J Allergy Clin Immunol. 2012;130:1049–62.
20. Poddighe D, Gelardi M, Licari A, Del Giudice MM, Marseglia GL. Non-allergic rhinitis in children: epidemiological aspects, pathological features, diagnostic methodology and clinical management. World J Methodol. 2016;6:200–13.
21. Carr TF, Zeki AA, Kraft M. Eosinophilic and Noneosinophilic asthma. Am J Respir Crit Care Med. 2018;197:22–37.
22. Brusselle GG, Maes T, Bracke KR. Eosinophils in the spotlight: Eosinophilic airway inflammation in nonallergic asthma. Nat Med. 2013;19:977–9.
23. Danvers L, Lo DKH, Gaillard EA. The role of objective tests to support a diagnosis of asthma in children. Paediatr Respir Rev. 2020;33:52–7.
24. Moral L, Vizmanos G, Torres-Borrego J, Praena-Crespo M, Tortajada-Girbés M, Pellegrini FJ, et al. Asthma diagnosis in infants and preschool children: a systematic review of clinical guidelines. Allergol Immunopathol (Madr). 2019;47:107–21.
25. Jayaram L, Pizzichini MM, Cook RJ, Boulet LP, Lemière C, Pizzichini E, et al. Determining asthma treatment by monitoring sputum cell counts: effect on exacerbations. Eur Respir J. 2006;27:483–94.
26. Fleming L, Wilson N, Regamey N, Bush A. Use of sputum eosinophil counts to guide management in children with severe asthma. Thorax. 2012;67:193–8.
27. Dweik RA, Boggs PB, Erzurum SC, Irvin CG, Leigh MW, Lundberg JO, et al. American Thoracic Society Committee on interpretation of exhaled nitric oxide levels (FENO) for clinical applications. An official ATS clinical practice guideline: interpretation of exhaled nitric oxide levels (FENO) for clinical applications. Am J Respir Crit Care Med. 2011;184:602–15.
28. Di Cicco M, Peroni DG, Ragazzo V, Comberiati P. Application of exhaled nitric oxide (FeNO) in pediatric asthma. Curr Opin Allergy Clin Immunol. 2021;21:151–8.
29. Wagener AH, de Nijs SB, Lutter R, Sousa AR, Weersink EJ, Bel EH, et al. External validation of blood eosinophils, FE(NO) and serum periostin as surrogates for sputum eosinophils in asthma. Thorax. 2015;70:115–20.
30. Bantz SK, Zhu Z, Zheng T. The atopic march: progression from atopic dermatitis to allergic rhinitis and asthma. J Clin Cell Immunol. 2014;5:202.
31. Yang YB, Gohari A, Lam J. Brief academic review and clinical practice guidelines for pediatric atopic dermatitis. Curr Pediatr Rev. 2021;17:229–37.

32. Chu CY. Treatments for childhood atopic dermatitis: an update on emerging therapies. Clin Rev Allergy Immunol. 2021;61:114–27.
33. de Bruin Weller MS, Knulst AC, Meijer Y, Bruijnzeel-Koomen CA, Pasmans SG. Evaluation of the child with atopic dermatitis. Clin Exp Allergy. 2012;42:352–62.
34. Lee J, Dierkhising R, Wu TT, Alexander J, Weiler C. Eosinophilic gastrointestinal disorders (EGID) with peripheral eosinophilia: a retrospective review at Mayo Clinic. Dig Dis Sci. 2011;56:3254–61.
35. Capucilli P, Hill DA. Allergic comorbidity in Eosinophilic esophagitis: mechanistic relevance and clinical implications. Clin Rev Allergy Immunol. 2019;57:111–27.
36. Dellon ES, Liacouras CA, Molina-Infante J, Furuta GT, Spergel JM, Zevit N, et al. Updated international consensus diagnostic criteria for eosinophilic esophagitis: proceedings of the AGREE conference. Gastroenterology. 2018;155:1022–1033.e10.
37. Ruffner MA, Kennedy K, Cianferoni A. Pathophysiology of eosinophilic esophagitis: recent advances and their clinical implications. Expert Rev Clin Immunol. 2019;15:83–95.
38. Jensen ET, Martin CF, Kappelman MD, Dellon ES. Prevalence of Eosinophilic gastritis, gastroenteritis, and colitis: estimates from a National Administrative Database. J Pediatr Gastroenterol Nutr. 2016;62:36–42.
39. Klein NC, Hargrove RL, Sleisenger MH, Jeffries GH. Eosinophilic gastroenteritis. Medicine (Baltimore). 1970;49:299–319.
40. Uppal V, Kreiger P, Kutsch E. Eosinophilic gastroenteritis and colitis: a comprehensive review. Clin Rev Allergy Immunol. 2016;50:175–88.
41. Walker MM, Potter M, Talley NJ. Eosinophilic gastroenteritis and other eosinophilic gut diseases distal to the oesophagus. Lancet Gastroenterol Hepatol. 2018;3:271–80.
42. Dalal AA, Duh MS, Gozalo L, Robitaille MN, Albers F, Yancey S, et al. Dose-response relationship between long-term systemic corticosteroid use and related complications in patients with severe asthma. J Manag Care Spec Pharm. 2016;22:833–47.
43. Volmer T, Effenberger T, Trautner C, Buhl R. Consequences of long-term oral corticosteroid therapy and its side-effects in severe asthma in adults: a focused review of the impact data in the literature. Eur Respir J. 2018;52:1800703.
44. Morita H, Matsumoto K, Saito H. Biologics for allergic and immunologic diseases. J Allergy Clin Immunol. 2022;150:766–77.

19 Mastocytosis in the Pediatric Patient

Arianna Giannetti, Iria Neri, and Giampaolo Ricci

Abstract

Mastocytosis is a group of hematopoietic disorders characterized by an abnormal increase and growth of mast cells (MCs) in the body's tissues. The World Health Organization (WHO) classifies mastocytosis into cutaneous mastocytosis (CM) and systemic mastocytosis (SM), with different variants of SM further distinguished. CM primarily affects the skin, while SM involves organs such as the bone marrow and liver.

Diagnosis of mastocytosis relies on specific features and criteria for different forms, and the International Classification of Diseases-10-Clinical Modification (ICD-10-CM) provides relevant codes for accurate diagnosis. Serum tryptase levels can be elevated in monomorphic mast cell proliferative disorders (MPCM) and diffuse cutaneous mastocytosis (DCM) but not necessarily in polymorphic MPCM and mastocytomas. In most cases, a skin biopsy is not required for mastocytoma diagnosis unless there is uncertainty.

Mastocytosis is associated with somatic gain-of-function mutations in the KIT gene, with the D816V mutation being the most common in both pediatric and adult cases. However, pediatric cutaneous mastocytosis can exhibit diverse KIT mutations. An elevated serum tryptase level (>20 ng/ml), along with abnormalities in blood tests and organ enlargement, can indicate systemic mastocytosis. It is crucial to consider hereditary alpha-tryptasemia (HAT) in the differential diagnosis.

Therapeutic interventions for mastocytosis focus on managing specific symptoms and preventing triggers. The treatment approach aims to improve the quality of life for individuals with mastocytosis by controlling symptoms such as itching, flushing, and gastrointestinal issues. Close monitoring and collaboration between patients and healthcare providers are essential for optimal management of the condition.

A. Giannetti (✉)
Paediatrics Unit, IRCCS Azienda Ospedaliero-Universitaria di Bologna, Bologna, Italy

I. Neri
Division of Dermatology, IRCCS Azienda Ospedaliero-Universitaria di Bologna, Bologna, Italy

Division of Dermatology, Department of Experimental, Diagnostic and Specialty Medicine (DIMES), University of Bologna, Bologna, Italy

G. Ricci
Department of Medical and Surgical Sciences (DIMEC), University of Bologna, Bologna, Italy
e-mail: giampaolo.ricci@unibo.it

C. Caffarelli, G. L. Marseglia (eds.), *Textbook of Pediatric Allergy*,
https://doi.org/10.1007/978-3-031-71283-8_19

Keywords

Mastocytosis · Cutaneous mastocytosis · Systemic mastocytosis · Indolent systemic mastocytosis · Smoldering systemic mastocytosis · Aggressive systemic mastocytosis · Systemic mastocytosis with associated hematological neoplasm · Mast cell leucemia · Mast cell · Diffuse cutaneous mastocytosis · Maculopapular cutaneous mastocytosis · Mastocytoma · Hereditary alpha-tryptasemia · Tryptase

Test your learning and check your understanding of this book's contents: use the "Springer Nature Flashcards" app to access questions using ▶ https://sn.pub/nspbjm. To use the app, please follow the instructions in Chap. 1.

19.1 Introduction

Mastocytosis is a group of heterogeneous hematopoietic disorders characterized by an abnormal increase and growth of MCs (MCs) in the body's tissues. Pediatric mastocytosis specifically refers to a group of disorders where there is an accumulation of MCs, especially in the skin, with different clinical presentations and outcomes [1, 2].

Only in 2016, the World Health Organization (WHO) introduced a classification system that divided mastocytosis into two main groups: cutaneous mastocytosis (CM) and systemic mastocytosis (SM) [2, 3] (Table 19.1). CM involves the skin with varying degrees of involvement, while SM affects organs such as the bone marrow, liver, and other internal organs. The WHO classification further distinguishes different variants of SM, including bone marrow mastocytosis, indolent SM, smoldering SM, aggressive SM (ASM), SM with an associated hematological neoplasm (SM-AHN), and MCs leukemia (MCL) (Table 19.1).

More recently, the International Classification of Diseases-10-Clinical Modification Code (ICD-10-CM) has addressed the diagnostic features and criteria of MCs activation disorders, including mastocytosis. It has defined specific codes for different forms of mastocytosis, particularly highlighting cutaneous mastocytosis in childhood. Additionally, the ICD-10-CM proposes an adjusted classification for disorders associated with MC activation, referred to as MC activation disorders (MCADs) [4].

Within this context, this chapter discusses pediatric mastocytosis, which typically manifests as a cutaneous disorder within the first 2 years of life. This condition is analyzed within the broader category of MC activation disorders.

Table 19.1 Modified WHO classification of mastocytoses 2016 to 2021 [2, 3]

Cutaneous mastocytoses (CM)	Maculopapular cutaneous mastocytosis (MPCM) = urticaria pigmentosa (UP)	*Monomorphic variant* Fig. 19.1.
		Polymorphic variant Fig. 19.2.
	Diffuse cutaneous mastocytosis (DCM) Fig. 19.3.	
	Mastocytoma of skin (cutaneous mastocytoma) Fig. 19.4.	*Isolated mastocytoma*
		Multilocalized mastocytomas
Systemic mastocytoses (SM)	Indolent mastocytosis (ISM)	
	Smoldering SM (SSM)	
	SM with associated hematological neoplasm (SM-AHM)	
	Aggressive SM (ASM)	
	MCs leucemia (MCL)	
MCs sarcome		

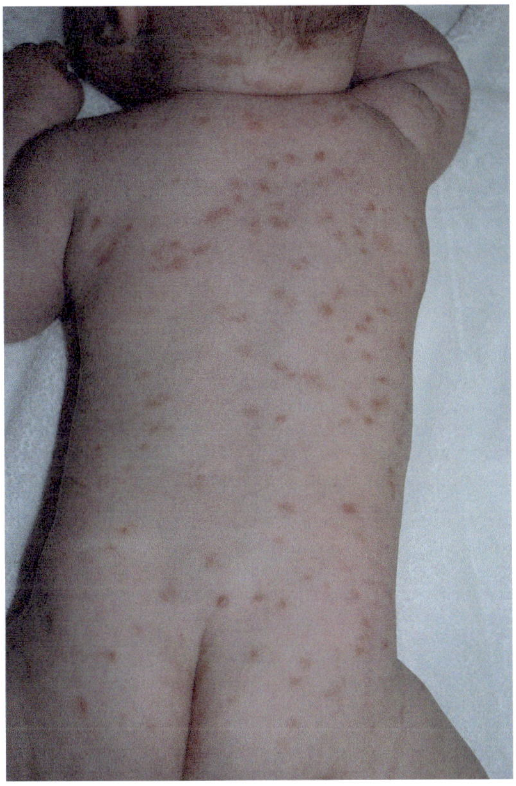

Fig. 19.1 MPCM monomorphic small lesions

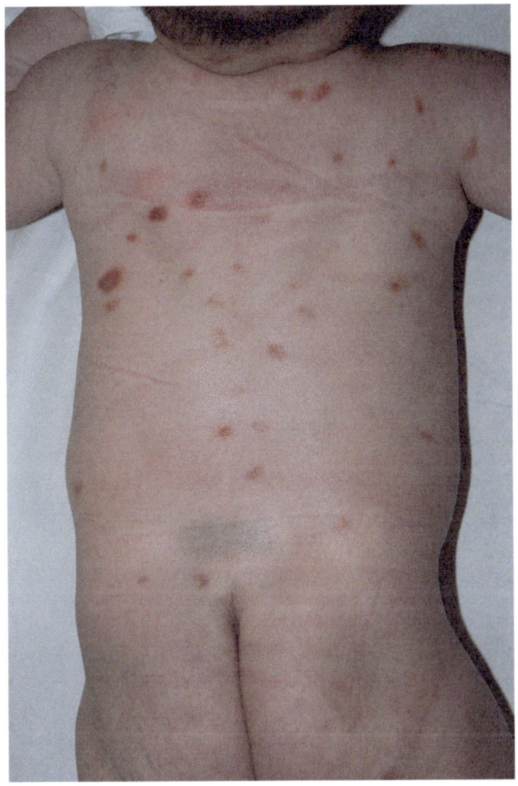

Fig. 19.2 MPCM polymorphic larger asymmetric lesions

19.2 The Biological Functions of Mast Cells

MCs, first described by Friedrich von Recklinghausen in 1863, are granulated cells found in connective tissues. However, it wasn't until 1878, when they were stained with basic aniline dyes, that they were named "Mastzellen" by Paul Ehrlich' thesis [5]and published the next year [6]. MCs originate from bone marrow hematopoietic progenitors and are primarily located within the connective tissue of vascularized organs, mucosal tissues (such as the respiratory and intestinal tracts, where they serve as "sentinels"), and predominantly in the skin [7].

MCs are the offsprings of CD34^{+} hematopoietic stem cells and have a stringent necessity for stem cell factor (SCF), the ligand for the c-kit receptor (CD117), for differentiation [8].

There are two anatomically distinct subtypes of MCs: MCTC (MCs co-expressing tryptase and chymase) and MCT (MCs expressing tryptase with little to no chymase) [9].

This strict classification, however, is somewhat outdated in humans, with the understanding that mast cell progenitors differentiate into mature cells below the effect of microenvironmental aspects that greatly increase mast cell heterogeneity [7].

MCTC cells are found in connective tissues, while MCT cells reside in the epithelium of mucosal tissues. These cells contain numerous cytoplasmic granules filled with pre-stored mediators, including histamine and tryptase. Upon activation, MCs release these mediators into the bloodstream, leading to clinical manifestations. MCs produce various pro-inflammatory mediators and cytokines, such as histamine, cysteinyl leukotrienes, prostaglandins, heparin, and various proteases. Tryptases, which are serine proteases, are preferentially produced and stored in MCs, accounting for more than 20% of the total protein content in tissue MCs [7].

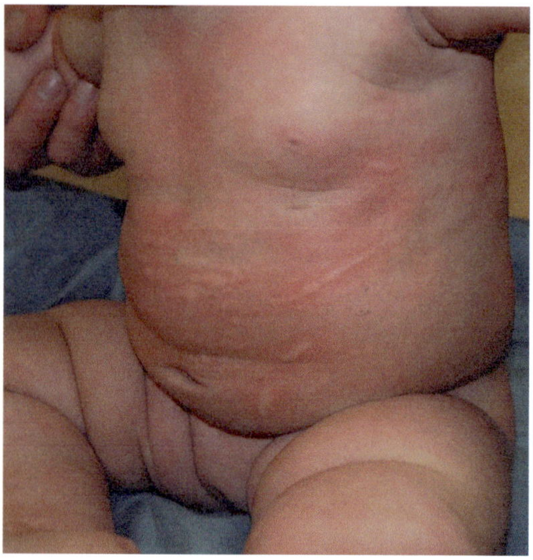

Fig. 19.3 Diffuse cutaneous mastocytosis(DCM)

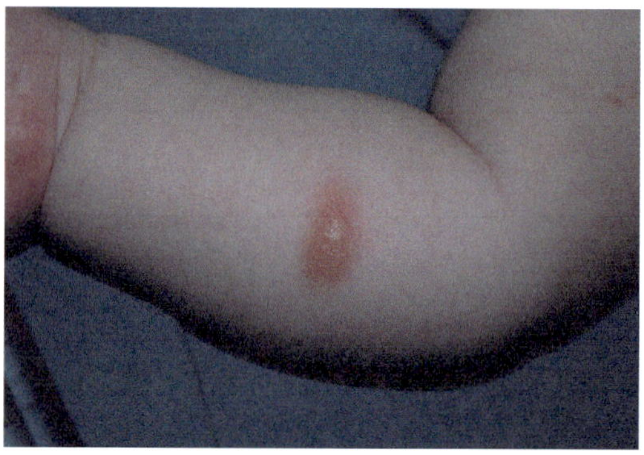

Fig. 19.4 Mastocytoma

While mature tryptases are mainly stored in metachromatic granules, precursor forms (pro-tryptases) are continuously released from resting MCs. The stable release rate of tryptases leads to an extremely constant basal serum tryptase level in healthy individuals. However, during severe anaphylactic events where MCs release large amounts of tryptase, the serum tryptase level significantly increases above the individual's baseline. The tryptase level returns to baseline within several hours (up to 24 h), providing a consistent diagnostic window of about 2–4 h for laboratory tests. Other chemical mediators like histamine, prostaglandin D2, and heparin may also serve as indicators. Tryptase is considered a reliable biomarker of severe systemic MCs activation [10]. While tryptase is also released by activated basophils, MCs contain much higher levels of tryptase, making it somewhat specific to their function.

The most well-known function of MCs is their key effector role in IgE-dependent allergic disorders. MC activation is classically induced by the binding of allergens to the high-affinity Fc epsilon receptor 1 (FcεRI) [11].

The severity of an anaphylactic reaction is influenced by the number of MCs involved, cytokine exposure, the nature and number of triggers, and the presence of cofactors. Severe or life-threatening episodes may occur when there is a high burden of MCs, when most or all MCs are in a "hyperactivated" state and release all their mediators massively and promptly, or when comorbidities such as cardiovascular or pulmonary diseases significantly contribute to the event. During an anaphylactic episode, there is a massive and rapid release of granular mediators and enzymes from MCs. Furthermore, during degranulation, the cell surface and cytoplasmic membranes of MCs undergo reorganization, and lipid membrane-derived mediators are produced and secreted de novo.

19.3 Definition of Mastocytosis Inside the Mastcells Activation Disorders

Mastocytosis is characterized by the abnormal expansion of clonal MCs, leading to their accumulation in various regions of the body, predominantly the skin and bone marrow. The prevalence rate of mastocytosis is estimated to be around 9 cases per 100,000 persons in the USA [12] and 13 cases per 100,000 persons in the Dutch region for individuals aged over 15 years [1].

In terms of pediatric mastocytosis, approximately 35 out of 100 cases are cutaneous mastocytosis, which primarily affects the skin, while systemic mastocytosis occurs in about 1.8 out of 100 cases [28]. Cutaneous mastocytosis is the most common form observed in children, whereas systemic forms are very rare in this age group.

Despite its long history, dating back to the first description of cutaneous mastocytosis in 1869

[13], it was only in 2016 that the World Health Organization (WHO) officially recognized mastocytosis as a distinct disease category separate from myeloproliferative neoplasms [3]. The term "mastocytosis" encompasses a wide range of clinical forms, ranging from the most benign to the rare but potentially life-threatening forms [14].

19.4 Genetic

Indeed, only a few antigens that are specifically expressed in MCs have been identified. One of these antigens is the stem cell factor (SCF) receptor KIT, also known as CD117. While KIT is a rather specific marker of MCs, it is also expressed in other cell types such as germ cells, bone marrow precursor cells, and plasma cells. KIT is encoded by the proto-oncogene c-Kit. Upon activation by its cytokine ligand (SCF), KIT plays a crucial role in the proliferation, differentiation, migration, and apoptosis of various cell types. It is involved in hematopoiesis, stem cell maintenance, gametogenesis, melanogenesis, as well as MCs development, movement, and function [1].

In mastocytosis, a disorder characterized by an abnormal accumulation of MCs, somatic gain-of-function mutations in the KIT gene have been identified. The most common mutation is an aspartic acid-to-valine substitution at position 816 (D816V) [15], which enhances the survival and autonomous growth of neoplastic MCs. These mutations are implicated in the development of mastocytosis in both pediatric and adult populations. The D816V mutation leads to intrinsic activation and phosphorylation of the stem cell factor, driving MC differentiation, survival, and infiltration into organs. It is found in over 80% of adult-onset mastocytosis cases associated with activating KIT mutations in exon 17. However, this mutation is only detected in approximately 35% of pediatric mastocytosis cases [1, 16].

In children with cutaneous mastocytosis, different variants of the KIT gene have been observed. In a study of pediatric cutaneous mastocytosis, 86% of children had various KIT mutations detected in lesional skin. Among the mutations found, 42% of children had mutations in codon 816 (including D816V, D816Y, and D816I), with the D816V mutation being present in only 36% of those cases [1, 16].

This indicates the presence of diverse KIT mutations in pediatric cutaneous mastocytosis.

19.5 Characterization of Pediatric Mastocytosis

- **Cutaneous mastocytosis (CM)** is the most common form of mastocytosis in the pediatric population. It is characterized by the local accumulation of MCs limited to the skin. CM has three different forms:
  - *MPCM*, also known as urticaria pigmentosa, which has two variants: monomorphic and polymorphic [17]. It is clinically characterized by the presence of small, monomorphic, red-brown macules/papules, typically found on the trunk and extremities, while face palms, soles, and scalp are usually spared [18].
  - *DCM* is relatively uncommon, accounting for no more than 2% of all forms of CM. It results from infiltration of MCs throughout the entire skin, often with a neonatal onset [19].
  - *Solitary/localized cutaneous mastocytoma* is another form of CM, accounting for up to 15% of all pediatric cases. This form of CM is characterized by a limited accumulation of MCs in a specific skin site, possibly triggered by the release of stem cell factor (SCF), nerve growth factor, and interleukin-5 [20].

In most cases, CM follows a benign course and often regresses by puberty. Recent data has shown that localized mastocytomas tend to regress at a rate of 10% per year, while MPCM has a slower regression rate of 1.9% per year [3, 17, 21].

- **Systemic mastocytosis (SM)** is very rare in pediatric age and is characterized by the involvement of multiple organs, requiring differentiation from MC activation syndrome

(MCAS). SM typically affects the bone marrow, spleen, liver, and gastrointestinal tract.

Based on the provided criteria, the diagnosis of systemic mastocytosis (SM) can be made if at least one major criterion and one minor criterion, or three minor criteria, are fulfilled [2]:

- *Major criterion:* Multifocal dense infiltrates of mast cells (≥15 mast cells in aggregates) in bone marrow biopsies and/or in sections of other extracutaneous organ(s).
- *Minor criteria:*
  a. ≥25% of all mast cells are atypical cells (type I or type II) on bone marrow smears or are spindle-shaped in mast cell infiltrates detected in sections of bone marrow or other extracutaneous organs.
  b. KIT-activating KIT point mutation(s) at codon 816 or in other critical regions of KIT in bone marrow or another extracutaneous organ.
  c. Mast cells in bone marrow, blood, or another extracutaneous organ express one or more of: CD2 and/or CD25 and/or CD30.
  d. Baseline serum tryptase concentration >20 ng/mL (in the case of an unrelated myeloid neoplasm, an elevated tryptase does not count as an SM criterion. In the case of a known HαT, the tryptase level should be adjusted).

The true incidence of SM in children is unknown. Some studies have reported a low prevalence of SM among children: a Spanish study recognized only 2 cases of SM out of 111 children with mastocytosis, an Australian study found SM in 2 out of 173 children, and a Polish study reported progression to SM in only 1 out of 101 children [22].

19.6 Main Clinical Findings

19.6.1 Maculopapular Cutaneous Mastocytosis

In approximately 70–80% of cases, the initial lesions of childhood-onset cutaneous mastocytosis develop within the first year of life. Typically, these lesions appear in the first few weeks or first half year of life [23] and rarely they can appear during toddler age or even in school age [23].

MPCM is characterized by the presence of yellow-brownish or red-brown papules and macules on the skin. The number of lesions can vary between <10 and >100.

The monomorphic variant of MPCM (Fig. 19.1) presents multiple small red-brown round maculopapular skin lesions. On the other hand, the polymorphic variant (Fig. 19.2), shows slightly larger lesions with different shapes. Plaques and nodules are reported, typically located on the trunk. The face and extremities are often spared.

Diagnosis of MPCM is often based on clinical findings, including characteristic skin lesions, age of onset, Darier's sign and a history suggestive of MC mediator release. Laboratory tests, such as serum tryptase, complete blood count with differential diagnosis, and liver function tests, may be performed to exclude systemic involvement. In unclear cases, skin biopsy is indicated to confirm the diagnosis. In the absence of systemic symptoms, hepatosplenomegaly (enlarged liver and spleen), lymphadenopathy (enlarged lymph nodes), and any laboratory evidence of systemic involvement, the patient can be followed longitudinally [24]. Bone marrow biopsy is not typically indicated unless tryptase levels are highly elevated (>20 ng/mL) [24].

19.6.2 Diffuse Cutaneous Mastocytosis

DCM is a rare variant of mastocytosis characterized by the infiltration of MCs throughout the entire skin. It accounts for no more than 2–5% of all forms of cutaneous mastocytosis [23].

DCM typically presents at birth or within the first few months of life. The skin may appear thick and leathery with a yellow-brown peau d'orange appearance.

The skin in DCM may also exhibit diffuse thickening (known as pachyderma), which gives it an "orange skin" appearance. Intense itching and episodes of diarrhea can also occur in individuals with DCM. Positive Darier sign (urticaria and erythema upon stroking or rubbing the skin) and strong dermographism (raised red lines or welts appearing with light scratching or pressure) are typical features of DCM [25].

The Darier's sign is typical for all forms of CM.

CM is often associated with systemic symptoms due to the release of mast cell mediators. Flushing, itching, blistering, diarrhea, abdominal pain, vomiting, hypotension, headache and bone pain are the most frequently reported symptoms [25].

19.6.3 Mastocytoma

Mastocytomas (Fig. 19.4) is a solitary (or up to three) lesion can appear as round or oval macules, papules, plaques, or nodules, typically ranging in size from 1 to 5 cm in diameter. The lesional margins may be either unclear or sharp. The lesion often shows a peau d'orange appearance [26].

Mastocytomas can be found on various body regions, including the trunk, extremities, flexural areas, head, and neck. The lesional margins may be either unclear or sharp. Initially, the mastocytoma tends to grow in size over several months or for a variable period of time before eventually regressing over time.

The main symptoms associated with mastocytoma include pruritus (itching), flushing (sudden reddening of the skin), and wheals (raised areas of skin) that occur upon stroking, rubbing, or scratching the lesion. These symptoms are caused by the spontaneous or induced activation of MCs, resulting in the release of vasoactive amines [20]. Common triggers include local or systemic causes (Table 19.2).

It's important to note that a positive Darier sign, which refers to the induction of localized urticaria and erythema upon rubbing or stroking the affected skin, can only be triggered in approximately 50–90% of patients [26].

However, the absence of a Darier sign does not exclude the diagnosis of mastocytoma. In cases of large mastocytomas, the Darier sign should not be vigorously elicited as it can lead to blistering of the lesion and the potential onset of systemic symptoms such as flushing, dyspnea (shortness of breath), hypotension (low blood pressure), nausea, vomiting, abdominal pain, and diarrhea. Organomegaly (enlarged organs) and lymphadenopathy (enlarged lymph nodes) are typically absent in mastocytoma cases [26].

19.6.4 Systemic Mastocytosis

Systemic mastocytosis (SM) is indeed rare in children and accounts for less than 10% of pediatric mastocytosis cases. In SM, there is an abnormal accumulation of MCs not only in the

Table 19.2 Local or systemic triggers in Mastocytosis

Mechanical irritation	Local friction, rubbing, massage, and stroking can trigger MCs degranulation. Surgical trauma, such as vaccinations, tooth extraction, or surgery, can also lead to MCs activation.
Physical stimuli	MCs can be activated by physical stimuli, such as exercise, emotional stress, and extremes of temperature (very cold or hot baths).
Foods ingestion	Certain foods can trigger MCs degranulation, including alcohol, hot beverages, spicy foods, and cheese.
Drugs	Various medications can induce MCs activation, including dextromethorphan, aspirin, nonsteroidal anti-inflammatory drugs (NSAIDs), anticholinergic medications, thiamine, procaine, certain antibiotics (e.g., penicillins, vancomycin, polymyxin B sulfate), opiates (e.g., codeine and morphine), and muscle relaxants (e.g., succinylcholine, rocuronium, atracurium).
Vaccines	Particularly live viral vaccines can trigger MC activation, which is more problematic in diffuse cutaneous mastocytosis.
Others	Additional triggers include exposure to iodinated radiocontrast agents, venomous snake bites, jellyfish stings, hymenoptera stings, and teething in young children.

Modified by Ref. [27]

skin but also in multiple organs throughout the body [24].

Children with SM typically have skin lesions that appear different from the typical maculopapular cutaneous mastocytosis (MPCM) seen in pediatric cases. The skin lesions in SM are described as small and uniform in appearance, which may distinguish them from MPCM.

In systemic disease, MCs can accumulate in various organs such as the bone marrow, gastrointestinal tract, liver, spleen, and lymph nodes. However, it's important to note that the majority of children with SM tend to have an indolent (slow-growing) form of the disease, which means that it progresses slowly and is less aggressive compared to other forms of systemic mastocytosis [24].

19.7 Laboratory

In monomorphic MPCM, serum tryptase levels can sometimes be increased. This suggests an association between mast cell proliferation and the underlying hematologic disorder. In polymorphic MPCM and mastocytomas, serum tryptase levels are usually not increased. This is because these conditions are typically characterized by localized mast cell proliferation without systemic involvement [23, 24]. Tryptase can be significantly higher in DCM even in the absence of systemic disease.

In mastocytoma and polymorphic MPCM patients typically do not show any significant laboratory alterations, and skin biopsy is usually not necessary for diagnosis unless there is doubt about the diagnosis. However, if a skin biopsy is performed, the specimen should be sent for histopathological examination to confirm the presence of MCs and, if necessary, for analysis of KIT mutations.

To minimize the adverse effects of a biopsy and potential MCs activation, it is recommended to administer premedication with an oral corticosteroid and antihistamines before the procedure.

On the other hand, baseline laboratory investigations are necessary for other CM or SM. These investigations typically include a complete blood cell count and liver function tests, which assess markers such as aminotransferases, alkaline phosphatase, gamma-glutamyl transpeptidase, bilirubin, albumin, and serum tryptase level.

An elevated serum tryptase level (>20 ng/ml) can suggest systemic mastocytosis, especially when accompanied by abnormalities in the complete blood count and liver function tests, as well as the presence of splenomegaly, hepatomegaly, or lymphadenopathy [1].

However, it's important to note that an elevated serum tryptase level and systemic symptoms/signs can also occur due to mechanical irritation of a solitary cutaneous mastocytoma. Therefore, it is advised to avoid any mechanical irritation, such as stroking, of a solitary cutaneous mastocytoma before blood samples are taken to prevent potential MCs activation and misleading results.

19.8 Differential Diagnosis

In the context of mastocytosis, one of the diseases that should be taken into consideration in the differential diagnosis is hereditary alpha-tryptasemia (HAT) (Table 19.3).

19.8.1 Hereditary Alpha-Tryptasemia

HAT is an autosomal dominant genetic feature characterized by an increase in the number of copies of one of the genes encoding for serum tryptase [28].

All individuals recognized with increased alpha-encoding copy number have basal serum tryptases above 8 ng/mL (average basal serum tryptase caused by duplication is 15 ± 5 ng/mL, and a triplication is 24 ± 6 ng/mL); the human tryptase locus consists of four paralogous genes, and an increase in the copies of one of these genes leads to elevated levels of serum tryptase. Pro-tryptases, which have not undergone enzymatic conversion into mature tetrameric tryptases, are secreted into serum in their monomeric form and deliver the huge bulk of measured basal serum tryptase in healthy individuals [29].

Table 19.3 Diseases in the Differential Diagnosis of Mastocytosis

Juvenile xanthogranuloma	Xanthoma	Postinflammatory hyperpigmentation
Bruise	Melanocytic nevus	Spitz nevus
Granuloma faciale	Hemangioma	Nodular scabies
Leukemia cutis	Chronic urticaria	Herpes simplex
Epidermolysis bullosa simplex	Allergic contact dermatitis	Café-au-lait macule
Amelanotic melanoma	Neurofibroma	Granuloma annulare
Arthropod bite	Drug-related eruption	Histiocytosis
Bullous impetigo	Hidrocystoma	Linear Iga bullous dermatosis
Hereditary alpha-tryptasemia		

Mature αβ-tryptases, which are increased in individuals with HAT, can contribute to MC degranulation in an autocrine manner. They also have the ability to selectively cleave and activate Protease Activated Receptor 2 (PAR2), which can potentially increase vascular permeability and neuroinflammation.

Elevated basal serum tryptase (at present defined as >11.4 ng/mL) appears to be quite common, being reported in 4–7% of the general population [30, 31].

This prevalence is significantly higher among individuals with severe anaphylaxis due to stinging insects or unknown causes (idiopathic), as well as among individuals with systemic mastocytosis. Studies have reported the presence of HAT in a range of 4.4–17.2% in various populations [32, 33].

Determining the normal value of serum tryptase is challenging. An increase in basal serum tryptase by approximately 9–10 ng/mL or >11.4 ng/mL may be suggestive of HAT, but definitive cut-off values have not yet been established. It is important to note that many individuals with HAT may be asymptomatic, with estimates suggesting that up to two-thirds of individuals with HAT may not manifest symptoms.

The clinical phenotypes associated with HAT are variable but often affect the skin and gastrointestinal tract.

The main clinical features reported in association with HAT are presented in Table 19.4 [28, 34, 35].

Common symptoms include gastroesophageal reflux disease, abdominal pain with diarrhea, and cutaneous manifestations such as flushing, pruritus, and urticaria [36]. There is a high frequency of association with atopy among HAT patients [28, 34, 35].

Table 19.4 Main clinical features reported in association with HAT [28, 34, 35]

Main clinical features	%
Basal serum tryptase >8 ng/mL	100%
Chronic gastroesophageal reflux symptoms	56–77%
Arthralgia	44–45%
Body pain/headache	33–47%
Flushing/pruritus	32–55%
Irritable bowel syndrome (Rome III)	28–49%
Sleep disruption	22–39%
Systemic immediate hypersensitivity reaction	21–28%
Retained primary dentition	20–33%
Systemic venom reaction	14–22%
Congenital skeletal abnormality	11–26%
Joint hypermobility	0–28%
Positive tilt-table test	0–11%

While HAT is present from birth, some individuals may experience symptom onset later in life, frequently after puberty. HAT has also been associated with more severe anaphylaxis among venom-allergic individuals and is nearly three times more common among individuals with idiopathic anaphylaxis [37].

19.9 Therapy

Therapeutic interventions for mastocytosis are aimed at controlling specific symptoms and preventing triggers [25]. Here is a summary of the therapeutic approaches:

1. **Preventive Measures:**
    - Avoidance of triggers such as mechanical or physical stimuli, infections, teething,

and allergens, especially hymenoptera venom stings.
- Identification and avoidance of drugs that can trigger MCs activation, including analgesics (such as aspirin and NSAIDs), opioids, muscle relaxants, cough suppressants, contrast media, and quinolone antibiotics.

2. **Pharmacological Treatment:**
   - Recurrent pruritus in solitary mastocytomas can be managed with topical application of potent corticosteroids, which can reduce symptoms and improve cosmetic issues. Topical calcineurin inhibitors like pimecrolimus or tacrolimus can also help alleviate symptoms [1].
   - If triggers cannot be avoided, covering the lesion with a plaster bandage or protective clothing may be beneficial. Surgical excision is rarely recommended.
   - Non-sedating antihistamines are the first-line treatment for diffuse pruritus. The dosage can be increased up to four times if symptoms persist, similar to the treatment of chronic spontaneous urticaria.
   - Leukotriene antagonists, such as montelukast, can be considered as an alternative or adjunctive support [22].
   - Gastrointestinal symptoms can be relieved with H2 blockers, proton pump inhibitors, and diarrhea, reflux or abdominal cramping. Oral cromolyn 5 mg/kg every 6 h is used for patients with gastrointestinal symptoms [38].
   - Oral methoxypsoralen therapy combined with long-wave psoralen plus ultraviolet A radiation (PUVA) has been reported as an effective treatment option for bullous DCM in children (over 12 years old), including those with life-threatening episodes of mast cell mediator release. However, it is important to note that the response to PUVA treatment is typically better in non-hyperpigmented DCM cases, while the effectiveness is usually poor in nodular or plaque forms of the condition [39, 40].
   - Oral corticosteroids are used in cases with associated angioedema or abdominal pain that is unresponsive to sodium cromolyn, with or without diarrhea [25].
   - There are no data on use of cytoreductive in pediatric mastocytosis. Off-label oral midostaurin (a multikinase inhibitor approved for adult ASM) has been used in an infant with ISM up to a maximal tolerated dose of 60 mg/m2 every 12 h with symptomatic improvement of skin lesions and cytopenias [41].
3. **Biological Drugs:**
   - Omalizumab has shown positive effects in individual cases of severe cutaneous mastocytosis in children [42, 43].
   - Nemolizumab, an anti-IL-31 antibody, is a potential therapeutic option for the treatment of pruritus in severe forms of cutaneous mastocytosis (CM). IL-31 is a cytokine that plays a role in mediating itching and inflammation. Increased levels of IL-31 have been associated with pruritus in various skin conditions, including mastocytosis [44]. Nemolizumab specifically targets IL-31 and can potentially reduce pruritus by blocking its activity. Although nemolizumab is not currently approved for use in mastocytosis, it may be considered as a therapeutic option in the future if it becomes available for this specific indication [45].
4. **Vaccination:**
   - Children with mastocytosis should receive regular vaccinations as recommended. Although there is some debate about a slightly higher risk of side effects after the first vaccination, the incidence of reactions is typically mild [46]. Patients with elevated tryptase levels may be suggested to take a daily antihistamine to control symptoms before vaccination [27].
5. **Educational Program:**
   - Detailed information about the clinical presentation, harmlessness of skin symptoms, and favorable prognosis should be provided to patients and their families.
   - Premedication is recommended before anticipated exposure to triggers, including surgery, vaccinations (especially live viral

vaccines in childhood), and radiological procedures.

- An action plan should be provided if urticaria, flushing, or blistering occurs, with instructions on how to manage symptoms.
- Patients at risk for anaphylactic reactions, such as those with elevated tryptase or previous anaphylactic symptoms, should be provided with an emergency kit that includes an adrenaline auto-injector [27].

Key Points

- Mastocytosis is a disorder characterized by an abnormal increase of mast cells in the body's tissues.
- It is classified as cutaneous mastocytosis or systemic mastocytosis.
- Diagnosis is based on specific criteria and codes.
- Serum tryptase levels can be elevated in some cases.
- In most cases, skin biopsy is unnecessary.
- Mastocytosis is associated with KIT gene mutations, with D816V being the most common.
- Elevated serum tryptase(>20 ng/ml), blood test abnormalities, and organ enlargement indicate systemic mastocytosis.
- Hereditary alpha-tryptasemia should be considered in the differential diagnosis.
- Treatment focuses on symptom management and trigger prevention.

Take-Home Messages

- Mastocytosis is a group of hematopoietic disorders characterized by an abnormal increase and growth of MCs in the body's tissues.
- The WHO classifies mastocytosis into CM and SM, with different variants of SM further distinguished. CM primarily affects the skin, while SM involves organs like the bone marrow and liver.
- Different forms of mastocytosis have specific diagnostic features and criteria, and the ICD-10-CM provides relevant codes for diagnosis. Serum tryptase levels can be elevated in monomorphic MPCM but not necessarily in polymorphic MPCM and mastocytomas. Mastocytoma diagnosis typically does not require skin biopsy unless there is doubt.
- Mastocytosis is associated with somatic gain-of-function mutations in the KIT gene, most commonly the D816V mutation. However, diverse KIT mutations are observed in pediatric cutaneous mastocytosis. An elevated serum tryptase level (>20 ng/ml), along with other abnormalities in blood tests and organ enlargement, can suggest systemic mastocytosis.
- Hereditary alpha-tryptasemia should be considered in the differential diagnosis.
- Therapeutic interventions for mastocytosis aim to control specific symptoms and prevent triggers.

References

1. Lange M, Hartmann K, Carter MC, Siebenhaar F, Alvarez-twose I, Torrado I, et al. Molecular background, clinical features and management of pediatric mastocytosis: status 2021. Int J Mol Sci. 2021;22:1–24.
2. Valent P, Akin C, Hartmann K, Alvarez-Twose I, Brockow K, Hermine O, et al. Updated diagnostic criteria and classification of mast cell disorders: a consensus proposal. Hema. 2021;5:e646.
3. Valent P, Akin C, Metcalfe DD. Mastocytosis: 2016 updated WHO classification and novel emerging treatment concepts [cited 2023 Jul 6];
4. Valent P, Hartmann K, Bonadonna P, Gülen T, Brockow K, Alvarez-Twose I, et al. Global classification of mast cell activation disorders: an ICD-10-CM–adjusted proposal of the ECNM-AIM consortium. J Allergy Clin Immunol Pract. 2022;10:1941–50.

5. Ehrlich P. Beitrage zur Theorie und Praxis der histologischen Farbung. 1878.
6. Ehrlich P. BBeiträge zur Kenntniss der granulirten Bindegewebszellen und der eosinophilen Leukocythen. Arch Anat Phys. 1879:166–9.
7. Valent P, Akin C, Hartmann K, Nilsson G, Reiter A, Hermine O, et al. Mast cells as a unique hematopoietic lineage and cell system: from Paul Ehrlich's visions to precision medicine concepts. Theranostics. 2020;10:10743–68.
8. Valent P. The riddle of the mast cell: kit(CD117)-ligand as the missing link? Immunol Today. 1994;15:111–4.
9. Irani AA, Schechtert NM, Craigt SS, Deblois G, Schwartz LB. Two types of human mast cells that have distinct neutral protease compositions (tryptase/chymotryptic proteinase). Proc Nati Acad Sci USA. 1986;83:4464–8.
10. Mukai K, Tsai M, Saito H, Galli SJ. Mast cells as sources of cytokines, chemokines, and growth factors. Immunol Rev. 2018;282:121–50.
11. Moon TC, Befus AD, Kulka M, Lacy P, Redegeld FA. Mast cell mediators: their differential release and the secretory pathways involved. 2014 [cited 2023 Jul 6].
12. Schuler Iv CF, Volertas S, Khokhar D, Yuce H, Chen L, Baser O, et al. Prevalence of mastocytosis and Hymenoptera venom allergy in the United States. J Allergy Clin Immunol. 2021;148:1316–23.
13. Nettleship E. Rare forms of urticaria. Br Med J. 1869;2:323–4.
14. Theoharides TC, Valent P, Akin C. Mast cells, mastocytosis, and related disorders. N Engl J Med. 2015;373:163–72.
15. Pardanani A. Systemic mastocytosis in adults: 2021 update on diagnosis, risk stratification and management. Am J Hematol. 2021;96:508–25.
16. Bodemer C, Hermine O, Palmérini F, Yang Y, Grandpeix-Guyodo C, Leventhal PS, et al. Pediatric mastocytosis is a clonal disease associated with D 816 V and other activating c-KIT mutations. J Invest Dermatol. 2010;130:804–15. [cited 2023 Jul 7].
17. Gurnee EA, Johansen ML, Phung TL, Guo EL, Fong A, Tollefson M, et al. Pediatric maculopapular cutaneous mastocytosis: retrospective review of signs, symptoms, and associated conditions. Pediatr Dermatol. 2021;38:159–63.
18. Macri A, Cook C. Urticaria pigmentosa. J Dermatol Nurses Assoc. 2022;5:190–4. [cited 2023 Jul 7].
19. Hosking AM, Makdisi J, Ortenzio F, de Feraudy S, Smith J, Linden K. Diffuse cutaneous mastocytosis: case report and literature review. Pediatr Dermatol. 2018;35:e348–52.
20. Leung AKC, Lam JM, Leong KF. Childhood solitary cutaneous mastocytoma: clinical manifestations, diagnosis, evaluation, and management. Curr Pediatr Rev. 2019;15:42–6.
21. Hartmann K, Escribano L, Grattan C, Brockow K, Carter MC, Alvarez-Twose I, et al. Cutaneous manifestations in patients with mastocytosis: Consensus report of the European Competence Network on Mastocytosis; the American Academy of Allergy, Asthma & Immunology; and the European Academy of Allergology and Clinical Immunology. J Allergy Clin Immunol. 2016;137:35–45.
22. Coltoff A, Mascarenhas J. Relevant updates in systemic mastocytosis. Leuk Res. 2019;81:10–8.
23. Nemat K, Abraham S. Cutaneous mastocytosis in childhood. Allergol Select. 2022;6:1–10.
24. Carter MC, Clayton ST, Komarow HD, Brittain EH, Scott LM, Cantave D, et al. Assessment of clinical findings, tryptase levels, and bone marrow histopathology in the management of pediatric mastocytosis. J Allergy Clin Immunol. 2015;136:1673–1679.e3.
25. Castells M, Metcalfe DD, Escribano L. Guidelines for the diagnosis and treatment of cutaneous mastocytosis in children. Am J Clin Dermatol. 2011;12:259–70.
26. Sławińska M, Kaszuba A, Lange M, Nowicki RJ, Sobjanek M, Errichetti E. Dermoscopic features of different forms of cutaneous mastocytosis: a systematic review. J Clin Med. 2022;11:4649.
27. Ertugrul A, Baskaya N, Cetin S, Bostanci I. Anaphylaxis and epinephrine autoinjector use in pediatric patients with cutaneous mastocytosis. Pediatr Dermatol. 2021;38:1080–5.
28. Lyons JJ, Sun G, Stone KD, Nelson CRNPC, Wisch MSNL, Bsn BR, et al. Mendelian inheritance of elevated serum tryptase associated with atopy and connective tissue abnormalities. J Allergy Clin Immunol. 2014;133:1471–4.
29. Schwartz LB, Sakai K, Bradford TR, Ren S, Zweiman B, Worobec AS, et al. The alpha form of human tryptase is the predominant type present in blood at baseline in normal subjects and is elevated in those with systemic mastocytosis. J Clin Invest. 1995;96:2702–10.
30. Fellinger C, Hemmer W, Wöhrl S, Sesztak-Greinecker G, Jarisch R, Wantke F. Clinical characteristics and risk profile of patients with elevated baseline serum tryptase. Allergol Immunopathol (Madr). 2014;42:544–52.
31. Gonzalez-Quintela A, Vizcaino L, Gude F, Rey J, Meijide L, Fernandez-Merino C, et al. Factors influencing serum total tryptase concentrations in a general adult population. Clin Chem Lab Med. 2010;48:701–6.
32. Sturm GJ, Kranzelbinder B, Schuster C, Sturm EM, Bokanovic D, Vollmann J, et al. Sensitization to hymenoptera venoms is common, but systemic sting reactions are rare. J Allergy Clin Immunol. 2014;133:1635–1643.e1.
33. Bonadonna P, Zanotti R, Müller U. Mastocytosis and insect venom allergy. Curr Opin Allergy Clin Immunol. 2010;10:347–53.
34. Valent P, Sperr WR, Sotlar K, Reiter A, Akin C, Gotlib J, et al. The serum tryptase test: an emerging robust biomarker in clinical hematology. Expert Rev Hematol. 2014;7:683–90.
35. Sabato V, Van De Vijver E, Hagendorens M, Vrelust I, Reyniers E, Fransen E, et al. Familial hypertryptasemia with associated mast cell activation syndrome. J Allergy Clin Immunol, 1448–1450.e3. 2014, 2014;134 [cited 2023 Jul 7].

36. Doong JC, Chichester K, Oliver ET, Schwartz LB, Saini SS. Chronic idiopathic urticaria: systemic complaints and their relationship with disease and immune measures. J Allergy Clin Immunol Pract. 2017;5:1314–8.
37. Sahiner UM, Yavuz ST, Buyuktiryaki B, Cavkaytar O, Yilmaz EA, Tuncer A, et al. Serum basal tryptase may be a good marker for predicting the risk of anaphylaxis in children with food allergy. Allergy. 2014;69:265–8.
38. Tiano R, Krase IZ, Sacco K. Updates in diagnosis and management of paediatric mastocytosis. Curr Opin Allergy Clin Immunol. 2023;23:158–63.
39. Mackey S. Diffuse cutaneous mastocytosis. Treatment with oral psoralen plus UV-A. Arch Dermatol. 1996;132:1429–30.
40. Smith ML, Orton PW, Chu H, Weston WL. Photochemotherapy of dominant, diffuse, cutaneous Mastocytosis. Pediatr Dermatol. 1990;7:251–5.
41. Liu MM, Kohn LA, Roach GD, Sun G, Garcia-Lloret MI, Butte MJ. Treatment of systemic mastocytosis in an infant with midostaurin. J Allergy Clin Immunol Pract. 2019;7:2929–2931.e1.
42. Maun HR, Jackman JK, Choy DF, Arron JR, Lazarus RA, Yi T. An allosteric anti-tryptase antibody for the treatment of mast cell-mediated severe asthma. [cited 2023 Jul 7].
43. Caimmi D, Barni S, Mastrorilli C, Arasi S, Chiera F, Comberiati P, et al. Le sindromi da attivazione mastocitaria. Riv Immunol Allergol Pediatrr. 2020;34.
44. Lange M, Gleń J, Zabłotna M, Nedoszytko B, Sokołowska-Wojdyło M, Rębała K, et al. Interleukin-31 polymorphisms and serum IL-31 level in patients with mastocytosis: correlation with clinical presentation and pruritus. Acta Dermato Venereologica. 2017;97:47–53.
45. Serra-Baldrich E, Santamaría-Babí LF, Francisco SJ. Nemolizumab: un innovador tratamiento biológico para el control de la interleuquina 31 (IL-31) clave en la dermatitis atópica y el prurigo nodular. Actas Dermosifiliogr. 2022;113:674–84.
46. Johansen ML, Lawley LP. Assessing vaccination reactions in pediatric patients with maculopapular cutaneous mastocytosis. Pediatr Dermatol. 2021;38:502–3.

Contact Dermatitis in Children

20

Anna Belloni Fortina, Anna Zambello, and Francesca Caroppo

Abstract

Contact dermatitis (CD) is a common skin condition that can also affect children. It occurs when the skin comes into direct contact with an irritant or an allergen, leading to an inflammatory reaction. The condition is characterized by redness, itching, and sometimes swelling or blistering of the affected area.It is estimated that 80% of contact dermatitis is Irritant Contact Cermatitis (ICD) and 20% of contact dermatitis is Allergic Contact (ACD). ICD develops because of a direct insult to the stratum corneum, causing alteration in pH or cellular lipids, leading to cell activation and a visible inflammatory reaction. The most common form of ICD in early infancy is diaper dermatitis or napkin dermatitis. ACD is an inflammatory skin disease which affects adults and children worldwide. ACD is an induced IV delayed-type hypersensitivity to a specific antigen, which occurs when a person's skin surface comes in contact with it, resulting in an allergic reaction. Diagnosis of ACD comes from the combination of clinical data and patch testing. The distribution of dermatitis is of diagnostic importance, but its polymorphic morphology doesn't usually help with the differential diagnosis among different allergens and between various types of CD. The association between AD and ACD has been studied and still presents controversial results: particularly, the relationship of atopic eczema to the predisposition of ACD has prompted much debate. AD children with ACD for more than one allergen and statistically more girls than boys. A significant difference in contact allergy frequency was demonstrated for those with hand or foot eczema compared to those without: for this reason, AD patients should always be patch tested to evaluate whether they have a relevant contact allergy and thus ACD. Differential diagnosis needs to consider in primis AD, seborrheic dermatitis, psoriasis, infections and infestations. The greater contact with an increasing number of environmental chemicals from jewelry, cosmetics, and personal hygiene products, to sporting gear and toys, made an increment in sensitization in pediatric population, which may be still on rise. They develop the condition from the usual offenders and even from exposure to diapers, baby wipes, sunscreens, clothing with snaps, dyes, etc. Acknowledge of a prevalence increase of this disease, have supported studies worldwide, to push on the patch test technique even at young age, for a quick diagnosis and a better treatment and prevention.

A. B. Fortina (✉) · A. Zambello · F. Caroppo
Pediatric Dermatology Referral Center – Department of Women's and Child's Health SDB and Department of Medicine DIMED, University of Padua, Padua, Italy
e-mail: anna.bellonifortina@unipd.it

C. Caffarelli, G. L. Marseglia (eds.), *Textbook of Pediatric Allergy*,
https://doi.org/10.1007/978-3-031-71283-8_20

Test your learning and check your understanding of this book's contents: use the "Springer Nature Flashcards" app to access questions using ▶ https://sn.pub/nspbjm. To use the app, please follow the instructions in Chap. 1.

Contact Dermatitis: Overview

There are two types of contact dermatitis, allergic contact dermatitis (ACD), and irritant contact dermatitis (ICD) and together they make-up more than 90% of occupational skin disorders.

They are readily distinguishable based on the characteristics of symptoms and mechanism of response. However, diagnosis is not always easy because there is not a specific pattern for each type.

Contact dermatitis is a common skin condition that can also affect children. It occurs when the skin comes into direct contact with an irritant or an allergen, leading to an inflammatory reaction. The condition is characterized by redness, itching, and sometimes swelling or blistering of the affected area.

It is estimated that 80% of contact dermatitis is ICD and 20% of contact dermatitis is ACD.

In the following paragraphs, the principal characteristics of ICD and ACD are explained.

20.1 Irritant Contact Dermatitis

Irritant contact dermatitis (ICD) is more frequent than the allergic forms: it is a nonimmune related physical and chemical modification of the skin due to pro-inflammatory and lethal effects of organic solvents, soaps, environmental factors, and acids, which are too aggressive, particularly in case of children with atopic dermatitis [1].

ICD develops because of a direct insult to the stratum corneum, causing alteration in pH or cellular lipids, leading to cell activation and a visible inflammatory reaction. Everyone exposed to the same irritating agent is potentially capable of responding in a certain manner, although specific factors such as the presence of ongoing dermatitis (i.e., AD), environmental factors, or skin traumas may facilitate onset. Main irritants in children include saliva, urine, feces (in infants), and personal care products [2].

The most common form of ICD in early infancy is diaper dermatitis or napkin dermatitis. The causes may be the pale blue, pink, or green dyes [3] or rubbers contained in nappies, as has been demonstrated by the recently described "Lucky Luke dermatitis"due to the use of derivatives of rubber and glues used in the manufacture of some types of nappies [4].

There has been recently reported an increase in the prevalence of both ACDs and ICDs due to textiles, especially clothing; the second one is probably caused by the excessive heat that may develop under certain conditions and by perspiration that collects in skin folds (which may also be irritated by rubbing), because of it favors the release of substances by the material, and thus induces sensitization [5].

The most widely known are dyes and fixing resins, but glues, rubber, and metal accessories of clothing can also lead to sensitization if they remain in contact with the skin [6].

Therapy is based on the use of mildly antiseptic packs followed by the application of emulsions. Topical corticosteroids should be avoided, particularly those that are fluoridated, because they can give rise to granulomas and atrophy [6].

20.2 Allergic Contact Dermatitis

Allergic contact dermatitis (ACD) is a common inflammatory skin disease which affects adults and children worldwide. Despite ACD being previously under-recognized among the pediatric population [7], thanks to the notable rise in investigative research in this field, ACD now accounts for up to 20% of all childhood dermatitis. It must be noted that this is in stark contrast to the predetermined belief that ACD was a rarity in children [6, 8].

ACD is an induced hypersensitivity to a specific antigen, which occurs when a person's skin surface comes in contact with it, resulting in an allergic reaction [1].

In other words, it is caused by the body's reaction to something that directly contacts the skin [9]. The inflammatory response takes place in the skin after percutaneous absorption of the antigen, resulting in recruitment of previously sensitized, antigen-specific T lymphocytes into the surface [10, 11].

ACD can be caused in children by many different substances, which are called "allergens," like fragrances and preservatives, usually innocuous for most people and may not even be noticed the first time the child is exposed. But once the skin becomes allergic to the allergen, any exposure will produce a reaction [12].

Diagnosis of allergic contact dermatitis comes from the combination of clinical data and patch testing, a sophisticated but very useful mean, although there is the possibility that the test gives false-positive and false-negative results, which can be correctly interpreted only by experienced dermatologists [12]. Nevertheless, different countries and centers usually have their own patch testing traditions, despite the efforts to standardize the procedure by international societies. Thus, makes it difficult to compare results obtained in different countries [13].

20.2.1 Epidemiology

In clinical practice, allergic contact dermatitis is a relatively common skin complaint whose prevalence has increased in recent years [10], with a great socioeconomic impact [14]. Its prevalence is currently estimated between 14.5% and 70%, depending on whether the population was selected or not, the method used and the size of the sample, and seems to have a tendency to increase with age [6].

In Europe, about 20% of the general population suffers from contact allergy to at least one contact allergen [15, 16], where the most common are allergies to metals, fragrances, and preservatives [15–17].

20.2.1.1 Prevalence in Children

Pediatric ACD has recently become a much more frequently entity, showing growth in frequency and reaching with age the prevalence as that of adult population [6].

During the last 10–20 years, several reports have described a considerable number of children with CA (patch testing without clinical correlation) and ACD, confirming that both may be frequent in children and cause considerable problems [18, 19]. The few studies investigating contact sensitivity (CS) in asymptomatic children, reported rates of positive patch test reactions between 13.3% and 30.7% [20]. The prevalence of contact sensitization, based on positive patch test reactions in children with a clinical suspicion of ACD, is between 14.5% and 95.6% [21].

In 2008, the first reported patch test studies in American populations were reported, confirming that contact dermatitis was equally prevalent in US children as it was in the adult population and that patch testing was safe and efficacious. Today, the United States accounts for an estimated 20% of all cases of dermatitis in this subgroup [22]; however, it is important to recognize that this type of dermatitis may be overlooked, especially in very young children and when it is a contributing factor in atopic dermatitis [23].

Although this was the case in the United States, a significant number of children were patch-tested over the last decade at many international centers and were.

found to have ACD mainly related to nickel-containing piercings, cosmetics, fragrances, and preservatives [24].

In Europe, the two most recent studies conducted on children aged between 0 and 15 years old with suspected CD have shown a prevalence of CS of 46.7–69.3%, of which 49.7–69.8% were relevant [25, 26].

In Italy, the prevalence of contact sensitization seems to vary between 27% and 96% of children with suspected CD.3 Different studies in fact recognized that contact dermatitis often starts at a young age, with a prevalence of 15% in 12- to 16-year-old children23 and occurs twice as frequently in females as in males [8].

20.2.2 Pathophysiology

Knowledge about the physiology of ACD is mainly derived from animal models in which the skin inflammation induced by hapten on the skin is referred to as contact sensitivity (CS) or contact hypersensitivity (CHS), defined by a hapten-specific T-cell-mediated respond [5, 27].

Three elements are necessary for the development of a CS reaction: antigen-presenting dendritic cells (DCs), which are the antigen-presenting cells (APCs) of the epidermis, hapten-specific T cells, and the hapten itself. The composition and nature of the compounds able to induce a CS reaction are very different, but they share some common features: contact allergens are low molecular weight chemicals (<500 Dalton) named haptens, which are not immunogenic by themselves, but they need to bind to epidermal proteins. These haptens act as carrier proteins to form the hapten-carrier complex that finally acts as the antigen. Most haptens bear lipophilic residues, which enable them to cross through the corneal barrier, and electrophilic residues, which account for covalent bonds to the nucleophilic residues of cutaneous proteins [28–30].

Haptens often derive from unstable chemicals, named *prohaptens*, which require an additional metabolization step in vivo in the epidermis to be converted into an electrophilic hapten endowed with antigenic properties. This is the case of urushiol (poison ivy) [31] and of photosensitizers, which must be activated by UV light in order to bind to epidermal proteins.

Metal salts do not bind covalently to cutaneous proteins but form complexes with these proteins through weak interactions. Some metal salts also undergo chemical. conversions in the skin, such as hexavalent chromium salts, which are turned into trivalent chromium, a highly reactive form binding to cutaneous proteins [32].

20.2.2.1 Sensitization Phase (See Fig. 20.1)

ACD can be thought of as occurring in two main stages: the first process and rate-limiting step being sensitization or induction and the second being elicitation. The induction phase involves all the steps, from the initial contact with the allergen to the development of sensitization. Elicitation starts after contact with the hapten in a previously sensitized individual and consequences in ACD [33]. As it involves a cell-mediated allergic response, ACD is considered an IV delayed-type hypersensitivity reaction that is caused by an allergen penetrating the skin.

The ability of a hapten to induce sensitization relies on two distinct properties. Firstly, through their pro-inflammatory properties, haptens trigger the skin innate immunity and send signals able to induce the migration and maturation of cutaneous dendritic cells (DC). Secondly, thanks to their binding with amino-acid residues, they modify self-proteins and allow the expression of new antigenic determinants in the skin. As stated before, skin cells are composed of molecules containing nucleophilic atoms, whereas allergens have electrophilic atoms and thank to their physic-chemical properties, the interaction between these two results in a strong covalent bond resulting in a "complete antigen." [34].

Proteins, to which the haptens bind, can be derived from keratinocytes, components of Langerhans cells (LC) or peptides previously processed and bound to MHC class I or II [35]. Therefore, haptens or haptenated proteins are loaded by cutaneous DC and are expressed as haptenated peptides in the groove of MHC class I and class II molecules [36], associating either directly or via antigen-peptide binding sites in the groove of MHC molecule [37]. This epicutaneously applied antigen associates with these antigen-presenting cells within 6 h [38].

Characteristics like the nature of the hapten, the type of binding to its carrier and the final

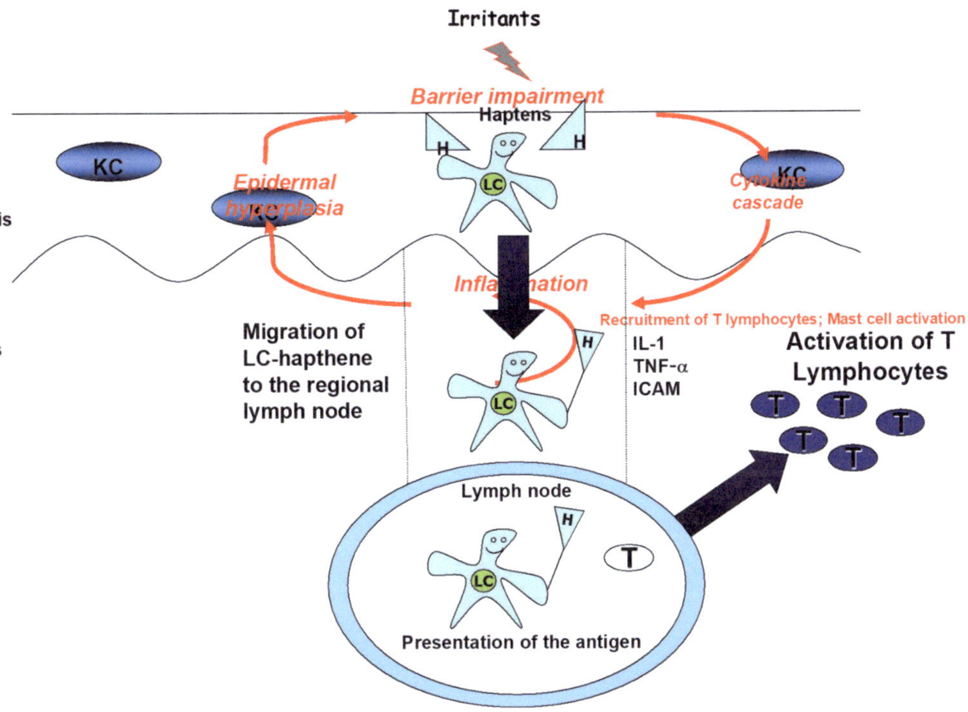

Fig. 20.1 Sensitization phase of ACD

three-dimensional configuration of the complex formed influence the immunogenicity of the hapten-protein complex [39]. Lipophilic haptens can penetrate LC and bind to cytoplasmic components of these cells, which are processed by proteasomes and bind to MHC class I to be presented to CD8 TL.

In contrast, hydrophilic haptens tend to combine with extracellular tissue proteins and are captured by LC, processed and bound to MHC class II molecules to be presented to CD4 TL [35]. The peptide-MHC complex is expressed on the surface of the dendritic cell (DC), enabling the presentation of the antigen to hapten-specific T lymphocytes in the regional lymph node [28].

Capture of antigens promotes a series of morphological and functional changes in the DCs. They become more dendritic, increase the number of Birbeck granules and costimulatory molecules, produce greater amounts of cytokines and change the profile of chemokine receptors in their membranes. So the innate immunity is activated through release of interleukin (IL)-1a, Interleukin-1β (IL-1b), tumor necrosis factor alpha (TNF-α), granulocytemacrophage-colony-stimulating factor(GM-CSF), ILs-8 and -18.37,38,39 IL-1b cytokines released by LC cause keratinocytes to produce TNF-α and GM-CSF, which together with IL-1β determine the maturation and migration of DC [40, 41].

Consequentially, Langerhans and dermal DCs uptake the allergen and migrate to the regional lymph nodes to activate antigen-specific T cells [42].

The allergen carried by Langerhans cells travels via the afferent lymphatics to the paracortical areas of regional lymph nodes, where they find “T” lymphocytes. This binding is assisted by physical factors and specialist cellular adhesion molecules (CAMs). With the recognition of the antigen, again many mediators or cytokines are released, such as IL-1 and IL-2, causing blast formation in the lymph node and present them to naive T cells, resulting in memory T-cell clonal expansion, antigen-specific CD8 and CD4 cells [42, 43].

At this point, after the process of clonal expansion and of cytokine-induced proliferation, T cells bearing unique T-cell receptors (TCRs), specific for the antigen, are created. The "T" cells disseminate via the efferent lymphatics throughout the body and interact with LCs and residual antigen in the skin [44]. Contact hypersensitivity is mediated through this subset of "T" cells that express Cutaneous Lymphocyte Associated antigen (CLA). CLA-positive lymphocytes express CCR1 the receptor for the chemokine CCL-27, produced by basal keratinocytes, which helps in localization [45]. Then, they can persist at site of original contact for some months [46].

The sensitization step lasts 10–15 days and at the end of this phase, the subject is sensitized to the hapten, in the most of cases without clinical consequences. However, theory of the first contact of a chemical being immunogenic for the host is true for the strong haptens but cannot be accepted for the vast majority of haptens responsible for ACD. Indeed, ACD to moderate or weak haptens almost never occurs after the first contact but may take years of permanent skin exposure to develop [36].

20.2.2.2 Elicitation Phase (See Fig. 20.2)

If a sensitized person is re-exposed to a specific allergen in determined concentration, the clinical reaction subsequently develops much more quickly and more aggressively, usually within 24–48 h. When recognition of the allergen occurs, cloning of memory T cells and inflammatory cytokines are released. Consequentially, when exposed to the allergen again, antigen-specific T cells are activated through this release of cytokines and induce an inflammatory process: antigen-presenting LCs passes to regional lymph nodes and bind specific "T" lymphocytes and also specific "T" lymphocytes in epidermis [47]. IL1-secreting keratinocytes may acquire Ia/HLA-DR status and also present antigen to the TDTH cells (T-cell-mediated delayed-type hypersensitivity), augmenting the cascade [47–49].

A delayed or late reaction describes a delayed elicitation response, following antigenic challenge in subjects who are already sensitized. Cytotoxic "T" cells induce keratinocyte death

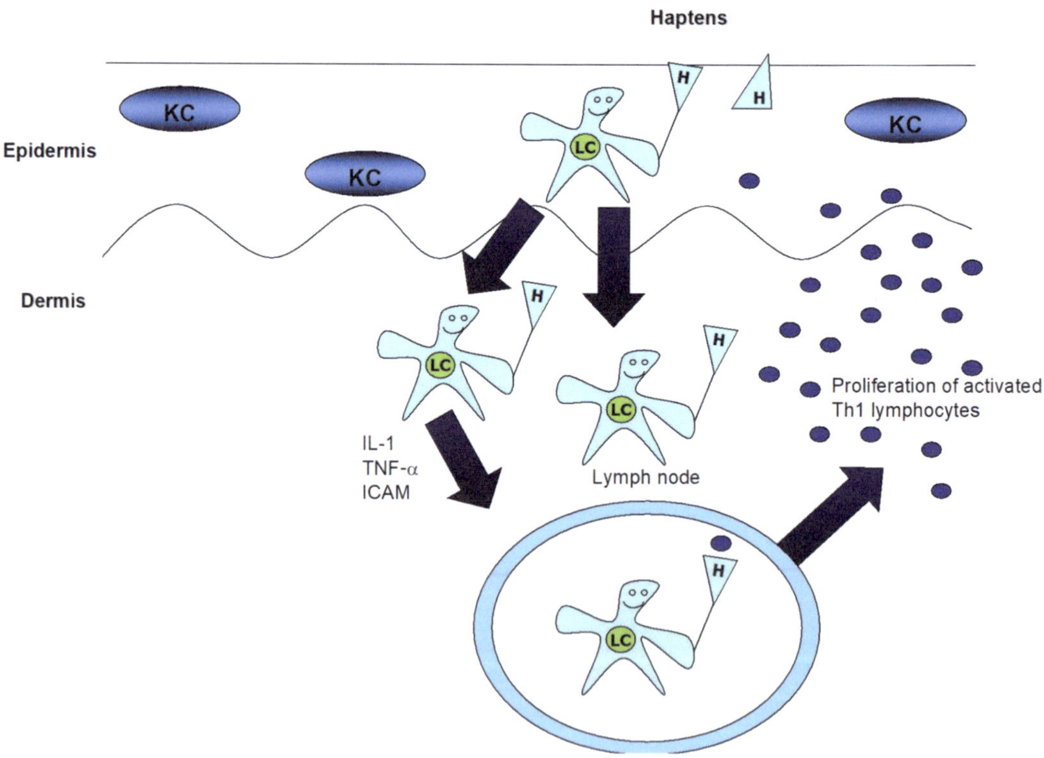

Fig. 20.2 Elicitation phase of ACD

through release of Fas ligand and Perforin mediated pathways and the inflammatory cytokines secreted activate the phagocytic cells, resulting in nonspecific tissue destruction and induce inflammation where symptoms usually take 24–72 h to develop [50].

The site of the inflammatory reaction, which came in contact with an allergen in a sensitized individual, results in redness, papules, and vesicles, followed by scaling and dry skin [51]. After a peak obtained at 24/48 h, the inflammation starts to resolve slowly by active down-regulatory mechanisms, which limit the tissue damage and maintain the skin integrity [36].

20.2.3 Primary Allergic Contact Sensitivity

Although the development of CS has been postulated to require two spatially and temporally dissociated phases, clinical evidence demonstrated that ACD could develop after a single skin contact with a strong hapten in previously nonsensitized patients. This phenomenon has been referred to as "primary ACD" [52, 53].

A recent study on a murine model demonstrated that the pathophysiology of this primary (one step) ACD is identical to the classical (two step) ACD reaction [52]. The afferent and efferent phases of primary ACD can be induced after a single skin contact with haptens due to the persistence of the hapten in the skin for a long period of time, allowing the skin recruitment and the activation of T cells, which have been primed in the lymphoid organs [36].

The Central Role of Dendritic Cells and Cytokines

The application of haptens to the skin induces successive extension and retraction of the dendrites of Langerhans cells (LC), as well as it induces the migration of these cells to regional lymph nodes [26, 27, 54].

These movements are stimulated by IL-1 and TNF alpha, cytokines produced by keratinocytes and by LC themselves after contact with the antigen [54, 55]. During the process of maturation, DC increase also the expression of costimulatory molecules such as CD40, CD80, and CD86, adhesion molecules such as ICAM-1 and cytokines such as IL-12, necessary for effector and memory TL activation [55].

Research published in 2014 identified increased levels even of IL-9 and the Th9-associated transcription factors, PU1, ETS-1, IRF4, and GcN5 at similar levels as these well-known ACD classically associated cytokines. This suggests that even Th9-derived IL-9 plays a role in human ACD, where recently also Th17 lymphocytes seem to exert an important effector role [56–58] (see Figs. 20.1 and 20.2).

Activation of Th17 cells occurs upon contact with allergens in subjects with DACs, and secretion of IL-17 increases local inflammation through the induction of pro-inflammatory cytokines, chemokines, and adhesion molecules. The potential role of Th17 was also demonstrated by an experimental study that showed that the DAC-type reactions had decreased in the absence of IL-17 [58, 59].

Dermal CDs play an essential part in educating naive T cells in the lymph node to become antigen-specific effector cells during cutaneous sensitization. This results in the appearance of dermatitis at the site of contact with the allergen, potentially at prior sites of reactivity [23, 48].

However, the role of LC is still not well understood: Langerhans cells have now been shown to interact with skin resident T cells and generally promote tolerance when encountering antigens by stimulating Treg cells [60–62].

LCs have been implicated in promoting adaptive T-cell immunity, innate immunity, or tolerance to self-antigens, but further studies are needed to clarify this mechanism.

Furthermore, recent studies have demonstrated that CD8+ cytotoxic T lymphocytes are the main effector cells of CS to strong haptens and that they are recruited before the massive infiltration of leucocytes, which contain the down-regulatory cells of CS, found in the CD4+ T-cell subset, by secreting an immune suppressive range of cytokines [48, 63].

Even if ACD was considered the prototype of delayed-type hypersensitivity (DHT) for a long time, the subpopulations of lymphocytes and the antigens involved in the pathological mechanism present peculiarities which individualize this reaction [35]. In DHT, the antigens are relatively large and soluble proteins, whereas in contact sensitization, the compounds are small, reactive, and lipophilic [63].

Furthermore, new works on CS to common allergens (e.g., nickel and fragrance) in human skin have shown that different allergens have distinct molecular fingerprinting. For example, nickel promotes strong Th1/Th17 polarization, whereas fragrance allergy causes Th2/Th22 skewing, which is like the phenotype of AD. While ACD has previously been constant across all allergens, largely based on mouse models involving strong sensitizers, these new data suggest that ACD differs mechanistically according to allergen. Additionally, house dust mite reactions in human skin have been profiled to show unique Th2, Th9, and Th17/22 activation compared to controls, which are similar to the phenotype of psoriasis and contact responses to nickel [18, 64] (see Fig. 20.2).

The emerging idea is that ACD patients should be treated based on their unique allergen polarity with personalized therapy in the next years. The advance in understanding cellular and molecular events seen in recent decades is still in ongoing. The mechanisms involved in loss of tolerance, the discovery of regulating and effector cells, the possible involvement of B cells, as well as the unveiling of the role of DCs and cytokines involved in the process will enable the development of new therapies.

20.2.4 Predisposing and Risk Factors

20.2.4.1 The Role of the Environment

Climate

Climate, UV exposure, heat and relative humidity, may partially contribute to contact allergy, in fact UVB exposure has been shown to reduce the skin's immune response to contact allergens [65]. Besides chapping of skin during winter predisposes to irritant contact dermatitis and false-positive patch test reactions.

Flora

Some tree substances can cause irritant or allergic contact dermatitis. Some commonly known forest plants causing ACD are members of the genus *Toxicodendron* (of the Anacardiaceae family) such as poison ivy (*T. radicans*), eastern poison oak (*T. quercifolium*), western poison oak, and so on. Urushiol, the chief allergenic component, is widely distributed throughout plants, including leaves, stems, and roots [66]. Allergic contact dermatitis results from direct contact with the sap from a portion of a bruised or injured plant, even though indirect contact using clothing, shoes, tools, and pets. Pollen from trees, shrubs, weeds, and grasses is one of the chief causes of allergy. Susceptible individuals can suffer from rhinitis, conjunctivitis, hay fever, asthma, dermatitis, and even anaphylactic shock upon exposure to pollen [67]. Other plants are *Primula obconica*, of the Primulaceae family, whose allergy varies with the changing of season and light, while the allergenic plants of Compositae family are destroyed by cold and frosty weather and return during warmer periods: distribution of 15 allergenic plant material, in fact, is facilitated by dry and windy climates. Pesticides used in agriculture and on plants can be the reason behind these reactions, even if they may seem to be caused by plants.

Cultural and Socioeconomic

Cultural and traditional differences as well as social class, living conditions and geography are involved in the prevalence of ACD and allergens [68]: pattern of perfume, cosmetic and jewelry are more common in upper classes and among the occidental world, whereas habits such as use of henna tattoos and specific dyes are more frequent in India and more generally Asia. Thus, ethnical differences exist, but it is most probably due to different environmental daily exposure rather than predisposition [69].

Stress

Physiological and infection states are indivisibly identified with overproduction of receptive oxygen and responsive nitrogen species nearby with the associative inadequacy against oxidative resistances of an individual. Introductory allergen refinement and in addition advancement of pathogenic insusceptible reaction has been determined with an ascent in foundational interleukin i.e., IL-6, IL-1, and tumor corruption factor (TNF and OxS), with the last one characterized as an overproduction of receptive oxygen. In hypersensitive contact dermatitis, hoisted fundamental levels of these factors are proposed to take an interest in the underlying allergen sharpening and in the advancement of pathogenic unfavorably susceptible reactions [70].

Dietary

A consistent number of studies have been performed to investigate the link between diet and dermatitis. Research has established that for some AD patients, specific foods can indeed lead to an exacerbation of dermatitis and in case of systemic contact dermatitis (SCD), specific foods can actually cause dermatitis. However, establishing which patients may be helped by the avoidance of some food, requires a thorough medical evaluation: research indicates that in a subset of 16 patients with ACD against specific allergens, dietary elimination of these substances will result in an improvement of their skin condition. Well-described allergens in foods that can exacerbate SCD include balsam of Peru (BOP) and nickel. Multiple reports have implicated other food allergens, including propylene glycol, chamomile, and formaldehyde [71].

20.2.4.2 The Role of Gender and Age

Sensitization presupposes individual susceptibility: certain individuals are in fact more prone for developing sensitivity to particular substances, e.g., nickel [72]. The capacity for sensitization varies in each subject and does not seem to follow the Mendelian model of inheritance [73]. However, the prevalence of contact sensitization seems also to vary according to age and gender.

Gender and Hormones

It is proved that women have stronger cell-mediated immunity responses than men. Not only this can be the reason for the prevalence of women with ACD, but this female preponderance in clinical patch test studies is probably due to the large number of greater exposures to fragrances, cosmetics, ear piercing, jewelry, and hair dyes inside this group, in which one of the main allergens involved is nickel, constantly used for the creation of these objects. As persistently shown in many studies, women are significantly more often patch test-positive to nickel sulfate than men [74].

Nonetheless, regardless of whether nickel is considered, women still have a higher pervasiveness for ACD, but the frequency varies also with the characteristics of the sample [75].

Hormonal impacts likely cause this higher powerlessness. Women have higher levels of immunoglobulin (IgM and IgG) than men, and more grounded cell-intervened immune reactions [75, 76]. Both in animal studies and in people, there is a prevalence of immune system illness in ladies contrasted with men, but the impact of sex hormones on enlistment and elicitation of CS is to a great extent still obscure.

In a pilot study, reaction to DNCB (dinitrochlorobenzene) was improved in ladies who got oral prophylactic hormones and a preliminary report shows that the cutaneous reactivity to fix testing varies inside the menstrual cycle. Pregnancy and menstrual cycle may influence the results of patch tests, but the restricted information in this field is uncertain, and merits encourage efficient assessment [77].

Although some studies disagree with this, this seems also to keep up a correspondence in children, where girls are found more frequently positive than boys.81 The increased number of published studies on patch test in children and adolescents has contributed vast knowledge on the subject: two recent Israeli studies found out that nickel sensitivity is more common in girls than in boys and that females were significantly more likely to show a positive response to at least one allergen [74, 78]. Girls are also frequently sensitized to perfumes contained in numerous products, often including those that are claimed to be "fragrance-free," in the form of essential oils or perfumed preservatives, such as benzyl alcohol [79, 80]. The corresponding hapten positivities are fragrance mix and balsam of Peru.

Allergens and Age Onset

Many studies show that the allergic form of dermatitis generally starts developing at the age of 2–3 years and sometimes even as early as 6 months because of the immaturity of the cell-mediated immune system during the first 2 years of life and the progressive exposure to sensitizing agents [81]. It has become a significant problem over the last few years during which greater attention from pediatricians and dermatologists has increased the use of patch tests and consequently the number of diagnoses. The growing number of case reports and cross-sectional studies through the past three decades have shown how allergic contact dermatitis in pediatric patients appears to be on increase, confirming that contact sensitization begins already in infancy.

However, despite some studies affirm there is no difference between ages groups and age does not influence the capacity of sensitization, on the contrary, recent studies found the highest sensitization rate in children aged 0–3 years [82], showing again the idea that contact sensitization may occur early in life [83].

The reason why this process may occur could be explained by the skin characteristics of the pediatric age: children have a thinner stratum corneum than adults, and the formation of the other layers of the epidermis is incomplete; it is only at the age of puberty that it acquires the thickness and trophism typical of adult skin. Consequentially, the absorption of substances in contact with the skin is greater in newborns and infants: their skin is thinner, there is a high ratio between skin surface area and body weight, and it is covered by a sort of down that increases the absorbent surface [84], even more in those subjects with impaired skin barrier, such as AD, where the entrance of allergens into the skin is facilitated.

Some systematic reviews found out age-related patterns which occur in relation to some allergens [85–89]. In early infancy, but also later, there is evidence of topical medicaments such as antibiotics [90] and topical cortisones [91], antiseptics and disinfectants, including mercurochrome [92] and neomycin, very important because of their relevant widespread use [93].

Contact with metals increases exponentially during school age: those responsible for the highest incidence of ACD during childhood are nickel, which is confirmed the most frequent contact allergen among all age-groups, chrome and cobalt, which can also induce co-sensitization to other metals [93]. Ear piercing is the main cause of nickel sulfate sensitization, and the risk increases with the number of piercings, while in adolescence, the substances used in hair dyes (such as *p*-phenylenediamine) can cause ACD of scalp, face, and eyelids. Working adolescents result more often positive to methyl(chloro) isothiazolinone, predominantly on their hands, when compared to nonworking peers [85].

In comparison to adults, in some studies, children and adolescents showed also significantly lower frequency for fragrance mix, methyldibromoglutaronitrile, methylisothiazolinone, and propolis, whereas to sorbitan sesquioleate and mercapto mix among children and to cobalt among adolescents were significantly higher than in adults.89 These results show that the incidence and hapten-pattern not only depends on the age of the subject, but even to habits [23]. However, regarding age onset and allergens, studies are not always concordant, suggesting they also may depend on country and lifestyle [94].

20.2.5 Clinical Features

The primary signs in ACD are rash or skin lesions at the site of exposure. They may include erythema, blisters, papules and papulovesicles or even just a simple red area. Depending on the degree of severity of the reaction, there may be only erythema, visible at the site of contact, or, in more severe cases, the development of bullae with a clear line of demarcation between normal and involved skin [8]. If contact dermatitis persists due to repeated exposure to the allergen, skin becomes dry, scaly, and thicker and lichenification and fissuring can develop later (Fig. 20.1) [95].

Other symptoms may include itching, skin redness or inflammation, localized swelling and the area can become more tender or warmer, with other symptoms like burning and pain. ACD arises from 24 to 72 h after contact with the responsible substance, and it settles down over some days, during which the skin is no longer in

Table 20.1 Major body sites of CS with typical allergen correlation

Distribution	Cause
Hands and upper limbs	Hand eczema is multifactorial, (101) but there is not a particular etiology for a characteristic hand eczema. Rubber gloves can induce a clear pattern of dermatitis over the sites where they are worn, whereas chromate in cement can induce a palmar pattern of ACD and a discoid pattern of allergy. Plants chiefly cause streaky dermatitis.
Face	Perfumes, preservatives, skin care products and cosmetics are commonly implicated (93)
Eyelids	Allergens affecting face can cause eyelid dermatitis; in addiction Primula obconica and poison ivy can cause acute edema. Hair dye, eye drops and ointments, contact lens solutions are commonly implicated (102)
Perioral area and lips	Lipsticks, toothpaste, flavors, and dentures are usually found responsible.
Ears	Medicaments in drops and topical forms, hairpins, hearing aids, spectacle frame, dyes, earrings are implicated.
Scalp	Hair dyes are the commonest sensitizers. Bleaches, hair styling products, shampoos are also found.
Neck	Textiles and necklaces can cause a collar like dermatitis, while airborne allergens, photosensitizers and perfumes can also be responsible.
Axillae	Deodorants, body sprays and antiseptics are common allergens.
Trunk	Clothing dermatitis involves trunk commonly. Photoallergic substances, detergents, fabric conditioners and perfumes are other causes.
Anogenital	Main causes are toilet tissues, nylon, soaps, sprays, (103) but it is also a common site for medicament sensitization.
Thighs	Nickel, rubber, textiles are common. belt and objects kept in pockets may provoke signs of dermatitis.
Lower legs	Medicaments and sportswear predominate. Rubber, colophony, nylon are other sensitizers.
Feet	Shoes, stockings, antiseptics are common allergens.
Exposed sites	Dust, pollens, volatile substances, medicaments, plants, natural resins, woods are common allergens.
Widespread	Medicaments and preservatives are often found.

contact with the allergen. It is generally confined to the site of contact with the allergen, but it may extend outside the contact area or generalize [8]. It can also lead to an infection if the affected area is repeatedly scratched, causing it to become wet and oozing. This creates a good place for bacteria or fungi to grow and may cause an infection and other complications.

20.2.5.1 Body Sites

The distribution of dermatitis is of diagnostic importance, but its polymorphic morphology doesn't usually help with the differential diagnosis among different allergens and between various types of CD. However, anatomical patterns of dermatitis can often suggest a specific cause: CS in typical sites, for example, the wrist, can be correlated with the contact of watches or bracelets, containing nickel parts. Legs and feet, hands and face are the sites most frequently affected by pediatric ACD, mainly caused by metals, footwear, topical medications and cosmetics. Furthermore, studies have shown that also genitals, for the repetitive use of irritating textile dyes in newborns, and eyelids, particularly due to the use of mascara, eyeliners, eye pencils, and eye shadow in girls, have become relevant sites.

Primary Patterns

The primary patterns are represented in Table 20.1.

Secondary Patterns

Not only there is the possibility of the reaction to be very distant from the site of exposure, but even to evolve in a systemic reaction, or again generate an idiopathic response. This can happen even delayed from the time of exposure, not helping consequentially with the right diagnosis. Contact dermatitis can begin at one site, but subsequently other sites are involved. Seriously contaminated areas, or those that were exposed last, tendentially react first,

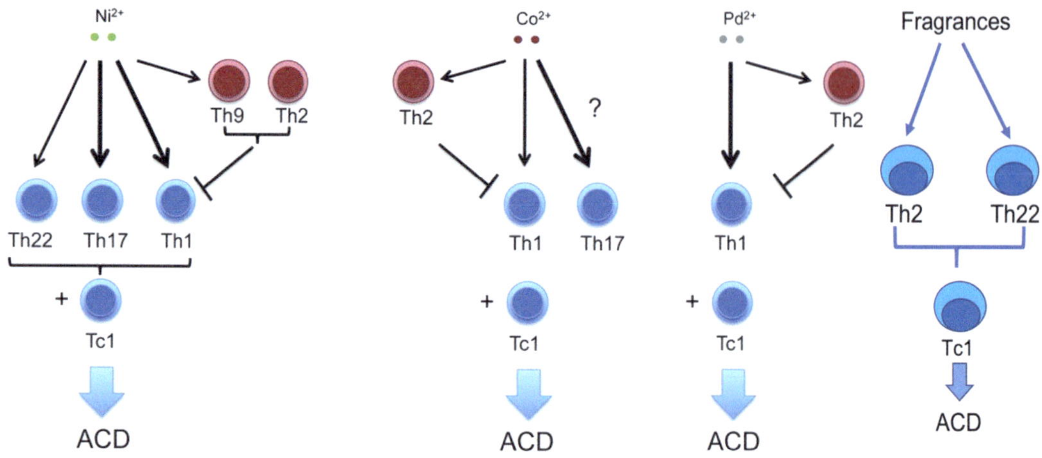

Fig. 20.3 Allergens polarity in the pathophysiology of ACD to metals and fragrances

whereas the other sites flare later. Regions close to the primary site of CS are easily contaminated by the allergen, while dissemination to distant regions has been termed an "id like" reactions, also known as disseminated eczema or generalized eczema: types of acute dermatitis developing after days or weeks at skin locations distant from the initial inflammatory or infectious site [1, 2].

The primary site largely determines the pattern of spread: dermatitis of the hands commonly spreads to arms and face, whereas if it is on feet generally go to legs and hands, transmission from the fingers can lead to dermatitis on the eyelids and genitals, whereas dissemination of leg eczema commonly involves arms and shoulders in a patchy fashion, before becoming generalized. Severe Nickel allergy may induce extensive patchy eczema [2].

20.2.5.2 Clinical Variety

Irritant Contact Dermatitis

They are readily distinguishable based on the characteristics of symptoms and mechanism of response for ICD and ACD. However, diagnosis is not always easy because there is not a specific pattern for each type. ICD is more frequent than the allergic forms: it is a nonimmune related physical and chemical modification of the skin due to proinflammatory and lethal effects of organic solvents, soaps, environmental factors, and acids, which are too aggressive, particularly in case of children with atopic dermatitis [1]. Irritant contact dermatitis (ICD) develops as a result of a direct insult to the stratum corneum, causing alteration in pH or cellular lipids, leading to cell activation and a visible inflammatory reaction. Everyone exposed to the same irritating agent is potentially capable of responding in a certain manner, although specific factors such as the presence of ongoing dermatitis (i.e., AD), environmental factors, or skin traumas may facilitate onset (Fig. 20.2) [2, 96].

Main irritants in children include saliva, urine, feces (in infants), and personal care products (Fig. 20.3) [96].

The most common form of ICD in early infancy is diaper dermatitis or napkin dermatitis. The causes may be the pale blue, pink, or green dyes [3] or rubbers contained in nappies, as has been demonstrated by the recently described "Lucky Luke dermatitis"due to the use of derivates of rubber (mercaptobenzothiazole) and glues (p-terbutylphenolformaldehyde resin) used in manufacture of some types of nappies (Fig. 20.4) [4].

There has recently been an increase in the prevalence of both ACDs and ICDs due to textiles, especially clothing. The second one probably is caused by the excessive heat that may develop under certain conditions and by perspiration that collects in skin folds (which may also be irritated by rubbing) because of it favors the release of substances by the material, and thus induces sensitization [5]. The most widely known are dyes and fixing resins, but glues, rubber, and metal acces-

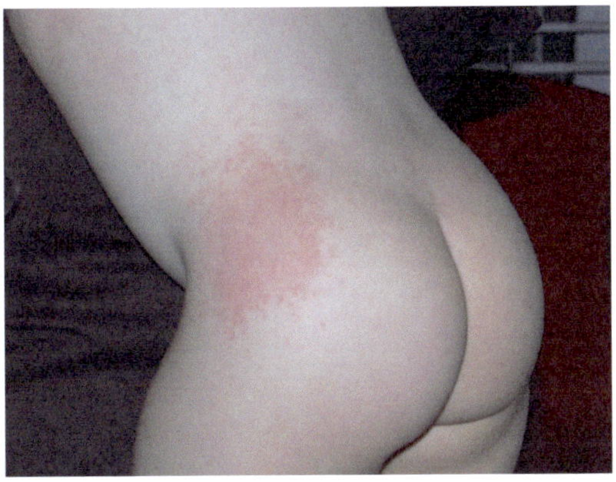

Fig. 20.4 Diaper dermatitis

sories of clothing can also lead to sensitization if they remain in contact with the skin [1, 2].

Therapy is based on the use of mild antiseptic packs followed by the application of emulsions. Topical corticosteroids should be avoided, particularly those that are fluoridated because they can give rise to granulomas and atrophy [6].

Photoallergic and Airborne Contact Dermatitis

Certain substances are transformed into photosensitizers after irradiation with UV or short-wave visible radiation (280–600 nm) and the wavelength required is usually the same as the absorption spectrum of the substance [97]. Photoallergic reactions are based on immunological mechanisms same as that of allergic contact dermatitis. Common photoallergens are UV filters (para-aminobenzoic acid (PABA), cinnamates, benzophenones), perfumes (musk ambrette), halogenated salicylanilides, topical NSAIDs (ketoprofen), phenothiazines, sulphonamides, and other allergens like eosin, quinines, and thiourea. They show the same spectrum of features seen with ACD, with dermatitis localized on the exposed areas of skin, sparing the part below the chin. There is a most distinctive sign for this type of dermatitis is the exempt "Wilkinson's triangle," localized behind earlobe; however, recent studies have shown that these crucial distinctions are often overlooked by medical professionals when evaluating dermatitis [98, 99].

Photoallergic reactions may progress to produce a light sensitivity that may persist a long time after the elimination of the sensitizer called

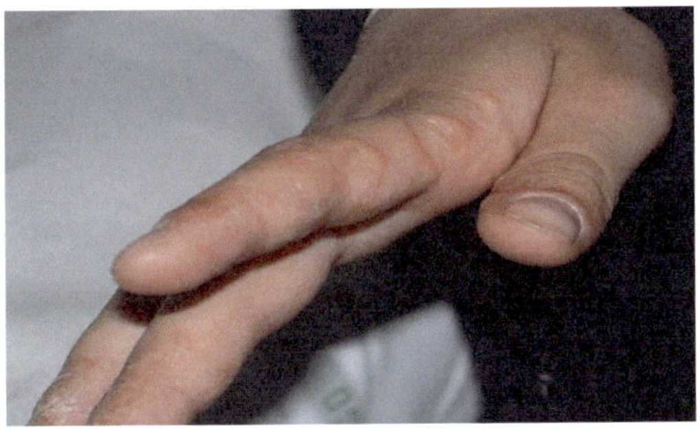

Fig. 20.5 Airborne allergene contact dermatitis

as "Persistent light reaction." [2] Combined airborne and photo-aggravated contact allergy are seen above all with compositae, and the investigation of photoallergy is done by photopatch test. Airborne ACD affects predominantly the air-exposed areas of the body, independently from sun exposure and it is caused by allergens suspended in air (Fig. 20.5) [100].

Noneczematous Forms

Unusual clinical features of ACD are not infrequent: the most common of these types is erythema multiform-like contact dermatitis, which can be elicited by a lot of substances (e.g., woods and plants, topical medicaments, and disperse blue). It is clinically characterized by eczematous lesions at the site of contact with the allergen, which after 15 days turn into target-like erythematic-vesicular or urticarial lesions. Another type is purpuric dermatitis, which is often undiagnosed: clinical features are characterized by classical eczematous foci alternating with papulo-purpuric and papulo-vesicular lesions, which evolve leaving on the skin surface an hyperpigmented outcome [101].

Lichenoid dermatitis is another unusual presentation of ACD, represented by clinical features similar to those of lichen planus. Lichenoid contact dermatitis can affect both skin and mucosa. In this case there are eczematous lesions that evolve together with other papular lesions, with a peculiar lilac red gradation. About the skin, the most frequent cause of this particular form of dermatitis is para-phenylenediamine (PPD), whereas in the mucous membranes, the main cause is metals contained in dental implants (e.g., copper, zinc, mercury, and gold) [102, 103].

Table 20.2 Non-eczematous responses and typical allergens involved

Type	Allergens
Contact urticaria	Natural rubber latex, food, sweat, semen, proteins.
Erythema multiform-like reactions	Quinones, tree tea oil, compositae, poison ivy, rubber, textile dyes, hair dyes, topical medicaments.
Purpuric reactions	Textile dyes, resins, hair dyes, balsam of Peru, rubber.
Pustular dermatitis	Nitrofurazone, black rubber, and medicaments (minoxidil).
Dyshidrosiform dermatitis	Metals, latter, medicaments.
Lichenoid reactions	PPD, metals, tattoo pigments.
Pigmented dermatitis	Fragments, pigments, dyes, medicaments (typically fungicides).
Depigmented dermatitis	PPD, perfumes, tattoos, plants, chloroxylenol, methacrylates.
Granulomatous lesions	Zirconium in deodorants, aluminum-absorbed vaccines, tattoo pigments.
Onycholosys	Hairdressing chemicals, nail varnish.
Systemic	Sulfones in lauryl, ethyl sulfate.

Finally, among the atypical forms of ACD, there is dyshidrosiform contact dermatitis, in which clinical features are typically characterized by pruritic and vesicular eruptions on fingers, palms, and soles, frequently for occupational causes. The main causative agents are metals (e.g., nickel, chrome, and cobalt) and other substances such as PPD, mercaptobenzothiazole and para-tert-butylphenol formaldehyde resin [101].

Other types of noneczematous responses with their common causes are included in Table 20.2.

20.2.5.3 Systemic Contact Dermatitis

Systemic contact dermatitis or systemically reactivated allergic contact dermatitis (SCD) can appear after ingestion or other systemic exposure to a contact allergen in an already sensitized person, possibly resulting in several different patterns of skin eruption. The threshold of reaction varies in each individual case and depends on the dose given and the level of sensitivity. Most frequent types of reaction are focal flares of previous patch tests and old sites of dermatitis, vesicular hand eczema or widespread eczema [2, 104].

ACD and SCD are related but have distinct immunological reactions. A subset of patients with ACD to a specific allergen will develop SCD after systemic exposure. Both reactions are T-cell mediated, and patch testing is used in both conditions to identify the causative allergens, but clinical presentation may differ markedly. ACD occurs due to external allergen exposure that results in a local inflammatory response at the site of skin contact, while SCD has multiple clinical presentations [105]. All contact allergens can cause systemic reactions provided the patient has a sufficient degree of preexisting sensitivity and the dose administered is sufficiently large [106].

SCD from medicaments is common: Neomycin, Quinolines, local anesthetics, ethylenediamine, and corticosteroids are common substances. Flares of vesicular hand eczema are caused generally by nickel, balsam of Peru, garlic, food colors, preservatives, and antioxidants [107].

20.2.6 Concomitant Diseases

Dermatological Diseases

Preexisting or concomitant constitutional dermatitis and ICD damage the skin, affecting its barrier function and producing increased opportunities for allergen absorption and secondary sensitization. In fact, CS is more easily acquired if an allergen is applied to damaged skin, concomitant ICD will promote sensitization and lower the threshold for elicitation of ACD in children exposed to associated allergens [100].

The enhanced risk of sensitization may be due to the increased absorption of allergen as a result of skin barrier disruption, priming of the immunological response with prior recruitment of immunocompetent cells like cytokines and accumulation of mononuclear cells. Furthermore, it has been suggested that ACD can only develop in the presence of cytokine release from nonimmune skin cells, principally composed by keratinocytes, provoked by a coexisting irritant or trauma. If there is no concomitant irritancy, then tolerance will follow rather than allergy. As an example, it is known that hand eczema predisposes to nickel sensitivity and vice versa, and that the prevalence of chromate, cobalt, and balsam sensitivity is increased in men with eczema. It is also time-dependent: longer is the duration of eczema, greater will be the chance of sensitization. Occlusion greatly promotes percutaneous absorption and probably contributes to the extremely high incidence of medicament dermatitis, i.e., in stasis eczema, otitis externa and perianal dermatitis, and is also a factor in dermatitis from shoes and rubber gloves [2].

Nondermatological Diseases
Patients with acute or debilitating diseases such as cancer, Hodgkin's disease, Mycosis fungoides and those with impaired T-lymphocyte function have been seen to have impaired capacity for CS. Experts believe this may also apply to patients who for other reasons, have impaired T-lymphocyte function, i. e., patients with sarcoidosis, lepromatous leprosy and parasitosis [108]. If on one hand, some diseases can be associated, on the other hand, some are not, researchers have found an inverse relationship between CA and type 1 diabetes in pediatric population. Thus, there may be a protective effect of having CA for the risk of type 1 diabetes, or vice versa; type 1 diabetes may lead to skin tolerance rather than hypersensitivity [109]. Alternatively, these two diseases may share common genetic factors, although at present these are unknown.

20.2.7 Contact Sensitization and Atopic Dermatitis

The association between atopy and ACD has been studied and still presents controversial results: particularly, the relationship of atopic eczema to the predisposition of ACD has prompted much debate [82, 110, 111]. For the past, the standard appreciation was that contact sharpening was less ceaseless in patients with AD, inferable from a prevented cell-safe response of the skin, provoking a lessened ability to fight skin defilements and raise type IV sensitivities [112].

Atopics are known to exhibit downregulation of Th1-cells, which should mean a decreased tendency of development of ACD [113].

On the other hand, AD is an inflammatory skin condition in which there are defects in the epidermal barrier, so the presence of AD could facilitate the penetration of contact allergens and promote immune activation [113, 114].

Although some studies showed similar rates of ACD in patients regardless of AD, also showing no associated differences on the gender basis [115–117], latest studies have demonstrated that contact sharpening may vary with the seriousness of AD, proposing an additionally complicated relationship. Difficult-to-treat AD patients frequently suffer from concomitant (multiple) contact allergies, and this may be a reason why the AD turns into a difficult-to-treat disease [118]. Indeed, moderate to severe atopic patients with chronic disease begin to express Th1-cytokines, and thus the development of ACD may be enhanced [119, 120].

Some studies have shown that children affected by AD are at higher risk for developing ACD because of skin barrier dysfunction [111] and they result to be highly sensitive for the external aggression, allowing for allergens to more easily penetrate the skin [121].

Other studies agree that even atopy is a general risk factor concluding that children with a personal or family history of atopy have an increased risk of ACD [122]. There can be also immunological shared pathways between AD and ACD, which include Th1, Th2, Th9, and Th17 responds [122]. Finally, from a pathogenetic point of view, it can be said that sensitization is more likely in periods of disease quiescence rather than exacerbation because of the shift toward a Th1-mediated reaction [123]. However, this is still a theme of debate.

Allergens and Risk Factors in Atopic Dermatitis
Some researchers have shown similar sensitization rates between the two categories of population [116], although AD patients have a higher sensitization to certain allergens, supposedly related to the inflammatory (IL-4) milieu. Studies report that children with AD have different reaction profiles than those without AD, above all to skin care products [124]: major frequency of

reactions to CAPB, wool alcohol lanolin, fragrance, tixocortol pivalate, parthenolide, compositae mix and disperse blue and lower frequency of reaction to MI, cobalt, and nickel, but they even show controversial results on potassium dichromate [122, 125].

It should be considered that all children with AD are chronically exposed to chemicals in topical products and, as a result, the prolonged use of medicaments can increase their sensitization to antibiotics as well as corticosteroids, especially if they no longer respond to treatment [126, 127].

In addition, the prolonged use of these agents could increase the risk of CS to some medicaments (i.e., neomycin, benzocaine, budesonide, and tixocortol pivalate) and to the vehicles (i.e., preservatives and fragrances), for similarity and cross-sensitization phenomena. The topical antibiotics used in the case of the bacterial supra-infection of AD lesions may cause the onset of ACD at the level of the ano-perineal area, eyelids, the auricles, and the legs. Topical antivirals, antimycotics, NSAIDs and antihistamines may also cause ACD: the last two may cause photodermatitis. Even emollients that are strongly recommended in the attack and maintenance therapy of AD can cause ACD because they contain albeit minimum amounts of surface-active agents and preservatives [6].

Mailhol et al. found, in order of frequency, emollients, antiseptics, and cortisones, the causes of onset of medicinal-induced ACD in AD subjects and that the factors related to a higher risk were the severity of the disease, the early onset (at the age of <6 months), and the presence of IgE-mediated sensitization.140 Allergens were emollients (47.5%), chlorhexidine (42.5%), hexamidine (7.5%), tixocortol pivalate, and bufexamac (2.5% each). Consequentially, testing children with AD with additional series besides the European and Italian baseline series may be necessary, as reactions may otherwise be missed [128].

Studies specifically on pediatric patients have shown that AD children have tested positive for more than one allergen and statistically more girls than boys1, whereas other studies did not have the same results, probably due to the sample characteristics. A statistically significant difference in contact allergy frequency was demonstrated for those with hand or foot eczema compared to those without: for this reason, these patients should always be patch tested to evaluate whether they have a relevant contact allergy and thus ACD [129].

20.2.8 Differential Diagnosis

Differential diagnosis needs to consider ICD, ACD, AD, seborrheic dermatitis, psoriasis, infections, and acrodermatitis enteropathica due to zinc deficiency. Sometimes, in children, psoriasis and ACD may present similar clinical features, moreover they can coexist. Examples of anatomical sites, in which it may be difficult to distinguish psoriasis from ACD, are the soles of feet and the palms of hands. Whereas histopathology is not very indicative, as in both diseases there are acanthosis, parakeratosis and spongiosis, the medical history of the patient and of his family may help to reach the correct diagnosis [131].

The differential diagnosis between ICD and ACD can be done by the patch test, the gold standard for differential diagnosis, and it is based on timeline. The patch test time of reading of the positive reactions can differentiate an irritant reaction from an allergic reaction. "Doubtful" reactions, showing only macular erythema, can at times be difficult to distinguish between irritant from allergic reactions, especially in patients with impaired skin barriers or chronic nonresponsive eczematous dermatitis (e.g., atopic dermatitis and xerosis). If in ICD the Patch test gives characteristically a decrescendo phenomenon, in which the reaction reaches a rapid peak and then starts to resolve, generally by 72–96 h, in ACD normally we can see the opposite: a crescendo phenomenon, keeps worsening and resolves more slowly.

In addition, ICD is usually confined to areas of contact exposure, will appear as a well-demarcated erythematous with sometimes follicular reaction, and tends to burn, whereas ACD often expands beyond the area of contact, is marked by induration and/or papulovesicular eruptions, and tends to itch (Table 20.3).

Table 20.3 Main characteristics and differences between ICD and ACD

Irritant contact dermatitis	Allergic contact dermatitis
Often acute onset.	Acute, subacute, or chronic in onset.
Appears after the first exposure.	Sensitization necessary before reaction occurs.
Decrescendo phenomenon: Reaches a rapid peak and starts to resolve.	Crescendo phenomenon: Keeps worsening and resolves more slowly.
Red swollen skin, sometimes ulcerated, in acute form.	Vesicles are typical, but ulceration or skin necrosis is rare in acute cases.
Thickening, erosion, fissuring, or shiny skin following chronic irritation.	Vesicles may not be found in chronic cases.
Sharply delimitated rash around contact.	More ill-defined boundaries, but lesions usually found in areas of contact.
Burning or stinging of the area, which is intensely tender.	Intensely pruritic lesions.

Besides the key factors that suggest irritant reactions, such as timing (earlier presentation) and clinical history, a technique which can be helpful to identify irritant reactions are the "pull test," which help to delineate irritant reactions and to differentiate it from ACD. To perform the test, gentle pressure is applied against the skin tension lines and then released. Upon release, there can be enhancement of the epidermal wrinkling and accentuation of a confluent scaled patch, when there is an irritant reaction, whereas doubtful allergic reactions don't enhance the same way [132]. Chronic ICD and chronic ACD, however, can be extremely difficult to distinguish from each other as the inflammatory areas become poorly demarcated and lichenified, and here, the patch test becomes a highly useful tool.

20.2.9 Diagnosis of ACD

Diagnosing ACD is primarily based on physical exam and medical history. After that, patch testing (PT) is the gold standard for a certain diagnosis. Eliciting a thorough history from the patient and their family to determine which allergens have the greatest potential to be culprits is the first step in evaluation. This includes information about the patient's medical history, personal hygiene, and home environment. A review of their caregiver's environment is also necessary, as patients may develop a connubial dermatitis from transfer from a caregiver, either directly or indirectly. The geographic locations of the reaction can also provide clues regarding allergens to which the patient may be reacting. Furthermore, examining and reviewing the products used by patients and their habits can help determine the allergens that may be repeating in the patients' environment, often from seemingly unrelated sources. An important clinical clue for the diagnosis of ACD and a diagnostic conundrum is that it may take several days after contact with the instigating substance to develop the hypersensitivity response. Because of this, patients may not be able to identify a temporal association with a source. Furthermore, the allergen may be something that the patient has been in contact with or has used repeatedly for years without problems. This can lead the patient to doubt the association. When the threshold, i.e., the point at which the skin's ability to "tolerate" the chemical has been surpassed, the dermatitis reaction occurs. Each exposure is additive, making avoidance necessary to get beneath the threshold and into the "rash-free zone." [130] All these factors explain why the diagnosis is not easy for the pediatrician, both for clinical investigations and for recognition of the offending substances.

20.2.9.1 Patch Test

The patch test is the gold standard for the diagnosis of contact dermatitis (Fig. 20.6).

Patch testing is a biological incitement test which attempts to recreate an allergic reaction to nonirritating concentrations of an allergen that is suspended in a vehicle. Recent data report that the sensitivity and specificity of patch testing in diagnosis of ACD are 70% and 80%, respectively [133].

Some authors have suggested using lower hapten concentrations in children in order to

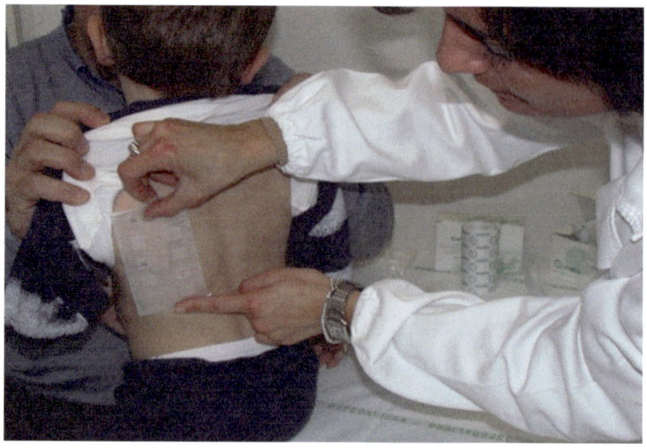

Fig. 20.6 Patch test

avoid false-positive reactions, but the majority now agree on using the same concentration as those used for adults and being more cautious in interpreting the responses [18]. However, irritant reactions may be reported in very young children or in patients with barrier deficiencies; in these cases, clinicians should adjust allergen concentration or reduce exposure interval [132–134].

Indications for Patch Testing in Children

General indications for doing patch tests are eczematous disorders where contact allergy is suspected or to be excluded; chronic hand and foot eczema; persistent or intermittent eczema of the face, eyelids, ears, and perineum [135].

Patch testing assessment guidelines in children include five key considerations: if a patient's dermatitis worsens, changes distribution, fails to improve with topical therapy, or immediately rebounds after removal of topical treatments; if a patient has a particular distribution of dermatitis; if a working adolescent has hand eczema that fails to improve with therapy; if the patient has AD that started in adolescence or adulthood with definitely no history of childhood eczema; and importantly, if a patient has severe or widespread AD that will require immunosuppressive systemic medication [136].

Materials and Technique

The most common system used to apply allergens is the Finn chamber on Scanpor tape. The chambers consist of small occlusive aluminum discs to ensure occluded contact with skin, mounted on nonocclusive tape. Other systems consist of square plastic chambers (Vanderbend chambers), oval plastic chambers (Epicheck) and older AL test system (a filter paper mounted on aluminized paper) [137]. Of late, there is a pre-packaged ready to use patch test system called TRUE (Thin layer Rapid Use Epicutaneous test), based on dispersion of allergen in a hydrophilic polymer. The amount of allergen is defined by its concentration in the vehicle and amount applied and the concentrations used for patch testing are usually much higher than those encountered during development of dermatitis [138].

The test substance should be soluble in the vehicle and the ideal one used is petrolatum, which rarely gives allergic reactions. In hot climates, petrolatum may not be ideal as it melts too quickly. If petrolatum is used as the vehicle and disposable syringes are the containers, a length of 5 mm of test substance will suffice. If vehicle is a fluid, a digital pipette should be used to deliver 15–20 μL to a filter paper in the chamber. Uniform dispersion and particle size are also important. Irritant solvents such as chloroform and benzene must not be employed.

Patch testing is, for practical reasons, performed on the upper back [139]. In the contact dermatitis literature, it is regularly stated that there are regional differences in reactivity [140]. The lower back has been said to have lower reactivity than the upper part of the back; however, the results of studies are divergent and recent studies didn't observed differences [141]. Both allergic and irritant reactions are most easily provoked on the upper back and this site is least likely to be disturbed; other sites used are

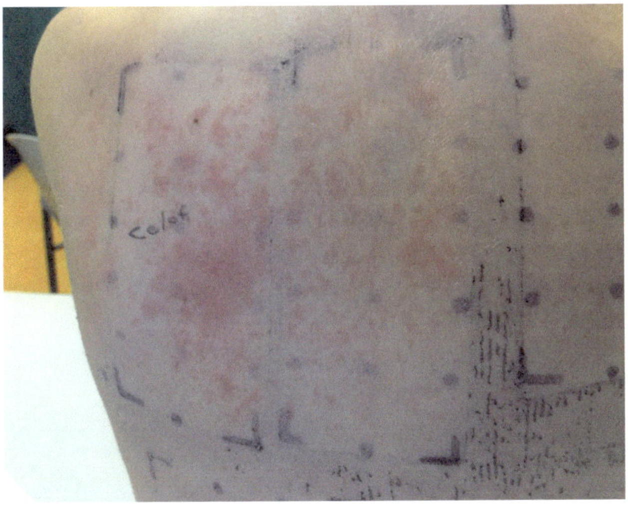

Fig. 20.7 Skin area marking in patch test procedure

lateral aspect of upper arm, abdomen, thighs. Then, test site must be marked with indelible ink or stratum corneum stains (Fig. 20.7) [37].

Exposure Time and Interpretation

Well-established allergens are conventionally tested in such concentration that a 48-h exposure, under an occlusive patch, will generally allow penetration of an amount sufficient to produce a reaction. After 24–48 h, these chambers should be removed to reduce irritant reactions and the initial reading is performed at this time, noting any erythema, induration, papules, or blistering. Some reactions may take up to 1 h to develop once the pressure of the strips has been released and the infiltration allowed to swell the dermis. The patient then returns for a 72- to 120-h delayed read, and again, this reading helps also to distinguish between allergic and irritant contact reactions. The accepted paradigm is that contact allergy reactions rise later during the course of the patch test procedure, while irritant contact reactions present earlier and decrease with time [142, 143]. ICD reactions, as mentioned above, are typically seen early and are usually in the healing resolution phase by 72–96 h [144]. ACD reactions, on the other hand, continue to worsen over the duration of the patch test procedure. A second retrospective history is obtained after the final patch test reading, preferably with the same observer performing each reading, to further delineate the clinical relevance of the positive reactions and to investigate for potential exposure sources. This is crucial to avoid unnecessarily restricting the patients' daily routine, as all positive patch test results may not be relevant to the patient's current dermatitis presentation.

Owing to geographical or organizational circumstances, the reading times may vary [141].

Ideally, readings should be performed at D2, D3 or D4, and around D7. Some studies investigate the role of adding a new later lecture of patch testing, at 4, 5 or 7 days after the exposure, finding out that D7 reading is probably of added value to identify new positive patch test reactions, especially for topicals and corticosteroids [133], with no associations found with gender, AD, and occupational dermatitis. These results were concordant with previous findings, and additional readings after day 7 were particularly useful for identifying reactions to metals (gold, cobalt, beryllium, palladium), specific preservatives (dodecyl gallate, propolis), and topical antibiotics such as neomycin [145]. For patients with therapy-resistant skin lesions affecting the face and hands, patch testing with an evaluation for 7 days is recommended [146]. Days 3, 5, and 7 or later should also be considered for acrylates but, if only a single reading is feasible, it is better performed on D4 than on D3, with less false-negative and false-positive reactions [147].

Recommendations

Precise instructions must be given to patients:

1. Patch test must be left in place for 2 days and two nights.
2. No bath or wash of the back is allowed during the period.
3. Tight garments must be avoided.
4. Exercise or any other activity causing sweating must be avoided.
5. Incorrect behaviors like friction or rubbing, lying on back, exposure to sunlight/UV light, and scratching the patch test site are not allowed.
6. Severe itching or irritation must be reported immediately.

Corticosteroids and other immunosuppressive drugs should be stopped before patch testing as they may reduce positive patch tests in sensitized subjects. It is a general clinical concern that systemic prednisolone in a dosage surpassing 15 mg/day may reduce or smother unfavorably susceptible patch test responses, as may topical corticoid treatment, bringing to false-negative patch test reactions, as well as immunomodulators, UVB, PUVA therapy which also reduce contact allergy reactions [148, 149].

A recent study reported that the total number of positive nickel patch test reactions decreased significantly in patients during prednisone treatment. The threshold concentration to elicit a patch test reaction increased and the overall degree of reactivity to nickel sulfate shifted toward weaker reactions [150]. However, the effect of prednisone treatment on the response to irritants was divergent with both increased and decreased numbers of reactions, concluding that oral treatment with prednisone suppresses patch test reactivity to nickel in nickel allergic patients, but not to the irritants tested.

Fixing tape should be nonocclusive, nonallergenic and nonirritant and ideally patch testing should not be carried out in patients with active eczema, as it reduces the threshold of activity: consequentially, any acute eruption has to disappear before testing the allergens, or false-positive reactions could occur. On the other side, immediately after removal of the patch test, there may be erythema from the stripping action of the tape, especially in dermographic subjects, and this must be allowed to settle.

False-Negative and False-Positive Reactions

It is essential that the technique method, including timing and specific instruction given to the patient, are respected, to avoid false reactions and consequentially false diagnosis or misdiagnosis. Lack of respect of rules can make tests invalidated and not reliable, creating false-negative or false-positive reactions.

Common causes of false-negative reactions are:

1. Insufficient concentration.
2. Insufficient amount applied.
3. Poor adhesion of patches.
4. Inappropriate vehicle.
5. Readings performed too early.
6. Pretreatment of patch test site with topical corticosteroids.
7. UV irradiation of patch test site.
8. Systemic treatment with immunosuppressant.

On the other hand, common causes of false-positive patch test reactions can be:

1. Excessive concentration of allergen applied.
2. Impure substances.
3. Irritant vehicle.
4. Uneven dispersion.
5. Current or recent dermatitis in patch test site or at distant sites.
6. Pressure effects.
7. Adhesive tape reactions.
8. Angry back reaction or the excited skin syndrome.
9. Artifact.

Generally, there is a delay in the recognition of this disease on children, which can be because patch testing above all in infants may be particularly difficult. In fact, the diagnostic procedure requires specific skills in diagnostic techniques, such as patch test, not always easy to achieve.

Complications

Possible complication during PT can be:

1. Pruritis.
2. Folliculitis.
3. Leakage of materials on to clothing.
4. Localized flare of dermatitis.

5. Generalized flare of dermatitis.
6. Irritant reactions.
7. Active sensitization.
8. Pigmentation or depigmentation.
9. Scarring.
10. Anaphylaxis.

Quinones, phenols, and acrylics can cause vitiligo. Anaphylactic reactions are a potential risk when patch testing with some substances such as rubber latex and penicillin. Systemic absorption in fact can even damage organs and cause asthma and bronchial obstruction, with IgE-respond.

Flare-up sensitization reactions are positive reactions that appear at least 7 days after the application of the test apparatus (usually around day 15). They are caused by the interaction of a hapten with newly sensitized tissue [137].

Multiple Patch Test Reactions

Nonspecific Hyperreactivity

The threshold at which false-positive irritant reaction develops differs from individual to individual. During active dermatitis, uninvolved skin, even at distant body sites, exhibits increased susceptibility to irritant reactions. This status eczematicus may lead to false-positive patch test results. When this affects adjacent patch test sites, it is referred to as "Excited skin." The "excited skin syndrome," also called "angry back" ("irritated back" syndrome), is a phenomenon attributed to hyperreactivity of the skin, especially in the presence of an intense positive reaction to a given substance, where other possible positive reactions can be observed which, in this case, must be deemed dubious.

Multiple Primary Hypersensitivities

Multiple primary specific sensitivities to substances that are unrelated chemically are frequent among patients with CD. Patients with a long history of dermatitis are those most likely to accumulate several primary sensitivities, because of the opportunities to encounter new allergens under conditions favorable for sensitization. This is commonly seen in leg ulcer patients and with chronic actinic dermatitis. One sensitivity may predispose to the acquisition of another, and there may be a genetic or constitutional predisposition to acquire sensitivities.

Cross-Reactions

It is a phenomenon where sensitization engendered by one compound, the primary allergen, extends to one or more other compounds, the secondary allergens because of structural similarity. The proposal is that the primary and secondary allergens are so closely related that sensitized "T" cells are unable to distinguish between them. Enantiospecificity or stereospecificity may lead to cross-reactivity with some isomers and not others.

20.2.9.2 Photopatch Test

Photopatch testing is done to investigate patients with eczematous eruptions, predominantly affecting light-exposed sites and who have worsening of lesions following sun exposure with UV-A source from 5 to 10 J/cm^2 dose [137]. Application of the allergens is performed in an identical manner to conventional patch tests, except that they must be applied in duplicate, where one set is irradiated and the control one is not. Usually, two sets of the tests are applied on either side of the midline on the upper back, at the same level: the control site and the rest of the skin must be covered by a opaque material during irradiation. The common method followed is to apply the allergens on D0, then patches are removed and results are read on D2. On the same day, allergens on one side are irradiated and results are again read on D4. If the same allergen provokes an equally strong reaction on both sides, it is an indication of ACD alone; if it is significantly strong on the irradiated side, then combined allergy and photocontact allergy are occurring [151].

20.2.9.3 Patch Test and Atopic Dermatitis

Patch testing is safe and effective in children even with atopic AD; nevertheless, the National Institute of Arthritis and Musculoskeletal and Skin Diseases estimates that 10–20% of all children experience AD, which is likely incorrect, as most children are not evaluated with PT and, thus, could potentially be classified as AD, when they may have ACD or overlap of both disorders when they coexist [152].

It is important to recognize that this type of dermatitis may be overlooked, especially in the very young and when it is a contributing factor in AD [128].

Along these same lines, distinguishing between ACD and AD can be challenging because of their similar morphologic presentation. PTs can be useful, particularly with attention on corticosteroids, cosmetic and antibiotic series, or on products used by the child.

AD lesions localized to typical sites (the face and convex surface in early infancy; the flexor surfaces, eyelids, and hands in school-age children and adults) that are resistant or worsened by topical treatments. In all other cases of AD, patch tests are indicated if the subject has a history of onset of lesions in a body region that is not characteristic of the disease but is site of contact with various substances (e.g., metals, footwear, textiles, and perfumes).

Included studies used different tools to diagnose AD, did not always provide information on current or past disease and patch test allergens varied between studies.

Several studies have been published aiming to shed light on this important question but results still are contradictory: investigation has been limited thus far by a paucity of data on the overlap of these disorders in pediatric patients [18, 41].

Atopy Patch Test

The APT (atopy patch test) for aeroallergens and trophoallergens was introduced in 1989 as a technique capable of inducing a type I IgE-mediated hypersensitivity reaction, and a delayed reaction in skin areas, tested to evaluate the role of allergens in maintaining or worsening the AD in the absence of any other known cause [153].

These aeroallergens are substances known to be responsible for allergic responses of type I. dermatophagoides mix is a mix of two species of house dust mites: the European house dust mite (*Dermatophagoides pteronyssinus*) and the American domestic dust mite (*Dermatophagoides farinae*). Domestic dust mites are a common cause of asthma and allergic symptoms and can be found in mattresses, carpets, furniture, and bedding.

On the contrary, is not well defined the role of *Dermatophagoides* in causing or perpetuating AD and other forms of dermatitis, particularly airborne contact dermatitis. In addition, the prevalence of APT positivity for dermatophagoides in general population is in large part unknown [154].

The clinical value of APT for dermatophagoides is still debated, mainly for two reasons: the high rate of irritant reactions in patients with AD and the difficulties to determine actual clinical relevance in some patients [154, 155]. For this reason, the relevance of this allergen and its role behind ACD is not well known, due to the high rate of reactivity even in common people. On the other side, other results confirm the high value of APT in patients with AD induced by dermatophagoides and suggest that its routine use may improve the diagnosis of respiratory allergies to these allergens [156, 157].

20.2.9.4 Pediatric Series of Patch Test

The standard series of a country is made up of haptens whose incidence of allergy is over 1%; in Italy we refer to AIFA recommended pediatric standard series. (Table 20.4) (www.aifa.gov).

Table 20.4 Italian recommended pediatric standard series (AIFA)

1	Balsamo del Perù 25% pet
2	Cobalto cloruro 1% pet
3	Coccoamidopropilbetaina 1% acq
4	Colofonia 20% pet
5	Composite mix II 5% pet
6	Dimetilaminopropilamina (DMAPA) 1% acq
7	Dispersi mix 6,6% pet
8	Formaldeide 1% acq
9	Alcoli della lanolina 30% pet
10	Mercapto mix 2% pet
11	Kathon CG (MCI/MI) 0,02% acq
12	Metil-isotiazolinone (MI) 0.2% acq
13	Neomicina solfato 20% pet
14	Nichel solfato 5% pet
15	Para-fenilendiamina 1% pet
16	Potassio bicromato 0,5% pet
17	Profumi mix I + sorbitan sesquioleato 8% + 5% pet
18	Profumi mix II (Mx-25) 14% pet
19	Resina 4-ter-butilfenolformaldeidica 1% pet
20	Sorbitan sesquioleato 20% pet
21	Tiuram mix 1% pet
22	Vaselina 100%

The greater contact with an increasing number of environmental chemicals from jewelry, cosmetics, and personal hygiene products, to sporting gear and toys, made an increment in sensitization in pediatric population, which may be still on rise [24]. They develop the condition from the usual offenders and even from exposure to diapers, baby wipes, sunscreens, clothing with snaps, dyes, etc. Acknowledge of a prevalence increase of this disease, have supported studies worldwide, to push on the patch test technique even at young age, for a quick diagnosis and a better treatment and prevention.

In pediatrics, 15–52% of patch tests on children with suspected ACD prove to be positive: approximately 20% of individuals younger than 18 years are affected by ACD, with another study reporting ACD prevalence as high as 52.1% [158–162]; data variability may be due in part to the use of different patch test.

Studies on younger patients prove that there are some substances which occur more frequently during childhood: Nickel is always the most common allergen in children [163, 164], followed by cobalt [165], mercurials (thimerosal and metallic mercury), rubber chemicals (thiuram mix, carba mix, mercapto mix and mercaptobenzothiazole, PPD) and fragrance mix [18, 166–168].

An Iranian study of 2016 showed that most common allergens were nickel sulfate, cobalt, methylisothiazolinone, and colophony; while an Australian research of this year shows that the most common relevant patch test substances were fragrance mix, MCI/MI and MI, Myroxylon pereirae, nickel sulfate, and colophonium [169]; whereas in a Spanish study of 2017 the allergens most frequently identified were in decreasing order thiomersal, cobalt chloride, colophony, PPD, potassium dichromate, mercury, and nickel [5]. This is proof of how changes occur depending on geographical basis and on selection of the sample.

20.2.9.5 Aptens Involved in Pediatric CD

Substances can be divided into different categories: the most common substances patch tested belonged to metals (e.g., nickel, cobalt, chromium, gold, and silver), gums (carbamix, thiuramix, I-PPD, MBT, and MBTmix), resins (epoxy resin), preservatives (thimerosal, formaldehyde, Kathon, MI, Parabens, and quaternium), fragrances (fragrance mix I and fragrance mix II, Balsam of Peru, Lyral) and topical medicaments (i.e., Neomycin, benzocaine, and budesonide). Besides the commercially available preconceived haptens in standard and additional series, other substances proposed or supplied by the patient could be tested if there was a specific suspicion of connection with the site of lesion. These are called extemporaneous preparations, i.e., substances proposed by the patient that can be set up at appropriate concentrations, which can successively be tested. Although patch testing methods used for adults are well standardized, currently, there is not a recognized and universally approved pediatric standard series: this changes among centers, and it is normally based on the most common allergens for children, which are:

- metals (nickel sulfate, potassium bichromate, cobalt chloride);
- topical medicaments (neomycin sulfate, benzocaine, corticosteroids);
- fragrances (fragrance mix, myroxylon pereirae);
- preservatives (thimerosal, methylisothiazolinone, methylchloroisothiazolinone);
- cocamidopropyl betaine;
- lanolin alcohols [24, 115].

Metals
Nickel Sulfate

Metals are the principal allergens and nickel is the most common of them, both in children and in adults [170, 171].

It is a silvery-white lustrous, hard, and ductile transition metal, widely used in alloys to improve resistance to corrosion, wear, and abrasion. It is one of the most frequent source of sensitization, due to the various amount of applications of nickel in daily life, such as in batteries, coins or keys, orthopedic plates, metal plating, wristwatch and costume jewelry, and for this last reason its sensitivity is more frequent among girls [48, 172, 173]. In fact, nickel-sensitive patients are significantly more likely to be female, young, and atopic (with eczema and asthma) and have dermatitis affecting face, scalp, ears, neck, arm, or trunk [173, 174].

Several data show that frequency of jewelry as source of nickel sensitivity in pediatric population increases with age CS to nickel in children may result also from toys, musical instruments and technological devices such as laptops, tablets, computers, mobile phones, metallic mobile telephone cases, other metal containers (such as make-up containers) [175].

In Europe, the prevalence of nickel allergy has slightly declined190 in several countries following implementation of the EU Nickel Directive, [174, 176] above all in the youngest population [177] and this is probably due to the new directive adopted, which limits the rate of nickel release from products [5, 115]. However, CS to nickel remains high, not only in adults, but also in children: not all the countries have a nickel directive to protect consumers from nickel sensitization consequentially in some regions there is significant increment, as in North America, which rises up from 14.3% to 20.1% in over 2 decades [178–180].

The usual prevalence of nickel sensitivity in a patch test clinic is 15–30%: positive patch test reactions to nickel are reported approximately of 8–19% in adults196 and 8–26.8% in children and adolescents [74, 180]; however, experts state that a lot of test reactions in infancy are probably of irritant or nonspecific nature [181, 182]. On the other hand, the prevalence may be higher in some selected occupational groups, such as hairdressers [183].

Even concomitant positive PT reactions to different transitional metals are frequently seen in patients with ACD, in which great value has the association palladium–nickel [176], but it can even be released from other materials containing it as alloying elements (such as white gold) [184].

Sensitization is chiefly the result of frequent skin contact with corroded objects containing nickel: commonly Nickel chloride (Nicl2) and Nickel sulfate (NiSo4) are readily soluble in water and sweat and have strong sensitizing properties [185].

Systemic exposure may take place from diet: in fact certain foods and plants contain much higher concentration of nickel (ingestion allergies with food cooked in aluminum pans and stainless steel, or even in fish, mushroom, and canned food).

The classical sites of nickel allergy are seen in places of contact with metal objects, most commonly the wrists from watches and bracelets, the neck from necklaces, ears from earring, central back and upper chest from bra components, central abdomen from studs and zips in trousers, especially jeans and dorsa of feet from the shoe buckles [143]. The eruption may be papular, nummular, diffuse or of only excoriated papules and a secondary spread of dermatitis to other areas can occur successively [186, 187].

Nickel sensitized women have a predilection for hand eczema203, whereas a recurrent vesicular palmar dyshidrotic pattern of eczema has been related to dietary intake of nickel. In the European baseline series of PT, nickel is tested in form of nickel sulfate (2.0 mg/cm^2) in petrolatum. False-negative tests are common with 2.5% nickel, used in North America, with whom irritant false-positive reactions can occur [40, 41, 187].

Cobalt Chloride

Cobalt is a grayish, hard, attractive, bendable, and to some degree moldable metal, very similar to nickel and iron and present in metal alloys. The cobalt salts are typically hued, so primarily used as shades for glass, ceramics, cosmetics, and hair dyes. There are occupational-related factors: manufactures (bond, paints, gums, and paint driers), metals (adornments and coins), medications (metal dental prostheses and joints, vitamin B12), but the most successive reason for sharpening to this metal is nickel-plated objects, which quite often contain cobalt. Cobalt is usually considered a co-reactor to nickel and patients may frequently have a positive reaction to patch tests to both allergens [188].

It is now currently a "hot topic," as it is increasingly being recognized as an independent sensitizer204 and new sources of exposure are coming to light [178, 189], but the actual knowledge about causative consumer exposure to cobalt is for now limited [190].

It is the second most common allergen, and the frequency of allergy to this metal is very high (5–10%), demonstrable with PTs; but because often it gives an irritative reaction, this must be distinguished from the real allergic reaction, in order to not overeating results. It is tested in the form of cobalt chloride 1%, and the prevalence of positive patch test reactions in children is reported to vary between 4.4% and 11.11% [167, 190].

CS to cobalt in children may result not only from jewelry but also from toys and leather footwear [169].

Potassium Dichromate

The metal itself is insoluble and seems not to be sensitizing as nickel. The prevalence of sensitivity seems to be more common in men, where occupational dermatitis predominate.

The main source of hexavalent chromium is cement [191]. Other sources are antirust paints, plating salts, metal alloys, printing materials, cutting oils, foundry sand, matches, photographic chemicals, welding fumes, wood ashes, glazing enamels, cat gut, violin strings, textiles, tire fitting solution and dental prosthesis. Trivalent agents are used as a tanning agent for leather. Chromate sensitivity tends to persist, and the prognosis of occupational dermatitis is poor, because of its continuation and associated social handicap, so chronicity and frequent relapses are not infrequent. Although knowledge on potassium dichromate exposure sources in children is relatively limited, the most common sources of exposure are leather shoes [5, 192, 193].

The prevalence of PT reactions to potassium dichromate in children is reported between 1.3% and 9.9% [25, 167].

The sensitivity is demonstrated by a PT with potassium dichromate 0.5% in petrolatum.

Topical Medicaments

Topical medicaments are frequent sources of ACD in children and, above all, as mentioned before, in those patients with prolonged applications for skin diseases (i.e., AD). Contact sensitivity to corticosteroids has been progressively perceived worldwide as an issue of extensive clinical and helpful significance. The rate of corticosteroid sensitivity goes from 0.5% to 5%, but differs in each report and relies upon a few factors, like mindfulness and testing for corticosteroid hypersensitivity, tolerant choice, going before skin infection, endorsing propensities, kind of corticosteroids chosen, and the test and perusing strategies utilized.

Budesonide and Tixocortol Pivalate

A glucocorticoid budesonide is an epiremic mixture of α- and β-propyl forms of 16α, 17 α-butylidenedioxy-11- β, 21-dihydroxypregna-1,4-diene-3,20-dione. It.

has been topically used for the treatment of various skin disorders, but is more often used by inhalation in the management of asthma in the form of a metered aerosol, even as a nasal spray for the prophylaxis and treatment of allergic rhinitis. It is tested as budesonide 0.01%.

The glucocorticoid tixocortol pivalate is 11β, 17α-dihydroxy-21-mercaptopregn-4-ene-3,20-dione21-pivalate. Tixocortol pivalate allergy has been detected in 0.9–4.4% of consecutive dermatitis patients. It does not produce irritant patch test reactions, and like budesonide, late readings should be performed [194]. It is tested as tixocortol pivalate 0.1%.

Studies on multiple-sensitization consider that contact allergies to tixocortol pivalate and hydrocortisone are associated, while reactions to budesonide are strongly correlated with reactions to both the acetonide group and ester group [195]

Neomycin Sulfate

Neomycin is a widely used aminoglycoside antibiotic [196]. In the United States, the frequency of neomycin sensitivity in the general population was 1.1% more than 20 years ago, but it has been ranked among the top 3 allergens in children for more than a decade, with a reported prevalence up to 5.2% in Italy and now up to 6.6% in the USA [197].

However, the frequency varies depending to a large extent on referral and prescription habits of the region. In Danish literature, the frequency of neomycin sensitivity was about 2.9% and even other several patch test studies demonstrated that there has been an upward trend in the occurrence of neomycin sensitivity over the years, probably due to an increased use of topical drugs containing neomycin.

Patients particularly at risk appear to be children with chronic and recurrent dermatitis in skin areas where occlusion or bandaging is prone to occur or is used, as in stasis dermatitis, but also those with otitis externa and perianal eczema, [168] but diagnosis of an allergy toward this allergen may be difficult, because the type of dermatitis is not vesicular or bullous, instead appears often as aggravation or simply chronicity of preexisting dermatitis.

The therapeutic concentration of neomycin is of 0.5%, while the patch test concentration is 20%, but even at this concentration, some positives may be missed and the positive reactions appear later, after 3–4 days in many cases. The cross-sensitization pattern of neomycin is complex: regular cross-sensitivity occurs between neomycin, framycetin, and paromomycin, which all contain neosamine group.

Fragrances

Fragrance Mix I and II

Contact dermatitis toward ingredients of cosmetics and toiletries is common, accounting for 10% of patients attending patch test clinics [198]. Commercial perfumes are complex mixtures of natural essential oils and synthetic compounds. They are part of the composition of many products including cosmetics, topical medications, detergents, air fresheners, and food.

Fragrance mix I was developed in the late 1970s, and consists of eight ingredients, each at a concentration of 1%: amyl cinnamal, cinnamal, cinnamyl alcohol, eugenol, evernia prunastri, geraniol, hydroxycitronellal, isoeugenol; fragrance mix II contains lyral, citral, citronellol, farne sol, coumarin, and hexyl cinnamic aldehyde. Fragrance mix II (FM II) was introduced in the patch test baseline series in Denmark in 2005 and contains six different fragrance chemicals, commonly present in cosmetic products and which are known allergens. If FM II had not been included as a screening marker in the baseline series, 15% of individuals with fragrance allergy would not have been identified by the other fragrance screening markers: so FM II contributes substantially to detecting fragrance allergy [199].

Fragrance substances are second only to metals as a cause of contact allergy: between 1.1% and 8% of the general population have a contact allergy to fragrance substances [200, 201]. The frequency of CS to fragrances, such as isothiazolinones, is increasing in children, because of their use in several personal perfumed hygiene products, even if specifically targeted to use in pediatric age as moisturizers, emollients, sunscreens. Another possible cause of CS to fragrance mix in children is the child's habit of playing with cosmetics and make-up [5, 18, 202]. It is important to underline that topical products listed as "*fragrance free*" may contain fragrance-related ingredients in the form of preservatives (such as eugenol, cinnamaldehyde, and benzyl alcohol) [171, 202]. Fragrance mix 8% and fragrance mix II pet 14% are the concentrations tested.

Balsam of Peru

Balsam of Peru (INCI name: *Myroxylon pereirae*) is the natural resinous balsam that exudes from the trunk of the Central American tree *Myroxylon pereirae* after scarification of the bark. The composition varies and standardization is based on physical characteristics and the identification of some major chemical constituents. Balsam of Peru contains 30–40% resins of unknown composition, while the remaining 60–70% consist of well-known chemicals: benzyl benzoate, benzyl cinnamate, cinnamic acid, benzoic acid, vanillin, farnesol (which is also increasingly being used in deodorants) and nerolidol [203]. Positive PT with one or more of these substances may be an indication of perfume allergy, because many perfumes and flavorings contain components either identical to, or cross-reacting with, materials contained in balsam of Peru and other natural resins. Even in medicinal preparations, Balsam of Peru is used for its dermatological effects, such as antimicrobial effects and be used as preservatives [204].

In a Danish epidemiological study the prevalence was at 4% both in males and females, while positive patch test reactions to balsam of Peru are reported in up to 8.4% of children [198].

Difference can be due to general habits, legislation and sample characteristics. Because of its sensitizing properties, crude balsam of Peru has been banned by the International fragrance Association from use since 1982, but extracts and distillates of balsam of Peru are still used up to a maximum level of 0.4% in consumer products. It is tested as Balsam of Peru 25%.

Preservatives

Preservatives are a group of substances used to prevent bacterial and fungal proliferation in topical medicaments, cosmetics, and personal care products. The main components of this group can be divided into formaldehyde releasers and non-formaldehyde agents. In some studies preservatives, such as MCI, formaldehyde, and formaldehyde releasers (quaternium-15, imidazolidinyl urea and MDBGN), emerge as the most frequent allergens in children who undergo patch testing because of ACD. This finding might be attributed to the increase in the utilization of these chemical compounds in personal hygiene products for children [205].

Formaldehyde

Formaldehyde is usually not added to products because it is classified by the International Agency for Research on Cancer as a known human carcinogen [206]. However, Formaldehyde is a ubiquitous and strong sensitizer: industrially, domestically, and medically. Formaldehyde exposure is difficult to estimate because the chemical, besides being manufactured and used as such, is incorporated into a huge variety of products and reactants in many chemical process, including formaldehyde releasers, polymerized plastics, medicaments, fabrics, cosmetics, detergents, clothing, cleaning products, glues, antiperspirants, disinfectants, and deodorizers. Shampoos may contain formaldehyde, but because they are quickly diluted and washed off, only exquisitely formaldehyde-sensitive consumers develop dermatitis on the scalp and face from their use, whereas hairdressers, because of their more intense exposure, may get hand dermatitis.

Formaldehyde dermatitis from textiles is rare today, because the manufactures have improved the fabric finish treatment and garments, made from 100% acrylic, polyester, linen, silk, nylon, and cotton, are generally considered to be formaldehyde free. Formaldehyde sensitivity is not necessary accompanied by simultaneous sensitivity to formaldehyde resins and its releasers, and vice versa, but some of its releasers might act as prohaptens.

The frequency of formaldehyde-positive patch tests in consecutive eczema patients is around 2–3%, but its epidemiology requires re-evaluation due to the irritant patch test concentrations used in studies. It is tested in our series as formaldehyde 1%, but sometimes 2% can be found in other series [207].

Methylchloroisothiazolinone (MCI) and Methylisothiazolinone (MI)

In the non-formaldehyde preservatives group, MCI and MI are utilized broadly in cement, stream motor fuel, latex emulsions and so forth. 226 MCI/MI (Kathon® CG), is a combination of MCI and MI, widely used as preservative in cosmetics, as well as in household cleaning products and industrial products such as paints and glues. From July 2015, the European Commission has banned MCI-MI in all leave-on body products227 whereas, regarding noncosmetic products such as paints, glues, and other chemical products, and since 2016 there has been an labeling obligation indicating concentration of MCI/MCI <0.0015% (15 ppm) and concentration of MI <300 ppm in rinse-off cosmetic products, with a mixture in the ratio of 3:1 of the two substances [209, 210].

Although, this limitation is not always observed, and there is no legislation about the industrially used limit concentration of MCI/MI.228 Despite these limitations, CS to isothiazolinones is increasing in Europe [211, 212].

Although the common thought was that MCI was a stronger sensitizer than MI, recent data reported some cases of CS following the use of products containing MI alone, such as wet wipes and moist toilet paper [213]. In fact, an American research of 2015 has shown the increasing prevalence of contact allergy to MI, by testing it alone and not in combination with MCI. As a result, MCI and MI are among the most frequent contact allergens in adult ACD [208].

Furthermore, MI has emerged as a significant allergen in the pediatric population, and is now among the top 5 allergens in children with dermatitis. This has also been observed in similar studies from other European countries, where prevalence of positive patch test reactions to mix MCI/MI is reported in up to 11.7% of children [214]. High positivity to Kathon CG suggests more attention to concentration of this substance, used in cosmetics and products for domestic use [215]. Researches still advice that MI of 2000 ppm needs to be patch tested on its own to not miss contact allergy [216]. In our series Kathon is tested as 0.01% and MI of 0.2%.

Methyldibromo Glutaronitrile (MDGN)

MDBGN is a bromine-containing preservative that is found in baby lotions and wipes, moist toilet paper, sunscreens, and other cosmetics and is a common cause of ACD [217]. In the mid-1980s, this preservative was approved for use in cosmetic products at a maximum concentration of 0.1%, and it was effective at low in-use concentrations and animal tests indicated that the preservative was a weak sensitizer. For this reason, MDBGN gradually became more widespread throughout the 1990s in household, industrial products, and cosmetics.

However, dermatological clinics in Europe found increasing numbers of eczema patients sensitized to the chemical. Patch test data from 16 European clinics showed an increasing average frequency of sensitivity in eczema patients from 0.7% to 3.5%, and based on these new frequency data, a change in the Cosmetics Directive was made in 2005, banning the use of MDBGN in stay-on products and later also from rinse-off products. Experts have recommended 0.2% as the optimal PT concentration due to the increased number of false-positive reactions with 0.5%.

Parabens

The most widely used preservatives in foods, drugs, and cosmetics are the parabens (alkyl esters of p-hydroxbenzoic acid) and most of the make-up registered at the FDA contain parabens. If used in combination, parabens have a synergistic antimicrobial effect. Cross-reactions between the four paraben esters methyl-, ethyl-, propryl-, and butylparaben are common, but exceptions occur. The paraben mix used these four esters, while benzyl paraben has been removed because it is no longer allowed for use in cosmetics and drugs as it is a suspected carcinogen [143].

The frequency of patch test reactions is approximately 1.0% and seems to be constant in spite of the extensive use of parabens: so they must be regarded as safe preservatives in topical products and ACD from them as relatively rare [218, 219].

Cross-reactions may occur to other para-compounds such as benzocaine, para-phenylenediamine and sulphonamides [220]. It has been suspected that paraben-sensitive patients may experience flare-ups of dermatitis from parabens in foods and systemic medicaments; however, a subsequent low-paraben diet had no effect on the dermatitis. Sometimes, the paraben mix produces an irritant-like patch test reaction, relative to the extensive use of these preservatives in cosmetics and medicaments, but they rarely sensitize. However, the paraben mix is important in the standard series because paraben allergy is difficult to suspect from the history or clinical appearance of dermatitis.

Thimerosal and Imidazolidinyl Urea

Thimerosal is a mercury-based preservative used, until the recent past, in multi-dose vials of medicines and vaccines. CS to thimerosal is very low in very young children (1%) and higher in older age-groups, probably due to the recent limitation of its use in vaccines since 2002 [140].

Imidazolidinyl urea is a very common preservative, frequently used in baby lotions, shampoos, and conditioners. However, the concentrations of formaldehyde released by this allergen is five parts per million (mg/kg), and this amount is usually tolerated by most of patients [221].

Cocamidopropyl Betaine (CAPB)

CAPB is the surfactant often used in shampoos, bath products, liquid shower gels, roll-on deodorants, eye and facial cleaners, liquid detergents, surface cleaners, pet care products, and other skin and hair care product. CD from CAPB may present as an eyelid, facial, scalp, and/or neck dermatitis. CS prevalence is estimated between 3.0% and 7.2%. The increasing rates of sensitization led to CAPB's being named "Allergen of the Year" in 2004. Related impurities rendered during the manufacturing process (such as amidoamine and dimethylaminopropylamine) are thought to play a role in sensitization [112] and an association between CAPB use and presence of AD on children was demonstrated [222].

Lanolin Alcohol

Lanolin is a natural product from sheep fleece and consists of a complex mixture of esters and polyesters of high-molecular-weight alcohols and fatty acids. The composition varies from time to time and from place to place. Wool wax alcohols (INCI name: Ianolin alcohol) are complex mixture of esters of alcohols and fatty acids derived from hydrolysis of the oily, waxy fraction of sheep fleece. The general incidence of Ianolin allergy in consecutively tested eczema patients is around 2–3%, showing an increment in the last years.

The use of lanolin extends from topical preparations to anticorrosives, printing inks, and paper constituents. Hjorth and Trolle Lassen described the clinical picture of lanolin allergy, emphasizing the frequency of its occurrence in elderly women with a long history of eczema, particularly in those with leg ulcer and stasis dermatitis, and spread of eczema in secondary sites was even common. Significant associations were found between AD and lanolin and lanolin alcohols allergy, whereas lanolin allergy is uncommon on normal skin and with cosmetic usage [223].

In several epidemiological studies of patients, most positive PT reactions are rather weak, with frequency of sensitization ranges from 1.1% to 6%, depending upon the selection of the sample and prescription habits. The allergy is increased by the simultaneous presence of detergent: in fact, removing free fatty alcohols and detergent from lanolin reduced the hypersensitivity by 96% in selected Ianolin-sensitive patients. The patch test preparation in the standard series is at 30% petrolatum. In the youngest children, the sensitization rates are between 1.3 and 1.5%, whereas lanolin can be found in 9% of cosmetics. Lanolin 30% is used in the patch test series [24, 134].

Other Allergens

Compositae Mix

The daisy or sunflower family Compositae (Asteraceae) is currently the most frequent cause of ACD by plants in Europe [224].

This chemical mix consists of extract from five different plants: Chamomile, Tansy, yarrow, Arnica, and Feverfew. Arnica, Chamomile, and Feverfew are flowers, and Yarrow and Tansy are herbs. These substances are usually found in conditioners, cosmetics, health care products, lip balms, medicines, oils, shampoos, skin creams, skin lotions, and herbal and natural products. The last ones have seen a big increment in the last decade. Anyone reacting to several herbs should consider checking for salicylate sensitivity as virtually as all herbs have a high salicylate content. This chemical may have cross-reactions with other types of plant family called Laurel (e.g., *Laurus nobilis*, family of Lauraceae) and members of the family Magnoliaceae. Occupational dermatitis to plants is common in farmers, gardeners, and florists, which is generally worse during the summer months and patterns vary from country to country [225, 226].

Anacardiaceae, Primulaceae, and Alliaceae are other common plant families implicated in plant dermatitis and the allergens are Sesquiterpene lactones including dehydrocastus lactone, alantolactone, costunolide, and parthenolide [227].

In most of cases patterns go from eczema to localized dermatitis and erythrodermatous or exfoliative. ACD to Compositae may occur in children who play among plants and flowers in the meadows or in children exposed to cosmetic products, and it is not uncommon in pediatric age with up to 2.6% of children prevalence, with a reported prevalence of positive PT reactions to compositae mix significantly higher in children with AD compared to children without the disease [227, 228].

Colophonium

Colophony (rosin) (INCI name: colophonium) is a widespread, naturally occurring material. It is the residue from the distillation of the volatile oil from the oleoresin, obtained from trees of the *Pinaceae* family. Its chemical composition is complex and variable depending on the manufacturing process, geographical area, and storage conditions. Beside contact eczema, it may also cause type I hypersensitivity and photosensitivity.

Concomitant and cross-reactions between colophonium (rosin), balsam of Peru, propolis, oil of turpentine, wood tar, pine resin, spruce resin, seqsquiterpane lactone mix, and Compositae plant extracts occur, often in the context of a fragrance allergy.

Exposure is likely in both work and leisure hours [229]: in cosmetics, colophonium occurs in depilatories, tonics, dressing, and hair grooming aids, make-up, mascara, and hair products, whereas in pharmaceutical products, it is used in topical medicaments, including surgical paints, and Chinese herbal medicine [230].

Mercaptobenzothiazole

2-Mercaptobenzothiazole (2-MBT) is tested inside the mercapto mix at a concentration of 0.5% or alone at a concentration of 2% pet. It is present in many rubbers, to which they are added as accelerators before vulcanization take place and are ubiquitous in rubber products. These include rubber handles, masks, elastic bands, tubing, elasticized garments, artificial limbs, and even cosmetic sponges. MBT is also present in a variety of nonrubber products, including cutting oils, greases, coolants, antifreezes, fungicides, adhesives, and veterinary medicaments.

On reviewing the sensitivity of patch test material, the German contact dermatitis Research group (DKG) has recommended testing with the components of the mercapto mix when there is a reaction to either the mix or MBT itself. Therefore, it has been concluded that both mercapto mix and MBT are required in the baseline series.

However, a review of 2013 has proved that MBT is the preferential screening allergen for mercapto compounds, because of the following: greater amount of missed reactions with MM; greater quantity of doubtful or mild reactions in the missed group for MM and in the group positive to both the low rate (2%) of moderate or strong reactions to MM and doubtful or mild reactions to MBT, as compared with the converse (21%). Mercapto mix may be useful in an auxiliary rubber series [231].

In a Swedish study of 2019 authors recommend replacing mercapto mix 2.0% pet. in the baseline series with mercapto mix 3.5% pet., since the latter also detected those patients who would have been missed, because MBT 2.0% is not included in the Swedish baseline series.251 Furthermore, results demonstrated that rubber accelerators have an important role in ACD in the northeast of Italy and their sensitization is associated significantly with occupations that wear gloves or use chemical substances. Between rubber accelerators tested, carba mix sensitization is prevalent and is increasing during last years [232].

Para-Phenylenediamine

Para-phenylenediamine (PPD) is an aniline derivative whose main use is for dyeing hair, but is also seen in rubber antioxidants, photography developing solution, petrol, oils, greases, and printing ink. CS to PPD in children is increasing and is often secondary to temporary black henna tattoos [233, 234].

There are several elements that can further promote CS, such as prolonged contact with the skin, the use of occlusive dressing to keep the henna attached to the skin or the use of syringes to apply the dye [245, 246]. However, it is important to consider that CS to PPD in very young children may also be due to contact of the child with the mother's dyed hair [113]. Once sensitized, children might experience ACD later in life because of contact with other several products containing PPD (leather shoes, fragrances, rubber, printing inks, paints) [233]. PPD and related hair dye allergy can result in extremely severe skin reactions. Scalp is often relatively spared, but edema and weeping of the scalp margin, ears, and eyes with extensive secondary eruptions can be seen. Hairdressers can also be sensitized by the dyeing process, resulting in hand dermatitis.

Cross-sensitivity to PPD has also been reported to topical anesthetics such as benzocaine, textile disperse dyes and sunscreen components (PABA and padimate O.). Patch testing is done with a concentration of PPD in 1% petrolatum.

Benzocaine (Ethylaminobenzoate)

Benzocaine is a para-aminobenzoic acid (PABA) derivative used as a local anesthetic. The incidence of CS reported varies widely from country to country, probably dependent on the level of use of benzocaine in the community. The incidence of positive reactions on topical anesthetics in eczema patients ranges from 0.8% to 1.5%. In some countries, such as the United States, it is widely used in over-the-counter preparations, whereas in others, like the United Kingdom, its use is much less frequent. While it does not have a high sensitizing potential, it is usually applied in the orefices of the body and to raw intertriginous areas, which render sensitization easier [235]. According to Wilkinson and co-workers, it would be better to include a "caine-mix" in the series, since benzocaine alone is inadequate; however, more work is required to determinate a nonirritant PT concentration.

Benzocaine can cross-react with other compounds: 25% of benzocaine-sensitive patients react to para-phenylenediamine and para-aminobenzoic acid esters used as sunscreens. It will also react with procaine, sulphonamides, and certain dyes; on the contrary benzocaine-sensitive individuals do not react to lidocaine. The standard patch test dilution of benzocaine is 5% pet.

Textile Dyes

Common allergens in clothing include textile dyes, formaldehyde, resins, rubber, chromate, and nickel. Disperse dyes are the class of dye most likely to sensitize. Disperse dyes are used to color artificial fibers, such as polyester, acetate, acrylic and nylon. The common sites of distribution of clothing dermatitis are areas of sweating and friction. The eruption typically starts in the axillae sparing the hairy part of the vault and forms a crescent patch on the anterior chest wall, sharply limited by the underwear. The dermatitis is located at the inner posterior thighs, popliteal fossae and lower legs may be involved when trousers and pants are responsible garments. Some fabrics provoke a purpuric, sometimes lichenoid dermatitis in areas of contact, as seen with uniforms. Cross-sensitivity to substances is seen with textile dermatitis. Standard series screening with four textile disperse dyes (Blue, Orange, Red and Yellow) allergens is advocated. All of them are tested separately in our series in 1% petrolatum. Specifically, the subtypes Disperse Blue 126, Yellow 3, Orange 3 and Red 1 were used.

Emerging Contact Allergens

Trends in allergens exposure are constantly in evolution: some allergens' sensitizations didn't seem to have changed over the years, such as to metals, which has been significant over the last 21 years, with few epidemiological changes. On the other side incidence of some substances seems to have increased in the recent period of time among children [236]. A 2016 research found that there were 10 most frequent allergens in some studies, representing emerging allergens, important when considering preventive measures: Kathon CG, tosylamide formaldehyde resin, gold thiosulfate, disperse dyes, cocamidopropylbetaine, tixocortol pivalate and propolis [237], with Isobornyl acrylate considered the allergen of the year 2020. However, as already stated, prevalence and causes can change with time and geographical area.

Implants

Metals are considered as the most common metals inspiring both cutaneous and extracutaneous unfavorably susceptible responses, as even some recent cases of surgical insertion of a metal implants show. Complex immune responses that occur around the implants may bring about torment, irritation, and relaxing of the implant. The most frequently incriminated haptens are in fact nickel, chrome, cobalt, and titanium, but such clinical pictures are rare in children, who, unlike adults, wear the appliances for just a few years.

It is also known that inclusion of metal alloys in orthopedic prostheses can have adverse effects on sensitized subjects, although these are less frequently encountered in children. Several studies have reported cases of metal allergy caused by titanium-containing materials, suggesting that pre-implant patients should be asked about a history of hypersensitivity reactions to metals and patch testing when recommended. Orthodontic appliances made of stainless steel, chrome-cobalt and nickel-titanium can cause perioral dermatitis (angular or other forms of cheilitis) and lesions of the oral mucosa [238].

Regarding the pediatric field, recent studies have shown an emerging issue: the association between ACD in pediatric patients with diagnosing of type 1 diabetes, who use technological devices for diabetes treatment, for monitoring of blood glucose levels, and its management, suggesting that the rate of sensitization to allergens included into diabetes devices, attached to the skin with adhesives, is higher than commonly assumed among pediatric patients [239].

New significant causes are found especially in acrylates, which may cause significant problems in nail polish and insulin pumps, used in treatment of diabetes. It is recommended that patients with rash related to use of medical devices, should be patch tested with IBOA [240, 241].

In fact, isobornyl acrylate (IBOA), ethyl cyanoacrylate, and N,N-dimethylacrylamide (DMAA) are used as monomeric diluents in ultraviolet curing adhesives and are often present in adhesives used for medical devices [242, 243]. However, there is a paucity of information regarding the prevalence of sensor-related dermatitis and detailed patient histories [244], but experts retain manufactures should supply detailed information about adhesives, in order to avoid dermatological complications and consequently a worsening of disease management and patients' quality of life [239].

Toys

A 2019 systemic review reported that there was a broad range of skin risks in the common toys [245]. Several toys were found to be associated with CD, including electronics, toy cars, costume jewelry, bicycles, electronics such as video game controllers, cellphones, iPads, computers and squash balls, Play-Doh, plasticine, and slime. This last one is typically made with household products (such as glue and borax) and is currently a popular childhood hobby that can cause ACD or ICD, particularly hand dermatitis due to MCI/MI and MI [246]. As result, there is still an unmet need for observation of this segment of industry for labeling of contents and ongoing surveillance [246–248].

Cosmetic Products

Analysis reveals that most of skincare products for neonates and infants contain haptens that can be responsible for ACD, even if they are labeled as hypoallergenic/dermatologically tested/safe. The most abundant sensitizers were CAPB, tocopherol, propylene glycol, fragrances, lanolin, and association of tocopheryl acetate (vitamin E) and cyclopentasiloxane, a silicone component, and sunscreen products [249–251]. Copolymers are substances widely used in sunscreens due to their film-forming, binding, viscosity-increasing, and enhancing water resistance properties. Polyvinylpyrrolidone (PVP)/eicosene, PVP/1-triacontene, and C30–38 olefin/isopropyl maleate/maleic anhydride are copolymers recently reported as responsible for ACD to sunscreens [250]. Regarding ACD to sunscreen products, octocrylene (a frequently used ultraviolet filter), benzoic acid and lauryl glucoside are other possibly involved allergens [252, 253].

Topical Treatment

Other relevant emerging contact allergens in children are topical antiseptics and panthenol. Panthenol is an alcohol analog of pantothenic acid, known as vitamin B5. It is a common ingredient in topical treatments, for rhinitis, conjunctivitis, sunburn, and it is widely used in several cosmetic products (hair lotions, wipes, moisturizers, sunscreens, make-up, nail polish). Panthenol represents an emerging relevant contact allergen, especially in adolescents [254, 255].

Products with a high content of propylene glycol and other substances contained in emollients, largely used in children with ACD or AD, can induce ICD, ACD, and nonimmunologic contact urticaria, and should not be used in children younger than 2 years [256]. Chlorhexidine and benzalkonium chloride have been reported as allergens frequently implicated in CD, from use of antiseptic products in very young children [257, 258]. Benzalkonium chloride is also used as preservative in health care and household products. Furthermore, the use of antiseptics for umbilical cord care could be the cause of CS reported in newborns [257, 258]. Diagnosis of ACD to chlorexidine is important because it can mimic other dermatoses common during childhood, and it can also lead to acute immediate hypersensitivity reactions following successive exposures [259].

The use of natural remedies is also increasing. In early infancy it is proved that natural products play an important role for ACD, because mothers are increasingly using herbal or other products containing active ingredients that are not classified as medicinal specialties, such as tea tree oil, propolis and marigold [260, 261].

Additional Series for Children

There are now many hapten batteries available: the standard series, the supplementary series, and the specific series standard and additional series of PT allergens are sold by companies working in close connection with the International Contact Dermatitis Research Group (ICDRG), as well as other international and national groups [262]. Different substances may be used in patch testing for different children ages [263]. The principle of screening all patients with a series of allergens commonly encountered in their environment is now well established, vary from one country to another, in general including in the battery substances which give positive reactions in more than 1% of those tested.

Main patch test allergen producers now market extra series, which must be adapted to local habits or occupational exposures. In addition, patients may bring a wide variety of materials of their own from home for testing, which must be thoroughly assessed and diluted appropriately before being tested, generally testing the substance in a low concentration if it is not well known. Expended and personalized patch tests should be recommended, because pediatric patients frequently have reactions to allergens not included in standard series, and these allergens are commonly found in household products, such as CAPB [222].

Comprehensive patch testing or custom-tailored individual allergen panels have the highest efficacy in determining the cause of a patient's ACD because the allergens are selected specifically based on the patient's environmental exposures and increase the rate of relevant patch test reactions. It should be considered that children have less body surface area on which to apply patches, and the patches need to be chosen thoughtfully [264].

20.3 Prevention and Treatment of CD in Children

Once the allergen has been identified, avoidance of contact with the substance is the key of a successful treatment in ACD. Compliance improves if a list of products with identified allergens is given to patients. Skin protection can be also useful, especially in occupational type of dermatitis. However, avoidance is not always possible: nickel is contained in many foodstuffs and found as an impurity in metallic and various objects, cosmetics often contain traces of fragrances that are not included in the published product specifications, and this can follow on chronic dermatitis and lichenification, with worse life expectation [265].

In some instances, use of specialized skin creams, such as barrier creams, can be considered: above all in the acute phase, mildly antiseptic solutions and emollient creams are recommended, and low-strength corticosteroids can be used locally for a brief period, in most instances to control the symptoms of the disorder. Use of optical or systemic steroids depends on the severity of the disease: in case of chronic forms, more potent and systemic corticosteroids can be useful because of their moisturizing properties, in greasy vehicles for thicker skins. On the contrary, oral hyposensitization is not routinely recommended.

Prognosis of allergic contact dermatitis depends on its cause and feasibility of avoiding repeated or continued exposure of the causative allergen. The prognosis is poor for patients allergic to nickel and chromate, because of their ubiquity in the environment and daily life [266].

Conflict of Interest No conflict of interest.

References

1. Jacob SE, Brankov N, Kerr A. Diagnosis, and management of allergic contact dermatitis in children: common allergens that can be easily missed. Curr Opin Pediatr. 2017;29:443–7.
2. Burns T, et al. Rook's textbook of dermatology, vol. 1. 8th ed. Wiley; 2010.
3. Alberta L, Sweeney SM, Wiss K. Diaper dye dermatitis. Pediatrics. 2005;116:e450–2.
4. Roul S, Ducombs G, Leaute-Labreze C, Taïeb A. 'Lucky Luke' contact dermatitis due to rubber components of diapers. Contact Dermatitis. 1998;38:363–4.
5. Ortiz Salvador JM, Esteve Martínez A, Subiabre Ferrer A, Victoria Martínez AM, de la Cuadra OJ, Zaragoza NV, Dermatitis alérgica de contacto pediátrica. Estudioclínico-epidemiológico en un hospital terciario. Actas Dermosifiliogr. 2017;108:571–8.
6. Pigatto P, Martelli A, Marsili C, Fiocchi A. Contact dermatitis in children. Ital J Pediatr. 2010;36:2. Published 2010 Jan 13.
7. Belloni Fortina A, Romano I, Peserico A. Contact sensitization in very young children. J Am Acad Dermatol. 2011;65:772–9.
8. Fontana E, Belloni FA. Allergic contact dermatitis in children. Giornale Italiano di Dermatologia e Venereologia. 2014;149:693–701.
9. Murphy PB, Hooten JN, Atwater AR, et al. Allergic contact dermatitis. Treasure Island. 2020.
10. Stoðkutë L, Dubakienë R. Allergic contact dermatitis and patch testing in children. Acta Medica Lituanica. 2005;12:71–4.
11. Dotterud LK, Falk ES. Metal allergy in north Norwegian schoolchildren and its relationship with ear piercing and atopy. Contact Dermatitis. 1994;31:308–13.
12. Zinkevičienė A, Kainov D, Lastauskienė E, Kvedarienė V, Bychkov D, Byrne M, et al. Serum biomarkers of allergic contact dermatitis: a pilot study. Int Arch Allergy Immunol. 2015;168:161–4.
13. Malinauskiene L, Isaksson M, Bruze M. Patch testing with the swedish baseline series in two countries. J Clin Exp Dermatol Res. 2015;6:189–90.
14. Bordel-Gómez MT, Miranda-Romero A, Castrodeza-Sanz J. Epidemiología de la dermatitis de contacto: prevalencia de sensibilización a diferentes alérgenos y factores asociados [Epidemiology of contact dermatitis: prevalence of sensitization to different allergens and associated factors]. Actas Dermosifiliogr. 2010;101:59–75.
15. Uter W, Schnuch A, Geier J, Frosch PJ. Epidemiology of contact dermatitis. The information network of departments of dermatology (IVDK) in Germany. Eur J Dermatol. 1998;8:36–40.
16. Peiser M, Tralau T, Heidler J, Api AM, Arts JH, Basketter DA, et al. Allergic contact dermatitis: epidemiology, molecular mechanisms, in vitro methods, and regulatory aspects. Cell Mol Life Sci. 2012;69:763–81.
17. Thyssen JP, Linneberg A, Menné T, Johansen JD. The epidemiology of contact allergy in the general population: prevalence and main findings. Contact Dermatitis. 2007;57:287–90.
18. Simonsen AB, Deleuran M, Johansen JD, Sommerlund M. Contact allergy and allergic contact dermatitis in children: a review of current data. Contact Dermatitis. 2011;65:254–65.
19. Pevny I, Brennenstuhl M, Razinskas G. Patch testing in children (I). Collective test results; skin testability in children. Contact Dermatitis. 1984;11:201–6.
20. Machovcova A. The frequency of contact allergy in children and adolescents in the Czech Republic. Acta Dermatovenerol Croat. 2012;20:75–9.
21. Jacob SE, Yang A, Herro E, Zhang C. Contact allergens in a pediatric population: association with atopic dermatitis and comparison with other North American referral centers. J Clin Aesthet Dermatol. 2010;3:29–35.
22. Jacob SE, Brod B, Crawford GH. Clinically relevant patch test reactions in children—a United States based study. Pediatr Dermatol. 2008;25:520–7.
23. Militello G, Jacob SE, Crawford GH. Allergic contact dermatitis in children. Curr Opin Pediatr. 2006;18:385–90.
24. Hogeling M, Pratt M. Allergic contact dermatitis in children: the Ottawa hospital patch-testing clinic experience, 1996 to 2006. Dermatitis. 2008;19:86–9.
25. Belloni Fortina A, Fontana E, Peserico A. Contact sensitization in children: a retrospective study of 2,614 children from a single center. Pediatr Dermatol. 2016;33:399–404.
26. Papagrigoraki A, Tessari G, Peroni A, Sabbadini C, Girolomoni P. Allergic contact dermatitis in children with and without atopic dermatitis. Dermatitis. 2012;23:275–80.
27. Krasteva M, Kehren J, Ducluzeau MT, Sayag M, Cacciapuoti M, Akiba H,et al. Contact dermatitis I. Pathophysiology of contact sensitivity. Eur J Dermatol. 1999;9:121.
28. Lepoittevin J, Leblond I. Hapten-peptide T cell receptor interactions: molecular basis for the recognition of haptens by T lymphocytes. Eur J Dermatol. 1997;7:151–4.
29. Dupuis GB. Nature of hapten-protein interactions. Chemically reactive function in haptens and proteins, in allergic contact dermatitis to simple chemicals. A molecular approach. New York: Ed Marcel Dekker, Inc.; 1982.

30. Berard F, Marty JP, Nicolas JF. Allergen penetration through the skin. Eur J Dermatol. 2003;13:324–3.
31. Dupuis G. Studies on poison ivy. In vitro lymphocyte transformation by urushiol-protein conjugates. Br J Dermatol. 1979;101:617–24.
32. Saloga J, Knop J, Kolde G. Ultrastructural cytochemical visualization of chromium in the skin of sensitized guinea pigs. Arch Dermatol Res. 1988;280:214–9.
33. Esser PR, Martin SF. Pathomechanisms of contact sensitization. Curr Allergy Asthma Rep. 2017;17:83.
34. Basketter D, Dooms-Goossens A, Karlberg AT. The chemistry of contact allergy: why is a molecule allergenic? Contact Dermatitis. 1995;32:65–73.
35. Blauvelt A, Hwang ST, Udey MC. Allergic and immunologic diseases of the skin. J Allergy Clin Immunol. 2003;111:S560–70.
36. Saint-Mezard P, Rosieres A, Krasteva M, Berard F, Dubois B, Kaiserlian D, et al. Allergic contact dermatitis. Eur J Dermatol. 2004;14:284–95.
37. Wolff K, Stingl G. The Langerhan's cell. J Invest Dermatol. 1983;80:17–21.
38. Carr MM, Botham PA, Gawkrodger DJ, McVittie E, Ross JA, Stewart IC, et al. Early cellular reactions induced by dinitrochlorobenzene in sensitized humans. Br J Dermatol. 1984;110:637–41.
39. Kohler J, Martin S, Pflugfelder U, Ruh H, Vollmer J, Weltzien HU. Cross-reactive trinitrophenylated peptides as antigens for class II major histocompatibility complex restricted T cells and inducers of contact sensitivity in mice. Limited T cell receptor repertoire. Eur J Immunol. 1995;25:92–101.
40. Enk AH. Allergic contact dermatitis: understaning the immune response and potential for targeted therapy using cytokines. Mol Med Today. 1997;3:122.
41. Steinman R, Hoffman L, Pope M. Maturation and migration of cutaneous dendritic cells. J Invest Dermatol. 1995;105:2S–7S.
42. Frey JR, Wenk P. Experimentelle Untersuchungen zur pathogenese des Kontaktekzems. Dermatologica. 1956;112:265–305.
43. Hoefakker S, Caubo M, Vant Erve EHM, Roggeveen MJ, Boersma WJ, van Joost T, et al. In vivo cytokine profiles in allergic and irritant contact dermatitis. Contact Dermatitis. 1995;33:258–67.
44. Kimber I, Dearman RJ. Allergic contact dermatitis: The cellular effects. Contact Dermatitis. 2002;46:1–5.
45. Silverberg I, Baer RL, Rosenthal SA. The role of Langerhan's cells in contact allergy. Acta derm Venereol. 1974;54:321–31.
46. Homey B, Alenius H, Muller A, Soto H, Bowman EP, Yuan W, et al. CCL 27—CCR 10 interactions regulate T-cell mediated skin inflammation. Nat Med. 2002;8:157–65.
47. Trautmann A, Akdis M, Kleemann D, Altznauer F, Simon HU, Graeve T, et al. T-cell mediated Fas—Induced keratinocyte apoptosis plays a key pathogenetic role in eczematous dermatitis. J Clin Invest. 2000;106:25–35.
48. Brandão MH, Gontijo B. Contact sensitivity to metals (chromium, cobalt and nickel) in childhood. Anais brasileiros de dermatologia. 2012;87:269–76.
49. Cresswell P. Antigen recognition by Lymphocytes. Immunol Today. 1987;8:67–9.
50. Breathnach SM, Katz SI. Cell mediated immunity and the skin. Hum Pathol. 1986;17:161–7.
51. Li LY, Cruz PD Jr. Allergic Contact Dermatitis: Pathophysiology applied to future therapy. Dermatol Ther. 2004;17:219–23.
52. Krasteva M, et al. Contact dermatitis II. Clinical aspects and diagnosis. Eur J Dermatol. 1999;9:144–59.
53. Vigan M, Girardin P, Adessi B, Laurent R. Late reading of patch tests. Eur J Dermatol. 1997;7:574–6.
54. Nishibu A, Ward BR, Jester JV, Ploegh HL, Boes M, Takashima A. Behavioral responses of epidermal Langerhans cells in situ to local pathological stimuli. J Invest Dermatol. 2006;126:787–96.
55. Hauser C. Cultured epidermal Langerhans cells activate effector T cells for contact sensitivity. J Invest Dermatol. 1990;95:436–40.
56. Liu J, Harberts E, Tammaro A, Girardi N, Filler RB, Fishelevich R, et al. IL-9 regulates allergen-specific Th1 responses in allergic contact dermatitis. J Invest Dermatol. 2014;134:1903–11.
57. Schmidt JD, Ahlström MG, Johansen JD, Dyring-Andersen B, Agerbeck C, Nielsen MM, et al. Rapid allergen-induced interleukin-17 and interferon-γ secretion by skin-resident memory CD8+ T cells. Contact Dermatitis. 2017;76:218–27.
58. Zhao Y, Balato A, Fishelevich R, Chapoval A, Mann DL, Gaspari AA. Th17/Tc17 infiltration and associated cytokine gene expression in elicitation phase of allergic contact dermatitis. Br J Dermatol. 2009;161:1301–6.
59. Nakae S, Komiyama Y, Nambu A, Sudo K, Iwase M, Homma I, et al. Antigen-specific T cell sensitization is impaired in IL-17-deficient mice, causing suppression of allergic cellular and humoral responses. Immunity. 2002;17:375–87.
60. Dieli F. Dendritic cells and the handling of antigen. Clin Exp Immunol. 2003;134:178–80.
61. Griffiths C, Barker J, Bleiker T, Chalmers R, Creamer D, editors. Rook's textbook of dermatology. John Wiley & Sons; 2016.
62. Seneschal J, Clark RA, Gehad A, Baecher-Allan CM, Kupper TS. Human epidermal Langerhans cells maintain immune homeostasis in skin by activating skin resident regulatory T cells. Immunity. 2012;36:873–84.
63. Vocanson M, Goujon C, Chabeau G, Castelain M, Valeyrie M, Floc'h F, et al. The skin allergenic properties of chemicals may depend on contaminants--evidence from studies on coumarin. Int Arch Allergy Immunol. 2006;140:231–8.
64. Leonard A, Guttman-Yassky E. The unique molecular signatures of contact dermatitis and implications for treatment. Clin Rev Allergy Immunol. 2019;56:1–8.

65. Cooper KD, Oberhelman L, Hamilton TA, Baadsgaard O, Terhune M, LeVee G, et al. UV exposure reduces immunization rates and promotes tolerance to epicutaneous antigens in humans; Relationship to doses, CD1a – DR+ epidermal macrophage induction, and Langerhan's cell depletion. Proc Natl Acad Sci USA. 1992;89:8497–501.
66. Rozas-Muñoz E, Lepoittevin JP, Pujol RM, Giménez-Arnau A. Allergic contact dermatitis to plants: understanding the chemistry will help our diagnostic approach. Actas Dermosifiliogr. 2012;103:456–77.
67. Barral P, Batanero E, Palomares O, Quiralte J, Villalba M, Rodríguez R. A major allergen from pollen defines a novel family of plant proteins and shows intra- and interspecies cross-reactivity. J Immunol. 2004;172:3644–51.
68. Schnuch A, Geier J, Uter W, Frosch PJ, Lehmacher W, Aberer W, et al. National rates and regional differences in sensitization to allergens of the standard series. Population-adjusted frequencies of sensitization (PAFS) in 40,000 patients from a multicenter study (IVDK). Contact Dermatitis. 1997;37:200–9.
69. Goh CL. Prevalence of contact allergy by sex, race and age. Contact Dermatitis. 1986;14:237–40.
70. Lee HY, Stieger M, Yawalkar N, Kakeda M. Cytokines and chemokines in irritant contact dermatitis. Mediators Inflamm. 2013;2013:916497.
71. Katta R, Schlichte M. Diet and dermatitis: food triggers. J Clin Aesthet Dermatol. 2014;7:30–6.
72. Menne T, Holm V. Nickel allergy in a female twin population. Int J Dermatol. 1983;22:22–8.
73. Menne T, Holm V. Genetic susceptibility in human allergic sensitization. Semin Dermatol. 1986;5:301–6.
74. Zafrir Y, Trattner A, Hodak E, Eldar O, Lapidoth M, Ben AD. Patch testing in Israeli children with suspected allergic contact dermatitis: A retrospective study and literature review. Pediatr Dermatol. 2018;35:76–86.
75. Dor-Wojnarowska A, Liebhart J, Miecielica J, Rabski M, Fal A, Samoliński B, et al. The impact of sex and age on the prevalence of clinically relevant sensitization and asymptomatic sensitization in the general population. Arch Immunol Ther Exp (Warsz). 2017;65:253–61.
76. Crisp HC, Quinn JM. Quantitative immunoglobulins in adulthood. Allergy Asthma Proc. 2009;30:649–54.
77. Desai MK, Brinton RD. Autoimmune disease in women: endocrine transition and risk across the lifespan. Front Endocrinol (Lausanne). 2019;10:265.
78. Mortazavi H, Ehsani A, Sajjadi SS, et al. Patch testing in Iranian children with allergic contact dermatitis. BMC Dermatol. 2016;16:10.
79. Simonsen A, Deleuran M, Gotthard Mortz C, Johansen JD, Sommerlund M. Allergic contact dermatitis in Danish children referred for patch testing—a nationwide multicentre study. Contact Dermatitis. 2013;70:104–11.
80. Fisher AA. Perfume dermatitis in children sensitized to balsam of Peru in topical agents. Cutis. 1990;45:21–3.
81. Simon AK, Hollander GA, McMichael A. Evolution of the immune system in humans from infancy to old age. Proc Biol Sci. 1821;2015:20143085.
82. Manzini BM, Ferdani G, Simonetti V, Donini M, Seidenari S. Contact sensitization in children. Pediatr Dermatol. 1998;15:12–7.
83. Mortz CG, Andersen KE. Allergic contact dermatitis in children and adolescents. Contact Dermatitis. 1999;41:121–30.
84. Carder KR. Hypersensitivity reactions in neonates and infants. Dermatol Ther. 2005;18:160–75.
85. Wojciech F, Johannes G, Steffen S, Worm M. A case-control analysis of skin contact allergy in children and adolescents. Pediatr Allergy Immunol. 2019;30:632–7.
86. Fernández Vozmediano JM, Armario Hita JC. Allergic contact dermatitis in children. J Eur Acad Dermatol Venereol. 2005;19:42–6.
87. Zug KA, McGinley-Smith D, Warshaw EM, Taylor JS, Rietschel RL, Maibach HI, et al. Contact allergy in children referred for patch testing: North American Contact Dermatitis Group data, 2001–2004. Arch Dermatol. 2008;144:126.
88. Czarnobilska E, Obtulowicz K, Dyga W, Wsolek-Wnek K, Spiewak R. Contact hypersensitivity and allergic contact dermatitis among school children and teenagers with eczema. Contact Dermatitis. 2009;60:264–9.
89. Czarnobilska E, Obtulowicz K, Dyga W, Spiewak R. The most important contact sensitizers in Polish children and adolescents with atopy and chronic recurrent eczema as detected with the extended European Baseline Series. Pediatr Allergy Immunol. 2011;22:252–6.
90. Morris SD, Rycroft RJ, White IR, Wakelin SH, McFadden JP. Comparative frequency of patch test reactions to topical antibiotics. Br J Dermatol. 2002;146:1047–51.
91. Oh-i T. Contact dermatitis due to topical steroids with conceivable cross reactions between topical steroid preparations. J Dermatol. 1996;23:200–8.
92. Riboldi A, Pigatto PD, Morelli M, Altomare GF, Polenghi MM. Allergy to mercurochrome and rifamycin. Contact Dermatitis. 1985;12:180.
93. Goh CL. Contact sensitivity to topical medicaments. Int J Dermatol. 1989;28:25–8.
94. Sharma VK, Mandal SK, Sethuraman G, Bakshi NA. Para-phenylenediamine induced lichenoid eruptions. Contact Dermatitis. 1999;41:40–1.
95. Kostner L, Anzengruber F, Guillod C, Recher M, Schmid-Grendelmeier P, Navarini AA. Allergic contact dermatitis. Immunol Allergy Clin North Am. 2017;37:141–52.
96. Maaks DLG, Dirks M, Driessnack M, Duderstadt K, Gaylordet NM. Burn's pediatric primary care. Elsevier; 2017. p. 127.
97. Frain-Bell W. Photodermatoses. In: Rook A, editor. Recent advances in dermatology. Wiley; 1973. p. 101–33.
98. Osmundsen PE. Contact photo allergy to tribromosalicylanilide. Br J Dermatol. 1968;31:429–34.

99. Jacob SE, Breithaupt AD. An important difference between "exposed" and "photodistributed" underscores the importance of identifying common reactions. J Clin Aesthet Dermatol. 2009;2:44–5.
100. De Groot AC. Labelling cosmetics with their ingredients. BMJ. 1990;300:1636–8.
101. Bonamonte D, Foti C, Vestita M, Angelini G. Noneczematous contact dermatitis. ISRN Allergy. 2013;15:361746.
102. Price A, Stone NM, Harding KG. An unusual presentation of a common condition: Allergic contact dermatitis. Int Wound J. 2018;15:645–8.
103. Ahlgren C, Bruze M, Moller H, Gruvberger B, Axéll T, Liedholm R, et al. Contact allergy to gold in patients with oral lichen lesions. Acta Derm Venereol. 2012;92:138–43.
104. Società Italiana Dermatologia. Linee guida e raccomandazioni SIDeMAST. Pacini editore, Pisa, Italy. 2011.
105. Rietschel RL, Fowler JF. Fisher's contact dermatitis. 2001. 728–729.
106. Cronin E. Ekzematose Reaktioner bei innerlicher Aufnahme von Kontaktallergenen. Hautarzt. 1975;26:68–71.
107. Christensen OB, Moller H. External and internal exposure to the antigen in the hand eczema of Nickel allergy. Contact Dermatitis. 1975;1:136–41.
108. Grossman J, Baum J, Gluckman J, Fusner J, Condemi JJ. The effect of aging and acute illness on delayed hypersensitivity. J Allergy Clin Immunol. 1975;55:262–75.
109. Engkilde K, Menné T, Johansen JD. Inverse relationship between allergic contact dermatitis and type 1 diabetes mellitus: a retrospective clinic-based study. Diabetologia. 2006;49:644–7.
110. Garner LA. Contact dermatitis to metals. Dermatol Ther. 2004;17:321–7.
111. Fowler JF, Fowler LM, Hunter JE. Allergy to cocamidopropyl betaine may be due to amidoamine: a patch test and product use test study. Contact Dermatitis. 1997;37:276–81.
112. Jacob SE, Amini S. Cocamidopropyl betaine. Dermatitis. 2008;19:157–60.
113. Hammonds LM, Hall VC, Yiannias JA. Allergic contact dermatitis in 136 children patch tested between 2000 and 2006. Int J Dermatol. 2009;48:271–4.
114. Seidenari S, Giusti F, Pepe P, Mantovani L. Contact sensitization in 1094 children undergoing patch testing over a 7-year period. Pediatr Dermatol. 2005;22:1–5.
115. Admani S, Jacob SE. Allergic contact dermatitis in children: review of the past decade. Curr Allergy Asthma Rep. 2014;14:421.
116. Thyssen JP, McFadden JP, Kimber I. The multiple factors affecting the association between atopic dermatitis and contact sensitization. Allergy. 2014;69:28–36.
117. Gittler JK, Krueger JG, Guttman-Yassky E. Atopic dermatitis results in intrinsic barrier and immune abnormalities: implications for contact dermatitis. J Allergy Clin Immunol. 2013;131:300–13.
118. Simonsen AB, Johansen JD, Deleuran M, Mortz CG, Sommerlund M. Contact allergy in children with atopic dermatitis: a systematic review. Br J Dermatol. 2017;177:395–405.
119. Uehara M, Sawai T. A longitudinal study of contact sensitivity in patients with atopic dermatitis. Arch Dermatol. 1989;125:366–8.
120. Jacob SE, Yang A, Herro E, Zhang C. Contact allergens in a pediatric population: association with atopic dermatitis and comparison with other north american referral centers. J Clin Aesthet Dermatol. 2010;3:29–35.
121. Belloni Fortina A, Cooper SM, Spiewak R, Fontana E, Schnuch A, Uter W. Patch test results in children and adolescents across Europe. Analysis of the ESSCA Network 2002–2010. Pediatr Allergy Immunol. 2015;26:446–55.
122. Uter W, Werfel T, White IR, Johansen JD. Contact allergy: a review of current problems from a clinical perspective. Int J Environ Res Public Health. 2018;15:1108.
123. Frsbeck M, Skog E, Ytterborn KH. Delayed type of allergy and atopic disease among twins. Acta Derm Venereol. 1968;48:192–7.
124. Boonstra M, Rustemeyer T, Middelkamp-Hup MA. Both children and adult patients with difficult-to-treat atopic dermatitis have high prevalences of concomitant allergic contact dermatitis and are frequently polysensitized. J Eur Acad Dermatol Venereol. 2018;32:1554–61.
125. Belhadjali H, Mohamed M, Youssef M, Mandhouj S, Chakroun M, Zili J. Contact sensitization in atopic dermatitis: results of a prospective study of 89 cases in Tunisia. Contact Dermatitis. 2008;58:188–9.
126. Oranje AP, Bruynzeel DP, Stenveld HJ, Dieges PH. Immediate- and delayed-type contact hypersensitivity in children older than 5 years with atopic dermatitis: a pilot study comparing different tests. Pediatr Dermatol. 1994;11:209–15.
127. Giordano Labadie F, Rance F, Pellegrin F, Bazex J, Dutau G, Schwarze HP. Frequency of contact allergy in children with atopic dermatitis: results of a prospective study of 137 cases. Contact Dermatitis. 1999;40:192Y195.
128. Gober MD, Gaspari AA. Allergic contact dermatitis. Curr Dir Autoimmun. 2008;10:1–26.
129. Pelletier JL, Perez C, Jacob SE. Contact dermatitis in pediatrics. Pediatr Ann. 2016;45:287–92.
130. Lagrelius M, Wahlgren CF, Matura M, Bergström A, Kull I, Lidén C. Atopic dermatitis at preschool age and contact allergy in adolescence: a population-based cohort study. Br J Dermatol. 2019;180:782–9.
131. Simonsen AB, Johansen JD, Deleuran M, Mortz CG, Skov L, Sommerlund M. Children with atopic dermatitis may have unacknowledged contact allergies contributing to their skin symptoms. J Eur Acad Dermatol Venereol. 2018;32:428–36.
132. Lammintausta K, Kamino K, Fagerlund VL. Patch test reactions in atopic patients. Contact Dermatitis. 1992;26:234Y240.

133. Gonul M, Gul U. Detection of contact hypersensitivity to corticosteroids in allergic contact dermatitis patients who do not respond to topical corticosteroids. Contact Dermatitis. 2005;53:67Y70.
134. Lubbes S, Rustemeyer T, Sillevis Smitt JH, Schuttelaar ML, Middelkamp-Hup MA. Contact sensitization in Dutch children and adolescents with and without atopic dermatitis - a retrospective analysis. Contact Dermatitis. 2017;76:151–9.
135. Isaksson M, Olhardt S, Rådehed J, Svensson Å. Children with atopic dermatitis should always be patch-tested if they have hand or foot dermatitis. Acta Derm Venereol. 2015;95:583–6.
136. Herro EM, Matiz C, Sullivan K, Hamann C, Jacob SE. Frequency of contact allergens in pediatric patients with atopic dermatitis. J Clin Aesthet Dermatol. 2011;4:39–41.
137. Kolesnik M, Franke I, Lux A, Quist SR, Gollnick HP. Eczema in psoriatico: an important differential diagnosis between chronic allergic contact dermatitis and psoriasis in palmoplantar localization. Acta Derm Venereol. 2018;98:50–8.
138. Jacob SE, Shehla A. The 'Pull Test' delineation of irritant patch test reactions. J Clin Exp Dermatol Res. 2014;5:4.
139. Diepgen TL, Coenraads PJ. Sensitivity, specificity and positive predictive value of patch testing: the more you test, the more you get? ESCD Working Party on Epidemiology. Contact Dermatitis. 2000;42:315–7.
140. Jacob SE, Steel T, Brod B, Crawford GH. Dispelling the myths behind pediatric patch testing-experience from our tertiary care patch testing centers. Pediatr Dermatol. 2008;25:296–300.
141. Cristophersen J, Menne T, Tanghof P, Andersen KE, Brandrup F, Kaaber K, et al. Clinical patch test data evaluated by multivariate analysis. Contact Dermatitis. 1989;21:291–9.
142. Borok J, Matiz C, Goldenberg A, Jacob SE. Contact dermatitis in atopic dermatitis children-past, present, and future. Clin Rev Allergy Immunol. 2019;56:86–98.
143. Thilak S. A study of 300 cases of allergic contact dermatitis. Int J Res Dermatol. 2017;3:20164409.
144. Nettis EN, Angelini G. Atlante e compendio: il patch test. 2017.
145. Johansen JD, Aalto-Korte K, Agner T, Andersen KE, Bircher A, Bruze M, et al. European Society of Contact Dermatitis guideline for diagnostic patch testing – recommendations on best practice. Contact Dermatitis. 2015;73:195–221.
146. Magnusson B, Hersle K. Patch test methods. II. Regional variations of patch test responses. Acta Derm Venereol. 1965;45:257–61.
147. Björk AK, Bruze M, Engfeldt M, Nielsen C, Svedman C. The reactivity of the back revisited. Are there differences in reactivity in different parts of the back? Contact Dermatitis. 2017;76:19–26.
148. Lachapelle JM. The Spectrum of diseases for which patch testing is recommended. In: Patch testing and prick testing. Berlin/Heidelberg: Springer; 2009.
149. Ale SI, Maibachet HI. Irritant contact dermatitis versus allergic contact dermatitis. Berlin: Springer; 2006. p. 11–8.
150. Nijhawen RI, Matiz C, Jacob SE. Contact dermatitis: From basics to allergodromes. Pediatric Annals. 2009;38:99Y108.
151. Chaudhry HM, Drage LA, El-Azhary RA, Hall MR, Killian JM, Prakash AV et al. Delayed patch-test reading after 5 days: an update from the Mayo Clinic Contact Dermatitis Group. Dermatitis. 2017;28:253–60.
152. Eszter B, Erzsébet T, Ilona N, Miklós S, Györgyi P. Contact hypersensitivity in adolescents. Pediatric Dermatol. 2018;35:769–73.
153. Cantwell HM, Drage LA, El-Azhary RA, Hall MR, Killian JM, Yiannias JA, et al. The final patch test read: day 5 or day >7? Dermatitis. 2020;31:42–52.
154. Feuerman E, Levy A. A study of the effect of prednisolone and antihistamine on patch test reactions. Br J Dermatol. 1972;86:68–71.
155. Thorvaldsen J, Volden G. PUVA—Induced diminution of contact allergic and irritant skin reactions. Clin Exp Dermatol. 1980;5:43–6.
156. Anveden I, Lindberg M, Andersen KE, Bruze M, Isaksson M, Liden C, et al. Oral prednisone suppresses allergic but not irritant patch test reactions in individuals hypersensitive to nickel. Contact Dermatitis. 2004;50:298–303.
157. Rai R, Thomas M. Photopatch and UV-irradiated patch testing in photosensitive dermatitis. Indian Dermatol Online J. 2016;7:12–6.
158. Jacob SE, Burk CJ, Connelly EA. Patch testing: another steroid-sparing agent to consider in children. Pediatr Dermatol. 2008;25:81–7.
159. Girolomoni G, Abeni D, Masini C, Sera F, Ayala F, Belloni-Fortina A, et al. The epidemiology of atopic dermatitis in Italian schoolchildren. Allergy. 2003;58:420–5.
160. Dou X, Kim J, Ni CY, Shao Y, Zhang J. Atopy patch test with house dust mite in Chinese patients with atopic dermatitis. J Eur Acad Dermatol Venereol. 2016;30:1522–6.
161. Davis MD, Richardson DM, Ahmed DD. Rate of patch test reactions to a Dermatophagoides mix currently on the market: a mite too sensitive? Am J Contact Dermat. 2002;13:71–3.
162. Fuiano N, Incorvaia C. Confronto tra skin prick test e atopy patch test nella diagnosi di allergia a Dermatophagoides in soggetti con patologia respiratoria e/o dermatite atopica. Minerva Pediatrica. 2004;56:537–40.
163. Kapur C, Shenoi SD, Prabhu SS, Balachandran C. Patch testing with dermatophagoides and its correlation with chronic eczema and atopic dermatitis. Indian J Dermatol. 2009;54:243–6.
164. Stables GI, Forsyth A, Lever RS. Patch testing in children. Contact Dermatitis. 1996;34:341–4.
165. Rademaker M, Forsyth A. Contact dermatitis in children. Contact Dermatitis. 1989;20:104–7.

166. Barros MA, Baptista A, Correia TM, Azevedo F. Patch testing in children: a study of 562 schoolchildren. Contact Dermatitis. 1991;25:156–9.
167. Goossens A, Neyens K, Vigan M. Contact allergy in children. In: Textbook of contact dermatitis. 3rd ed. Berlin: Springer; 2001. p. 581–603.
168. de Waard-van der Spek FB, Oranje AP. Patch tests in children with suspected allergic contact dermatitis: a prospective study and review of the literature. Dermatology. 2009;218:119–25.
169. Ascha M, Irfan M, Bena J, Taylor JS, Sood A. Pediatric patch testing: a 10-year retrospective study. Ann Allergy Asthma Immunol. 2016;117:661–7.
170. Felmingham C, Davenport R, Bala H, Palmer A, Nixon R. Allergic contact dermatitis in children and proposal for an Australian Paediatric Baseline Series. Australas J Dermatol. 2020;61:33–8.
171. Warshaw EM, Zhang AJ, DeKoven JG, Maibach HI, Belsito DV, Sasseville D, et al. Epidemiology of nickel sensitivity: Retrospective cross-sectional analysis of North American Contact Dermatitis Group data 1994–2014. J Am Acad Dermatol. 2019;80:701–13.
172. Rosholm Comstedt L, Dahlin J, Bruze M, Åkesson A, Hindsén M, Pontén A, et al. Prevalence of contact allergy to metals: nickel, palladium, and cobalt in Suthern Sweden from 1995–2016. Contact Dermatitis. 2020;82:218–26.
173. Ahlström MG, Thyssen JP, Menné T, Johansen JD. Prevalence of nickel allergy in Europe following the EU Nickel Directive—a review. Contact Dermatitis. 2017;77:193–200.
174. Warshaw EM, Aschenbeck KA, DeKoven JG, Maibach HI, Taylor JS, Sasseville D et al. Epidemiology of pediatric nickel sensitivity: retrospective review of North American Contact Dermatitis Group (NACDG) data 1994–2014. J Am Acad Dermatol. 2018;79:664–771.
175. Bordel-Gómez MT, Miranda-Romero A, Castrodeza-Sanz J. Isolated and concurrent prevalence of sensitization to transition metals in a Spanish population. J Eur Acad Dermatol Venereol. 2008;22:1452–7.
176. Cristaudo A, Petrucci F, Giannarelli D, Cercato MC, Orsini D, Morrone A, et al. Nickel dermatitis from earrings 15 years after EU directive implementation: a clinical-epidemiological study and a market survey in Rome, Italy. J Eur Acad Dermatol Venereol. 2019;33:1928–34.
177. Ahlström MG, Thyssen JP, Wennervaldt M, Menné T, Johansen JD. Nickel allergy and allergic contact dermatitis: a clinical review of immunology, epidemiology, exposure, and treatment. Contact Dermatitis. 2019;81:227–41.
178. Simonsen A, Foss-Skiftesvik MH, Thyssen JP, Deleuran M, Mortz CG, Zachariae C, et al. Contact allergy in Danish children: current trends. Contact Dermatitis. 2018;79:295–302.
179. Thyssen JP, Uter W, McFadden J, Menné T, Spiewak R, Vigan M, et al. The EU Nickel Directive revisited - future steps towards better protection against nickel allergy. Contact Dermatitis. 2011;64:121–5.
180. Uter W, Aberer WW, Armario-Hita JC, Fernandez-Vomediano JM, Ayala F, Balato A, et al. Current patch test results with the European baseline series and extensions to it from the 'European Surveillance System on Contact Allergy' network, 2007–2008. Contact Dermatitis. 2012;67:9–19.
181. Schena D, Papagrigoraki A, Tessari G, Peroni A, Sabbadini C, Girolomoni P. Allergic contact dermatitis in children with and without atopic dermatitis. Dermatitis. 2012;23:275–80.
182. Mortz GC, Kjaer HF, Eller E, Osterballe M, Norberg LA, Høst A, et al. Positive nickel patch tests in infants are of low clinical relevance and rarely reproducible. Pediatr Allergy Immunol. 2013;24:84–7.
183. Jøhnke H, Norberg LA, Vach W, Bindslev-Jensen C, Høst A, Andersen KE. Reactivity to patch tests with nickel sulfate and fragrance mix in infants. Contact Dermatitis. 2004;51:141–7.
184. Liden C, Menne T, Burrows D. Nickel containing alloys and plating and their ability to cause dermatitis. Br J Dermatol. 1996;134:193–8.
185. Midander K, Kettelarij J, Julander A, Lidén C. Nickel release from white gold. Contact Dermatitis. 2014;71:109–11.
186. Nielsen NH, Menne T. Allergy contact sensitization in an unselected Danish population. Acta Derm Venereol. 1992;72:456–60.
187. Calnan CD. Nickel dermatitis. Br J Dermatol. 1956;68:229–36.
188. Menne T, Borgan O, Green A. Nickel allergy and hand dermatitis. Acta Derm Venereol. 1982;62:35–41.
189. Fowler JF Jr. Cobalt. Dermatitis. 2016;27:3–8.
190. Lidén C, Andersson N, Julander A, Matura M. Cobalt allergy: suitable test concentration, and concomitant reactivity to nickel and chromium. Contact Dermatitis. 2016;74:360–7.
191. Bregnbak D, Thyssen JP, Zachariae C, et al. Association between cobalt allergy and dermatitis caused by leather articles—a questionnaire study. Contact Dermatitis. 2014;72:106–14.
192. Irvine C, Pugh CE, Hansen EJ. Cement dermatitis in underground workers. Occup Med. 1994;44:17–23. Seishima M, Oyama Z, Oda M. Cellular phone dermatitis with chromate allergy. Dermatology 2003;207:48–50.
193. Richardson C, Hamann CR, Hamann D, Thyssen JP. Mobile phone dermatitis in children and adults: a review of the literature. Pediatr Allergy Immunol Pulmonol. 2014;27:60–9.
194. Lutz ME, el Azhary RA, Gibson LE, Fransway AF. Contact hypersensitivity to tixocortol pivalate. J Am Acad Dermatol. 1998;38:691–5.
195. Lepoittevin JP, Drieghe J, Dooms-Goossens A. Studies in patients with corticosteroid contact allergy. Understanding cross-reactivity among different steroids. Arch Dermatol. 1995;131:31–7.

196. Goldenberg A, Mousdicas N, Silverberg N, Powell D, Pelletier JL, Silverberg JI,et al. Pediatric contact dermatitis registry inaugural case data. Dermatitis. 2016;27:293–302.
197. Yu J, Atwater AR, Brod B, Chen JK, Chisolm SS, Cohen DE, et al. Pediatric baseline patch test series: pediatriccontact dermatitis workgroup. Dermatitis. 2018;29:206–12.
198. Adams RM, Maibach I. A five year study of cosmetic reactions. J Am Acad Dermatol. 1985;13:1062–9.
199. Heisterberg MV, Andersen KE, Avnstorp C, Kristensen B, Kristensen O, Kaaber K, et al. Fragrance mix II in the baseline series contributes significantly to detection of fragrance allergy. Contact Dermatitis. 2010;63:270–6.
200. Thyssen JP, Menné T, Linneberg A, Johansen JD. Contact sensitization to fragrances in the general population: a Koch's approach may reveal the burden of disease. Br J Dermatol. 2009;160:729–35.
201. Rossi M, Coenraads PJ, Diepgen T, Svensson Å, Elsner P, Gonçalo M, et al. Design and feasibility of an international study assessing the prevalence of contact allergy to fragrances in the general population: the European Dermato-Epidemiology Network Fragrance Study. Dermatology. 2010;221:267–75.
202. Johansen JD. Fragrance contact allergy: a clinical review. Am J Clin Dermatol. 2003;4:789–98.
203. Tichy M, Karlova I. Allergic contact dermatitis and changes in the frequency of the causative allergens demonstrated with patch testing in 2008–2012. Biomed Pap Med Fac Univ Palacky Olomouc Czech Repub. 2015;159:480e488.136–8.
204. de Groot AC. Myroxylon pereirae resin (balsam of Peru) - A critical review of the literature and assessment of the significance of positive patch test reactions and the usefulness of restrictive diets. Contact Dermatitis. 2019;80:335–53.
205. Kundak S. Patch test results of contact sensitization in children without atopic dermatitis: a single tertiary center experience. Dermatitis. 2020;31:153–6.
206. de Groot A, Flyvholm M, Lensen G, Menné T, Coenraads P. Formaldehyde-releasers: relationship to formaldehyde contact allergy. Contact allergy to formaldehyde and inventory of formaldehyde-releasers. Contact Dermatitis. 2009;61:63–85.
207. Trattner A, Johansen JD, Menné T. Formaldehyde concentration in diagnostic patch testing: comparison of 1% with 2%. Contact Dermatitis. 1998;38:9–13.
208. Zaragoza-Ninet V, Blasco Encinas R, Vilata-Corell J, Pérez-Ferriols A, Sierra-Talamantes C, Esteve-Martínez A, et al. Dermatitis alérgica de contacto a cosméticos, estudio clínico-epidemiológico en un hospital terciario. Actas Dermosifiliogr. 2016;107:329–36.
209. Yu SH, Sood A, Taylor JS. Patch testing for methylisothiazolinone and methylchloroisothiazolinone-methylisothiazolinone contact allergy. JAMA Dermatol. 2016;152:67–72.
210. Aerts O, Goossens A, Lambert J, Lepoittevin JP. Contact allergy caused by isothiazolinone derivatives: an overview of non-cosmetic and unusual cosmetic sources. Eur J Dermatol. 2017;27:115–22.
211. Dusefante A, Mauro M, Belloni Fortina A, Corradin MT, Larese FF. Contact allergy to methylchloroisothiazolinone/methylisothiazolinone in north-easternItaly: a temporal trend from 1996 to 2016. J Eur Acad Dermatol Venereol. 2019;33:912–7.
212. DeKoven JG, Warshaw EM, Zug KA, Maibach HI, Belsito DV, Sasseville D, et al. North American contact dermatitis group patch test results: 2015–2016. Dermatitis. 2018;29:297–309.
213. Chang MW, Nakrani R. Six children with allergic contact dermatitis to methylisothiazolinone in wet wipes (baby wipes). Pediatrics. 2014;133:e434–8.
214. Toledo F, Garcıa-Bravo B, Fernandez-Redondo V, De la Cuadra J, Giménez-Arnau AM, Borrego L, et al. Patch testing in children with hand eczema. A 5-year multicentre study in Spain. Contact Dermatitis. 2011;65:213–9.
215. Silva EA, Bosco MRM, Lozano RR, Latini ACP, Souza VNB. High rate of sensitization to Kathon CG, detected by patch tests in patients with suspected allergic contact dermatitis. An Bras Dermatol. 2020;95:194–9.
216. Isaksson M, Ale I, Andersen KE, Elsner P, Goh CL, Goossens A, et al. Multicenter patch testing with methylisothiazolinone and methylchloroisothiazolinone/methylisothiazolinone within the international contact dermatitis research group. Dermatitis. 2017;28:210–4.
217. Johansen JD, Veien N, Laaurberg G, Avnstorp C, Kaaber K, Andersen KE, et al. Decreasing trend in methylbromo glutaronitrile contact allergy following regulatory intervention. Contact Dermatitis. 2008;59:48–51.
218. Menné T, Hjorth N. Routine patch testing with paraben esters. Contact Dermatitis. 1988;19:189–91.
219. Fransway AF, Fransway PJ, Belsito DV, et al. Parabens. Dermatitis. 2019;30:3–31.
220. Turchin I, Moreau L, Warshaw E, Sasseville D. Cross-reactions among parabens, para-phenylenediamine, and benzocaine: a retrospective analysis of patch testing. Dermatitis. 2006;17:192–5.
221. Sasseville D. Hypersensitivity to preservatives. Dermatol Ther. 2004;17:251–63.
222. Collis RW, Morris GM, Sheinbein DM, Coughlin CC. Expanded series and personalized patch tests for children: a retrospective cohort study. Dermatitis. 2020;31:144–6.
223. Fransen M, Overgaard LEK, Johansen JD, Thyssen JP. Contact allergy to lanolin: temporal changes in prevalence and association with atopic dermatitis. Contact Dermatitis. 2018;78:70–5.
224. Paulsen E, Andersen KE. Clinical patterns of Compositae dermatitis in Danish monosensitized patients. Contact Dermatitis. 2018;78:185–93.
225. Belloni Fortina A, Marciani Magno F, Cappelletti EM, Peserico A. Contact dermatitis from Vernonia noveboracensis. Contact Dermatitis. 2002;46:357–8.

226. Paulsen E. Contact sensitization from Compositae-containing herbal remedies and cosmetics. Contact Dermatitis. 2002;47:189–98.
227. Rietschel RL, Fowler JF. Fisher's contact dermatitis. 5th ed. Baltimore: Lippincott, Williams and Wilkins; 1995. 351–95, 715–21.
228. Heine G, Schnuch A, Uter W, Worm M. Frequency of contact allergy in German children and adolescents patch tested between 1995 and 2002: results from the Information Network of Departments of Dermatology and the German Contact Dermatitis Research Group. Contact Dermatitis. 2004;51:111–7.
229. Pesonen M, Suuronen K, Suomela S, Aalto-Korte K. Occupational allergic contact dermatitis caused by colophonium. Contact Dermatitis. 2019;80:9–17.
230. Hausen BM, Mohnert J. Contact allergy due to colophony. (V). Patch test results with different types of colophony and modified-colophony products. Contact Dermatitis. 1989;20:295–301.
231. Warshaw EM, Raju SI, Mathias CG, DeKoven JG, Belsito DV, Maibach HI, et al. Concomitant patch test reactions to mercapto mix and mercaptobenzothiazole: retrospective analysis from the North American Contact Dermatitis Group, 1994–2008. Dermatitis. 2013;24:321–7.
232. Engfeldt M, Isaksson M, Glas B, Hagvall L, Löfnertz Petersson A, et al. Patch testing with a new composition of mercapto mix: a multi-centre study by the Swedish contact dermatitis research group. Acta Derm Venereol. 2019;99:960–3.
233. Panfili E, Esposito S, Di Cara G. Temporary Black Henna Tattoos and Sensitization to para-Phenylenediamine (PPD): two paediatric case reports and a review of the literature. Int J Environ Res Public Health. 2017;14:421.
234. Di Prisco MC, Puig L, Alomar A. Contact dermatitis due to paraphenylenediamine (PPD) on a temporal tattoo with henna. Cross reaction to azoic dyes. Investig Clin. 2006;47:295–9.
235. Rycroft RJG, Menné T, Frosch PJ, Lepoittevinet J-P. Textbook of contact dermatitis. Berlin, Heidelberg: Springer; 2001.
236. Duarte I, Mendonça RF, Korkes KL, Lazzarini R, Hafner MFS. Nickel, chromium and cobalt: the relevant allergens in allergic contact dermatitis. Comparative study between two periods: 1995–2002 and 2003–2015. An Bras Dermatol. 2018;93:59–62.
237. Rodrigues DF, Goulart EM. Patch-test results in children and adolescents: systematic review of a 15-year period. An Bras Dermatol. 2016;91:64–72.
238. Cobb HK, Shinohara MM, Huss JT, Welch MP, Gardner JM. Systemic contact dermatitis to a surgical implant presenting as red decorative tattoo reaction. JAAD Case Rep. 2017;3:348–50.
239. Lombardo F, Salzano G, Crisafulli G, Panasiti I, Alibrandi A, Messina MF, et al. Allergic contact dermatitis in pediatric patients with type 1 diabetes: An emerging issue. Diabetes Res Clin Pract. 2020;162:108089.
240. Romita P, Foti C, Barlusconi C, Hansel K, Tramontana M, Stingeni L. Contact allergy to (meth) acrylates in gel nail polish in a child: An emerging risk for children. Contact Dermatitis. 2020;83:39–40.
241. Johansen JD, Werfel T. Highlights in allergic contact dermatitis 2018/2019. Curr Opin Allergy Clin Immunol. 2019;19:334–40.
242. Mowitz M, Herman A, Baeck M, Isaksson M, Antelmi A, Hamnerius N, Pontén A, Bruze M. N,N-dimethylacrylamide-A new sensitizer in the FreeStyle Libre glucose sensor. Contact Dermatitis. 2019;81:27–31.
243. Mine Y, Urakami T, Matsuura D. Allergic contact dermatitis caused by isobornyl acrylate when using the FreeStyle(®) Libre. J Diabetes Investig. 2019;10:1382–4.
244. Hyry HSI, Liippo JP, Virtanen HM. Allergic contact dermatitis caused by glucose sensors in type 1 diabetes patients. Contact Dermatitis. 2019;81:161–6.
245. Fenner J, Hadi A, Yeh L, Silverberg N. Hidden risks in toys: a systematic review of pediatric toy contact dermatitis. Contact Dermatitis. 2020;82:265–71.
246. Anderson LE, Treat JR, Brod BA, Yu J. "Slime" contact dermatitis: Case report and review of relevant allergens. Pediatr Dermatol. 2019;36:335–7.
247. Mainwaring W, Zhao J, Hunt R. Allergic contact dermatitis related to homemade slime: a case and review of the literature. Dermatol Online J. 2019;25:140.
248. Zhang AJ, Boyd AH, Asch S, Warshaw EM. Allergic contact dermatitis to slime: The epidemic of isothiazolinone allergy encompasses school glue. Pediatr Dermatol. 2019;36:e37–8.
249. Milanesi N, Gola M, Francalanci S. Allergic contact dermatitis caused by VEA(®) lipogel: compound allergy? Contact Dermatitis. 2016;75:243–4.
250. Waas RLV, Hill G. Allergic contact dermatitis caused by vinylpyrrolidone/eicosene copolymer in a sunscreen. Contact Dermatitis. 2019;80:63.
251. Dumycz K, Kunkiel K, Feleszko W. Cosmetics for neonates and infants: haptens in products' composition. Clin Transl Allergy. 2019;9:15.
252. Uter W, Lessmann H, Geier J, IVDK. Is octocrylene a frequent contact allergen? Contact Dermatitis. 2017;77:127–8.
253. Martínez-González MI, González-Pérez R, García-Rio I, Heras-González S. Allergic contact dermatitis caused by benzoic acid and lauryl glucoside in a sunscreen. Contact Dermatitis. 2017;77:186–7.
254. Miroux-Catarino A, Silva L, Amaro C, Viana I. Allergic contact dermatitis caused dexpanthenol-But is that all? Contact Dermatitis. 2019;81:391–2.
255. Clerens I, Goossens A. Allergic contact dermatitis caused by panthenol: a rare but relevant sensitizer. Contact Dermatitis. 2017;76:122–3.
256. Funk JO, Maibach HI. Propylene glycol dermatitis: re-evaluation of an old problem. Contact Dermat. 1994;31:236–41.
257. Darrigade AS, Léauté-Labrèze C, Boralevi F, Taïeb A, Milpied B. Allergic contact reaction to antisep-

tics in very young children. J Eur Acad Dermatol Venereol. 2018;32:2284–7.

258. Isaac J, Scheinman PL. Benzalkonium chloride: an irritant and sensitizer. Dermatitis. 2017;28:346–52.
259. Magdaleno-Tapial J. Allergic contact dermatitis to chlorhexidine in pediatric patients. Pediatr Dermatol. 2019;36:549–60.
260. Hausen BM. Evaluation of the main contact allergens in oxidized tea tree oil. Dermatitis. 2004;15:213–4.
261. Jacob SE, Chimento S, Castanedo-Tardan MP. Allergic contact dermatitis to propolis and carnauba wax from lip balm and chewable vitamins in a child. Contact Dermat. 2008;58:242–3.
262. Fonacier L, Noor I. Contact dermatitis and patch testing for the allergist. Ann Allergy Asthma Immunol. 2018;120:592–8.
263. Herro EM, Jacob ES. Allergic contact dermatitis in children. J Dermatol Nurse Assoc. 2011;3:142–7.
264. Brod BA, Treat JR, Rothe MJ, Jacob SE. Allergic contact dermatitis: kids are not just little people. Clin Dermatol. 2015;33:605–12.
265. Kutting B, Brehler R, Traupe H. Allergic contact dermatitis in children: strategies of prevention and risk management. Eur J Dermatol. 2004;14:80–5.
266. Ayala F, Balato N, Lembo G, et al. Statistical evaluation of the persistence of acquired hypersensitivity by standardized patch tests. Contact Dermatitis. 1996;34:354–8.

21 Allergic Manifestations of Inborn Errors of Immunity

Viviana Moschese, Emilia Cirillo, Giorgio Costagliola, Simona Graziani, Maria Felicia Mastrototaro, Lucia Pacillo, Caterina Cancrini, and Baldassarre Martire

Abstract

Allergic disorders are increasingly recognized in patients with inborn errors of immunity (IEI), with predominance of bronchial asthma and atopic dermatitis. On the other hand, urticaria is more rarely described in patients with IEI, in most of the cases in patients with autoinflammatory disorders. Distinguishing classical allergic disorders from IEI is very important since the onset of allergic manifestations can lead to a significant diagnostic delay. Atopic phenotypes have been observed in several IEI, such as Omenn syndrome, hyper-IgE syndromes, Wiskott-Aldrich syndrome, IPEX and related disorders, STAT6 mutations, and CBM-opathies due to mutations in CARD, BCL10, and MALT1. Clinical red flags including autoimmunity, infections, lymphoproliferation, malignancy, growth failure, connective tissue abnormalities, high IgE levels, eosinophilia, family history or consanguinity, and early age at onset associated with atopic phenotypes should arise the suspicion for considering IEI. Indeed, only the early suspicion of an immune defect may lead to carry out immunological and genetic investigations to make a timely and correct diagnosis. Therefore, early diagnosis with the knowledge of the genetic/functional defect could allow to adopt targeted or semi-targeted therapies as well as to improve the quality and the expectancy of life of IEI patients.

Keywords

Asthma · Atopic dermatitis · Cryopyrin-associated periodic syndromes · Common variable immunodeficiency · Hyper-IgE syndrome · IgA deficiency · Immune dysregulation · Inborn errors of immunity · IPEX · Omenn syndrome · Primary atopic disorders · Primary immunodeficiency · Urticaria · Wiskott-Aldrich syndrome

V. Moschese (✉) · S. Graziani
Pediatric Immunopathology and Allergology Unit, Policlinico Tor Vergata, University of Rome Tor Vergata, Rome, Italy
e-mail: moschese@med.uniroma2.it; simona.graziani@infinito.it

E. Cirillo
Department of Translational Medical Sciences, Pediatrics Section, Federico II University of Naples, Naples, Italy

G. Costagliola
Division of Pediatric Oncology and Hematology, Santa Chiara Hospital, Pisa, Italy

M. F. Mastrototaro · B. Martire
Pediatrics and Neonatology Unit, Maternal-Infant Department, Monsignor A. R. Dimiccoli Hospital, Barletta, Italy

L. Pacillo · C. Cancrini
Research Unit of Primary Immunodeficiencies, Unit of Clinical Immunology and Vaccinology, IRCCS Bambino Gesù Children Hospital, Rome, Italy

Department of System Medicine, University of Rome Tor Vergata, Rome, Italy
e-mail: lucia.pacillo@opbg.net; cancrini@med.uniroma2.it

C. Caffarelli, G. L. Marseglia (eds.), *Textbook of Pediatric Allergy*,
https://doi.org/10.1007/978-3-031-71283-8_21

Test your learning and check your understanding of this book's contents: use the "Springer Nature Flashcards" app to access questions using ▶ https://sn.pub/nspbjm. To use the app, please follow the instructions in Chap. 1.

21.1 Introduction

Atopy is defined as a tendency to become sensitized and express IgE to environmental allergens after "ordinary exposure" [1]. Atopic diseases, in particular food and environmental allergies, such as atopic dermatitis, allergic rhinitis, allergic conjunctivitis, and asthma, are growing chronic conditions estimated to affect approximately 20–30% of the global population [2]. These disorders result in reduced quality of life, increased morbidity and mortality, and remarkable socioeconomic burden on the affected individuals and their families. Although commonly considered as polygenic multifactorial disorders caused by the interaction of several genes with the environment, it is now clear that allergic diseases can also be caused by monogenic variants affecting the immune system and the skin epithelial barrier, and as such, be manifestations of an underlying immune deficiency.

Recent advances in immunogenetics have led to the discovery of approximately 500 novel monogenic causes of inborn errors of immunity (IEI) to date [3]. It is now well known that different types of immune dysregulation as autoimmunity, autoinflammatory diseases, bone marrow failure, malignancy, and allergic inflammation disorders occur frequently in patients with IEI. In the context of monogenic disorders leading to allergic inflammation, the term *inborn errors of immunity associated with atopy* (IEIs-A), also defined *primary atopic disorders* (PADs), has been coined for the first time in 2018 as a subgroup of IEIs to classify genetic disorders presenting with dysregulated pathogenic allergic effector responses irrespective of sensitization [4].

The diagnosis of IEIs-A may be challenging in the context of atopic disorders. Indeed, to dissect these forms from other atopic phenotypes and decipher the role of polymorphisms in target genes is crucial to ensure prompt diagnosis and appropriate treatments that may be profoundly different from the ones reported for typical allergic conditions [5]. So far, there are limited studies that evaluate the burden of allergic diseases across the spectrum of IEI, with variable results. Indeed, the true prevalence of atopic disorders in this setting is not well known [6].

The identification of monogenic allergic diseases by advanced genetic technologies might dramatically improve the outcome of these disorders, allowing the development of precision medicine and use of treatments targeting a specific defect [7]. To date, at least 40 monogenic disorders can be subcategorized as PAD [8]. The study of these conditions has provided important insights into human immunity and the pathogenesis of allergic diseases. The main pathways implicated in the development of atopy range from defects in immune components and epithelial barrier dysfunction to changes in metabolism. In particular, they include impaired T-cell receptor (TCR) signaling and cytoskeletal remodeling, TCR restriction, altered cytokine signaling, tolerance failure, cellular metabolic disturbance, mast cell dysregulation, and epithelial barrier dysfunction [8]. Among IEI with atopic phenotype, according to the predominant clinical and laboratory characteristics, PAD can be generally classified into the following different phenotypes [3]:

1. Hyper-IgE syndromes (HIES)
2. Omenn syndrome (OS)
3. Wiskott-Aldrich syndrome (WAS) and WAS-like conditions
4. Immune dysregulation, polyendocrinopathy, enteropathy, X-linked (IPEX) and IPEX-like conditions
5. CBM-opathies due to mutations in genes encoding for caspase recruitment domain (CARD) proteins—B-cell CLL/lymphoma 10 (BCL10)—MALT1 paracaspase (MALT1), altogether known as CBM complexes

6. Skin barrier defects
7. A miscellanea of other IEI presenting with allergic phenotype

21.2 Atopic Dermatitis and Inborn Errors of Immunity

Atopic dermatitis (AD) represents the most common chronic inflammatory skin disease that typically occurs in early childhood. The pathogenesis of AD is extremely complex since several genetic and environmental factors contribute to the imbalance of immune response, the impairment of epidermal function, and the cutaneous dysbiosis, resulting in the development of a Th2 inflammatory response. However, as recently reported, the pathogenesis of different AD endotypes is also affected by the contribution of other immune axes involving Th17, Th22, and Th1 [9–12]. According to the United States Immunodeficiency Network (USIDNET), AD has been observed in 24% of IEI patients [13]. Dissecting common polygenic AD from IEI with an initial AD presentation is very important since a diagnostic delay can affect disease course and optimal management.

Clinically, AD of PADs presents some differences compared to classic AD, such as earlier onset, the different localization and extension, no response to classical treatment, and association with other clinical features (bone and connective tissue abnormalities, facial and hair abnormalities, enteropathy, vascular abnormalities, endocrinopathies, recurrent viral and/or fungal infections). Moreover, in the presence of a positive family history for IEI or consanguinity, the suspicion of PADs is warranted [14, 15].

Indeed, seven clinical red flags, including autoimmunity, malignancy, atopy, infections, growth failure, connective tissue abnormalities, and elevated IgE levels and eosinophils, have been suggested for suspicion of PADs [14–19]. In these cases, referral to a clinical immunologist for immunological work-up, including genetic analysis, is recommended.

Main IEI associated with atopic phenotypes are Omenn syndrome (OS), Hyper-IgE syndromes (HIES), Wiskott-Aldrich syndrome (WAS) and WAS-like conditions, immune dysregulation, polyendocrinopathy, enteropathy, X-linked (IPEX) and IPEX-like conditions, and CBM-opathies due to mutations in CARD, BCL10, and MALT1 and other IEI presenting with atopic phenotypes (Fig. 21.1) [14, 18, 20]. Omenn syndrome was first described in 1965 in infants who presented with generalized erythroderma, lymphadenopathy, eosinophilia, and combined immunodeficiency (CID). This condition has been initially described in SCID/CID due to mutations in the recombination activating gene 1 and 2 (RAG1 and RAG2), involved in the VDJ recombination. It is an exaggerated inflammatory condition that significantly reduces, but does not abrogate, T-cell development, resulting in an oligoclonal expansion of CD4+ T cells. However, mutations of other genes, including ARTEMIS, DNA ligase IV, IL-2Rg, ZAP-70, and IL-7Ra, have been associated with clinical phenotypes resembling the OS [14, 15, 18]. Other diseases, such as cartilage hair hypoplasia (CHH), CHARGE syndrome, adenosine deaminase deficiency (ADA-SCID), EXTL3 deficiency, and the atypical complete DiGeorge syndrome, may present the same clinical features of the OS at the onset. Skin lesions usually appear in the first months of life with a neonatal eczematous rash or a diffuse erythroderma involving more than 90% of the body surface. The skin manifestations are usually associated with alopecia, chronic diarrhea, failure to thrive, lymphadenopathy, hepatosplenomegaly, and increased susceptibility to viral and fungal infections [14, 18–21].

Hyper-IgE syndromes (HIES) represent an heterogeneous group of immune diseases mainly characterized by the triad of eczema, recurrent infections, and elevated IgE levels. Initially, only three forms of HIES were described, caused by STAT3 gene mutations with an autosomal dominant transmission and by PGM3 and DOCK8 genes mutations with an autosomal recessive transmission, respectively [22]. Recently, new monogenic disorders affecting some genes involved in the STAT3 pathway (ZNF341, IL6ST, IL6R, ERBIN, and TGFBR), BCL11B, SPINK5, and CARD11 have been included in the group of

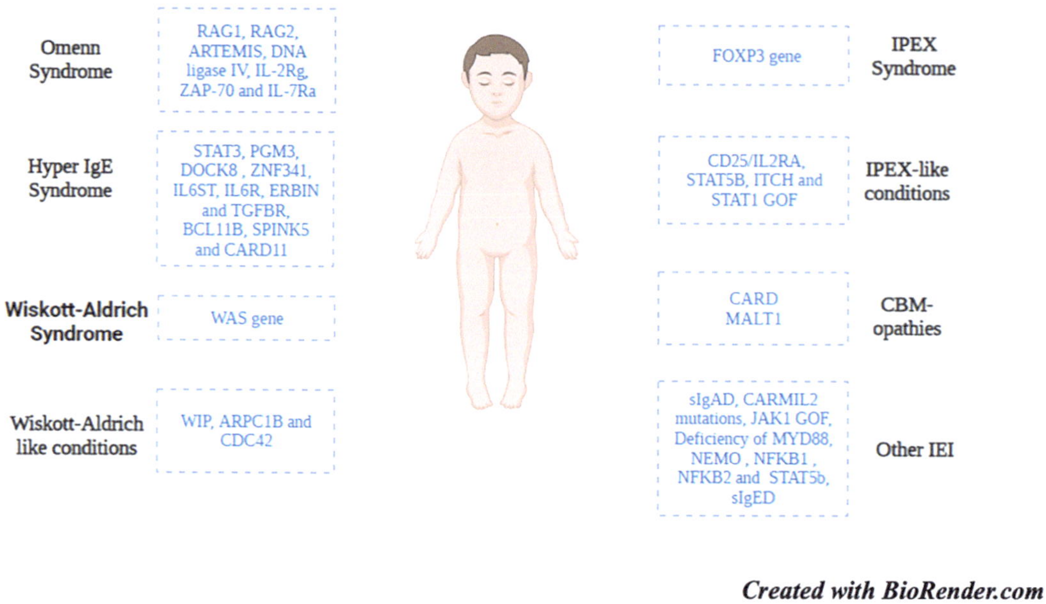

Fig. 21.1 IEI with atopic dermatitis

HIES. The prototypic HIES syndrome, caused by STAT-3 mutations (AD-HIES or STAT3-HIES), is characterized by early-onset eczema, chronic mucocutaneous candidiasis, cold skin abscesses, and recurrent pneumonia leading to pneumatoceles, and skeletal and connective tissue abnormalities such as bone fragility, scoliosis, and decidual tooth retention. Typically, the eczematous dermatitis, preceded by a papulopustular rash occurring in the first few weeks of life, appears during the first year of life and usually involves the face and the scalp with an increased risk of *Staphylococcus aureus* infections [22]. Other HIES, caused by mutations of genes involved in the STAT3 pathway, may present recurrent infections, high IgE values, eczema, excoriated skin lesions, dermatitis, skin infections, eosinophilia, and a lower incidence of skeletal and connective tissue abnormalities. PGM3 deficiency is extremely heterogeneous as it may present thc classical features of STAT3-HIES or those of a combined immune deficiency (SCID) with a neurocognitive impairment that occurs in early life. Conversely, moderate-to-severe allergic manifestations with early onset associated with viral infections, high IgE, and eosinophilia characterize the clinical phenotype of patients with CARD11 mutation. Even if DOCK8 deficiency is currently considered a SCID, its clinical phenotype includes the classical HIES manifestations, food allergies, asthma, and viral skin infections caused by herpes simplex virus (HSV), human papillomavirus (HPV), and molluscum contagiosum with consequently a greater risk for malignancy.

Wiskott-Aldrich syndrome (WAS) is an IEI characterized by thrombocytopenia with small platelets (mean platelet volume < 6 fL), eczema, infections, and an increased risk of autoimmune diseases and malignancies. WAS is caused by WAS gene mutations located on the short arm of the X chromosome (Xp11.23), encoding Wiskott-Aldrich syndrome protein (WASp), expressed exclusively in hematopoietic cells. WASp is involved in the actin remodeling of the cytoskeleton, in the signal transduction and apoptosis [23, 24]. An attenuated form of WAS, known as X-linked thrombocytopenia (XLT), is caused by hypomorphic mutations of WAS, while a mutation in the WIPF1 gene, coding for a WAS-interacting protein (WIP) that stabilizes and prevents the degradation of WAS, was recently related to a WAS-like phenotype, just as mutations in the actin-related protein complex 1B (ARPC1B) and in cell division cycle 42 (CDC42) that are involved in actin branching and in several cellular processes, respectively [23, 24]. The first clinical signs are hemorrhagic, such as petechiae, ecchymosis, purpura, epistaxis, hematemesis, melena, and intracranial hemorrhage. Eczema represents the second hallmark and occurs during the first year of life. Due to combined immunodeficiency, most patients have respiratory, intestinal, and skin infections, caused by regular or opportunistic pathogens. Autoimmune manifestations include autoimmune hemolytic anemia, neutropenia, vasculitis, inflammatory bowel disease, IgA nephropathy, and arthritis. WAS patients have also an increased risk of developing malignancy, especially EBV-associated lymphoma, at all ages [23, 24].

IPEX is an X-linked recessive disorder characterized by a triad of polyendocrinopathy, enteropathy, and dermatitis, although the clinical signs and severity may vary considerably. The disease affects males being X-linked recessive and has an estimated incidence below 1:1,000,000. IPEX is caused by mutations of Forkhead box protein 3 (FOXP3) gene, involved in the maintenance of immune tolerance regulating Treg cell development and function [25, 26]. Moreover, clinical phenotypes resembling IPEX syndrome, caused by monogenic defects involving CD25/IL2RA, STAT5B, STAT1 gain-of-function (STAT1 GOF), and itchy E3 ubiquitin protein ligase (ITCH), have been recently observed and defined as IPEX-like conditions [27, 28].

The clinical onset of IPEX is generally in the first months of life. The severe autoimmune enteropathy occurs as intractable secretory diarrhea, resulting in malabsorption, electrolyte imbalance, and growth delay. Autoimmune manifestations usually include type 1 diabetes mellitus, thyroiditis, hemolytic anemia, neutropenia, nephropathy, myopathy, and hepatitis. Skin involvement consists of a widespread eruption manifesting as severe eczema, erythroderma, psoriasiform dermatitis, exfoliative dermatitis, pemphigoid nodularis, alopecia, onychodystrophy, cheilitis, or urticaria [25, 26]. Moreover, the immune defect along with impaired cutaneous and gut barriers leads to an increased incidence of local or systemic infections due to several pathogens such as *Enterococcus*, *Staphylococcus*, *Candida*, and *Cytomegalovirus* [25, 26]. IPEX-like syndromes have clinical manifestations similar to those of IPEX patients but with a later onset, an higher incidence of infections and a variability of allergic disorders [27]. Specific clinical features of distinct genetic defects may aid in the differential diagnosis of IEI patients with AD. Indeed, an higher incidence of chronic mucocutaneous candidiasis may be found in STAT1 GOF individuals, whereas growth delay, dysmorphic facial features, and an increased incidence of infections may suggest STAT5 deficiency, ITCH deficiency, and CD25/IL2RA deficiency, respectively [27].

Recently, a variety of new disorders, due to mutations of the signalosome or CBM complex and known as CBM-opathies, have been described. The CBM complex consists of different proteins such as caspase recruitment domain (CARD), B-cell CLL/lymphoma 10 (BCL10), and MALT1 paracaspase (MALT1) involved in the process of the immune and inflammatory responses [29]. Germline mutations of these proteins are extremely heterogeneous and cause a broad spectrum of clinical phenotypes ranging from atopic disorders to combined immune deficiency. Not only the mutated gene but also the type of mutation and altered protein function are factors that greatly affect the clinical phenotype of these diseases. The clinical phenotype of CARD11 deficiency ranges from a combined immunodeficiency to an immunodeficiency with B-cell expansion and NF kB and T-cell anergy (BENTA) due to a complete loss of protein function (LOF) and to heterozygous gain-of-function mutations (GOF), respectively [29, 30]. Moreover, a clinical entity characterized by atopic disorders, mainly eczema and asthma, combined to recurrent respiratory and viral skin infections and caused by heterozygous mutations with dominant negative effect, has been defined CARD11-associated atopy with dominant interference of NF-kB signaling (CADINS).

CARD14 mutations may lead to clinical phenotypes ranging from severe atopic disorders with recurrent respiratory and skin infections to psoriasis and pityriasis rubra pilaris due to LOF and GOF mutations, respectively. On the other hand, recurrent respiratory, gastrointestinal and cutaneous infections associated with dermatitis, growth delay, inflammatory bowel disease, and periodontal disorders have been related to MALT1 LOF mutations [29, 30].

Other IEI may present with moderate/severe atopic dermatitis variously associated with immunodysregulatory, autoimmune, and/or infectious manifestations. The different clinical phenotypes are closely related to the underlying genetic defect. Defects such as selective IgA deficiency (sIgAD), the capping protein regulator and myosin 1 linker 2 (CARMIL2) mutations, Janus kinase 1 (JAK1) gain-of-function, myeloid differentiation primary response protein 88 (MYD88) deficiency, ectodermodysplasia with immunodeficiency due to IKBKG deficiency (NEMO deficiency), NFKB1 deficiency, NFKB2 deficiency, as well as hypereosinophilic syndrome due to somatic mutations in STAT5b are included in this group [29–31]. A new entity named selective IgE deficiency (SIgED) is increasingly being described even if it has not yet been officially recognized as an inborn error of immunity [32]. It is characterized by low serum IgE levels with normal values of the other Ig isotypes and skin manifestations such as eczema, urticaria, and angioedema. Furthermore, lichen planus, anaphylactoid purpura, thrombocytopenic purpura, bullous pemphigoid, bullous pyoderma gangrenosum, and atypical cutaneous lymphoproliferative infiltrate together with autoimmune diseases and malignancies have been observed in SIgED, thus suggesting an underlying immune dysregulation [32]. Recently, a new human disorder caused by germline AD GOF STAT6 (signal transducer and activator of transcription 6) variants has been described and proposed as a PAD since its clinical phenotype is characterized by severe allergic disease with onset in first years of life, severe treatment-resistant atopic dermatitis, food allergies, recurrent skin, respiratory and viral infections, eosinophilia, and elevated IgE values [33].

Mutations of genes that regulate NF-κB pathway may induce heterogeneous clinical phenotypes due to the involvement of this pathway in the regulation of the immune and inflammatory response. Particularly, hypomorphic mutations in the coding region of the IKBKG or NEMO gene cause hypohidrotic ectodermal dysplasia with immunodeficiency, an IEI characterized by atrichosis/hypotrichosis, anodontia/hypodontia, anhidrosis/hypohidrosis and typical facies, increased susceptibility to opportunistic infections, hypogammaglobulinemia, reduced antibody response to polysaccharides, or NK cell activity [18, 19, 34].

In conclusion, a growing list of IEI may onset with atopic dermatitis or appear over time. Early recognition of monogenic allergic diseases (Fig. 21.2) and outcomes will definitively con-

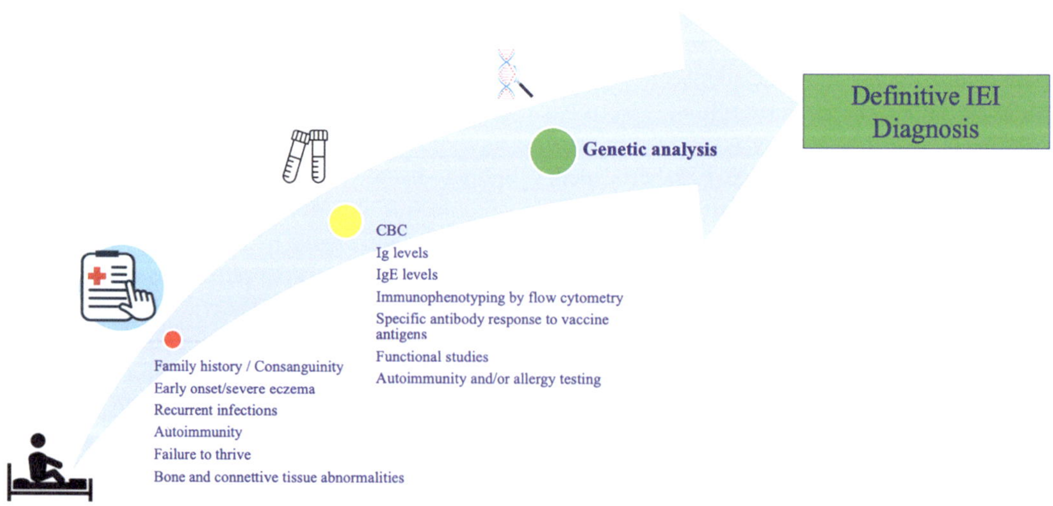

Fig. 21.2 Evaluation of atopic dermatitis patients with a suspicion of IEI

tribute to our understanding of pathogenic mechanisms underlying AD and to the identification of novel molecular targets for the prevention and treatment of common allergic disease with better control of adverse events due to chronic treatments [35–37]. A multidisciplinary approach will allow optimal management of these complex cases.

21.3 Asthma and Inborn Errors of Immunity

Asthma is a chronic airway inflammatory disease, affecting more than 300 million people worldwide, characterized by airway hyperresponsiveness, reversible airflow limitation, mucus overproduction, and airway wall remodeling [38]. The pathogenesis of childhood asthma is multifactorial including interactions among endogenous stimuli, and genetic and environmental factors [39, 40].

Pulmonary complications are common in patients affected with inborn errors of immunity (IEI) and can significantly contribute to increased morbidity and mortality [41]. In addition to recurrent, severe respiratory infections, patients with IEIs are at increased risk for non-infectious pulmonary manifestations, including asthma, bronchiectasis, interstitial lung disease, malignancy, and autoimmune disease. Pathophysiology of asthma among patients affected with IEI has not been clearly defined and more needs to be understood with regard to asthma clinical phenotypes.

Bronchial hyperreactivity has been reported in about 40–60% of children affected by different primary antibody disorders including selective IgA deficiency (sIgAD), common variable immunodeficiency (CVID), and IgG subclass deficiency [13, 42, 43], even though only a limited number of CVID had proven IgE-mediated allergy [44]. Furthermore, a few studies showed a positive impact of Ig replacement therapy in improving asthma, and reducing the frequency of acute exacerbations in asthmatic patients with hypogammaglobulinemia [45]. In these patients, asthma should be differentiated from bronchiolitis obliterans (BO), which is common also in patients with combined immunodeficiency. BO is characterized by non-reversible airflow obstruction, which helps to distinguish it from asthma. With few exceptions, the main forms of monogenic IEI associated with significant allergic inflammation are inherited in an autosomal recessive manner and lack a family history of disease. Genes responsible of disease pathogenesis are involved in multiple functions including the control of protease/antiprotease balance (*SPINK5*), epithelial barrier function (*SPINK5*, *CARD14*), TCR signaling and cytoskeletal remodeling (*CARMIL2*, *ARPC1B*) altered cytokine signaling (e.g., *STAT3*^{DN}, *STAT5B*^{GOF}), T-cell repertoire restriction (e.g., *ADA*, *22q11del*), tolerance failure (e.g., *IL2RA*), and glycosylation (*PGM3*) [46, 47]. Impairments of most of these processes have been observed in patients with severe asthma, and several of these genes have been directly implicated in the pathogenesis of severe asthma [47]. SPINK5 is an important molecule in asthma, which regulates production of cytokines and chemokines, such as IL-6, IL-8, and RANTES by airway epithelial cells, and stimulating the involvement of B and T lymphocytes, neutrophils, and eosinophils in the airway inflammatory process [48].

Moderate-persistent asthma has been reported in a few patients with rare dominant negative mutation in caspase recruitment domain-containing protein 14 gene (*CARD14*), which encodes for a molecule that can signal downstream of C-type lectin receptor in keratinocytes [49, 50]. CARD14 contributes to house dust mite-associated allergic asthma by inducing cytokines that promote airway immune cell infiltration [51]. One-third of patients affected with loss-of-function biallelic mutations in capping protein regulator and myosin 1 linker 2 (*CARMIL2*) suffered from allergic asthma. These patients had a combined immunodeficiency characterized by susceptibility to viral, bacterial, mycobacterial, and fungal infections, immune dysregulation involving in particular gut and skin and a susceptibility to EBV+ smooth muscle tumors [52]. These patients also had reduced numbers of Tregs. ARPC1B is a key molecule driving the dynamics of the cytoskeleton. Homozygous mutations in the *ARPC1B* gene cause a combined immune deficiency characterized by impaired T-cell migration and proliferation, increased levels of IgE and IgA, asthma, and thrombocytopenia [53].

About 30% of patients affected with autosomal-recessive-HIES due to *DOCK8* mutations (AR-HIES), an inherited condition characterized by highly elevated serum levels of IgE, eczema, recurrent staphylococcal abscesses, and hypereosinophilia, have asthma, even though not severe or difficult to manage [54]. On the contrary, patients with dominant negative *STAT3* variants are usually free from allergic manifestations with only 7% of them suffering from asthma [55]. Asthma, seasonal allergy, and allergic bronchopulmonary aspergillosis have also been reported in patients affected with hypomorphic mutations in phosphoglucomutase 3 (*PGM3*) [18]. These patients showed a multisystem disorder characterized by infection, immune dysregulation, connective tissue abnormalities, and neurodevelopmental defects. PGM3 is a critical enzyme in the hexosamine pathway which is essential for normal glycosylation in certain tissues, in particular naive T cells. How this leads to allergic disease is not understood.

Abnormal TGF-β signaling has been implicated in a series of human allergic diseases including severe asthma and eosinophilic gastrointestinal disease. Heterozygous mutations in transforming growth factor beta receptor 1 and 2 (*TGFBR1* and *TGFBR2*) found in Loeys-Dietz syndrome led to vascular and connective tissue abnormalities similar to those observed in patients affected with STAT3 pathway disorders [4, 56]. Allergic asthma associated with IgE-mediated food allergy, eosinophilic gastrointestinal disorders, and atopic dermatitis has been reported. T-bet or T-box transcription factor protein 21 encoded by the *TBX21* gene is crucial for naive T lymphocyte development, interferon-γ production, airway hyperresponsiveness, and regulation of corticosteroid response in asthmatics [57]. Recently, its association with susceptibility to mycobacteria has been reported [58]. Patients with gain-of-function heterozygous mutation in *JAK1* or *STAT5b* patients had marked peripheral and tissue eosinophilia and allergic asthma. In these patients, treatment with ruxolitinib, a JAK inhibitor, led to marked clinical improvement and resolution of eosinophilia [4].

Variant in *IL6R* that leads to diminution of function can predispose to asthma, elevated IgE levels, and persistent atopic dermatitis [4]. The same variant seems to protect from inflammatory disease such as rheumatoid arthritis and type 1 diabetes. This is especially of interest since IL-6 receptor blockade is utilized in a number of inflammatory diseases but does not lead to allergic disease [59]. Recently, germline gain-of-function variants in signal transducer and activator of transcription 6 (*STAT6*), involved in the biological effects of IL-4, a key cytokine necessary for type 2 differentiation of T cells, B-cell survival, proliferation, and class switching to IgE, have been described as responsible of a monogenic early-onset severe allergic disorders associated with asthma, anaphylaxis, severe atopic dermatitis, and eosinophilic gastrointestinal disorders [33].

Among severe combined immunodeficiency (SCID), atopy and eosinophilia are frequently reported in adenosine deaminase (ADA)-SCID. Adenosine deaminase-deficient mice manifest an asthma phenotype with mucus hypersecretion, bronchial hyperresponsiveness, mast cell degranulation, eosinophilia reversed by enzyme replacement therapy, and attenuated by theophylline [60]. Asthma is also reported in 7% of patients affected with 22q11.2 deletion syndrome, being more frequent among older children and lowest CD3+ T-cell levels [61].

Heterozygous dominant negative mutations of *CARD11* are responsible for a distinctive clinical entity called CARD11-associated atopy with dominant interference of NF-kB signaling (CADINS). The most typical clinical manifestations reported in patients with CADINS include atopic disease, respiratory tract infections, and cutaneous viral infections. Nearly 90% of patients with CADINS present atopic diseases, with atopic dermatitis and asthma being the most frequent, followed by allergic rhinoconjunctivitis, food allergy, and eosinophilic esophagitis.

In conclusion, asthma is a frequent manifestation of both common and uncommon IEI. A better understanding of common pathogenic pathways involved in these disorders may help patients to benefit from personalized treatments in addition to those suggested by the Global Initiative for Asthma (GINA).

21.4 Urticaria/Angioedema and Inborn Errors of Immunity

The potential etiologies of urticaria and angioedema are multiple and include allergic diseases, infectious diseases, and endocrine and metabolic disorders, but in most of cases, they are classified as idiopathic. However, during the last years, an increasing interest has been posed on the role of urticaria as the first or leading sign of different disorders of the immune and inflammatory response. Differently, angioedema is only rarely the presenting sign of IEI. In the wide spectrum of IEI associated with urticaria, the pathogenesis of this clinical sign is different, as well as its course and the associated manifestations. As a general rule, urticaria caused by an underlying IEI usually presents with a chronic course with multiple relapses and shows refractoriness to common treatment, such as H1/H2 antihistamines.

The most well-recognized IEIs associated with urticaria are autoinflammatory disorders, specifically those caused by alterations in the cryopyrin pathway, known as cryopyrin-associated periodic syndromes (CAPS). CAPS are mostly caused by activating mutations of the NLRP3 (CIAS1) gene, which encodes for cryopyrin, a pivotal component of the NLRP3 inflammasome. The uncontrolled activation of the inflammasome results in an enhanced caspase-dependent release of IL-1β, with consequent systemic inflammation [62]. The historical classification of CAPS includes three conditions with different disease severity: familial cold associated syndrome (FCAS), Muckle-Wells syndrome, and chronic infantile neurological cutaneous articular (CINCA) syndrome [2]. In all diseases, the main clinical sign is represented by chronic urticaria, which is usually triggered by cold exposure. Other signs include periodic episodes of fever and elevation of inflammatory markers, often associated with other symptoms including arthralgia, lymphadenopathy, and abdominal pain [63, 64].

Patients with CINCA syndrome, which is the most severe presentation of CAPS, could develop chronic sequelae resulting from hyperinflammation, including deforming arthropathy, sensorial hearing loss, and neurodevelopmental delay [65]. As treatment with IL-1 blockade (anakinra, canakinumab) could reduce the incidence of these complications, providing a correct diagnosis of CAPS in a patient presenting with urticaria could significantly improve the clinical outcome [65]. Therefore, it should be highlighted that the association between cold-triggered urticaria and recurrent episodes of fever represents a warning sign for an underlying CAPS. Moreover, in patients with CINCA syndrome, the early onset of urticaria (usually in the neonatal period) and the association with skeletal abnormalities (such as frontal bossing) should contribute to raising the diagnostic suspicion. Beyond NLRP3-associated diseases, other autoinflammatory disorders could present with the features of CAPS, including the NLRP12-associated disease [66].

Urticaria can also be observed in patients with IEIs involving the humoral response. Indeed, it is not rarely described in patients with sIgAD [67], and there are some reports of urticaria or angioedema as the presenting sign of CVID [68–70]. The prevalence of urticaria in sIgAD has been scarcely investigated, and the disease is often featured by a benign disease course, in the absence of a severe infectious phenotype [71, 72]. However, as some patients with sIgAD could progress to CVID [72], identifying these patients is of clinical relevance, since they could benefit from an immunological assessment and follow-up. Therefore, the determination of serum immunoglobulin should be performed in the diagnostic work-up of patients with urticaria.

Differently from sIgAD, isolated IgE deficiency is not currently classified as an IEI. However, recent cohort studies support the hypothesis that patients with IgE deficiency could present with a disease spectrum featured by allergic diseases, pulmonary involvement, and immune dysregulation [32]. Apart from the nosological definition of IgE deficiency, evidencing low IgE levels in a patient with chronic refractory urticaria could be of clinical relevance, since those patients are less likely to respond to the anti-IgE monoclonal antibody omalizumab.

The pathogenesis of urticaria in CVID is complex and comprehends multiple mechanisms. Indeed, previous studies demonstrate the involvement of the infection-dependent complement activation and the development of antibodies against IgE molecules or targeting the high-affinity IgE receptors FcεRIα (that cause the cross-linking of adjacent receptors), causing in both cases the degranulation of mast cells and basophils [68, 73]. In patients with CVID presenting with urticaria, an accurate personal and family history should be performed to search signs of immune dysfunction (recurrent or severe infections) and other signs of immune dysregulation, including autoimmune diseases, lymphoproliferation, and other atopic diseases. As the genetic background of CVID is in continuous expansion [74], it is possible that patients with a high prevalence of atopic diseases and urticaria could further be better characterized from the genetic and pathogenic point.

Some specific entities with distinct phenotypic features are identified every year. A paradigmatic condition of CVID-like disorder associated with urticaria is represented by the phospholipase C gamma 2–(PLCγ2) antibody deficiency and immune dysregulation (PLAID), which is caused by mutations in PLCG2 gene [75]. PLAID is clinically featured by cold-induced urticaria, hypogammaglobulinemia with susceptibility to upper and lower respiratory infections, and immune dysregulation (cutaneous granulomas, enteropathy, autoimmunity). In this condition, urticaria is typically triggered by evaporative cooling [75]. The pathogenesis of PLAID relies on the spontaneous activation of mast cells carrying mutant PLCγ2 after exposure to lower temperatures [76]. As frequently the CVID-like symptoms (infections, bronchiectasis, autoimmunity) develop only in later life, careful monitoring of patients with PLAID is required, as well as the initiation of intravenous immunoglobulin (IVIG) replacement treatment based on the clinical phenotype and serum immunoglobulin levels.

For what specifically concerns angioedema, its association with autoinflammatory disorders or antibody deficiencies is poorly documented. However, it is well known that patients carrying C1q inhibitor (C1-INH) deficiency develop hereditary angioedema, as a consequence of the spontaneous activation of the complement system with an elevated generation of bradykinin from high-molecular-weight kininogen (HMWK) [77]. Patients with hereditary angioedema develop recurrent episodes of swelling localized in the facial or abdominal area or at extremities in the absence of urticarial rash, and the disease could potentially be associated with life-threatening complications deriving from airway obstruction [78]. Therefore, a positive family history in patients presenting with an episode of angioedema should promptly raise the suspicion of a C1-INH deficiency, to identify patients that could benefit from specific prophylaxis.

Finally, although disorders of regulatory T cells (Tregopathies) present more frequently with severe eczema, in some cases they can be associated with severe refractory urticaria. Urticaria has been reported in patients with IPEX syndrome, often in association with endocrine autoimmune disorders [79]. Moreover, Tregopathies are associated with an increased incidence of food allergies, which are usually multiple (as recently described also in patients with STAT6 gain of function) [33], and thus could potentially present with urticaria or angioedema. Therefore, the knowledge of the spectrum of signs and symptoms associated with Tregopathies (eczema, endocrinopathies, enteropathy, autoimmune cytopenia, lymphoproliferation, infectious susceptibility) [80] could help in the diagnostic approach to patients with urticaria/angioedema and food allergies.

To conclude, current knowledge about IEI associated with urticaria or, more rarely, angioedema, highlights that a critical approach to urticaria or angioedema is necessary to identify an underlying IEI. In particular, the cold trigger, the association with severe or recurrent infections, and the presence of other signs of immune or inflammatory dysregulation should promptly raise the diagnostic suspicion of an underlying IEI, especially in the presence of a positive family history.

21.5 A Clinical Approach to the Diagnosis of IEI/PADs

Identification of IEI/PADs may be extremely challenging due to the high prevalence of polygenic allergic disease. To date, we do not have sufficient evidence to create a diagnostic algorithm with predicted sensitivity and specificity to identify which patients should undergo genetic testing for a PAD. Current clinical guidelines for diagnosing IEIs, such as the Jeffrey Modell Foundation's warning signs of primary immunodeficiency (Table 21.1), mostly focus on infectious phenotypes omitting other important features of IEIs delaying appropriate recognition of PADs [14]. On the other hand, although the phenotypes of PADs are related to defects in single genes, environmental and host factors such as skin and gut microbiome, diet, psychological stress, and skin infections, may contribute to clinical heterogeneity even in individuals with the same gene defect, resulting in variable penetrance. In addition, the atopic features of patients with PADs can also vary or emerge over their lifetime. Currently, some clinical and laboratory red flags, including atopy, infections, autoimmunity, malignancy, growth failure, connective tissue abnormalities, and elevated IgE levels and eosinophils, should arise the suspicion of considering PADs/IEI and, consequently, lead to basic laboratory investigations to establish whether a patient should be referred to a clinical immunologist for work-up including genetic analysis (Fig. 21.3).

Standard assessments and investigations should include:

21.5.1 Family and Patient History

At first, personal history (atopic diathesis and recurrent/severe infections, especially due to opportunistic pathogens and herpesviridae), family history (presence of other affected family members and/or familial severe atopic diathesis), and consanguinity should be assessed.

21.5.2 Clinical Features

- Chronic skin disease is one of the main clinical manifestations in IEIs-As and may manifest with eczema, erythroderma, and urticaria. Clinical findings of AD significantly overlap with several IEIs including eczema, elevated serum IgE, and eosinophilia. Eczema is the

Table 21.1 Jeffrey Modell Foundations' 10 warning signs of primary immunodeficiency

Warning signs in children	Warning signs in adults
1. ≥4 new ear infections within 1 year	1. ≥2 new ear infections within 1 year
2. ≥2 serious sinus infections within 1 year	2. ≥2 new sinus infections within 1 year, in the absence of allergy
3. ≥2 months on antibiotics with little effect	3. 1 pneumonia per year for >1 year
4. ≥2 pneumonias within 1 year	4. Chronic diarrhea with weight loss
5. Failure of an infant to gain weight or grow normally	5. Recurrent viral infections (colds, herpes, warts, condyloma)
6. Recurrent, deep skin, or organ abscesses	6. Recurrent need for IV antibiotics to clear infections
7. Persistent thrush in mouth or fungal infection on skin	7. Recurrent, deep abscesses of the skin or internal organs
8. Need for IV antibiotics to clear infections	8. Persistent thrush or fungal infection on skin or elsewhere
9. ≥2 deep-seated infections including septicemia	9. Infection with normally harmless tuberculosis-like bacteria
10. A family history of PID	10. A family history of PID

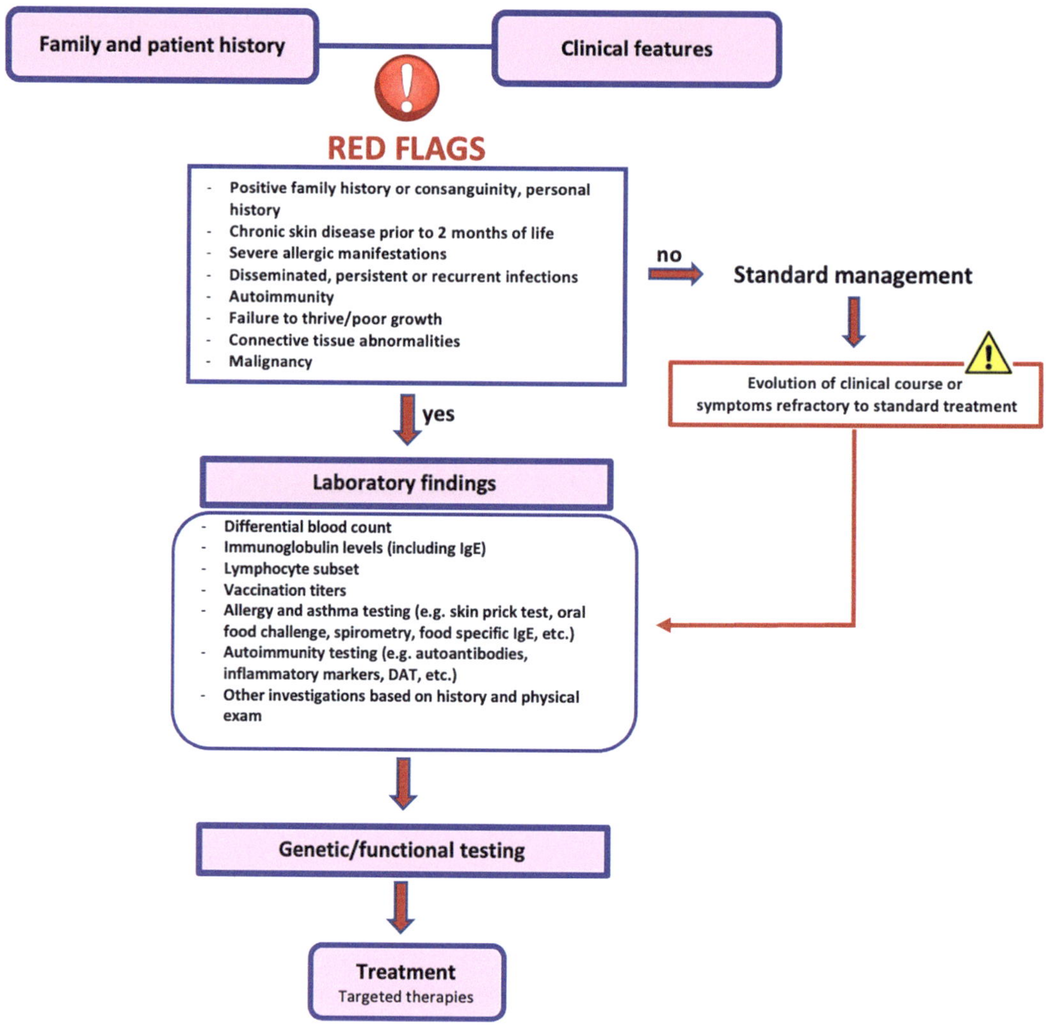

Fig. 21.3 Standard assessments and investigations of patients with suspected PADs. (Modified from Vaseghi-Shanjani et al. [14])

most frequent manifestation, and it is reported in 13–22% of IEIs patients [81]. In most cases, the skin involvement is similar to that found in non-immunocompromised patients, but when observed in IEIs-As, it tends to have an earlier onset, prior to 2 months of life , great severity, and infectious complications [82]. Another features of eczema in patients with IEIs-A are their unresponsiveness to conventional treatment. Severe AD may be the initial and sole manifestation of an inborn errors of immunity (i.e., caspase recruitment domain family member 11, CARD11-associated atopy with dominant interference of nuclear factor-kB signaling, CADINS), thus leading to a relevant diagnostic delay with an average frequency of 7.5% [83]. In particular, eczematous skin lesions in STAT3-HIES may resemble AD but are often present within 6 weeks of life. Generalized inflamed skin comparable with a graft-versus-host disease may develop in IPEX or Omenn syndrome immediately after birth [84, 85]. The WAS syndrome may show slightly inflamed eczema and petechiae owing to the associated thrombocytopenia [86]. Patients with Comèl-Netherton syndrome and DOCK8 deficiency may present with a generalized ichthyosiform dermatitis different from AD [87].

- Infectious history is another crucial tool to PAD evaluation. The spectrum and severity of infections provides useful clues regarding the potential molecular etiology of the patient's immune disorder. Persistent candidiasis unresponsive to common treatment, or if generalizes or affects nails, may hint to STAT3-HIES or another IEI such as chronic mucocutaneous candidiasis (CMC) [88, 89]. Disseminated viral infections with herpes simplex virus or coxsackie virus are a relevant complication of AD, but extensive warts, molluscum contagiosum, or other viral skin infections may be also suggestive for actinopathies such as DOCK8 deficiency and T-cell defects· [90]. Recurrent *S. aureus* skin infections are commonly limited to the skin in AD, whereas extracutaneous *S. aureus* infections such as abscesses in the lung or other visceral organs are frequently observed in STAT3-HIES patients, as well as fungal infections, mostly from *Aspergillus* spp. Patients with DOCK8 deficiency or Comèl-Netherton syndrome and many of the others PADs/IEI frequently report food allergy or even anaphylactic reactions to food [91], whereas STAT3 pathway patients rarely show any sensitization or reactivity to common aeroallergens or food allergens, which may be explained by an impaired B-cell development, as well as defects in mast cell activation and vascular responses to histamine [92, 93].
- Connective tissue abnormalities are observed in many PADs secondary to increased TGF-b signaling. Patients affected by STAT3 HIES may have abnormal dentition, joint hyperextensibility, osteopenia, bone fractures, scoliosis, facial dysmorphism, and vascular abnormalities [94].
- Autoimmunity (hemolytic anemia, vasculitis, uveitis, hypothyroidism, nephritis, systemic lupus erythematosus) often coexists with allergic manifestations in patients with PADs and is particularly relevant in T-cell receptor signaling defects and actinopathies such as dedicator of cytokinesis 8 (DOCK8) deficiency [95], and IPEX [96].
- Short stature and growth failure in the context of allergic inflammation are red flags for PADs, and they can be seen in IPEX syndrome, mucosa-associated lymphoid tissue lymphoma translocation gene1 (MALT1) deficiency [97], DOCK8 deficiency [98], JAK1 GOF [99], and STAT5B GOF [100], following to chronic allergic inflammation, or secondary to molecular defect affecting signaling pathways shared between growth factors and cytokines involved in allergic inflammation. Clinicians must therefore suspect PADs when assessing patients with impaired growth and laboratory and/or clinical features of allergic inflammation.
- Increased risk of malignancy is described in patients with DOCK8 deficiency [101], CADINS [102], and WAS [103], mostly leukemia and lymphoma but also solid tumors, such as squamous cell carcinoma associated with HPV- and EBV-associated smooth muscle neoplasms. Thus, a history of malignancy, in particular with childhood onset, a viral association or hematologic malignancies in a patient with underlying atopy should prompt consideration of an underlying PAD.

21.6 Laboratory Findings

If the clinical presentation suggests a monogenic allergic disease, patients should undergo an immune evaluation, and if laboratory values are abnormal or in the case of a persistent clinical suspicion, genetic testing should be performed. The basic work-up should include differential blood count, serum IgG, IgM, IgA, and IgE levels, lymphocyte subsets, as well as vaccination titers for diphtheria, tetanus, *H. influenzae*, and pneumococcus and allergy testing according to patient's history. A differential blood count may point toward IEIs such as Omenn syndrome or DOCK8 deficiency in case of low lymphocyte counts or toward WAS if thrombocytopenia with low mean platelet volume is detected. Flow cytometric analysis of B and T cells is recommended because low levels of memory B cells are present in the majority of IEIs. Low Th17 cell counts are useful to distinguish STAT3-HIES from AD in children older than 12 months, whereas lymphopenia and low IgM serum levels might be a diagnostic hallmark of DOCK8 deficiency [90].

Even though AD is the most common chronic inflammatory skin disease in infancy, red flags of IEIs should be prompted recognized because of therapeutic and life-changing implications for the affected patients. It is important to keep in mind that distinct findings of IEIs may be present at birth or shortly after but may also develop over time. Consequently, patients should be monitored periodically in order to reconsider the possibility of a monogenic condition, involving several healthcare providers (i.e., pediatricians, allergologists/immunologists and dermatologists) in the evaluation for a PAD condition.

21.7 Molecular Diagnosis

With the advent of new diagnostic techniques like next-generation sequencing (NGS), the field of IEI has exploded in the last years. Approximately 500 monogenic IEI have been discovered to date [3, 104] in which at least 40 could be subcategorized as PADs, as previously discussed [8]. Severe atopic immune dysregulation symptoms are the main clinical manifestations.

Early-onset severe atopic dermatitis refractory to standard therapies, severe and multiple food allergies with anaphylactic shock, severe refractory asthma, high IgE level, and eosinophilia could represent the warning signs of PADs requiring prompt molecular investigations.

Targeted gene sequencing is recommended if the clinical suspicion is very specific, while in other cases, clinical exome sequencing (CES) or whole exome sequencing (WES) are warranted. In selected cases, whole genome sequencing (WGS) might be indicated.

A pitfall of NGS is the discovery of a large number of variants of uncertain significance (VUS) that are often difficult to interpret and require functional investigations. Genetic variants cause disease by altering expression and/or function of gene products such as proteins or noncoding RNAs. When a mutation occurs, the function of the protein may be lost or reduced. These mutations which are generally termed LOF (loss-of-function) mutations, according to the degree, are further classified as null or hypomorphic mutations. When a mutation produces a protein with new or increased functions, we refer to gain-of-function (GOF) mutations. The nature of the variants as well as the mode of inheritance may affect the mechanisms of IEI diseases. Indeed, monoallelic variants can cause disease by haploinsufficiency, negative dominance, or GOF. In contrast, biallelic genetic lesions (homozygous, compound heterozygous) cause autosomal recessive (AR) traits by loss of expression, LOF, or even neomorphic function of the encoded protein, X-linked recessive traits arise from LOF variants on the X chromosome, either in hemizygosity in males, or rarely in homozygosity in females. Rare X-linked dominant traits can also arise from LOF or GOF variants. The discovery of novel IEI continues to demonstrate that distinct types of variants (recessive or dominant GOF/LOF) in the same gene can cause disparate clinical conditions (i.e., STAT3, CARD11).

The main molecular mechanisms involved in PAD pathogenesis [46, 105] include:

1. Skin Barrier Dysfunction: Although they involve non-hematopoietic cells, mutations in genes encoding skin components may increase the risk of infections secondary to a disrupted barrier to microbial penetration and the risk of atopy due to higher skin permeability to allergens. They include mutations in *FLG*, *SPINK5* (Netherton syndrome), *CDSN*, *DGS1*, and *DSM*.
2. Actin Cytoskeletal/Immune Synapse Disruption: Actin polymerization is essential for the immunological synapse formation between CD4+ T cells and dendritic cells for T-cell activation. Many proteins are involved in the actin cytoskeleton and therefore may affect this interaction. They include *WAS* [106], *WIP*, *DOCK8*, *CDC42*, and *ARPC1B* [107].
3. Aberrant TCR Signaling. Alterations in T-cell receptor (TCR) signaling affect the generation of Th2 cells and type 2 inflammation. The CARD11–BCL10–MALT1 (CBM) complex

links T- and B-cell receptor engagement with nuclear factor-kappa B (NF-kB) and mTOR signaling pathways. Therefore, mutations in these genes (*CARD11*, *BCL10*, *MALT1*, *ZAP70*, and *LAT*) are responsible of different clinical phenotypes, including those associated with atopic dysregulation [29].

4. Altered Cytokine Signaling Pathways: Cytokines produced by innate cells constitute another important signal for T-cell differentiation. Alteration in their production can disrupt the equilibrium promoting a Th2 skewing, responsible of atopic manifestations. Genes involved in this mechanism are *STAT3*, *ZNF341*, IL6ST [108], *IL6RA*, and *STAT6* [33].
5. Decreased TCR Diversity: Oligoclonal T-cell expansion in Omenn syndrome is associated with Th2 differentiation, secretion of type 2 cytokines, elevated total serum IgE, and eosinophilia. Histologically, the erythrodermic skin inflammation of Omenn syndrome very closely resembles that of severe atopic dermatitis. The genes involved in Omenn syndrome include *RAG1/*RAG2 [109–111], *DCLRE1C*, *ADA*, *IL7RA*, *LIG4*, *ZAP70*, *AK2*, and *CARD11*. Thymic defects, in DiGeorge syndrome (22q11del), CHARGE syndrome (CHD7), and FOXN1 deficiency can also present with an Omenn phenotype.
6. Regulatory T-Cell (Treg) Dysfunction: It is well known that Treg cells have a central role in turning off autoimmune or atopic activations. Therefore, mutations in genes involved in their production and function are responsible for primary immune dysregulation disorders. These genes include *FOXP3* (IPEX syndrome), *IL2RA*, and *STAT5B*, but also other already described IEIs can affect Treg diversity or function like mutations in *WAS*, *DOCK8*, *CBM* complex components, *CARMIL2* and *RAG1/2*.
7. Altered Innate Cell Effector Mechanisms: Monogenic disorders primarily affecting innate immune cells and with unique atopic features have also been described, like *PCLG2* (PLAID).

The identification of the genetic cause and of the pathogenic mechanisms involved in PADs (summarized in Table 21.2) [14, 33, 51, 83, 94, 97, 99, 112–150] is essential for the diagnosis and the development of targeted personalized therapies.

Table 21.2 Currently defined human monogenic primary atopic disorders (PADs)

Disorder	Gene	Key clinical features	Inheritance molecular mechanism	Mechanism	Year of report
HIES-STAT6 GOF	*STAT6*	Severe early onset and treatment-resistant atopic dermatitis, severe food allergies (anaphylactic shock), asthma, hyper eosinophilia with eosinophilic enteropathy, ↑ IgE level	AD, GOF	Altered cytokine signaling and Th2 skewing	2023 [33]
T-bet deficiency	*TBX21*	Mycobacterial disease, persistent airway inflammation, eosinophilia	AR, LOF	Altered cytokine signaling	2021 [112]
HIES-IL6 signal transducer deficiency	*IL6ST*	Recurrent infections, eczema, bronchiectasis, ↑ IgE level, eosinophilia, connective tissue abnormalities	AD, DN	Altered cytokine signaling	2020 [108]
CBM-opathies CARD14 deficiency	*CARD14*	Asthma, allergy, atopic dermatitis, ↑ IgE level	AD, LOF	Skin barrier dysfunction	2019 [51]
HIES-IL6 receptor deficiency	*IL6R*	Eczema, eosinophilia, ↑ IgE level, recurrent infections	AR, LOF	Altered cytokine signaling	2019 [113]

(continued)

Table 21.2 (continued)

Disorder	Gene	Key clinical features	Inheritance molecular mechanism	Mechanism	Year of report
HIES-ZNF341 deficiency	*ZNF341*	Severe allergy and ↑ IgE level, chronic mucocutaneous candidiasis	AR, LOF	Altered cytokine signaling	2018 [94]
Arp2/3-mediated filament branching defect	*ARPC1B*	Severe atopy, eosinophilia, poor growth, infections	AR, LOF	Impaired T-cell receptor signaling and cytoskeletal remodeling	2017 [114]
CBM-opathies CADINS	*CARD11*	Severe atopic dermatitis, eosinophilia, infections	AD, DN	Impaired T-cell receptor signaling	2017 [83]
HIES-IL6 signal transducer deficiency	*IL6ST*	Recurrent infections, eczema, bronchiectasis, ↑ IgE level, eosinophilia, connective tissue abnormalities	AR, LOF	Altered cytokine signaling	2017 [115]
HIES-ERBIN deficiency	*ERBIN*	Atopic dermatitis, ↑ IgE level, eosinophilic esophagitis, connective tissue abnormalities	AD, LOF	Altered cytokine signaling	2017 [116]
JAK1 deficiency	*JAK1*	Severe atopy, eosinophilia, poor growth	AD, GOF	Altered cytokine signaling	2017 [99, 117]
STAT5b deficiency	*STAT5B* (GOF)	Severe atopy, eosinophilia, urticaria, diarrhea	Somatic, GOF	Altered cytokine signaling	2017 [118]
RLTPR deficiency	*CARMIL2*	Combined immunodeficiency associated with severe atopic dermatitis, ↑ IgE level, allergic asthma, food allergy, and cold urticaria	AR, LOF	Impaired T-cell receptor signaling and cytoskeletal remodeling	2016 [119]
STAT3 GOF mutation	*STAT3* (GOF)	Lymphadenopathy, multiorgan autoimmunity, infections, short stature, eczema	AD, GOF	Altered cytokine signaling	2014 [120, 121]
HIES-PGM3 deficiency	*PGM3*	Bronchiectasis, skin abscesses, developmental delay, ↑ IgE level	AR, LOF	Metabolic disturbance	2014 [122]
CBM-opathies MALT1 deficiency	*MALT1*	Severe dermatitis, ↑ IgE level, poor growth, infections	AR, LOF	Impaired T-cell receptor signaling	2013 [97]
Desmoglein1 deficiency	*DSG1*	Severe dermatitis and food allergies, ↑ IgE level, metabolic wasting	AR, LOF	Skin barrier dysfunction	2013 [123]
Loeys-Dietz syndrome	*TGFBR1*	Vascular and connective tissue abnormalities, atopy	AD	Altered cytokine signaling	2013 [124]
Loeys-Dietz syndrome	*TGFBR2*	Vascular and connective tissue abnormalities, atopy	AD	Altered cytokine signaling	2013 [124]
STAT1 GOF mutation	*STAT1*	CMC, autoimmunity, enteropathy, eczema, short stature, vascular abnormalities	AD, GOF	Altered cytokine signaling	2013 [125]
WIP deficiency	*WIPF1*	Eczema, infections, thrombocytopenia, ↑ IgE level	AR, LOF	Impaired T-cell receptor signaling and cytoskeletal remodeling	2012 [126]
PLAID-PLCG2 deficiency	*PLCG2*	Cold urticaria, bacterial infection, autoimmunity, skin granulomas	AD, GOF	Mast cell deregulation	2012 [127]

(continued)

Table 21.2 (continued)

Disorder	Gene	Key clinical features	Inheritance molecular mechanism	Mechanism	Year of report
Corneodesmosin deficiency	*CDSN*	Peeling skin, diffuse ichthyosis, erythroderma, pruritus, food allergies, ↑ IgE level	AR, LOF	Skin barrier dysfunction	2010 [128]
CID/HIES-DOCK8 deficiency	*DOCK8*	Severe atopy, eosinophilia, infections, ↑ IgE level	AR, LOF	Impaired T-cell receptor signaling and cytoskeletal remodeling	2009 [129]
CID-ZAP70 deficiency	*ZAP70*	Erythroderma, eosinophilia, enteropathy, infections, ↑ IgE level	AR, LOF	T-cell repertoire restriction	2009 [130]
SCID-DNA ligase 4 deficiency	*LIG4*	Erythroderma, eosinophilia, enteropathy, infections, ↑ IgE level	AR, LOF	T-cell repertoire restriction	2008 [131]
CHARGE syndrome	*CHD7*	Erythroderma, eosinophilia, enteropathy, infections, ↑ IgE level	AR, likely LOF	T-cell repertoire restriction	2008 [132]
IL2RG deficiency	*IL2RG*	Erythroderma, eosinophilia, enteropathy, infections, ↑ IgE level	XL	T-cell repertoire restriction	2008 [133]
HIES-STAT3 deficiency (Job Syndrome)	*STAT3* (LOF)	Eczema, eosinophilia, ↑ IgE level, CMC, connective tissue abnormalities	AD, DN LOF	Altered cytokine signaling	2007 [134]
IL2RA deficiency	*IL2RA*	Severe autoimmune enteritis, viral infections, lymphoproliferation, eczema	AR, LOF	Tolerance failure	2007 [135, 136]
STAT5B deficiency	*STAT5B* (LOF)	Growth failure, autoimmunity, eczema, ↑ IgE level	AD or AR, LOF	Altered cytokine signaling	2006 [137] 2018 [138]
SCID-IL7 receptor deficiency	*IL7R*	Erythroderma, eosinophilia, enteropathy, infections, ↑ IgE level	AR, LOF [140]	T-cell repertoire restriction	2006 [140]
Systemin mastocytosis	*KIT*	Systemic mastocytosis	AD, GOF	Mast cell deregulation	2005 [141]
SCID-Artemis deficiency	*DCLRE1C*	Erythroderma, eosinophilia, enteropathy, infections, ↑ IgE level	AR, LOF	T-cell repertoire restriction	2005 [142]
Thymus defects-TBX1 deficiency	*TBX1*	Erythroderma, eosinophilia, enteropathy, infections, ↑ IgE level	Haploinsufficiency	T-cell repertoire restriction	2004 [143, 144]
IPEX syndrome	*FOXP3*	Severe atopy, autoimmunity, enteropathy, eosinophilia, ↑ IgE level	XL, LOF [146]	Tolerance failure	2001 [146]
Comel-Netherton syndrome	*SPINK5*	Trichorrhexis invaginatum, ichthyosis, ↑ IgE level, atopy	AR, LOF	Skin barrier dysfunction	2000 [147]
SCID-RAG deficiency	*RAG1*	Erythroderma, eosinophilia, enteropathy, infections, ↑ IgE level	AR, LOF	T-cell repertoire restriction	1998 [148]
SCID-RAG deficiency	*RAG2*	Erythroderma, eosinophilia, enteropathy, infections, ↑ IgE level	AR, LOF	T-cell repertoire restriction	1998 [148]
Wiskott-Aldrich syndrome	*WAS*	Eczema, infections, thrombocytopenia, ↑ IgE level	XL, LOF	Impaired T-cell receptor signaling and cytoskeletal remodeling	1994 [149]
SCID-adenosine deaminase deficiency	*ADA*	Diarrhea, dermatitis, infections, ↑ IgE level, multiorgan abnormalities	AR, LOF	T-cell repertoire restriction	1972 [150]

Modified from Vaseghi-Shanjani et al. [14] with updates

21.8 Disease Management and Treatment

General management of atopic manifestations is based upon patient's symptoms and the underlying disease.

Standard therapies include the following:

- Topical and/or systemic steroids and moisturizer creams for atopic dermatitis.
- Topical steroids/antihistamines and systemic antihistamines for atopic rhinitis and conjunctivitis.
- Inhaled and/or systemic steroids, inhaled short-acting beta agonists (SABA) when needed for asthma flares.
- Preventive therapy based on antihistamines, inhaled steroids, and/or long-acting beta agonists (LABA), antileukotrienes for chronic asthma.
- Exclusion diet for food allergies.
- Adrenaline, steroids, and antihistamines for anaphylactic shock (often with access to the emergency department).

Patients with IEIs-A or PADs are often refractory to standard therapies and require alternative therapeutic options such as immunosuppressive agents or semi-targeted/targeted therapies.

Immunosuppressive drugs like systemic corticosteroids and cyclosporine that are often used to control immune dysregulation may expose to a higher infectious risk and to substantial side effects, especially in the pediatric age.

The identification of specific gene defects in IEIs-A/PADs patients allows personalized approaches and therapeutic targets with relative advantage due to the higher specificity and lower toxicity compared to other systemic therapies [7, 18].

Dupilumab is currently the most studied biological for atopic dermatitis. It binds IL-4Rα inhibiting the IL-13/IL-4/STAT6 axis that promotes Th2 skewing, IgE production, and other mechanisms involved in atopic dysregulation. Dupilumab has been licensed for the treatment of atopic dermatitis in children older than 6 months with good results and safety profile [37, 151]. It is also effective in asthma and chronic rhinosinusitis with nasal polyps [152]. Only few cases have been reported so far, and more knowledge is required in IEIs [153].

Omalizumab is a monoclonal Ab binding IgE with reduction of their peripheral levels and better control of allergic manifestations. It is currently licensed for allergic asthma and chronic spontaneous urticaria [152]. Only few case reports are described, mostly in the context of hyper-IgE syndrome (HIES) with good response in terms of IgE level decline, although with no skin improvement [154].

In selected refractory cases, some patients have been treated with a combination therapy of both dupilumab and omalizumab [155].

JAK inhibitors (*Upadacitinib/Ruxolitinib/Baricitinib/Tofacitinib*) block the transduction of the JAK-STAT signaling which plays a central role for Th2 cytokine production [156]. They can be used topically or systemically (oral administration) to treat severe atopic dermatitis or other immune dysregulation manifestations. In the context of IEIs-A, their use should be evaluated in selected cases where the axis is upregulated (i.e., STAT1 GOF, STAT3 GOF, STAT6 GOF), taking into consideration the high infectious risk [33, 157].

In different forms of congenital ichthyosis, the use of anti-IL-17A antibody and of IL-12/IL-23 antagonists (*Ustekinumab/Secukinumab*) has been proposed with promising results, based on an IL-17–skewed inflammatory signature observed in these patients [158]. Ustekinumab has been successfully used in a patient with leukocyte adhesion deficiency type 1 (LAD1) to control inflammatory mucosal and cutaneous lesions [159] as well as in chronic granulomatous disease (CGD)-related IBD [160] (Fig. 21.4).

In severe diseases affecting the hematopoietic stem cells, a definitive treatment with hematopoietic stem cell transplant (HSCT) or gene therapy (GT) may be indicated. In particular, GT has been explored for a limited number of IEI, including ADA-SCID and Wiskott-Aldrich syndrome (WAS), and several clinical studies are ongoing for a variety of IEI [161, 162]. The increasing identification of pathogenic genetic variants of

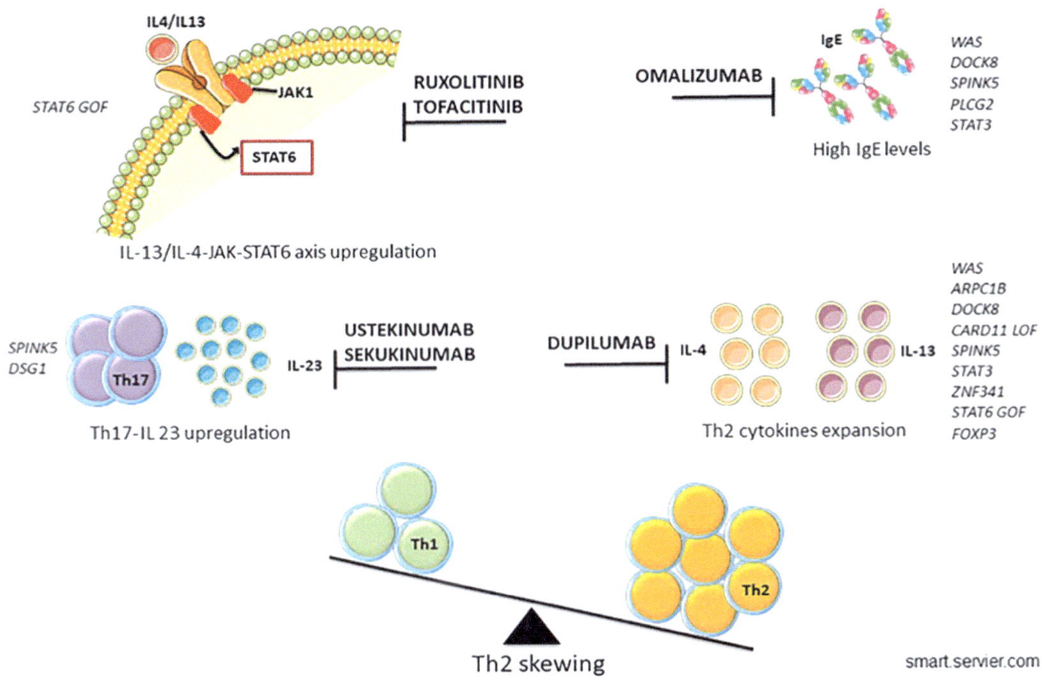

Fig. 21.4 Examples of tailored therapies for IEI-A/PADs. (From Giancotta et al. [7])

IEI conditions will allow the development of novel targeted treatments or their use as bridge therapy for candidates to HSCT/GT.

In conclusion, the management of atopic manifestations in the context of IEIs is often challenging, but the discovery of the molecular pathways underpinning these disorders could direct targeted/tailored therapy that can totally or partially control the immune dysregulation or represent a bridge to definitive therapies.

Key Points

Atopic dermatitis and inborn errors of immunity

- The earlier onset of dermatitis associated with atypical localization and extension, no response to classical treatment, other clinical features (bone and connective tissue abnormalities, facial and hair abnormalities, enteropathy, vascular abnormalities, endocrinopathies, recurrent viral and/or fungal infections), and a positive family history for IEI or consanguinity should arise the suspicion of PADs.

Asthma and inborn errors of immunity

- More than 40–60% of children with primary antibody disorders show bronchial hyperreactivity, although proven IgE-mediated allergy is more rarely described.
- Asthma is reported in about one-third of patients with hyper-IgE syndrome and is also described in several combined and syndromic immunodeficiencies.

Urticaria/angioedema and inborn errors of immunity

- Urticaria can be the presenting sign of several IEI, and the most frequent association is with autoinflammatory disorders, such as cryopyrin-associated periodic syndromes.

(continued)

- Also predominantly antibody deficiencies and immune dysregulation disorders could present with urticaria.
- The suspicion of an underlying IEI should be posed for patients with chronic urticaria with multiple relapses and refractoriness to common treatments, when other signs of immune dysfunction or dysregulation are found.

Take-Home Messages

- Allergic diseases can be caused by monogenic variants affecting the immune system and the skin epithelial barrier, and as such, be manifestations of an underlying immune deficiency.
- To dissect *inborn errors of immunity associated with atopy* from other isolated atopic phenotypes and decipher the role of polymorphisms in target genes is crucial to ensure prompt diagnosis and appropriate treatments.
- The discovery of the molecular pathways underpinnings *inborn errors of immunity associated with atopy* could direct targeted/tailored therapy that can totally or partially control the immune dysregulation or represent a bridge to definitive therapies.

References

1. Johansson SG, Bieber T, Dahl R, Friedmann PS, Lanier BQ, Lockey RF, et al. Revised nomenclature for allergy for global use: report of the Nomenclature Review Committee of the World Allergy Organization, October 2003. J Allergy Clin Immunol. 2004;113:832–6.
2. Dierick BJH, van der Molen T, Flokstra Blok BMJ, Muraro A, Postma MJ, Kocks JWH, et al. Burden and socioeconomics of asthma, allergic rhinitis, atopic dermatitis and food allergy. Expert Rev Pharmacoecon Outcomes Res. 2020;20:437–53.
3. Tangye SG, Al-Herz W, Bousfiha A, Cunningham-Rundles C, Franco JL, Holland SM, et al. Human inborn errors of immunity: 2022 update on the classification from the International Union of Immunological Societies Expert Committee. J Clin Immunol. 2022;42:1473–507.
4. Milner JD. Primary atopic disorders. Annu Rev Immunol. 2020;38:785–808.
5. Vaseghi-Shanjani M, Snow AL, Margolis DJ, Latrous M, Milner JD, Turvey SE, et al. Atopy as immune dysregulation: offender genes and targets. J Allergy Clin Immunol Pract. 2022;10:1737–56.
6. Sokol K, Milner JD. The overlap between allergy and immunodeficiency. Curr Opin Pediatr. 2018;30:848854.
7. Giancotta C, Colantoni N, Pacillo L, Santilli V, Amodio D, Manno EC, et al. Tailored treatments in inborn errors of immunity associated with atopy (IEIs-A) with skin involvement. Front Pediatr. 2023;11:1129249.
8. Lyons JJ, Milner JD. Primary atopic disorders. J Exp Med. 2018;215:1009–22.
9. Kondratuk K, Netravali IA, Castelo-Soccio L. Modern interventions for pediatric atopic dermatitis: an updated pharmacologic approach. Dermatol Ther (Heidelb). 2023;13:367–89.
10. Lehman H, Gordon C. The skin as a window into primary immune deficiency diseases: atopic dermatitis and chronic mucocutaneous candidiasis. J Allergy Clin Immunol Pract. 2019;7:788–98.
11. Bieber T. Atopic dermatitis: an expanding therapeutic pipeline for a complex disease. Nat Rev Drug Discov. 2022;21:21–40.
12. Fania L, Moretta G, Antonelli F, Scala E, Abeni D, Albanesi C, et al. Multiple roles for cytokines in atopic dermatitis: from pathogenic mediators to endotype-specific biomarkers to therapeutic targets. Int J Mol Sci. 2022;23:2684.
13. El-Sayed ZA, El-Ghoneimy DH, Ortega-Martell JA, Radwan N, Aldave JC, Al-Herz W,et al. Allergic manifestations of inborn errors of immunity and their impact on the diagnosis: a worldwide study. World Allergy Organ J. 2022;15:100657.
14. Vaseghi-Shanjani M, Smith KL, Sara RJ, Modi BP, Branch A, Sharma M, et al. Inborn errors of immunity manifesting as atopic disorders. J Allergy Clin Immunol. 2021;148:1130–9.
15. Costagliola G, Peroni DG, Consolini R. Beyond infections: new warning signs for inborn errors of immunity in children. Front Pediatr. 2022;10:855445.
16. Cinicola BL, Corrente S, Castagnoli R, et al. Primary atopic disorders and chronic skin disease. Pediatr Allergy Immunol. 2022;33(Suppl 27):65–8.
17. Candotti F, Eigenmann P. Inborn errors of immunity: an expanding horizon through a multitude of biological pathways. Pediatr Allergy Immunol. 2023;34:e13908.
18. Castagnoli R, Lougaris V, Giardino G, Volpi S, Leonardi L, La Torre F, et al. Inborn errors of immunity with atopic phenotypes: a practical guide for allergists. World Allergy Organ J. 2021;14:100513.

19. Stadler PC, Renner ED, Milner J, Wollenberg A. Inborn error of immunity or atopic dermatitis: when to be concerned and how to investigate. J Allergy Clin Immunol Pract. 2021;9:1501–7.
20. Bousfiha A, Moundir A, Tangye SG, Picard C, Jeddane L, Al-Herz W, et al. The 2022 update of IUIS phenotypical classification for human inborn errors of immunity. J Clin Immunol. 2022;42:1508–20.
21. Pan C, Zhao A, Li M. Atopic dermatitis-like genodermatosis: disease diagnosis and management. Diagnostics (Basel). 2022;12:2177.
22. Tsilifis C, Freeman AF, Gennery AR. STAT3 hyper-IgE syndrome—an update and unanswered questions. J Clin Immunol. 2021;41:864–80.
23. Candotti F. Clinical manifestations and pathophysiological mechanisms of the Wiskott-Aldrich syndrome. J Clin Immunol. 2018;38:13–27.
24. Rivers E, Worth A, Thrasher AJ, Burns SO. How I manage patients with Wiskott Aldrich syndrome. Br J Haematol. 2019;185:647–55.
25. Jamee M, Zaki-Dizaji M, Lo B, Abolhassani H, Aghamahdi F, Mosavian M,et al. Clinical, immunological, and genetic features in patients with immune dysregulation, polyendocrinopathy, enteropathy, X-linked (IPEX) and IPEX-like syndrome. J Allergy Clin Immunol Pract. 2020;8:2747–60.
26. Barzaghi F, Passerini L. IPEX syndrome: improved knowledge of immune pathogenesis empowers diagnosis. Front Pediatr. 2021;9:612760.
27. Paparella R, Menghi M, Micangeli G, Leonardi L, Profeta G, Tarani F, et al. Autoimmune polyendocrine syndromes in the pediatric age. Children (Basel). 2023;10:588.
28. Ding F, Wu C, Li Y, Mukherjee S, Ghosh S, Arrossi AV, et al. A case of hypereosinophilic syndrome with STAT5b N642H mutation. Oxf Med Case Rep. 2021;2021:omaa129.
29. Lu HY, Bauman BM, Arjunaraja S, Dorjbal B, Milner JD, Snow AL, et al. The CBM-opathies—a rapidly expanding spectrum of human inborn errors of immunity caused by mutations in the CARD11-BCL10-MALT1 complex. Front Immunol. 2018;9:2078.
30. Lu HY, Biggs CM, Blanchard-Rohner G, Fung SY, Sharma M, Turvey SE. Germline CBM-opathies: from immunodeficiency to atopy. J Allergy Clin Immunol. 2019;143:1661–73.
31. Chiriaco M, Di Matteo G, Conti F, Petricone D, De Luca M, Di Cesare S, et al. First case of patient with two homozygous mutations in MYD88 and CARD9 genes presenting with pyogenic bacterial infections, elevated IgE, and persistent EBV viremia. Front Immunol. 2019;10:130.
32. Picado C, García-Herrera AP, Hernández-Rodríguez J, Pascal M, Bartra J, Mascaró JM. Skin manifestations in patients with selective immunoglobulin E deficiency. J Clin Med. 2022;11:6795.
33. Sharma M, Leung D, Momenilandi M, Jones LCW, Pacillo L, James AE, et al. Human germline heterozygous gain-of-function STAT6 variants cause severe allergic disease. J Exp Med. 2023;220:e20221755.
34. Thalhammer J, Kindle G, Nieters A, Rusch S, Seppänen MRJ, Fischer A, et al. Initial presenting manifestations in 16,486 patients with inborn errors of immunity include infections and noninfectious manifestations. J Allergy Clin Immunol. 2021;148:1332–41.
35. David E, Ungar B, Renert-Yuval Y, Facheris P, Del Duca E, Guttman-Yassky E. The evolving landscape of biologic therapies for atopic dermatitis: present and future perspective. Clin Exp Allergy. 2023;53:156–72.
36. Pinto LM, Chiricozzi A, Calabrese L, Mannino M, Peris K. Novel therapeutic strategies in the topical treatment of atopic dermatitis. Pharmaceutics. 2022;14:2767.
37. Napolitano M, Fabbrocini G, Neri I, Stingeni L, Boccaletti V, Piccolo V, et al. Dupilumab treatment in children aged 6–11 years with atopic dermatitis: a multicentre, real-life study. Paediatr Drugs. 2022;24:671–8.
38. King-Biggs MB. Asthma. Ann Intern Med. 2019;171:Itc49–itc64.
39. Reddel HK, Bacharier LB, Bateman ED, Brightling CE, Brusselle GG, Buhl R, et al. Global Initiative for Asthma Strategy 2021: executive summary and rationale for key changes. Eur Respir J. 2021;59:2102730.
40. Bush A, Cutrera R, Piacentini G, Santamaria F, Ullmann N. Editorial: Difficult and severe asthma in children. Front Pediatr. 2019;7:205.
41. Romano R, Borrelli M, Cirillo E, Giardino G, Spadaro G, Crescenzi L, et al. Respiratory manifestations in primary immunodeficiencies: findings from a pediatric and adult cohort. Arch Bronconeumol. 2021;57:712–4.
42. Cinicola BL, Brindisi G, Capponi M, Gori A, Loffredo L, De Castro G, et al. The allergic phenotype of children and adolescents with selective IgA deficiency: a longitudinal monocentric study. J Clin Med. 2022,11.5705.
43. Cinetto F, Scarpa R, Rattazzi M, Agostini C. The broad spectrum of lung diseases in primary antibody deficiencies. Eur Respir Rev. 2018;27:180019.
44. Agondi RC, Barros MT, Rizzo LV, Kalil J, Giavina-Bianchi P. Allergic asthma in patients with common variable immunodeficiency. Allergy. 2010;65:510–5.
45. Cowan J, Gaudet L, Mulpuru S, Corrales-Medina V, Hawken S, Cameron C, et al. A retrospective longitudinal within-subject risk interval analysis of immunoglobulin treatment for recurrent acute exacerbation of chronic obstructive pulmonary disease. PLoS One. 2015;10:e0142205.
46. Nelson RW, Geha RS, McDonald DR. Inborn errors of the immune system associated with atopy. Front Immunol. 2022;13:860821.
47. Raby BA. Asthma severity, nature or nurture: genetic determinants. Curr Opin Pediatr. 2019;31:340–8.
48. Birben E, Sackesen C, Turgutoğlu N, Kalayci O. The role of SPINK5 in asthma related physiological events in the airway epithelium. Respir Med. 2012;106:349–55.

49. DeVore SB, Khurana Hershey GK. The role of the CBM complex in allergic inflammation and disease. J Allergy Clin Immunol. 2022;150:1011–30.
50. Freeman AF, Milner JD. The child with elevated IgE and infection susceptibility. Curr Allergy Asthma Rep. 2020;20:65.
51. Peled A, Sarig O, Sun G, Samuelov L, Ma CA, Zhang Y, et al. Loss-of-function mutations in caspase recruitment domain-containing protein 14 (CARD14) are associated with a severe variant of atopic dermatitis. J Allergy Clin Immunol. 2019;143:173–181.e10.
52. Lévy R, Gothe F, Momenilandi M, Magg T, Materna M, Peters P, et al. Human CARMIL2 deficiency underlies a broader immunological and clinical phenotype than CD28 deficiency. J Exp Med. 2023;220:e20220275.
53. Papadatou I, Marinakis N, Botsa E, Tzanoudaki M, Kanariou M, Orfanou I, et al. Case report: A novel synonymous ARPC1B gene mutation causes a syndrome of combined immunodeficiency, asthma, and allergy with significant intrafamilial clinical heterogeneity. Front Immunol. 2021;12:634313.
54. Pieniawska-Śmiech K, Pasternak G, Lewandowicz-Uszyńska A, Jutel M. Diagnostic challenges in patients with inborn errors of immunity with different manifestations of immune dysregulation. J Clin Med. 2022;11:4220.
55. Carrabba M, Dellepiane RM, Cortesi M, Baselli LA, Soresina A, Cirillo E, et al. Long term longitudinal follow-up of an AD-HIES cohort: the impact of early diagnosis and enrollment to IPINet centers on the natural history of Job's syndrome. Allergy Asthma Clin Immunol. 2023;19:32.
56. MacCarrick G, Black JH III, Bowdin S, El-Hamamsy I, Frischmeyer-Guerrerio PA, Guerrerio AL, et al. Loeys-Dietz syndrome: a primer for diagnosis and management. Genet Med. 2014;16:576–87.
57. Sharma N, Jaiswal I, Mandal RK, Phadke SR, Awasthi S. Genetic variation of TBX21 gene increases risk of asthma and its severity in Indian children. J Hum Genet. 2014;59:437–43.
58. Errami A, Baghdadi JE, Ailal F, Benhsaien I, Bakkouri JE, Jeddane L, et al. Mendelian susceptibility to mycobacterial disease (MSMD): clinical, immunological, and genetic features of 22 patients from 15 Moroccan kindreds. J Clin Immunol. 2023;43:728–40.
59. Choy EH, De Benedetti F, Takeuchi T, Hashizume M, John MR, Kishimoto T. Translating IL-6 biology into effective treatments. Nat Rev Rheumatol. 2020;16:335–45.
60. Blackburn MR, Volmer JB, Thrasher JL, Zhong H, Crosby JR, Lee JJ, et al. Metabolic consequences of adenosine deaminase deficiency in mice are associated with defects in alveogenesis, pulmonary inflammation, and airway obstruction. J Exp Med. 2000;192:159–70.
61. Deshpande DR, Demirdag YY, Marsh RA, Sullivan KE, Orange JS; USIDNET Consortium. Relationship between severity of T cell lymphopenia and immune dysregulation in patients with DiGeorge syndrome (22q11.2 deletions and/or related TBX1 mutations): a USIDNET study. J Clin Immunol. 2021;41:29–37.
62. Gattorno M, Tassi S, Carta S, Delfino L, Ferlito F, Pelagatti MA, et al. Pattern of interleukin-1beta secretion in response to lipopolysaccharide and ATP before and after interleukin-1 blockade in patients with CIAS1 mutations. Arthritis Rheum. 2007;56:3138–48.
63. Welzel T, Kuemmerle-Deschner JB. Diagnosis and management of the cryopyrin-associated periodic syndromes (CAPS): what do we know today? J Clin Med. 2021;10:128.
64. Levy R, Gérard L, Kuemmerle-Deschner J, Lachmann HJ, Koné-Paut I, Cantarini L, et al. Phenotypic and genotypic characteristics of cryopyrin-associated periodic syndrome: a series of 136 patients from the Eurofever Registry. Ann Rheum Dis. 2015;74:2043–9.
65. Finetti M, Omenetti A, Federici S, Caorsi R, Gattorno M. Chronic infantile neurological cutaneous and articular (CINCA) syndrome: a review. Orphanet J Rare Dis. 2016;11:167.
66. Wang HF. NLRP12-associated systemic autoinflammatory diseases in children. Pediatr Rheumatol Online J. 2022;20:9.
67. Frossi B, De Carli S, Bossi F, Pucillo C, De Carli M. Co-occurrence of chronic spontaneous urticaria with immunoglobulin A deficiency and autoimmune diseases. Int Arch Allergy Immunol. 2016;169:130–4.
68. Comberiati P, Costagliola G, Carli N, Legitimo A, D'Elios S, Consolini R, et al. Refractory chronic spontaneous urticaria treated with omalizumab in an adolescent with common variable immunodeficiency. Front Immunol. 2019;10:1700.
69. Altschul A, Cunningham-Rundles C. Chronic urticaria and angioedema as the first presentations of common variable immunodeficiency. J Allergy Clin Immunol. 2002;110:664–5.
70. Smith AA, Humphrey J, McAuley JB, Tharp MD. Common variable immunodeficiency presenting as chronic urticaria. J Am Acad Dermatol. 2008;59(2 Suppl 1):S40–1.
71. Yazdani R, Azizi G, Abolhassani H, Aghamohammadi A. Selective IgA deficiency: epidemiology, pathogenesis, clinical phenotype, diagnosis, prognosis and management. Scand J Immunol. 2017;85:3–12.
72. Morawska I, Kurkowska S, Bębnowska D, Hrynkiewicz R, Becht R, Michalski A, et al. The epidemiology and clinical presentations of atopic diseases in selective IgA deficiency. J Clin Med. 2021;10:3809.
73. Greaves M. Chronic urticaria. J Allergy Clin Immunol. 2000;105:664–72.
74. Ameratunga R, Edwards ESJ, Lehnert K, Leung E, Woon ST, Lea E, et al. The rapidly expanding genetic spectrum of common variable immunodeficiency-like disorders. J Allergy Clin Immunol Pract. 2023;11:1646–64.

75. Milner JD. PLAID: a syndrome of complex patterns of disease and unique phenotypes. J Clin Immunol. 2015;35:527–30.
76. Aderibigbe OM, Priel DL, Lee CC, Ombrello MJ, Prajapati VH, Liang MG, et al. Distinct cutaneous manifestations and cold-induced leukocyte activation associated with PLCG2 mutations. JAMA Dermatol. 2015;151:627–34.
77. Zafra H. Hereditary angioedema: a review. WMJ. 2022;121:48–53.
78. Wilkerson RG, Moellman JJ. Hereditary angioedema. Emerg Med Clin North Am. 2022;40:99–118.
79. Bacchetta R, Barzaghi F, Roncarolo MG. From IPEX syndrome to FOXP3 mutation: a lesson on immune dysregulation. Ann N Y Acad Sci. 2018;1417:5–22.
80. Cepika AM, Sato Y, Liu JM, Uyeda MJ, Bacchetta R, Roncarolo MG. Tregopathies: monogenic diseases resulting in regulatory T-cell deficiency. J Allergy Clin Immunol. 2018;142:1679–95.
81. Moin A, Farhoudi AAH, Moein M, Pourpak Z, Bazargan N. Cutaneous manifestations of primary immunodeficiency diseases in children. Iran J Allergy Asthma Immunol. 2006;5:121–6.
82. Berron-Ruiz A, Berron-Perez R, Ruiz-Maldonado R. Cutaneous markers of primary immunodeficiency diseases in children. Pediatr Dermatol. 2000;17:91–6.
83. Ma CA, Stinson JR, Zhang Y, Abbott JK, Weinreich MA, Hauk PJ, et al. Germline hypomorphic CARD11 mutations in severe atopic disease. Nat Genet. 2017;49:1192–201.
84. Gambineri E, Perroni L, Passerini L, Bianchi L, Doglioni C, Meschi F, et al. Clinical and molecular profile of a new series of patients with immune dysregulation, polyendocrinopathy, enteropathy, X-linked syndrome: inconsistent correlation between forkhead box protein 3 expression and disease severity. J Allergy Clin Immunol. 2008;122:1105–1112. e1.
85. Villa A, Notarangelo LD, Roifman CM. Omenn syndrome: inflammation in leaky severe combined immunodeficiency. J Allergy Clin Immunol. 2008;122:1082–6.
86. Ochs HD, Thrasher AJ. The Wiskott-Aldrich syndrome. J Allergy Clin Immunol. 2006;117:725–38.
87. Renner ED, Hartl D, Rylaarsdam S, Young ML, Monaco-Shawver L, Kleiner G, et al. Comel-Netherton syndrome defined as primary immunodeficiency. J Allergy Clin Immunol. 2009;124:536–43.
88. Wollenberg A, Renner E, Hagl B. Atopic eczema in childhood or primary immunodeficiency—what needs to be considered? MMW Fortschr Med. 2017;159:59–63.
89. Puel A. Human inborn errors of immunity underlying superficial or invasive candidiasis. Hum Genet. 2020;139:1011–22.
90. Schimke LF, Sawalle-Belohradsky J, Roesler J, Wollenberg A, Rack A, Borte M, et al. Diagnostic approach to the hyper-IgE syndromes: immunologic and clinical key findings to differentiate hyper-IgE syndromes from atopic dermatitis. J Allergy Clin Immunol. 2010;126:611–617.e1.
91. Boos AC, Hagl B, Schlesinger A, Halm BE, Ballenberger N, Pinarci M, et al. Atopic dermatitis, STAT3- and DOCK8-hyper-IgE syndromes differ in IgE based sensitization pattern. Allergy. 2014;69:943–53.
92. Hox V, O'Connell MP, Lyons JJ, Sackstein P, Dimaggio T, Jones N, et al. Diminution of signal transducer and activator of transcription 3 signaling inhibits vascular permeability and anaphylaxis. J Allergy Clin Immunol. 2016;138:187–99.
93. Siegel AM, Stone KD, Cruse G, Lawrence MG, Olivera A, Jung MY, et al. Diminished allergic disease in patients with STAT3 mutations reveals a role for STAT3 signaling in mast cell degranulation. J Allergy Clin Immunol. 2013;132:1388–96.
94. Beziat V, Li J, Lin J-X, Bousfiha A, Pellier I, Zoghi S, et al. A recessive form of hyperIgE syndrome by disruption of ZNF341-dependent STAT3 transcription and activity. Sci Immunol. 2018;3:eaat4956.
95. Biggs CM, Keles S, Chatila TA. DOCK8 deficiency: insights into pathophysiology, clinical features and management. Clin Immunol. 2017;181:75–82.
96. Aydin SE, Kilic SS, Aytekin C, Kumar A, Porras O, Kainulainen L, et al. DOCK8 deficiency: clinical and immunological phenotype and treatment options—a review of 136 patients. J Clin Immunol. 2015;35:189–98.
97. McKinnon ML, Rozmus J, Fung SY, Hirschfeld AF, Del Bel KL, Thomas L, et al. Combined immunodeficiency associated with homozygous MALT1 mutations. J Allergy Clin Immunol. 2014;133:1458–62. e1–7.
98. Momtazmanesh S, Rayzan E, Zoghi S, Shahkarami S, Molatefi R, Mohammadzadeh I, et al. Novel variants of DOCK8 deficiency in a case series of Iranian patients. Endocr Metab Immune Disord Drug Targets. 2022;22:159–68.
99. Del Bel KL, Ragotte RJ, Saferali A, Lee S, Vercauteren SM, Mostafavi SA, et al. JAK1 gain-of function causes an autosomal dominant immune dysregulatory and hypereosinophilic syndrome. J Allergy Clin Immunol. 2017;139:2016–20.e5.
100. Hwa V, Camacho-Hubner C, Little BM, David A, Metherell LA, El-Khatib N, et al. Growth hormone insensitivity and severe short stature in siblings: a novel mutation at the exon 13-intron 13 junction of the STAT5b gene. Horm Res. 2007;68:218–24.
101. Pillay BA, Avery DT, Smart JM, Cole T, Choo S, Chan D, et al. Hematopoietic stem cell transplant effectively rescues lymphocyte differentiation and function in DOCK8-deficient patients. JCI Insight. 2019;5:e127527.
102. Desjardins M, Arjunaraja S, Stinson JR, Dorjbal B, Sundaresan J, Niemela J, et al. A unique heterozygous CARD11 mutation combines pathogenic features of both gain- and loss-of-function patients in a four-generation family. Front Immunol. 2018;9:2944.

103. Ochs HD, Filipovich AH, Veys P, Cowan MJ, Kapoor N. Wiskott-Aldrich syndrome: diagnosis, clinical and laboratory manifestations, and treatment. Biol Blood Marrow Transplant. 2009;15:84–90.
104. Perez E. Future of therapy for inborn errors of immunity. Clin Rev Allergy Immunol. 2022;63:75–89.
105. Smith KL, Dai D, Modi BP, Sara R, Garabedian E, Marsh RA, et al. Inborn errors of immunity associated with type 2 inflammation in the USIDNET Registry. Front Immunol. 2022;13:831279.
106. Sereni L, Castiello MC, Marangoni F, Anselmo A, di Silvestre D, Motta S, et al. Autonomous role of Wiskott-Aldrich syndrome platelet deficiency in inducing autoimmunity and inflammation. J Allergy Clin Immunol. 2018;142:1272–84.
107. Volpi S, Cicalese MP, Tuijnenburg P, Tool ATJ, Cuadrado E, Abu-Halaweh M, et al. A combined immunodeficiency with severe infections, inflammation, and allergy caused by ARPC1B deficiency. J Allergy Clin Immunol. 2019;143:2296–9.
108. Béziat V, Tavernier SJ, Chen YH, Ma CS, Materna M, Laurence A, et al. Dominant-negative mutations in human IL6ST underlie hyper-IgE syndrome. J Exp Med. 2020;217:e20191804.
109. Cifaldi C, Rivalta B, Amodio D, Mattia A, Pacillo L, Di Cesare S, et al. Clinical, immunological, and molecular variability of RAG deficiency: a retrospective analysis of 22 RAG patients. J Clin Immunol. 2022;42:130–45.
110. Villa A, Notarangelo LD. RAG gene defects at the verge of immunodeficiency and immune dysregulation. Immunol Rev. 2019;287:73–90.
111. Delmonte OM, Villa A, Notarangelo LD. Immune dysregulation in patients with RAG deficiency and other forms of combined immune deficiency. Blood. 2020;135:610–9.
112. Yang R, Weisshaar M, Mele F, Benhsaien I, Dorgham K, Han J, et al. High Th2 cytokine levels and upper airway inflammation in human inherited T-bet deficiency. J Exp Med. 2021;218:e20202726.
113. Spencer S, Köstel Bal S, Egner W, Lango Allen H, Raza SI, Ma CA, et al. Loss of the interleukin-6 receptor causes immunodeficiency, atopy, and abnormal inflammatory responses. J Exp Med. 2019;216:1986–98.
114. Kuijpers TW, Tool ATJ, van der Bijl I, de Boer M, van Houdt M, de Cuyper IM, et al. Combined immunodeficiency with severe inflammation and allergy caused by ARPC1B deficiency. J Allergy Clin Immunol. 2017;140:273–7.e10.
115. Schwerd T, Twigg SRF, Aschenbrenner D, Manrique S, Miller KA, Taylor IB, et al. A biallelic mutation in IL6ST encoding the GP130 co-receptor causes immunodeficiency and craniosynostosis. J Exp Med. 2017;214:2547–62.
116. Lyons JJ, Liu Y, Ma CA, Yu X, O'Connell MP, Lawrence MG, et al. ERBIN deficiency links STAT3 and TGF-β pathway defects with atopy in humans. J Exp Med. 2017;214:669–80.
117. Gruber CN, Calis JJA, Buta S, Evrony G, Martin JC, Uhl SA, et al. Complex autoinflammatory syndrome unveils fundamental principles of JAK1 kinase transcriptional and biochemical function. Immunity. 2020;53:672–684.e11.
118. Ma CA, Xi L, Cauff B, DeZure A, Freeman AF, Hambleton S, et al. Somatic STAT5b gainoffunction mutations in early onset nonclonal eosinophilia, urticaria, dermatitis, and diarrhea. Blood. 2017;129:650–3.
119. Wang Y, Ma CS, Ling Y, Bousfiha A, Camcioglu Y, Jacquot S, et al. Dual T cell- and B cell intrinsic deficiency in humans with biallelic RLTPR mutations. J Exp Med. 2016;213:2413–35.
120. Milner JD, Vogel TP, Forbes L, Ma CA, Stray-Pedersen A, Niemela JE, et al. Early-onset lymphoproliferation and autoimmunity caused by germline STAT3 gain-of-function mutations. Blood. 2015;125:591–9.
121. Flanagan SE, Haapaniemi E, Russell MA, Caswell R, Allen HL, De Franco E, et al. Activating germline mutations in STAT3 cause early-onset multi-organ autoimmune disease. Nat Genet. 2014;46:812–4.
122. Sassi A, Lazaroski S, Wu G, Haslam SM, Fliegauf M, Mellouli F, et al. Hypomorphic homozygous mutations in phosphoglucomutase 3 (PGM3) impair immunity and increase serum IgE levels. J Allergy Clin Immunol. 2014;133:1410–9, 1419.e1–13.
123. Samuelov L, Sarig O, Harmon RM, Rapaport D, Ishida-Yamamoto A, Isakov O, et al. Desmoglein 1 deficiency results in severe dermatitis, multiple allergies and metabolic wasting. Nat Genet. 2013;45:1244–8.
124. Frischmeyer-Guerrerio PA, Guerrerio AL, Oswald G, Chichester K, Myers L, Halushka MK, et al. TGFβ receptor mutations impose a strong predisposition for human allergic disease. Sci Transl Med. 2013;5:195ra94.
125. Uzel G, Sampaio EP, Lawrence MG, Hsu AP, Hackett M, Dorsey MJ, et al. Dominant gain-of function STAT1 mutations in FOXP3 wild-type immune dysregulation-polyendocrinopathyenteropathy-X-linked-like syndrome. J Allergy Clin Immunol. 2013;131:1611–23.
126. Lanzi G, Moratto D, Vairo D, Masneri S, Delmonte O, Paganini T, et al. A novel primary human immunodeficiency due to deficiency in the WASP-interacting protein WIP. J Exp Med. 2012;209:29–34.
127. Ombrello MJ, Remmers EF, Sun G, Freeman AF, Datta S, Torabi-Parizi P, et al. Cold urticaria, immunodeficiency, and autoimmunity related to PLCG2 deletions. N Engl J Med. 2012;366:330–8.
128. Oji V, Eckl K-M, Aufenvenne K, Nätebus M, Tarinski T, Ackermann K, et al. Loss of corneodesmosin leads to severe skin barrier defect, pruritus, and atopy: unraveling the peeling skin disease. Am J Hum Genet. 2010;87:274–81.
129. Zhang Q, Davis JC, Lamborn IT, Freeman AF, Jing H, Favreau AJ, et al. Combined immunodeficiency associated with DOCK8 mutations. N Engl J Med. 2009;361:2046–55.

130. Turul T, Tezcan I, Artac H, de Bruin-Versteeg S, Barendregt BH, Reisli I,et al. Clinical heterogeneity can hamper the diagnosis of patients with ZAP70 deficiency. Eur J Pediatr. 2009;168:87–93.
131. Grunebaum E, Bates A, Roifman CM. Omenn syndrome is associated with mutations in DNA ligase IV. J Allergy Clin Immunol. 2008;122:1219–20.
132. Gennery AR, Slatter MA, Rice J, Hoefsloot LH, Barge D, McLean-Tooke A, et al. Mutations in CHD7 in patients with CHARGE syndrome cause T-B + natural killer cell + severe combined immune deficiency and may cause Omenn-like syndrome. Clin Exp Immunol. 2008;153:75–80.
133. Wada T, Yasui M, Toma T, Nakayama Y, Nishida M, Shimizu M, et al. Detection of T lymphocytes with a second-site mutation in skin lesions of atypical X-linked severe combined immunodeficiency mimicking Omenn syndrome. Blood. 2008;112:1872–5.
134. Holland SM, DeLeo FR, Elloumi HZ, Hsu AP, Uzel G, Brodsky N, et al. STAT3 mutations in the hyper-IgE syndrome. N Engl J Med. 2007;357:1608–19.
135. Goudy K, Aydin D, Barzaghi F, Gambineri E, Vignoli M, Ciullini Mannurita S, et al. Human IL2RA null mutation mediates immunodeficiency with lymphoproliferation and autoimmunity. Clin Immunol. 2013;146:248–61.
136. Caudy AA, Reddy ST, Chatila T, Atkinson JP, Verbsky JW. CD25 deficiency causes an immune dysregulation, polyendocrinopathy, enteropathy, X-linked–like syndrome, and defective IL-10 expression from CD4 lymphocytes. J Allergy Clin Immunol. 2007;119:482–7.
137. Bernasconi A, Marino R, Ribas A, Rossi J, Ciaccio M, Oleastro M, et al. Characterization of immunodeficiency in a patient with growth hormone insensitivity secondary to a novel STAT5b. Pediatrics. 2006;118:e1584–92.
138. Klammt J, Neumann D, Gevers EF, Andrew SF, Schwartz ID, Rockstroh D, et al. Dominant negative STAT5B mutations cause growth hormone insensitivity with short stature and mild immune dysregulation. Nat Commun. 2018;9:2105.
139. Lev A, Simon AJ, Barel O, Eyal E, Glick-Saar E, Nayshool O, et al. Reduced function and diversity of T cell repertoire and distinct clinical course in patients with IL7RA mutation. Front Immunol. 2019;10:1672.
140. Giliani S, Bonfim C, de Saint BG, Lanzi G, Brousse N, Koliski A, et al. Omenn syndrome in an infant with IL7RA gene mutation. J Pediatr. 2006;148:272–4.
141. Hartmann K, Wardelmann E, Ma Y, Merkelbach-Bruse S, Preussner LM, Woolery C, et al. Novel germline mutation of KIT associated with familial gastrointestinal stromal tumors and mastocytosis. Gastroenterology. 2005;129(3):1042–6.
142. Ege M, Ma Y, Manfras B, Kalwak K, Lu H, Lieber MR, Schwarz K, et al. Omenn syndrome due to ARTEMIS mutations. Blood. 2005;105:4179–86.
143. Markert ML, Alexieff MJ, Li J, Ozaki DA, Devlin BH, Sempowski GD, et al. Complete DiGeorge syndrome: development of rash, lymphadenopathy, and oligoclonal T cells in 5 cases. J Allergy Clin Immunol. 2004;113:734–41.
144. Yagi H, Furutani Y, Hamada H, Sasaki T, Asakawa S, Minoshima S, et al. Role of TBX1 in human del22q11.2 syndrome. Lancet. 2003;362:1366–73.
145. Van Gool F, Nguyen MLT, Mumbach MR, Satpathy AT, Rosenthal WL, Giacometti S, et al. A mutation in the transcription factor Foxp3 drives T helper 2 effector function in regulatory T cells. Immunity. 2019;50:362–377.e6.
146. Bennett CL, Christie J, Ramsdell F, Brunkow ME, Ferguson PJ, Whitesell L, et al. The immune dysregulation, polyendocrinopathy, enteropathy, X-linked syndrome (IPEX) is caused by mutations of FOXP3. Nat Genet. 2001;27:20–1.
147. Chavanas S, Bodemer C, Rochat A, Hamel-Teillac D, Ali M, Irvine AD, et al. Mutations in SPINK5, encoding a serine protease inhibitor, cause Netherton syndrome. Nat Genet. 2000;25:141–2.
148. Villa A, Santagata S, Bozzi F, Giliani S, Frattini A, Imberti L, et al. Partial V(D)J recombination activity leads to Omenn syndrome. Cell. 1998;93:885–96.
149. Derry JM, Ochs HD, Francke U. Isolation of a novel gene mutated in Wiskott-Aldrich syndrome. Cell. 1994;78:635–44.
150. Giblett E, Anderson J, Cohen F, Pollara B, Meuwissen HJ. Adenosine-deaminase deficiency in two patients with severely impaired cellular immunity. Lancet. 1972;2:1067–9.
151. Siegfried EC, Cork MJ, Katoh N, Zhang H, Chuang CC, Thomas RB, et al. Dupilumab provides clinically meaningful responses in children aged 6–11 years with severe atopic dermatitis: post hoc analysis results from a phase III trial. Am J Clin Dermatol. 2023;24:787.
152. Scioscia G, Nolasco S, Campisi R, Quarato CMI, Caruso C, Pelaia C, et al. Switching biological therapies in severe asthma. Int J Mol Sci. 2023;24:9563.
153. Matucci-Cerinic C, Viglizzo G, Pastorino C, Corcione A, Prigione I, Bocca P, et al. Remission of eczema and recovery of Th1 polarization following treatment with Dupilumab in STAT3 hyper IgE syndrome. Pediatr Allergy Immunol. 2022;33:e13770.
154. Gomes N, Miranda J, Lopes S, Carneiro-Leão L, Torres Costa J, Baudrier T, et al. Omalizumab in the treatment of hyper-IgE syndrome: 2 case reports. J Investig Allergol Clin Immunol. 2020;30:191–2.
155. Arasu A, Sharma N, Yazdabadi A, Sladden M. Dual biologic therapy with Omalizumab and Dupilumab for refractory atopic disease. Australas J Dermatol. 2022;63:110–1.
156. O'Shea JJ, Schwartz DM, Villarino AV, Gadina M, McInnes IB, Laurence A. The JAK-STAT pathway: impact on human disease and therapeutic intervention. Annu Rev Med. 2015;66:311–28.

157. Forbes L, Vogel TP, Cooper MA, Castro-Wagner J, Schussler E, Weinacht KG, et al. Jakinibs for the treatment of immune dysregulation in patients with gain-of-function signal transducer and activator of transcription 1 (STAT1) or STAT3 mutations. J Allergy Clin Immunol. 2018;142:1665–9.
158. Godsel LM, Roth-Carter QR, Koetsier JL, Tsoi LC, Huffine AL, Broussard JA, et al. Translational implications of Th17-skewed inflammation due to genetic deficiency of a cadherin stress sensor. J Clin Invest. 2022;132:e144363.
159. Moutsopoulos NM, Zerbe CS, Wild T, Dutzan N, Brenchley L, DiPasquale G, et al. Interleukin-12 and Interleukin-23 blockade in leukocyte adhesion deficiency type 1. N Engl J Med. 2017;376:1141–6.
160. Bhattacharya S, Marciano BE, Malech HL, Quezado M, Holland SM, De Ravin SS, et al. Safety and efficacy of ustekinumab in the inflammatory bowel disease of chronic granulomatous disease. Clin Gastroenterol Hepatol. 2022;20:461–464.e2.
161. Aiuti A, Roncarolo MG, Naldini L. Gene therapy for ADA-SCID, the first marketing approval of an ex vivo gene therapy in Europe: paving the road for the next generation of advanced therapy medicinal products. EMBO Mol Med. 2017;9:737–40.
162. Magnani A, Semeraro M, Adam F, Booth C, Dupré L, Morris EC, et al. Long-term safety and efficacy of lentiviral hematopoietic stem/progenitor cell gene therapy for Wiskott-Aldrich syndrome. Nat Med. 2022;28:71–80.

22 Laboratory Tests in Pediatric Allergy

Serena Gracci and Roberto Bernardini

Abstract

In vitro tests are part of the diagnostic pathway of allergic diseases. Circulating eosinophils are a marker of type 2 inflammation. Mild and transient eosinophilia can be due to atopic diseases, asthma, drug hypersensitivity, helminthic infections, or be idiopathic; instead, hypereosinophilia (moderate to severe and persistent or marked tissue eosinophilia) should be promptly investigated. The eosinophil cationic protein, evaluable in various biological fluids, is an index of eosinophil activity that can be increased in atopic and non-atopic conditions. Total serum IgE are a marker of atopy, influenced by many factors and increased also in non-allergic conditions, and should always be evaluated when specific IgE are tested. The latter are a marker of sensitization to a specific allergen that can be dosed individually or with multi-allergen tests. The basophil activation test is a functional assay that evaluates IgE function through the activation of basophils by a specific allergen. Nasal cytology is a simple tool that helps to characterize rhinitis, distinguishing allergic rhinitis from non-allergic rhinitis.

Keywords

Allergy diagnosis · In vitro tests · Circulating eosinophils · Eosinophil cationic protein · Immunoglobulin E · Basophil activation test · Nasal cytology

Test your learning and check your understanding of this book's contents: use the "Springer Nature Flashcards" app to access questions using ▶ https://sn.pub/nspbjm. To use the app, please follow the instructions in Chap. 1.

S. Gracci · R. Bernardini (✉)
Paediatric Unit, "San Giuseppe" Hospital, Empoli, Italy
e-mail: serena.gracci@uslcentro.toscana.it; roberto.bernardini@uslcentro.toscana.it

C. Caffarelli, G. L. Marseglia (eds.), *Textbook of Pediatric Allergy*,
https://doi.org/10.1007/978-3-031-71283-8_22

Key Points

In vitro test	Key Points
Circulating eosinophils	• Mild and transient eosinophilia (<1500/μL): atopic disease, asthma, drug hypersensitivity, helminth infection, idiopathic • Hypereosinophilia: moderate to severe (>1500/μL) and persistent eosinophilia, detected on ≥2 occasions at ≥2 weeks apart or marked tissue eosinophilia • Non-specific marker of type 2 inflammation/allergy
Eosinophil cationic protein	• Measurable in many biological fluids, serum normal values <20 μg/L • Marker of eosinophil activity • Increased in atopic conditions (asthma, AR, AD) and eosinophil-related diseases (infective, respiratory and gastrointestinal diseases, malignances)
Total serum IgE	• Marker of atopy, overlap between normal population and allergic subjects • IgE levels are influenced by age, race, gender, geographic area, seasons, and exposure to environmental pollutants • Other causes of increased IgE: helminthic infections, primary immunodeficiencies (including HIES), IgE multiple myeloma
Specific IgE	• Marker of sensitization to a specific allergen • More expensive and time-consuming, but safer than SPT, useful in patients with skin inflammation, uncooperative children and patients with high risk of anaphylaxis, no need to interrupt antihistamines • Multi-allergen screen tests available
Basophils activation test	• Functional assay that measures IgE response to an allergen (useful if other tests are ambiguous or discordant with the clinic, drug, and venom allergy) • Within 6–12 months of the reaction, not influenced by antihistamines, discontinue oral steroids 3 weeks before • Specific cut-off for allergen; if not available: 5% $CD63^+$ basophils (2.5% for drugs)
Nasal cytology	• Point-of-care instrument useful in the phenotyping of rhinitis • In allergic rhinitis: useful to perform nasal provocation tests, optimize and individualize the treatment, identify "overlapped" rhinitis

22.1 Introduction

There are many available tools in the diagnosis of allergic pathologies. They aim to identify the causative allergen of the given allergic pathology, but also to better characterize the clinical picture, for an appropriate management and treatment of the condition. Traditional in vivo skin tests and provocation tests are still relevant, but next to them new investigations have emerged over the years, especially in vitro tests [1]. In vitro tests include both non-specific allergy markers, useful in distinguish atopic from non-atopic conditions, and allergen-specific markers of sensitization. We will then analyze the diagnostic tools available, looking at their clinical significance, strengths, and limitations.

22.2 Circulating Eosinophils

Eosinophils are granulocytic leukocytes distinguished by their bilobed nuclei and large acidophilic cytoplasmic granules [2]. They grow and develop in the bone marrow, stimulated by IL-5, eotaxins, IL-4, IL-13, and IL-9. Under homeostatic condition, they are found primarily in the gastrointestinal tract and, responding to signals from cytokines, chemokines, and other proinflammatory mediators, they are released into the bloodstream and migrate through the endothelia to the tissues [3]. Hence, blood eosinophils reflect the balance between their production in the bone marrow, trafficking from the bone marrow into the tissues, and apoptosis.

They represent only a small minority (<5–6%) of the circulating leukocyte population and should be evaluated as absolute eosinophil counts (AEC), classifying the degree of eosinophilia as mild (AEC 500–1500/μL), moderate (AEC 1500–5000/μL), or severe (AEC >5000/μL) [4]. Mild and transient eosinophilia, frequently observed in the pediatric population, usually without clinical relevance, can be caused by atopic disease, asthma, drug hypersensitivity, and helminth infections [5]. Hypereosinophilia (HE) refers to moderate to severe and persistent eosinophilia, detected on at least two occasions at least 4 weeks apart, or marked tissue eosinophilia [6]. It is relatively rare, and an underlying cause and organ manifestations caused by eosinophilia, which characterize hypereosinophilic syndromes (HES), should be promptly sought [5]. Primary HE is rare, caused by myeloid and stem cell neoplasms, grouped under myeloproliferative HE/HES (M-HE or M-HES), and results from abnormal expansion of an eosinophilic clone in the bone marrow. Secondary (or reactive) HE is much more common and results from conditions leading to polyclonal expansion of eosinophils listed in Table 22.1. Concerning allergic disorders, they can be associated with HE, especially in children, but in the presence of AEC $\geq 5.0 \times 10^9$/L, other causes should be considered [5].

Eosinophils are characteristic of type 2 inflammation, considered a focal risk factor for persistent wheezing and poor asthma control in children, with increased symptoms, impaired lung function, increased airway hyperresponsiveness, frequent exacerbations, and increased response to steroids [8–10]. Therefore, its identification may be useful to target the therapy. Elevated blood eosinophils were also associated with increased odds and shorter times for the first acute visit and for hospitalizations [11].

Recently, higher blood eosinophils have also been associated with greater response to biological therapies, as anti-IL-5 (mepolizumab, reslizumab) [12, 13], anti-IL-5 receptor α (benralizumab) [14], and anti-IL-4 receptor α (dupilumab) [15]. However, eosinophil levels are not constant over time; therefore, multiple measurements over time are recommended to identify the patient's real eosinophilic status and guide treatment [16].

Table 22.1 Causes of secondary hypereosinophilia

Condition	Examples
Atopic diseases	Asthma, allergic rhinitis, atopic dermatitis
Helminthic infections	Strongyloidiasis, schistosomiasis, hookworm, filariasis, ascariasis, toxocariasis, trichinosis
Fungal infections	Coccidioidomycosis, allergic bronchopulmonary aspergillosis, histoplasmosis
Viral infections	HIV
Drugs	Antibiotics, NSAIDs, antiepileptics, DRESS syndrome
Gastrointestinal disorders	Eosinophilic gastrointestinal disease, eosinophilic esophagitis, inflammatory bowel disease
Hematologic diseases	Lymphocyte malignancy, aberrant lymphocyte clone, sickle cell disease
Immunodeficiencies	STAT3 deficiency, IPEX syndrome, DOCK8 deficiency, autoimmune lymphoproliferative syndrome, LRBA deficiency, Wiskott-Aldrich syndrome, Omenn SCID
Rheumatic diseases	Eosinophilic granulomatosis with polyangiitis, systemic lupus erythematosus, dermatomyositis, arthritis
Adrenal insufficiency	
Graft-versus-host disease	
Solid organ transplant rejection	

Adapted from Schwartz 2018 [7]

22.3 Eosinophil Cationic Protein

Eosinophil cationic protein (ECP) is a basic protein of eosinophil granules [17], released after the eosinophils leave the circulation, in an antibody-dependent and antibody-independent manner, with a 65-min turnover time in the blood [18, 19]. It is considered a marker of eosinophil activation and therefore of type 2 inflammation [20].

ECP can be measured in various body fluids as serum, plasma, sputum, saliva, nasal lavage fluid, broncho-alveolar lavage fluid, and urine, with different normal ranges [21]. Serum ECP is the most used in clinical practice, reflecting circulating ECP and the propensity of active eosinophils to release it ex vivo. Its sampling is extremely sensitive to the storage temperature, and close standardization of sampling procedure is necessary [22]. Serum ECP normal level for adults and children is <20 μg/L, while asthmatic subjects have higher values [21]. Sputum concentration of ECP (20–1280 μg/L) is higher and reflects the local inflammatory process in the airways [23]. There are some issues in its collection: some people must be induced to expectorate, sputum needs a preanalytical management, there may be saliva contamination, and its sampling should be standardized before use in clinical routine [23]. The measurement of ECP in other biological fluids is not well standardized, and it is used for research purposes [21].

Being a marker of type 2 inflammation [24], elevated serum ECP can be detected 6–24 h after exposure to the allergen, indicating acute allergen exposure [17]. As only activated eosinophils degranulate, ECP is a more specific index of eosinophil inflammation than blood eosinophil count [23]. Serum ECP is increased in atopic diseases as asthma, allergic rhinitis (AR), and atopic dermatitis (AD) [21, 25, 26], but also in other eosinophil-related conditions as infective, respiratory, and gastrointestinal diseases and malignances [27–29].

In asthmatic patients, it correlates with activated eosinophils in bronchial mucosa [30], virus-induced airway inflammation [31], severity, respiratory function [32, 33], and skin prick tests (SPT) [34]. It is higher in children at highest risk for recurrent exacerbations who could benefit from corticosteroid treatment [24], and it may guide tapering of inhaled corticosteroid therapy [35] and assess the compliance, as it decreases after anti-inflammatory treatment [36, 37], however, being increased in other atopic conditions [38], recurrent wheeze [39], and infections [40, 41]. In young patients with recurrent wheeze, the eosinophil activity may predict childhood asthma: among hospitalized children for wheezing in respiratory infections, the ones with higher ECP had an increased risk of asthma at school age [42].

Serum ECP is also a predictor of AR with low sensibility and specificity, so it cannot be used as a single diagnostic tool, but as a support in diagnosis [43]. Moreover, it is associated with the eosinophil count and the disease activity both in AR and non-allergic rhinitis (NAR) [44, 45].

Elevated ECP can be observed in AD, but there is not a correlation with its severity [46]. It can help to differentiate allergic contact dermatitis from non-allergic dermatitis, together with other diagnostic tests [47].

Finally, in the evaluation of HE, in which the eosinophil count does not relate with tissue infiltration and eosinophil activity, serum ECP is helpful in differential diagnosis, as highest values of ECP and ECP/eosinophil count are found in HES and reactive eosinophilia with malignancy [28, 29].

22.4 Total Serum IgE

The IgE molecule is a single four-chain unit with a molecular weight close to 190,000 D [48]. It is produced by B cells and plasma cells after an antigenic stimulus [49, 50, 51]. Once produced, it is released into the circulation and can bind to many cell types through the Cε2–3 region to their surface receptors. The activation by allergens of mast cell high-affinity receptors (FcεRI) is the basis of immediate hypersensitivity reactions [52].

The level of total serum IgE (tIgE) is usually expressed in kilo international units per liter (kIU/L) as recommended by the 75/502 IgE stan-

Table 22.2 Cut-off values of total serum IgE to distinguish atopic from non-atopic children

Age (years)	Cut-off (kIU/L)	Sensitivity (%)	Specificity (%)
<1	20.2	95.0	91.5
1	30.4	89.6	95.2
2	38.6	95.7	94.0
3	57.0	99.0	92.7
4	57.2	89.6	97.1
5	65.4	89.2	96.7
6	73.0	95.8	90.5
7	82.6	98.5	87.6
8	76.4	96.0	92.6
9	98.4	100.0	84.4
10	102.6	99.3	84.2
11	104.8	99.3	87.5
12	101.4	98.0	86.8
13	97.4	98.1	86.2
14	94.2	83.8	97.3
15	105.2	98.1	81.7
16	100.0	98.3	97.2

Adapted from Dodig et al. [57]

dard from the World Health Organization (WHO). By multiplying the kIU/L value by 2.4, it is possible to convert into units of mass per volume (μg/L) [53]. In healthy children, tIgE increase in the first decade of life, reaching a plateau at the beginning of adolescence, and slightly decline in the later ages [54].

It is considered a traditional marker of atopy, but about half of patients with atopy have normal tIgE [55] and there is a great overlap between the normal population and allergic subjects [56]. To distinguish atopic from non-atopic individuals, instead of using the normal values for age based on non-atopic subjects provided by each laboratory, it is more useful to use cut-off values determined by ROC analysis with optimal sensitivity and specificity, with an optimal cut-off which gradually increases from 20.2 kIU/L under 1 year of age, reaching 65.4 kIU/L at 5 years and 102.6 kIU/L at 10 years, to remain almost stable at subsequent ages [57] (Table 22.2). It is also important to remember that conditions other than allergies may be associated with high tIgE: helminthic infections [58], primary immunodeficiencies including hyper-IgE syndromes [59], and IgE multiple myeloma [60]. The serum tIgE level is also influenced by race, gender, geographic area, seasons, and exposure to environmental pollutants [61].

In the context of atopic diseases, a relationship has been observed between the level of tIgE and the severity of AD [62, 63] and allergic bronchopulmonary aspergillosis [64], while in asthma, the results are controversial [65, 66].

22.5 Specific IgE

Allergen-specific IgE antibody (sIgE) measurement is the most important in vitro test to confirm the sensitization to an allergen.

The first available in vitro test for sIgE was a radioallergosorbent test (RAST), introduced in 1967 [67]. The allergen extract, fixed on a solid phase, bound the specific antibody from human serum, which was then detected by radiolabeled human anti-human IgE. These first-generation qualitative methods have been replaced by second-generation semiquantitative IgE assays. They are quantitative enzyme immunoassays employing enzyme substrates and photometry or fluorimetry for signal detection, with a measuring range of 0.35–100 kU/L. They use new solid-phase matrices with high binding capacity, non-isotopic labels for the detection of antibodies and calibrators traceable to the WHO IgE reference standard 75/502. The cut-off of 0.35 kU/L distinguishes positive and negative results [53, 68].

Third-generation quantitative self-analyzers are chemiluminescent enzyme immunoassays performed on autoanalyzers having a true zero calibrator with a detection limit and functional sensitivity of 0.1 and 0.2 kU/L, respectively. The three most widely used third-generation assays are ImmunoCAP by Phadia, Immulite System from Siemens, and HYTEC-288 system from Hycor/Agilent Technologies [69, 70]. A key aspect of the sIgE assay is the used allergen. The use of extractive allergens, unlike molecular diagnostics that use single molecular components, requires a standardization of the extraction process to allow for consistency and reproducibility of the test [71].

The evaluation of sIgE has a sensitivity comparable to SPT for respiratory and food allergy, but it is complementary to the intra-dermal skin test for drug and venom allergy diagnosis [1]. Compared to SPT, sIgE assays are more expensive and results are not immediate, but they are useful in patients with skin inflammation, during antihistamine therapy which cannot be interrupted, uncooperative children and with high risk of anaphylaxis. There can be some discrepancies between skin tests and sIgE assays, because different proteins or IgE binding sites are represented [72].

A correct interpretation of the test is essential: the finding of sIgE denotes the state of sensitization, not equivalent to a diagnosis of allergy, for which a correlation with the clinical history is necessary. Patients with sIgE might have no clinical manifestations when exposed to the allergen; hence, it is unnecessary to test for a tolerated allergen [72]. IgE level should be also considered: high tIgE can be associated with numerous "positive" sIgE that may have no clinical meaning, while low sIgE may be relevant when tIgE are low [72].

Multi-allergen screen tests are also available and allow to measure sIgE antibodies to multiple allergens in a single blood specimen, with panels of aeroallergens and food allergens [74–76]. They have a high negative predictive value, allowing to rule out sensitization in patients without a significant history of allergy, but, if positive, they must be interpreted with an extensive clinical history and further diagnostic tests if needed.

Concerning food allergy, many factors must be considered in the interpretation of sIgE, as it is greatly influenced by the pretest probability, increased by clinical history of immediate hypersensitivity, younger age and relative prevalence of the atopic condition in the population, reduced by AD, inhalant allergies, and black ethnicity [77]. It is possible to establish a relationship between a level of sIgE and the probability of a clinically relevant allergic reaction in the patient following allergen exposure, as assessed in a double-blinded placebo-controlled food challenge. The threshold differs by the kind of food and the age of the patient [78].

In the diagnosis of immediate hypersensitivity reactions to drugs, sIgE assays are available only for a few drugs and often are not clinically validated. The most studied ones are β-lactam antibiotics, neuromuscular blocking agents (NMBA), and morphine [79].

22.6 Basophil Activation Test (BAT)

Basophils are important effector cells in immediate hypersensitivity responses: through FcεRI, they carry sIgE antibodies on their surface and degranulate when the allergen cross-links sIgE/FcεRI complexes. The BAT is a functional assay that measures IgE function, in terms of ability to induce the activation of basophils when the allergen is present. It uses flow cytometry to evaluate the expression of activation markers (mainly CD63) that are upregulated after the cross-linking of IgE to FcεRI, resulting from allergen stimulation, compared to a negative control [80, 81]. A positive control is also performed to verify the ability of the basophils to respond to a non-IgE stimulus [82]. A successful execution of the test requires well-trained operators and proper materials [80]. Allergen source is a critical factor, as it can range from crude extracts to single recombinants or purified allergenic sources; hence, standardized preparations are recommended in

Table 22.3 Optimal BAT cut-off in different allergy conditions

Allergic disease		Allergen stimulation	Cut-off
Food allergy	Peanut	Peanut extract 0.1–10,000 ng/mL	8.11% CD63$^+$ basophils
	Egg	Ovalbumin 0.1–100 μg/mL	5% CD63$^+$ basophils
Drug allergy	Beta-lactams	Various	5% CD63$^+$ basophils
	NMBA	Rocuronium	4% CD63$^+$ basophils
Insect venom allergy	Wasp venom	Wasp venom 0.0001–1 μg/mL	10% CD63$^+$ basophils
	Bee venom	Bee venom 0.0001–1 μg/mL	10% CD63$^+$ basophils
Respiratory allergy	Grass pollen	Grass pollen extract 100–0.0001 SQU/mL	2.5% CD63$^+$ basophils
	Aspergillus	*A. fumigatus* extract (10 μL) or rAsp f 1	ND

Adapted from Santos et al. [82]

comparing results between laboratories or over time [83].

Basophil reactivity represents the proportion of activated basophils compared to the negative control. It can be expressed as % CD63$^+$ basophils at a given allergen concentration or as the ratio of % CD63$^+$ basophils to allergen and the positive control [82]. There is no international agreement on the cut-off to establish the positivity of the test, and it should be calculated using the ROC curves of specific studies, available only for some allergens, as peanut, egg, beta-lactams, NMBA, wasp and bee venom, grass pollen and aspergillus [82] (Table 22.3). For rare allergens or in the absence of studies, an empirical cut-off of 5% CD63$^+$ basophils can be used, reduced to 2.5% in drug allergies [84].

BAT should be performed within 6–12 months of the clinical reaction, although it can remain positive even much longer. It is not affected by antihistamines, and oral steroids should be discontinued 3 weeks before [85].

It can be used if cutaneous test and sIgE are ambiguous or discordant with the clinic. Compared to a provocation test, it is less invasive, less expensive, and safer, avoiding the direct exposure of the patient to the allergen [82]. A limitation of BAT is that the basophils of about 10% of individuals do not respond to IgE-mediated allergenic FcεRI stimulation, even expressing surface IgE and normally activating to IgE-independent stimuli [86].

The use of BAT in food allergies is complicated by the source of the allergen, as results can differ according to the variety employed [87] and are not very reliable in plant-derived food allergy. However, its usefulness has been demonstrated in various food allergies and was highly sensitive and specific in diagnosis and assessment of tolerance [88, 89].

BAT is also used in drug allergy, where both in vitro tests are frequently lacking, and skin tests have limitations [90]. It has been applied to reactions to NMBA, antibiotics, nonsteroidal anti-inflammatory drugs, iodinated contrast media, and opiate with a sensitivity ranging from 50% to 60% and a specificity of 80%, except for with quinolones and NSAIDs [90–92].

In the context of hymenoptera venom allergy, where molecular diagnostics currently allow diagnosis even in the most difficult cases, BAT may be useful in patients showing double positive results for sIgE and at risk of inappropriate venom immunotherapy [93, 94], in patients with negative results and in treatment monitoring [95].

22.7 Nasal Cytology

Nasal cytology is an easy, cheap, non-invasive, and point-of-care instrument useful in the phenotyping of rhinitis.

Nasal cell specimens can be obtained with pre-weighted sinus packs or filter papers, direct aspiration with microsuction tubes, nasal brushing, nasal scraping, nasal swab, or nasal biopsy. Nasal scraping is the most routinely used, beside nasal swab in children and newborns. Nasal cytology should be performed after 7-day discontinuation of nasal and oral steroids [96]. The samples must be stained with May-Grünwald-Giemsa [97] and read at optical microscopy with

Table 22.4 Different cytological presentation of rhinitis

Disease	Eosinophils	Mast cells	Neutrophils	Bacteria	Fungal spores
Healthy	0	0	0/1+	0	0
AR	2+/4+	2+/4+	2+/4+	0	0
NARES	2+/4+	0	Variable	0	0
NARESMA	2+/4+	2+/4+		0	0
NARNE	0	0	3+/4+	0	0
Common cold	0	0	1+/4+	0	0
Bacterial	0/1+	0	3+/4+	3+/4+	0
Fungal	0	0	Variable	0	2+/4+
Atrophic	0	0	Variable	0	0

Adapted from Gelardi et al. [97]

oil immersion at 1000× magnification: white blood cell nuclei and basophil granulocyte granules are colored blue, red blood cells and eosinophil granules appear red, and white blood cell cytoplasm is light blue. At least 50 fields should be evaluated, and there should be more than 200 cells to be considered an adequate sample. The count of each cell type can be expressed in % or semi-quantitatively, according to a grading reported in the literature [98], defining different cellular patterns (Table 22.4). In the healthy subject, cells are absent or rare neutrophils are present; in RA, there are eosinophils, mast cells, and neutrophils; in NAR with eosinophils (NARES), eosinophils are found with variable presence of neutrophils; in NAR with eosinophils and mast cells (NARESMA), eosinophils and mast cells prevail; in NAR with neutrophils (NARNE), neutrophils are found; neutrophils may be present in viral rhinitis; in the bacterial one, neutrophils, bacteria, and sometimes eosinophils are found; in fungal rhinitis, fungal spores and sometimes neutrophils are observed; and neutrophils may be present in atrophic rhinitis [97].

In AR, an early histamine-mediated phase [99] and a late cell-mediated phase [100] are observed. Nasal cytology shows the presence of inflammatory cells, especially eosinophils, mast cells, neutrophils, and lymphocytes. The low level but persistent exposure, typical of perennial rhinitis, leads to a "minimal persistent inflammation," characterized by neutrophils, rare eosinophils, and mast cells, leading to a sub-chronic symptomatology [101]. In AR from mites, the months of April and October represent peak moments, and, in these periods, the eosinophilic component tends to increase [102]. In seasonal AR, during the pollen season the rhinocytogram is characterized by neutrophils, lymphocytes, and mast cells, while out of season, it will be normal [103]. Nasal cytology can be used in nasal provocation tests with the allergen [104] and in optimizing and individualizing AR treatment, as not all cell subtypes of AR respond in the same way to traditional treatments and to specific immunotherapy [105, 106].

Non-allergic vasomotor chronic rhinitis (NARNE, NARES, NARMA, and NARESMA), on a cellular basis, can only be diagnosed by cytological examination of the nasal mucosa. Furthermore, there are also "overlapped" rhinitis, due to the association of AR with non-allergic vasomotor rhinitis, in which, despite the presence of sensitization to seasonal allergens, the symptoms persist outside the typical season [107]. In these situations, nasal cytology allows to highlight the inflammatory basis of the condition and then to set a correct therapy.

22.8 Conclusions and Take-Home Messages

There are various in vitro tests available in allergy diagnosis, and none of them alone leads to the diagnosis, but they must be known and correctly inserted within the diagnostic path of the individual patient. Circulating eosinophils and ECP are non-specific markers of type 2 inflammation, associated with allergy but also with other conditions. Total serum IgE are a marker of atopy that should always be evaluated together with specific

IgE that represent a marker of sensitization to a specific allergen. The BAT is a functional assay that evaluates the IgE function, useful when the other tests are ambiguous or discordant with the clinic. Finally, nasal cytology is a point-of-care instrument that helps in phenotyping of rhinitis, essential for identifying non-allergic vasomotor chronic rhinitis and overlapped rhinitis.

References

1. Ansotegui IJ, Melioli G, Canonica GW, Caraballo L, Villa E, Ebisawa M, et al. IgE allergy diagnostics and other relevant tests in allergy, a World Allergy Organization position paper. World Allergy Organ J. 2020;13:100080.
2. Rothenberg ME, Hogan SP. The eosinophil. Annu Rev Immunol. 2006;24:147–74.
3. Weller PF. The immunobiology of eosinophils. N Engl J Med. 1991;324:1110–8.
4. Burris D, Rosenberg CE, Schwartz JT, Zhang Y, Eby MD, Abonia JP, et al. Pediatric hypereosinophilia: characteristics, clinical manifestations, and diagnoses. J Allergy Clin Immunol Pract. 2019;7:2750–2758.
5. Klion AD. How I treat hypereosinophilic syndromes. Blood. 2015;126:1069–77.
6. Valent P, Klion AD, Horny HP, Roufosse F, Gotlib J, Weller PF, et al. Contemporary consensus proposal on criteria and classification of eosinophilic disorders and related syndromes. J Allergy Clin Immunol. 2012;130:607–612.
7. Schwartz JT, Fulkerson PC. An approach to the evaluation of persistent hypereosinophilia in pediatric patients. Front Immunol. 2018;9:1944.
8. Pijnenburg MW, Fleming L. Advances in understanding and reducing the burden of severe asthma in children. Lancet Respir Med. 2020;8:1032–44.
9. Grunwell JR, Gillespie S, Morris CR, Fitzpatrick AM. Latent class analysis of school-age children at risk for asthma exacerbation. J Allergy Clin Immunol Pract. 2020;8:2275–2284.
10. Busby J, Khoo E, Pfeffer PE, Mansur AH, Heaney LG. The effects of oral corticosteroids on lung function, type-2 biomarkers and patient-reported outcomes in stable asthma: a systematic review and meta-analysis. Respir Med. 2020;173:106156.
11. Shah SP, Grunwell J, Shih J, Stephenson S, Fitzpatrick AM. Exploring the utility of noninvasive type 2 inflammatory markers for prediction of severe asthma exacerbations in children and adolescents. J Allergy Clin Immunol Pract. 2019;7:2624–2633.
12. Ortega HG, Yancey SW, Mayer B, Gunsoy NB, Keene ON, Bleecker ER, et al. Severe eosinophilic asthma treated with mepolizumab stratified by baseline eosinophil thresholds: a secondary analysis of the DREAM and MENSA studies. Lancet Respir Med. 2016;4:549–56.
13. Castro M, Zangrilli J, Wechsler ME, Bateman ED, Brusselle GG, Bardin P, et al. Reslizumab for inadequately controlled asthma with elevated blood eosinophil counts: results from two multicentre, parallel, double-blind, randomised, placebo-controlled, phase 3 trials. Lancet Respir Med. 2015;3:355–66.
14. FitzGerald JM, Bleecker ER, Nair P, Korn S, Ohta K, Lommatzsch M, et al. Benralizumab, an anti-interleukin-5 receptor α monoclonal antibody, as add-on treatment for patients with severe, uncontrolled, eosinophilic asthma (CALIMA): a randomised, double-blind, placebo-controlled phase 3 trial. Lancet. 2016;388:2128–41.
15. Castro M, Corren J, Pavord ID, Maspero J, Wenzel S, Rabe KF, et al. Dupilumab efficacy and safety in moderate-to-severe uncontrolled asthma. N Engl J Med. 2018;378:2486–96.
16. Chipps BE, Jarjour N, Calhoun WJ, Iqbal A, Haselkorn T, Yang M, et al. A comprehensive analysis of the stability of blood eosinophil levels. Ann Am Thorac Soc. 2021;18:1978–87.
17. Bernstein IL, Li JT, Bernstein DI, Hamilton R, Spector SL, Tan R, et al. Allergy diagnostic testing: an updated practice parameter. Ann Allergy Asthma Immunol. 2008;100(3 Suppl 3):S1–S148.
18. Malm-Erjefält M, Greiff L, Ankerst J, Andersson M, Wallengren J, Cardell LO, et al. Circulating eosinophils in asthma, allergic rhinitis, and atopic dermatitis lack morphological signs of degranulation. Clin Exp Allergy. 2005;35:1334–40.
19. Peterson CG, Enander I, Nystrand J, Anderson AS, Nilsson L, Venge P. Radioimmunoassay of human eosinophil cationic protein (ECP) by an improved method. Establishment of normal levels in serum and turnover *in vivo*. Clin Exp Allergy. 1991;21:561–7.
20. Bystrom J, Amin K, Bishop-Bailey D. Analysing the eosinophil cationic protein—a clue to the function of the eosinophil granulocyte. Respir Res. 2011;12:10.
21. Koh GC, Shek LP, Goh DY, Van Bever H, Koh DS. Eosinophil cationic protein: is it useful in asthma? A systematic review. Respir Med. 2007;101:696–705.
22. Björk A, Venge P, Peterson CG. Measurements of ECP in serum and the impact of plasma coagulation. Allergy. 2000;55:442–8.
23. Topic RZ, Dodig S. Eosinophil cationic protein—current concepts and controversies. Biochem Med (Zagreb). 2011;21:111–21.
24. Shah SN, Grunwell JR, Mohammad AF, Stephenson ST, Lee GB, et al. Performance of eosinophil cationic protein as a biomarker in asthmatic children. J Allergy Clin Immunol Pract. 2021;9:2761–2769.
25. Peona V, De Amici M, Quaglini S, Bellaviti G, Castellazzi AM, Marseglia G, et al. Serum eosinophilic cationic protein: is there a role in respiratory disorders? J Asthma. 2010;47:131–4.
26. Kämpe M, Stolt I, Lampinen M, Janson C, Stålenheim G, Carlson M. Patients with allergic rhi-

nitis and allergic asthma share the same pattern of eosinophil and neutrophil degranulation after allergen challenge. Clin Mol Allergy. 2011;9:3.
27. Hogan SP, Rothenberg ME. Eosinophil function in eosinophil-associated gastrointestinal disorders. Curr Allergy Asthma Rep. 2006;6:65–71.
28. Park YJ, Oh EJ, Park JW, Kim M, Han K. Plasma eosinophil cationic protein, interleukin-5, and ECP/Eo count ratio in patients with various eosinophilic diseases. Ann Clin Lab Sci. 2006;36:262–6.
29. Martinelli-Kläy CP, Mendis BR, Lombardi T. Eosinophils and oral squamous cell carcinoma: a short review. J Oncol. 2009;2009:310132.
30. Hoshino M, Nakamura Y. Relationship between activated eosinophils of the bronchial mucosa and serum eosinophil cationic protein in atopic asthma. Int Arch Allergy Immunol. 1997;112:59–64.
31. Yasuda H, Suzuki T, Zayasu K, Ishizuka S, Kubo H, Sasaki T, et al. Inflammatory and bronchospastic factors in asthma exacerbations caused by upper respiratory tract infections. Tohoku J Exp Med. 2005;207:109–18.
32. Bartoli ML, Bacci E, Carnevali S, Cianchetti S, Dente FL, Di Franco A, et al. Clinical assessment of asthma severity partially corresponds to sputum eosinophilic airway inflammation. Respir Med. 2004;98:184–93.
33. Badar A, Saeed W, Hussain MM, Aslam M. Correlation of eosinophil cationic protein with severity of asthma. J Ayub Med Coll Abbottabad. 2004;16:66–71.
34. Joseph-Bowen J, de Klerk N, Holt PG, Sly PD. Relationship of asthma, atopy, and bronchial responsiveness to serum eosinophil cationic proteins in early childhood. J Allergy Clin Immunol. 2004;114:1040–5.
35. Prehn A, Seger RA, Torresani T, Molinari L, Sennhauser FH. Evaluation of a clinical algorithm involving serum eosinophil cationic protein for guiding the anti-inflammatory treatment of bronchial asthma in childhood. Pediatr Allergy Immunol. 2000;11:87–94.
36. Basyigit I, Yildiz F, Kacar Ozkara S, Boyaci H, Ilgazli A, Ozkarakas O. Effects of different antiasthmatic agents on induced sputum and eosinophil cationic protein in mild asthmatics. Respirology. 2004;9:514–20.
37. Kandil AA, Hasan A, Taha O, El-Mesallamy H. Eosinophil cationic protein as a diagnostic marker for asthmatic children treated by immunotherapy. Egypt J Immunol. 2003;10:67–76.
38. Ahlstrom-Emanuelsson CA, Greiff L, Andersson M, Persson CG, Erjefält JS. Eosinophil degranulation status in allergic rhinitis: observations before and during seasonal allergen exposure. Eur Respir J. 2004;24:750–7.
39. Yu J, Yoo Y, Kim DK, Kang H, Koh YY. Bronchial responsiveness and serum eosinophil cationic protein levels in preschool children with recurrent wheezing. Ann Allergy Asthma Immunol. 2005;94:686–92.
40. Niehaus MD, Gwaltney JM Jr, Hendley JO, Newman MJ, Heymann PW, Rakes GP, et al. Lactoferrin and eosinophilic cationic protein in nasal secretions of patients with experimental rhinovirus colds, natural colds, and presumed acute community-acquired bacterial sinusitis. J Clin Microbiol. 2000;38:3100–2.
41. Grunberg K, Smits HH, Timmers MC, de Klerk EP, Dolhain RJ, Dick EC, et al. Experimental rhinovirus 16 infection. Effects on cell differentials and soluble markers in sputum in asthmatic subjects. Am J Respir Crit Care Med. 1997;156(2 Part 1):609–16.
42. Hyvärinen MK, Kotaniemi-Syrjänen A, Reijonen TM, Piippo-Savolainen E, Korppi M. Eosinophil activity in infants hospitalized for wheezing and risk of persistent childhood asthma. Pediatr Allergy Immunol. 2010;21(1 Pt 1):96–103.
43. Jung YG, Kim KH, Kim HY, Dhong HJ, Chung SK. Predictive capabilities of serum eosinophil cationic protein, percentage of eosinophils and total immunoglobulin E in allergic rhinitis without bronchial asthma. J Int Med Res. 2011;39:2209–16.
44. Min HJ, Hong YH, Yang HS, Kim KS. The correlation of serum eosinophil cationic protein level with eosinophil count, and total IgE level in Korean adult allergic rhinitis patients. Asian Pac J Allergy Immunol. 2016;34:33–7.
45. Hsu PY, Yang YH, Lin YT, Chiang BL. Serum eosinophil cationic protein level and disease activity in childhood rhinitis. Asian Pac J Allergy Immunol. 2004;22:19–24.
46. Murat-Susić S, Lipozencić J, Zizić V, Husar K, Marinović B. Serum eosinophil cationic protein in children with atopic dermatitis. Int J Dermatol. 2006;45:1156–60.
47. Kim J, Kim S, Lee YI, Kim J, Lee JH, Park CO. Eosinophil cationic protein is a potential surrogate marker of allergic contact dermatitis: a single-center, retrospective study of 216 patients. J Am Acad Dermatol. 2020;83:1819–21.
48. Johansson SG. The history of IgE: from discovery to 2010. Curr Allergy Asthma Rep. 2011;11:173–7.
49. Lebman DA, Coffman RL. Interleukin 4 causes isotype switching to IgE in T cell-stimulated clonal B cell cultures. J Exp Med. 1988;168:853–62.
50. Punnonen J, de Vries JE. IL-13 induces proliferation, Ig isotype switching, and Ig synthesis by immature human fetal B cells. J Immunol. 1994;152:1094–102.
51. Gould HJ, Sutton BJ, Beavil AJ, Beavil RL, McCloskey N, Coker HA, et al. The biology of IGE and the basis of allergic disease. Annu Rev Immunol. 2003;21:579–628.
52. Hamilton RG, Adkinson NF Jr. Clinical laboratory assessment of IgE-dependent hypersensitivity. J Allergy Clin Immunol. 2003;111(2 Suppl):S687–701.
53. Sacco C, Perna S, Vicari D, Alfò M, Bauer CP, Hoffman U, et al. Growth curves of "normal" serum total IgE levels throughout childhood: a quantile analysis in a birth cohort. Pediatr Allergy Immunol. 2017;28:525–34.

54. Novak N, Bieber T. Allergic and nonallergic forms of atopic diseases. J Allergy Clin Immunol. 2003;112:252–62.
55. Saarinen UM, Juntunen K, Kajosaari M, Björkstén F. Serum immunoglobulin E in atopic and non-atopic children aged 6 months to 5 years. A follow-up study. Acta Paediatr Scand. 1982;71:489–94.
56. Dodig S, Richter D, Benko B, Zivcić J, Raos M, Nogalo B, et al. Cut-off values for total serum immunoglobulin E between non-atopic and atopic children in north-west Croatia. Clin Chem Lab Med. 2006;44:639–47.
57. Luker AJ, Lownik JC, Conrad DH, Martin RK. A new look at IgE beyond allergies. F1000Res. 2019;8:736.
58. Ozcan E, Notarangelo LD, Geha RS. Primary immune deficiencies with aberrant IgE production. J Allergy Clin Immunol. 2008;122:1054–64.
59. Nafría Jiménez B, Oliveros Conejero R. IgE multiple myeloma: detection and follow-up. Adv Lab Med. 2021;3:79–90.
60. Berciano FA, Crespo M, Bao CG, Alvarez FV. Serum levels of total IgE in non-allergic children. Influence of genetic and environmental factors. Allergy. 1987;42:276–83.
61. Hu Y, Liu S, Liu P, Mu Z, Zhang J. Clinical relevance of eosinophils, basophils, serum total IgE level, allergen-specific IgE, and clinical features in atopic dermatitis. J Clin Lab Anal. 2020;34:e23214.
62. Kiiski V, Karlsson O, Remitz A, Reitamo S. High serum total IgE predicts poor long-term outcome in atopic dermatitis. Acta Derm Venereol. 2015;95:943–7.
63. Asano K, Hebisawa A, Ishiguro T, Takayanagi N, Nakamura Y, Suzuki J, et al. New clinical diagnostic criteria for allergic bronchopulmonary aspergillosis/mycosis and its validation. J Allergy Clin Immunol. 2021;147:1261–1268.
64. Davila I, Valero A, Entrenas LM, Valveny N, Herráez L, SIGE Study Group. Relationship between serum total IgE and disease severity in patients with allergic asthma in Spain. J Investig Allergol Clin Immunol. 2015;25:120–7.
65. Naqvi M, Choudhry S, Tsai HJ, Thyne S, Navarro D, Nazario S, et al. Association between IgE levels and asthma severity among African American, Mexican, and Puerto Rican patients with asthma. J Allergy Clin Immunol. 2007;120:137–43.
66. Wide L, Bennich H, Johansson SG. Diagnosis of allergy by an in-vitro test for allergen antibodies. Lancet. 1967;2:1105–7.
67. Goldstein MD, Hamilton RG. AAAAI Work Group Report: Allergy diagnosis in clinical practice. 2006.
68. Hamilton RG, Franklin Adkinson N Jr. In vitro assays for the diagnosis of IgE-mediated disorders. J Allergy Clin Immunol. 2004;114:213–26.
69. Yunginger JW, Ahlstedt S, Eggleston PA, Homburger HA, Nelson HS, Ownby DR, et al. Quantitative IgE antibody assays in allergic diseases. J Allergy Clin Immunol. 2000;105(6 Pt 1):1077–84.
70. Larsen JN, Dreborg S. Standardization of allergen extracts. Methods Mol Biol. 2019;2020:63–76.
71. Cox L, Williams B, Sicherer S, Oppenheimer J, Sher L, Hamilton R, et al. Pearls and pitfalls of allergy diagnostic testing: report from the American College of Allergy, Asthma and Immunology/American Academy of Allergy, Asthma and Immunology Specific IgE Test Task Force. Ann Allergy Asthma Immunol. 2008;101:580–92.
72. Federly TJ, Jones BL, Dai H, Dinakar C. Interpretation of food specific immunoglobulin E levels in the context of total IgE. Ann Allergy Asthma Immunol. 2013;111:20–4.
73. Duc J, Peitrequin R, Pécoud A. Value of a new screening test for respiratory allergy. Allergy. 1988;43:332–7.
74. Ballardini N, Nilsson C, Nilsson M, Lilja G. ImmunoCAP Phadiatop Infant—a new blood test for detecting IgE sensitisation in children at 2 years of age. Allergy. 2006;61:337–43
75. Wood RA, Schuberth KC, Sampson HA. Value of a multiantigen radioallergosorbent test in diagnosing atopic disease in young children. J Pediatr. 1990;117:882–5.
76. Santos AF, Brough HA. Making the most of in vitro tests to diagnose food allergy [published correction appears in J Allergy Clin Immunol Pract. 2017;5:875]. J Allergy Clin Immunol Pract. 2017;5:237–48.
77. LaHood NA, Patil SU. Food allergy testing. Clin Lab Med. 2019;39:625–42.
78. Decuyper II, Ebo DG, Uyttebroek AP, Hagendorens MM, Faber MA, Bridts CH, et al. Quantification of specific IgE antibodies in immediate drug hypersensitivity: more shortcomings than potentials? Clin Chim Acta. 2016;460:184–9.
79. Bridts CH, Sabato V, Mertens C, Hagendorens MM, De Clerck LS, Ebo DG. Flow cytometric allergy diagnosis: basophil activation techniques. Methods Mol Biol. 2014;1192:147–59.
80. Hemmings O, Kwok M, McKendry R, Santos AF. Basophil activation test: old and new applications in allergy [published correction appears in Curr Allergy Asthma Rep. 2019 Nov 27;19(12):58]. Curr Allergy Asthma Rep. 2018;18:77.
81. Santos AF, Alpan O, Hoffmann HJ. Basophil activation test: mechanisms and considerations for use in clinical trials and clinical practice. Allergy. 2021;76:2420–32.
82. Hoffmann HJ, Santos AF, Mayorga C, Nopp A, Eberlein B, Ferrer M, et al. The clinical utility of basophil activation testing in diagnosis and monitoring of allergic disease. Allergy. 2015;70:1393–405.
83. Pascal M, Nopp A, Mayorga C, Edelman S, Santos AF, Ebo D et al. Building confidence in the basophil activation test: standardization and external quality assurance—an EAACI task force. 2020. Paper presented at European-Academy-of-Allergology-and--Clinical-Immunology Digital Congress (EAACI), London.

84. Sturm GJ, Kranzelbinder B, Sturm EM, Heinemann A, Groselj-Strele A, Aberer W. The basophil activation test in the diagnosis of allergy: technical issues and critical factors. Allergy. 2009;64:1319–26.
85. Puan KJ, Andiappan AK, Lee B, Kumar D, Lai TS, Yeo G, et al. Systematic characterization of basophil anergy. Allergy. 2017;72:373–84.
86. Sabato V, van Hengel AJ, De Knop KJ, Verweij MM, Hagendorens MM, Bridts CH, et al. Basophil activation reveals divergent patient-specific responses to thermally processed peanuts. J Investig Allergol Clin Immunol. 2011;21:527–31.
87. Sato S, Tachimoto H, Shukuya A, Ogata M, Komata T, Imai T, et al. Utility of the peripheral blood basophil histamine release test in the diagnosis of hen's egg, cow's milk, and wheat allergy in children. Int Arch Allergy Immunol. 2011;155(Suppl 1):96–103.
88. Glaumann S, Nopp A, Johansson SG, Rudengren M, Borres MP, Nilsson C. Basophil allergen threshold sensitivity, CD-sens, IgE-sensitization and DBPCFC in peanut-sensitized children. Allergy. 2012;67:242–7.
89. Mangodt EA, Van Gasse AL, Decuyper I, Uyttebroek A, Faber MA, Sabato V, et al. In vitro diagnosis of immediate drug hypersensitivity: should we go with the flow. Int Arch Allergy Immunol. 2015;168(1):3–12.
90. Van Gasse AL, Sabato V, Uyttebroek AP, Elst J, Faber MA, Hagendorens MM, et al. Immediate moxifloxacin hypersensitivity: is there more than currently meets the eye? Allergy. 2017;72(12):2039–43.
91. Van Gasse AL, Hagendorens MM, Sabato V, Bridts CH, De Clerck LS, Ebo DG. IgE to poppy seed and morphine are not useful tools to diagnose opiate allergy. J Allergy Clin Immunol Pract. 2015;3:396–9.
92. Nemsovska J, Waczulikova I, Svecova D. Basophil activation test in the diagnostics of hymenoptera venom allergy. Bratisl Lek Listy. 2021;122:778–84.
93. Schmidle P, Blank S, Altrichter S, Hoetzenecker W, Brockow K, Darsow U, et al. Basophil activation test in double-sensitized patients with hymenoptera venom allergy: additional benefit of component-resolved diagnostics. J Allergy Clin Immunol Pract. 2023;11:2890–99.
94. Nullens S, Sabato V, Faber M, Leysen J, Bridts CH, De Clerck LS, et al. Basophilic histamine content and release during venom immunotherapy: insights by flow cytometry. Cytometry B Clin Cytom. 2013;84:173–8.
95. Ciprandi G, Ricca V, Paola F, Alessandra B, Riccio AM, Milanese M, et al. Duration of antiinflammatory and symptomatic effects after suspension of intranasal corticosteroid in persistent allergic rhinitis. Eur Ann Allergy Clin Immunol. 2004;36:63–6.
96. Gelardi M, Iannuzzi L, Quaranta N, Landi M, Passalacqua G. NASAL cytology: practical aspects and clinical relevance. Clin Exp Allergy. 2016;46:785–92.
97. Meltzer EO, Jalowayski AA. Nasal cytology in clinical practice. Am J Rhinol. 1988;2:47–54.
98. Pelikan Z, Pelikan-Filipek M. Cytologic changes in the nasal secretions during the immediate nasal response [published correction appears in J Allergy Clin Immunol 1989 May;83(5):870]. J Allergy Clin Immunol. 1988;82:1103–12.
99. Pelikan Z, Pelikan-Filipek M. Cytologic changes in the nasal secretions during the late nasal response. J Allergy Clin Immunol. 1989;83:1068–79.
100. Ciprandi G, Buscaglia S, Pesce G, Pronzato C, Ricca V, Parmiani S, et al. Minimal persistent inflammation is present at mucosal level in patients with asymptomatic rhinitis and mite allergy. J Allergy Clin Immunol. 1995;96(6 Pt 1):971–9.
101. Gelardi M, Peroni DG, Incorvaia C, Quaranta N, De Luca C, Barberi S, et al. Seasonal changes in nasal cytology in mite-allergic patients. J Inflamm Res. 2014;7:39–44.
102. Heffler E, Landi M, Caruso C, Fichera S, Gani F, Guida G, et al. Nasal cytology: methodology with application to clinical practice and research. Clin Exp Allergy. 2018;48:1092–106.
103. Hellings PW, Scadding G, Alobid I, Bachert C, Fokkens WJ, Gerth van Wijk R, et al. Executive summary of European Task Force document on diagnostic tools in rhinology. Rhinology. 2012;50:339–52.
104. Chen J, Zhou Y, Zhang L, Wang Y, Pepper AN, Cho SH, et al. Individualized treatment of allergic rhinitis according to nasal cytology. Allergy Asthma Immunol Res. 2017;9 :403–9.
105. Gelardi M, Russo C, Fiorella ML, Fiorella R, Canonica GW, Passalacqua G. When allergic rhinitis is not only allergic. Am J Rhinol Allergy. 2009;23:312–5.
106. Jiang H, Harris MB, Rothman P. IL-4/IL-13 signaling beyond JAK/STAT. J Allergy Clin Immunol. 2000;105(6 Pt 1):1063–70.
107. Jura-Szołtys E, Gawlik R, Branicka O, Stryjewska-Makuch G, Glück J. Nasal cytology can predict clinical efficacy of subcutaneous immunotherapy in intermittent allergic rhinitis. Postepy Dermatol Alergol. 2022;39:1110–5.

Molecular Diagnosis in Pediatric Allergy

23

Paolo Maria Matricardi and Alexandra Santos

Abstract

The advent of molecular biology has had a great impact on our understanding of IgE-mediated allergic diseases. In particular, new tests have been developed for in vitro diagnostics of respiratory and food allergies, some of which specifically suited to the pediatric age. In this chapter, we first review the most important basic concepts and definitions of molecular allergology; then, we specifically talk about molecular advances in diagnostics of allergic rhinitis and asthma and of atopic dermatitis and other diseases associated with allergic reactions to foods. After having discussed how IgE and allergen molecules interact on the surface of degranulating cells (basophils, mast cells), we present the evolution of total IgE levels and of specific IgE responses in childhood. In particular, we describe how the IgE response expands from one to more molecules of the same allergen source and discuss how this observation has modified our understanding of immunological intervention, pointing our attention on earlier diagnosis, immunotherapy, and even allergen-specific immunoprophylaxis. We also give some examples of how molecular IgE tests not only address biomarkers of specific phenotypes of allergic rhinitis, disease severity, and comorbidities (oral allergy syndrome, asthma) but also how they help in the identification of the culprit allergen for a more precise prescription of allergen immunotherapy. Then, we present the evolution of IgE responses to food allergens in childhood, and we illustrate the biomarkers of primary food allergy and other molecules, associated with less severe allergic reactions. Last, we focus on the trends of IgE antibody levels during spontaneous resolution of food allergy and on the role of IgG4 antibodies in accompanying this process.

P. M. Matricardi (✉)
Department of Pediatric Pulmonology, Immunology and Intensive Care Medicine, Charité—University Medicine Berlin, Berlin, Germany

Institute of Allergology, Charité-Universitätsmedizin Berlin, Berlin, Germany

Fraunhofer Institute for Translational Medicine and Pharmacology ITMP, Berlin, Germany
e-mail: paolo.matricardi@charite.de

A. Santos
Department of Women and Children's Health (Pediatric Allergy), School of Life Course Sciences, Faculty of Life Sciences and Medicine, King's College London, London, UK

Peter Gorer Department of Immunobiology, School of Immunology and Microbial Sciences, King's College London, London, UK

Children's Allergy Service, Evelina London Children's Hospital, Guy's and St Thomas' Hospital, London, UK
e-mail: alexandra.santos@kcl.ac.uk

C. Caffarelli, G. L. Marseglia (eds.), *Textbook of Pediatric Allergy*,
https://doi.org/10.1007/978-3-031-71283-8_23

Keywords

B-cell epitopes · Cross-reactive molecules · Allergen family · Inducer and elicitor molecules · Panallergens · Genuine molecules · Initiator molecules · Molecular spreading · Major and minor allergenic molecules · Specific activity · Very low IgE producers · Component resolved diagnostics (CRD) · Singleplex and multiplex IgE tests · Allergen microarrays · IgE antibodies · Basophil degranulation · Mast-cell activation · Fc-epsilon receptors · Allergen molecules · Molecular spreading · Allergen-specific immunotherapy · Sensitization stages · Cross-reactivity

Test your learning and check your understanding of this book's contents: use the "Springer Nature Flashcards" app to access questions using ▶ https://sn.pub/nspbjm. To use the app, please follow the instructions in Chap. 1.

23.1 Molecular Diagnosis in Allergology: A Short Introduction

23.1.1 Historical Background

Since over two decades, the in vitro diagnostics of IgE-mediated diseases, previously based mostly on serological assays measuring IgE antibodies against allergen extracts, has been expanded to include serological IgE tests against allergenic molecules. While the former include allergenic and non-allergic molecules "extracted" from an allergenic source, the latter includes the allergenic molecules only, either in a native form or produced with recombinant DNA technology [1]. This "component resolved diagnostics" [1, 2] has several advantages, being more precise, standardized, and informative [3]. More precise, as the quantitative information obtained by molecular assays is more reliable; more standardized, as different extraction and purification procedures are used by different manufacturers, so that the content in allergenic molecules of extracts is highly variable; more informative, as the information obtained allows distinguishing between genuine form cross-reactive sensitization to an allergen source [4].

The first pollen allergenic molecule whose primary sequence has been fully characterized and examined is Lol p 1 [5], while the first publication on allergen molecules produced with recombinant DNA technology appeared in 1988 [6]. Since then, the number and diversity of allergenic molecules available in commercial IgE assays has increased in the last 20 years from a few dozens to over 200, while the allergen molecules produced with rDNA technology are over 1600, of which about 1000 were already recognized by IUIS in 2021 [7]. The first international Symposium on Molecular Allergology was organized by Adriano Mari in Rome in 2005 and the first textbook of molecular allergology was produced and published in 2016 by EAACI [8] and recently upgraded and updated in its second edition [9]. The first IgE assays based on individual allergenic molecules were radioallergosorbent test (RAST) (Pharmacia, Uppsala, Sweden) and limited mainly to native molecules purified from milk, such as beta-lactoglobulin [10], while the first allergen microarray for IgE antibody testing was conceived in 2002 [11]. Many other singleplex, multiplex, micro- or macro-array, standard, or customized tests based on allergenic molecules have been developed in the last 10 years and a growing users' market is accompanied by a parallel expansion of product diversification [12].

23.2 Molecular Allergology: A Few Basic Concepts

A few immunological concepts must be concisely recapitulated before talking of molecular IgE tests for respiratory and food allergies in childhood: B-cell epitopes, cross-reactivity, genuine molecule, panallergen, molecular biomarkers, initiator molecule, molecular spreading, major and minor allergen molecules, specific activity, and others.

- **B-Cell Epitopes**—B-cell epitopes are small shapes, mostly at the surface of the tridimensional structure of the allergenic molecule, which are recognized by the antigen-binding sites of the membrane-bound B-cell receptor and of the respective soluble immunoglobulin [13].
- **Cross-Reactive Molecules**—Molecules containing similar B-cell epitopes are called also cross-reactive molecules, as antibodies induced by the B-cell epitopes of one of them can bind the same B-cell epitope on the others [14].
- **Allergen Family**—Molecules playing important roles and function for life are more frequently conserved during the evolution and can be found, with modifications in the primary sequence, in other species and they form a so-called "family" [15].
- **Inducer and Elicitor Molecules**—Hence, for IgE antibodies, sensitization induced by a molecule (inducer) may trigger reactions also when the patient is exposed to the molecules (elicitors) members of the same family [16].
- **Panallergens**—In general, cross-reactivity between two molecules of the same family and the similarity of their B-cell epitopes is the highest when the respective species are very close in the evolutionary tree. Allergen molecules highly spread over a relevant number of unrelated species are called "panallergens" [17].
- **Genuine Molecules**—At the other extreme, "genuine" molecules are those belonging only to a restricted number of species so that IgE antibodies to one of them is a marker of sensitization induced by its respective allergenic source [18].
- **Initiator Molecules**—Some allergen molecules are able to start an IgE response against an allergen source and are therefore called "initiators" or "initiator molecule" [19].
- **Molecular Spreading**—In many patients, the IgE response against an allergen source start monomolecular with an initiator and spread with time by involving other allergenic molecules of the same allergenic source, becoming oligomolecular (2–4 molecules are recognized by the patient's IgE antibodies) and finally polymolecular (5 or more molecules are recognized by IgE antibodies) [20].
- **Major and Minor Allergenic Molecules**—Major and minor allergenic molecules are those recognized by the IgE antibodies of more or less of 50% of the patients sensitized to the allergen source these molecules belong to [21].
- **Specific Activity**—Specific activity of the IgE antibodies is the percentage of the serum concentration of IgE toward a molecule and the concentration of serum total IgE. Together with the absolute IgE-Ab concentration, specific activity is the most important parameter in determining whether the mast cells or the basophils of a sensitized patient will degranulate once exposed to sufficient amount of that molecule [22, 23].
- **Very Low IgE Producers**—A tiny fraction of people live with very low total serum levels of IgE and have been called "very low IgE producers." When these patients become sensitized, even very low levels of specific IgE antibodies may be of high clinical relevance, as their specific activity will be high due to a low level of their total serum IgE [24].
- **Component Resolved Diagnostics (CRD)**—The concept of examining the sensitization profile of a patient at a molecular resolution level, i.e., at the level of the individual, different components contained in an allergen extract [1].
- **Singleplex and Multiplex IgE Tests**—IgE tests for one single or multiple reagent (extracts and/or molecules) [25].
- **Allergen Microarrays**—Nanotechnological IgE tests based on many dozens or hundreds of reagents (extracts and/or molecules) printed or spotted on a small surface. This technique allows to test with a few microliters of serum the presence of IgE antibodies against a very large panel of allergens [26].

23.2.1 IgE and Allergen Molecules for Basophil and Mast-Cell Degranulation: A Complex Interaction

IgE are antibodies interacting through their third domain of their two constant heavy chains (CH_3) with the high- and low-affinity fragment C (Fc) receptors on basophils and mast cells [27, 28]. Each basophil or mast cell can carry up to hundred thousands IgE molecules bound on its surface, whose repertoire is largely dependent by the local and systemic (bone marrow) IgE production by IgE-producing cells of the B lineage [29]. Basophil and mast cell degranulation is a quantitative, progressive phenomenon whose intensity is dependent on cross-linking of Fc-epsilon receptors on their membrane [30]. By simultaneously linking through their B-cell epitopes the antigen-binding sites of contiguous IgE antibodies, allergens cause activation of the Fce receptor and signal transduction ending up in degranulation [31]. The activation and the intensity of the degranulation is dependent on a series of factors, the most important ones being the absolute concentration of IgE to a given allergen molecule and their specific activity, followed by the affinity and clonal diversity of the IgE antibodies [22]. IgG or other antibodies interfering in the allergen-IgE interaction (e.g., blocking IgG1 or IgG4 antibodies) also interfere and regulate the intensity of basophil and mast cell degranulation upon their exposure to the allergen molecule [32].

This textbook knowledge premise is essential to introduce the high complexity of the function of IgE antibodies and to recognize how the simple measure of the serum concentration of IgE antibodies against an individual allergen molecule is only an indirect predictor of their biological and clinical relevance. In particular, it should be reminded that multiple bridging of IgE antibodies on the degranulating cell membrane, given a certain absolute concentration, is inversely proportional to their total IgE levels. IgE not recognizing the molecule(s) of the culprit allergen compete for the same Fce receptors on the membrane of the degranulating cell and, by sterically interfering with the bridging phenomenon, inhibit degranulation [33]. On the other hand, even very low amount of IgE antibodies specific for a given allergen molecule may trigger degranulation if the overall amount of IgE is also low and the IgE antibody-specific activity is high [23, 34]. A logic consequence of this phenomenon is that the level of total IgE in the serum is one of the predictors of the biological and clinical relevance of IgE antibodies [24].

23.2.2 The Evolution of Total and Specific IgE in Childhood

Opposite to IgG levels, total serum IgE levels may vary up to 10,000 times in the general population of westernized, helminth-free humans [35]. Non-atopic subjects can live well with 1 or with 1000 kU/l of total IgE levels [36]. Growth charts of total IgE levels in childhood show their increasing trend in the first decade of life, a plateau at adolescence, followed by a slight decline [37]. While trajectories of never-atopic children tend to maintain the same shape, their levels vary according to their percentile; the onset of an atopic response also determines a upward deviation out of the child's own percentile [37]. Consequently, a "very low IgE producer" child (e.g., <10th percentile) may become atopic even with total IgE levels considered "normal" for the general population. In this category of children, very low level of IgE-specific antibodies to a certain allergen molecule may trigger degranulation. Such a condition is not infrequent in childhood and it is very important for the interpretation of molecular IgE tests in very low IgE producing but allergic children (see below) [24, 38] (Fig. 23.1).

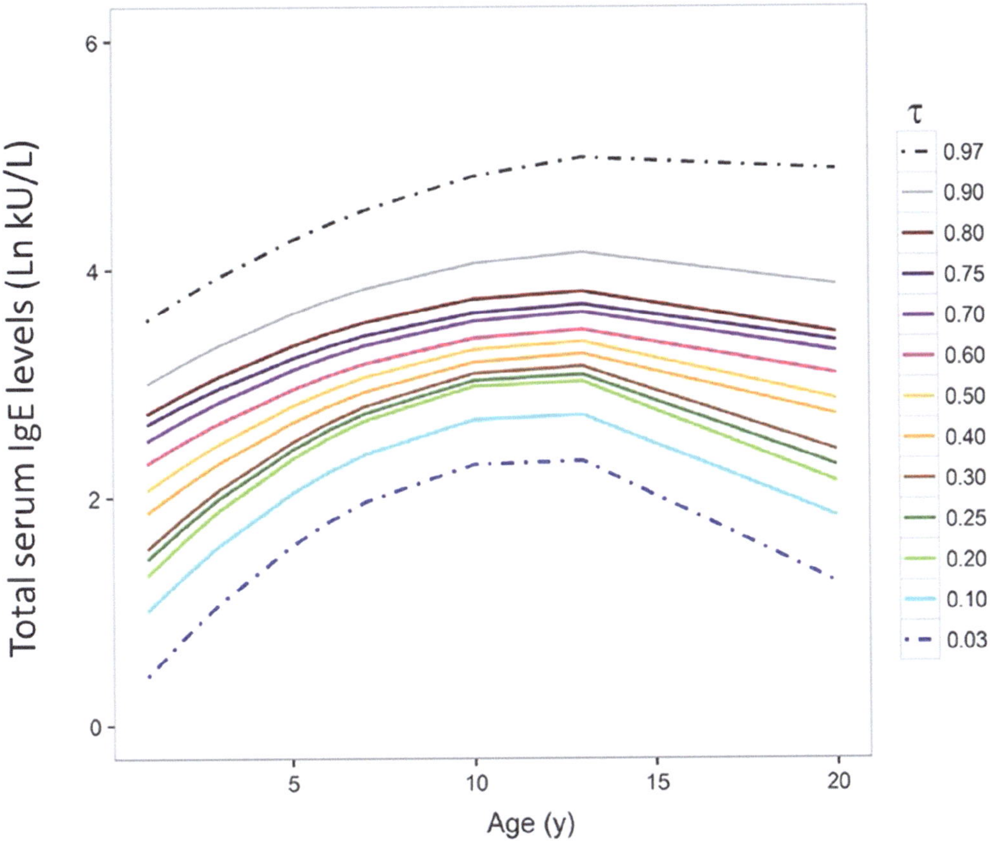

Fig. 23.1 Growth chart IgE. Quantile trajectories of predicted log-transformed t-IgE levels (kU/L) by age estimated in the population of "never atopic" subjects ($n = 466$) after the evaluation of quantile regression model for longitudinal data applied considering 13 quantiles (0.03, 0.10, 0.20, 0.25, 0.30, 0.40, 0.50, 0.60, 0.70, 0.75, 0.80, 0.90, 0.97). Quantile trajectories of absolute t-IgE levels (log (kU/L) between two consecutive follow-ups are shown, where the values 0, 2, 4, 6 of t-IgE levels in log-units (kU/L) correspond to 1.00, 7.39, 54.60, 403.43 kU/L. (Adapted from [37], under OA Creative Common CC BY license)

23.3 Molecular Allergology in Pediatrics

23.3.1 The Evolution of IgE Responses to Airborne Allergens in Childhood

23.3.1.1 Specific IgE, Initiators, Molecular Spreading, and Its Clinical Implications

Sero-epidemiological studies in birth cohorts have shown that the IgE sensitization to grass pollen starts extremely frequently with a response to Phl p 1, alone or in combination with other molecules, then involves Phl p 5 and Phl p 4, then Phl p 2, Phl p 6 and Phl p 11, last Phl p Phl p 12 and Phl p 7 [20]. While some sensitized humans remain at the monomolecular sensitization stage, others pass through the oligomolecular to reach the polymolecular one, especially if they are generated by atopic parents [39]. A similar evolution has been described in the same cohort for mite-allergic children [40]. IgE sensitization to Dermatophagoides pteronyssinus almost invariably starts with IgE sensitization to Der p 1, to Der p 2 or Der p 23 (alone or in combination) (molecules of the group "A"), then move to Der p 4, Der p 5, Der p 7, Der p 21 (group "B" molecules), to end up to Der p 11, Der p 14, Der p 15,

Der p 16, Der p 18, and other molecules (Group "C" molecules) [41]. Again, some patients do not make any progress and remain at stage "A" of sensitization, while other move until stage "AB" and some of these even to stage "ABC" [41]. The sensitization stage has diagnostic value, as those patients reaching a stage "ABC" are also more frequently affected by allergic asthma. Like for grass pollen, progression from one stage to the following one is influenced by atopic background (parents with hay fever). However, a higher exposure to mite allergens in early childhood is also facilitating molecular spreading [41]. This process has been confirmed in independent studies in other cohorts. For example, early sensitization to multiple molecules was associated with allergic asthma in the BAMSE cohort [42]. Similarly, a spreading in molecular IgE sensitization has been observed in the MAAS cohort [43]. A comprehensive testing of the MAS cohort with the ISAC microarray technique has also allowed confirmed of a list of expected initiators, including Fel d 1 for cat, Bet v 1 for birch, and others [44]. An obvious implication of the molecular spreading phenomenon is the need of earlier therapeutic ore even preventive intervention with allergen-specific approaches in early childhood [45] (Fig. 23.2).

23.3.1.2 Dual Function, Inverse Relation Grass Mites

One would expect that subjects undergoing molecular spreading to one allergen source also develop a polymolecular, intensive response to other allergens source. A recent study is showing that in the majority of the cases this is not the case. In particular, cross-sectional studies in childhood have shown that pollen-allergic children with a molecularly spread response to grass pollen tend to develop only low level, oligo or monomolecular response to Dermatophagoides pteronyssinus [46]. This pattern of response is confirming observations of different cluster of patients separating subjects with predominant response to grass pollen from those with predominant response to mites [47]. This apparently

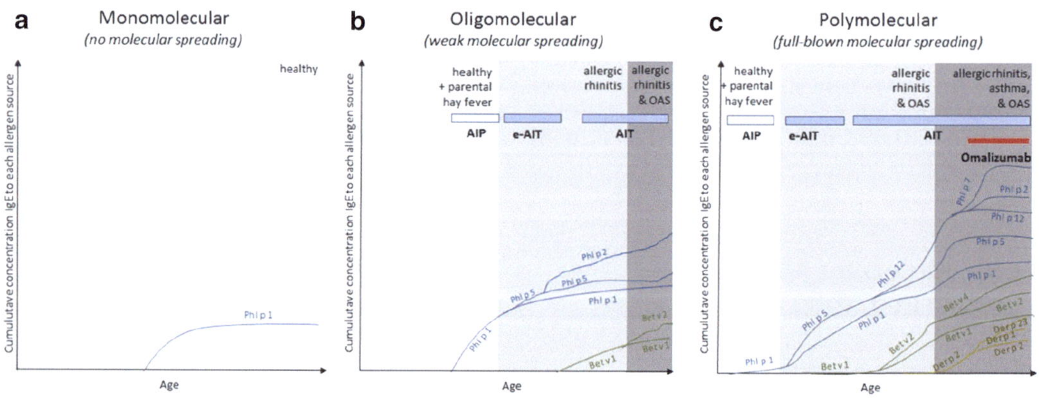

Fig. 23.2 Molecular spreading and its therapeutic implications in pediatric allergy. Timing and targets of immunologic intervention according to the stage of the IgE response. (**a**) Patient with persistent monomolecular sensitization (not undergoing molecular spreading). (**b**) Patient with modest molecular spreading, reaching an oligomolecular sensitization to 1 allergen source only. (**c**) Patient with intensive molecular spreading to three different allergen sources. In clinical practice, AIT would be normally prescribed at an advanced stage after some years of symptoms. An interesting hypothesis is that AIT would be more efficient if started much earlier, ideally at disease onset (early AIT [e-AIT]). Moreover, it could be investigated whether an immune intervention at the earliest preclinical stages of disease could even better change the natural history of the sensitization and prevent or delay disease onset (AIP). Finally, in patients with extreme polysensitization and comorbidities, AIT might have less chance of success, and experimental use anti-IgE therapy, addressing simultaneously multiple IgE responses and comorbidities, could be considered. (Reproduced from [45], with permission)

strange observation might be explained by the above-described dual role of IgE antibodies, i.e., aggressive in the presence of their allergen, and protective in their absence, according to a receptor saturation phenomenon already described in the 70s [48]. The development and expansion of an IgE response to mite allergen may be inhibited by an already established broad and intensive response to grass pollen. In other words, the first response would always have a higher specific activity than the second. Interestingly, some children escape this rule and develop broad responses to both, grass pollen allergen and mite allergen, indicating that in a minority of cases other factors are also relevant. The group of children polymolecularly sensitized to both grass pollen and mite allergens constitute a separate and well-differentiated cluster confirmed in other birth cohort studies [47, 49].

23.3.1.3 Testing IgE to Allergen Molecules in Children with Allergic Rhinitis and Asthma

The observation that initiator molecules start the IgE response has a lot of implications for screening, early diagnosis, and prevention of respiratory allergic diseases in childhood. First, it has been possible to design a novel screening test for respiratory allergies, specifically dedicated to early childhood, based on a mix of initiator molecules [49] (Fig. 23.3). Although the molecular composition was still suboptimal, the test has already demonstrated at a first evaluation a very high sensitivity and optimal specificity in identifying sensitization to airborne allergens in childhood [49]. In addition, the test (NOVEOS, HYCOR, USA) is using only 4 μL of serum, thus facilitating its use in a pediatric environment [50, 51].

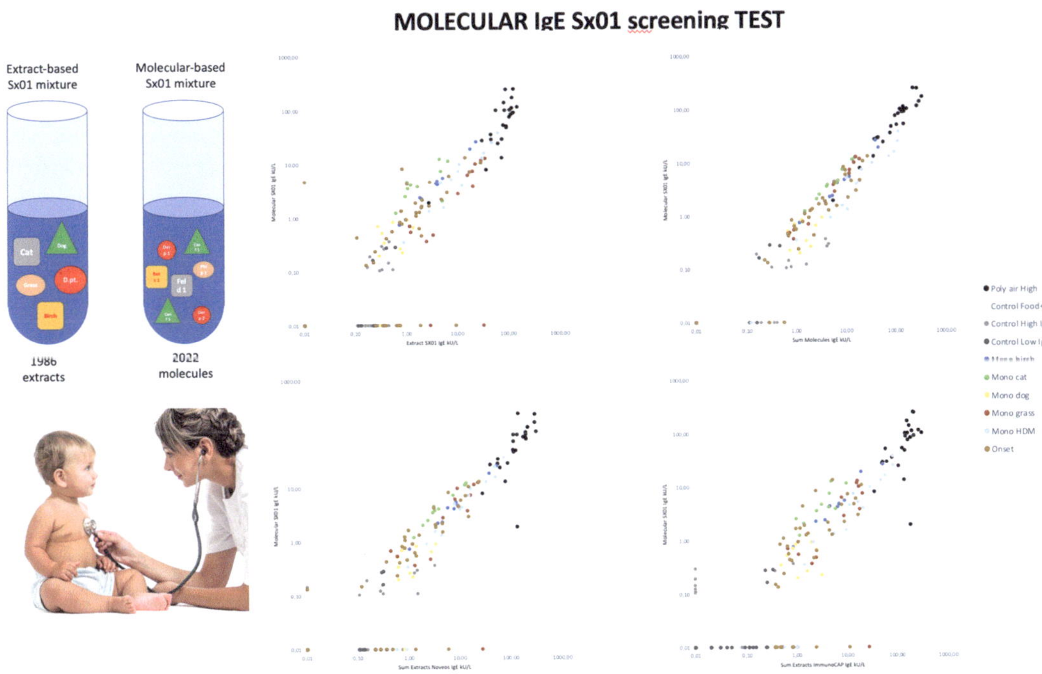

Fig. 23.3 Molecular SX01 screening test for respiratory allergies in childhood. The figure shows the prototype of a novel molecular, in vitro, singleplex test for the screening of IgE sensitization to respiratory allergies in childhood based on a mix of major allergen molecules from different and locally relevant airborne allergen sources, combined in a singleplex test. The results show that the new test is sensitive, specific, and quantitatively accurate in early detection of IgE sensitization at preschool age. Correlation between molecular SX01 and other methodologies: Scatter diagrams showing the correlation between IgE levels detected with molecular SX01 mix (y axis), and IgE levels detected with: (upper left) extract SX01 mix; (upper right) molecules (cumulative); (lower left) extracts (NOVEOS); (lower right) extracts (ImmunoCAP). (Adapted from [50], under OA Creative Common CC BY license)

IgE sensitization to certain molecules is not only a predictive biomarker of comorbidities associated with hay fever. For example, by testing IgE to profilins, PR10s, and nsLTPs is possible to characterize the sensitization profile and predict foods triggering oral allergy syndrome in patients with hay fever accompanied by pollen-food syndrome [52]. The presence of sensitization to Phl p 12 and other profilins [53], Bet v 1 and other PR.10 molecules [54], or to Pru p 3 and other nsLTPs [55], has been shown to predict reactions to a series of foods, in children not differently than in adults. IgE sensitization to other panallergens, like polcalcins, is a strong biomarker of asthma in pollen-allergic patients [56]. Similarly, IgE sensitization to Der p 23 is also a biomarker of asthma in mite-allergic patients [41, 57, 58].

Molecular diagnosis is also essential to precisely prescribe allergen immunotherapy in children with allergic rhinoconjunctivitis and/or asthma [2], by discriminating—among patients reacting with SPT or IgE tests to extracts, those with and those without IgE sensitization to the species-specific or "genuine" allergenic molecules [18, 59]. For example, in grass pollen-allergic patients, AIT should be prescribed almost exclusively to patients with IgE sensitization to Phl p 1 and/or Phl p 5 [9]. Similarly AIT to birch, cypress, ragweed, mugwort, pellitory, dermatophagoides pteronyssinus, or cat should be prescribed only in the presence of IgE sensitization to Bet v 1, Cup a 1, Amb a 1, Art v 1, Par j 2, Der p 1/2/23, or Fel d 1, respectively [9]. Studies have already shown that this molecular diagnosis is very important in temperate climatic area (e.g., Mediterranean) where patients are frequently polysensitized to many pollen or fungi sharing their peak season [60]. On the other hand, molecular diagnosis can be useful in predicting both, local and systemic adverse allergic reactions in patients receiving allergen immunotherapy [61].

The list of highly cross-reacting allergenic molecules or panallergens with diagnostic relevance in childhood respiratory allergies is never completed. Perhaps due to the allergy epidemic and the continuous increase in atopic susceptibility in the general population, more and more allergic patients are becoming sensitized also to components previously not considered relevant as allergenic molecules. For example, the pathogenetic role of gibberellin-regulated proteins in the cypress extract and in many vegetables and fruits has been discovered about 10 years ago [62] and repeatedly confirmed thereafter [63, 64]. Similarly, the diagnostic relevance of cyclophilins, a panallergen already characterized over 20 years ago [65], has been recently re-evaluated [66, 67]. Over 13% of a large population of Italian pollen-allergic children have IgE to Cyclophilin, indicating a relevance superior to that of polcalcins and approaching that of profilins. [68] Patients with IgE sensitization to cyclophilins, but not to profilins and polcalcins, react positively in vivo (SPT) and in vitro (IgE assays) to extracts of many different trees, grasses, and weeds [68]. The disturbing role of IgE to cyclophilins in the allergy diagnosis of pollen-allergic patients is therefore to be considered.

Last but not least, allergic children, especially those sensitized to grass pollen, are frequently developing also IgE to cross-reacting carbohydrate determinants (CCD) [69]. These IgE antibodies do not provoke degranulation but can induce false-positive reactions in IgE assays with allergen extracts or native glycoprotein allergens, such as Phl p 4 [70, 71], bearing CCD epitopes accessible on their 3D structure. Recent studies in the MAS cohort have shown that IgE to CCD can be observed in allergic children even at 2 years of age and that once they appear, their presence in the serum is in most cases persistent until adulthood [69].

23.3.2 The Evolution of IgE Responses to Food Allergens in Childhood

23.3.2.1 Patterns of Food-Specific IgE Levels Over Time

In atopic children, IgE to foods often develops in the first year of life, before IgE to airborne allergens develop. Children with atopic dermatitis are particularly prone to high IgE levels [72]. However, most children with food-specific IgE do not develop clinical reactions to foods. This discrepancy between the presence of IgE and clinical reactivity to foods is well documented in birth cohort studies and in studies of children seen in specialized outpatient clinics [73–76]. For instance, only about 1 in 5 peanut-sensitized children develops peanut allergy when challenged [38]. This difference in ability of IgE to covey an effector cell response following allergen stimulation could be due to difference in the IgE characteristics between allergic and sensitized tolerant children. In a peanut allergy model, peanut-specific IgE levels, IgE-specific activity (i.e., ratio of allergen to total IgE), diversity of peanut allergens recognized by IgE, and avidity of IgE for peanut all independently contributed to basophil and mast cell activation, which ultimately are responsible for allergic reactions to peanut [38, 75, 77, 78]. However, IgE diversity and specific activity were the greatest contributors for degranulation (Fig. 23.4).

Longitudinal studies show that, in food-allergic patients, sensitization to foods, like with airborne allergens, usually starts with sensitization to one initiator allergen and progresses to poly-sensitization over time. For instance, in the LEAP study, Ara h 1 seemed to be the initiator allergen closely followed by Ara h 2 with Ara h 3-specific IgE raising later in time (Fig. 23.5) [79]. In peanut-allergic children, the levels of IgE to the three major peanut allergens increased over time as did total peanut-specific IgE. In children who were sensitized but never developed peanut allergy, the levels of IgE to Ara h 2 and Ara h 1 decreased with Ara h 3-specific IgE remaining stationary. Total IgE to peanut increased in tolerant children between the 30 and 60 months of time points. This was likely to be due to the emergence of pollen allergy and increase in IgE to cross-reactive allergens, like PR-10 or Ara h 5 proteins from peanut, Ara h 8 and Ara h 5. IgE to these allergens are often not clinically relevant or cause at most pollen-food syndrome [80, 81]. Carbohydrate determinants can also induce falsely elevated IgE to peanut, which does not cause skin test reactivity, basophil activation or clinical reactions [82].

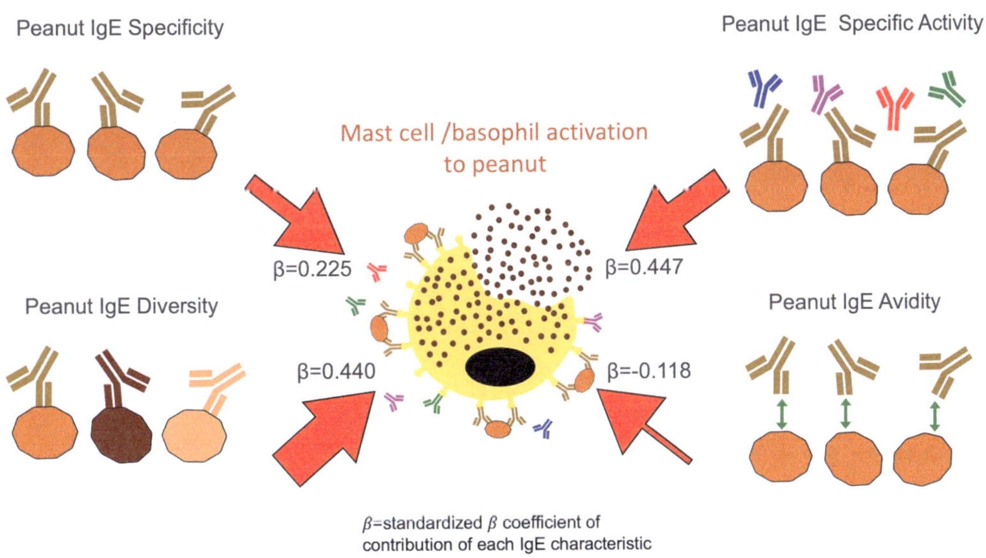

Fig. 23.4 Characteristics of IgE influence effector cell response to peanut. Specificity, specific activity, diversity, and avidity independently contribute for basophil and mast cell activation to peanut, with diversity and specific activity being the greatest contributors according to results of a multivariate logistic regression model (standardized beta coefficient of such model reflects the relative contribution of each factor). (Adapted from [38], under OA Creative Common CC BY license)

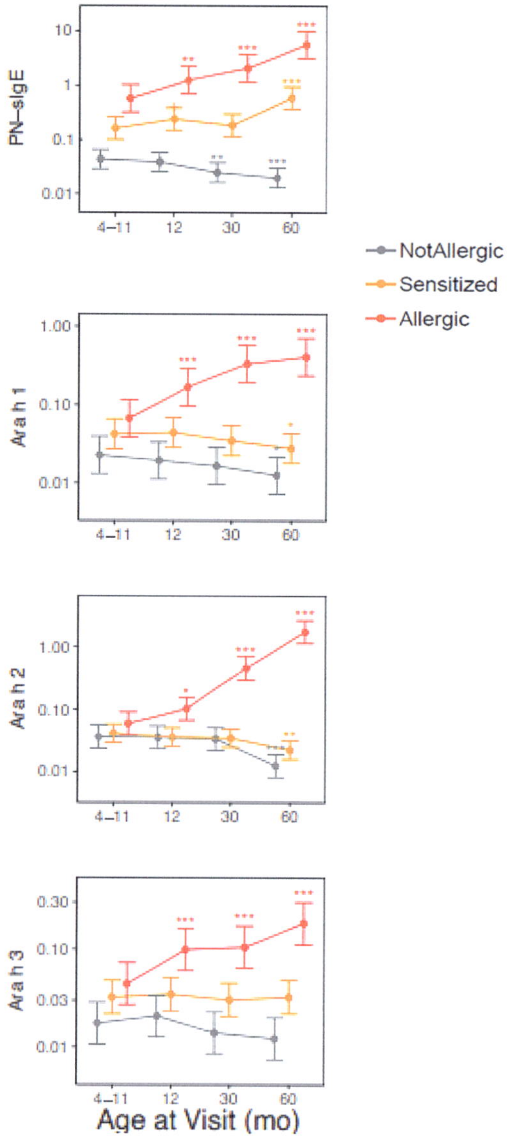

Fig. 23.5 Peanut-specific IgE over time during the first 5 years of life of a high-risk cohort. Levels of IgE to peanut and to peanut allergens Ara h 1, Ara h 2, and Ara h 3 in peanut-allergic, peanut-sensitized tolerant and non-sensitized children over the course of the LEAP study. (Reproduced from [79], with permission)

23.3.2.2 Biomarkers of Primary Food Allergy and Cross-Reactivity

Certain protein families are typical primary food allergens, such as seed storage proteins like vicilin (e.g., Ara h 1 from peanut, Cor a 11 and 16 from hazelnut, Ana o 1 from cashew nut), 2S albumins (e.g., Ara h 2 from peanut, Cor a 14 from hazelnut, Ana o 3 from cashew nut), and legumins (e.g., Ara h 3 from peanut, Cor a 9 from hazelnut, Ana o 2 from cashew nut) [9]. Other allergens that are important inducers of systemic reactions and anaphylaxis but are often absent from allergen extracts and not available for testing are lipophilic allergens oleosins and defensins (e.g., Ara h 10–15 from peanut and Cor a 12, 13 and 15 from hazelnut) [83–85]. Lipid transfer proteins are allergens responsible for primary allergy to plant foods like peach and apple (e.g., Pru p 3 and Mal d 3, respectively) in non-birch endemic areas, like Italy, Spain, and Portugal [86]. However, in birch endemic areas, individuals sensitized to these plant foods are usually sensitized to PR-10 proteins (e.g., Pru p 1 and Mal d 1) rather than LTP and either are asymptomatic or have pollen-food syndrome but do not typically develop systemic reactions or anaphylaxis [87].

The use of IgE to support the diagnosis of food allergy is based on the principle that the higher the levels of food-specific IgE, the higher the likelihood of clinical food allergy [88]. However, there can be significant overlap in food-specific IgE levels between allergic and tolerant children. IgE directed to primary food allergens can be particularly informative to support the diagnosis of food allergy. With a higher specificity compared to IgE to the whole extract, IgE to these informative allergens can help confirm the presence of clinical food allergy. A recent systematic review of the literature and meta-analyses demonstrated a particularly good diagnostic performance for certain allergens, such as Ara h 2 from peanut, Cor a 14 from hazelnut, and Ana o 3 from cashew nut [89]. Table 23.1 indicates the diagnostic performance of the cut-offs reported in the studies included in these meta-analyses.

23.3.2.3 Levels of IgE During Spontaneous Resolution of Food Allergy

Food allergy can resolve spontaneously during childhood [90]. This is particularly the case for allergies to cow's milk, egg, wheat, and soya. Allergies to peanut, tree nuts, seeds, fish, and

Table 23.1 IgE to individual allergens and their utility in the diagnosis of IgE-mediated allergies to peanut, hazelnut, and cashew nut

Allergen	Cut-off (95% CI)	Sensitivity (95% CI)	Specificity (95% CI)
Ara h 2	0.44 (0.3–1.3)	0.82 (0.77; 0.86)	0.92 (0.87; 0.95)
Cor a 14	0.64 (0.35–3.5)	0.73 (0.53; 0.87)	0.95 (0.90; 0.98)
Ana o 3	0.4 (0.2; 0.6)	0.96 (0.91; 0.98)	0.94 (0.88; 0.97)

shellfish tend to be more persistent with about 80% of peanut allergies and 10% of tree nut and seed allergies remaining lifelong. Levels of allergen-specific IgE decrease during the process of spontaneous resolution, being often used as an indicator of when reintroduction of the food can be attempted. Often allergen-specific IgE remains detectable when the food is tolerated raising questions about why this might be. Over time, in tolerant patients, IgE tends to progressively decrease until it is no longer detectable, unless it is directed to cross-reactive allergens, namely homologues to pollen allergens.

During spontaneous resolution of food allergy, and also in tolerance despite sensitization to major allergens, allergen-specific IgG4 has been reported to increase, particularly in transient food allergies like milk and egg [91, 92]. It has been postulated that IgG4 could have a protective role in food allergy. There is evidence from in vitro studies that IgG4 can reduce IgE-mediated reactivity of basophils and mast cells following allergen stimulation in children sensitized to peanut major allergens who are tolerant and in peanut-allergic children who were treated with peanut oral immunotherapy [93]. IgG4/IgE ratios were higher in these groups compared with peanut-allergic children and when IgG4 was removed there was an increase in reactivity of mat cells in response to peanut. In the LEAP study, IgG4 levels were higher in the intervention arm than in the avoidance arm, in which peanut allergy was more prevalent [94]. However, the intervention arm, who had less peanut allergy, was also the group of children who were consuming peanut; thus, the increase in IgG4 could have been driven by consumption rather than tolerance per se.

References

1. Valenta R, Lidholm J, Niederberger V, Hayek B, Kraft D, Gronlund H. The recombinant allergen-based concept of component-resolved diagnostics and immunotherapy (CRD and CRIT). Clin Exp Allergy. 1999;29:896–904.
2. Valenta R. The future of antigen-specific immunotherapy of allergy. Nat Rev Immunol. 2002;2:446–53.
3. Kleine-Tebbe J, Jakob T. Molecular allergy diagnostics using IgE singleplex determinations: methodological and practical consideration for use in clinical routine—Part 18 of the Series Molecular Allergology. Allergo J Int. 2015;24:185–97.
4. Matricardi PM, Kleine-Tebbe J. Molecular allergology between Precision Medicine and the Choosing Wisely initiative. Clin Exp Allergy. 2016;46:664–7.
5. Marsh DG, Milner FH, Johnson P. The allergenic activity and stability of purified allergens from the pollen of common rye grass (Lolium perenne). Int Arch Allergy Appl Immunol. 1966;29:521–35.
6. Fang KS, Vitale M, Fehlner P, King TP. cDNA cloning and primary structure of a white-face hornet venom allergen, antigen 5. Proc Natl Acad Sci USA. 1988;85:895–9.
7. Sudharson S, Kalic T, Hafner C, Breiteneder H. Newly defined allergens in the WHO/IUIS Allergen Nomenclature Database during 01/2019–03/2021. Allergy. 2021;76:3359–73.
8. Matricardi PM, Kleine-Tebbe J, Hoffmann HJ, Valenta R, Hilger C, Hofmaier S, et al. EAACI molecular allergology user's guide. Pediatr Allergy Immunol. 2016;27(Suppl 23):1–250.
9. Dramburg S, Hilger C, Santos AF, de Las Vecillas L, Aalberse RC, Acevedo N, et al. EAACI molecular allergology user's guide 2.0. Pediatr Allergy Immunol. 2023;34(Suppl 28):e13854.
10. Turner KJ, Baldo BA, Hilton JM. RAST studies: IgE antibodies to Dermatogoides pteronyssinus (house dust mite), Aspergillus fumigatus and beta-lactoglobulin in sudden death in infancy syndrome (SDIS). Dev Biol Stand. 1975;29:208–16.
11. Hiller R, Laffer S, Harwanegg C, Huber M, Schmidt WM, Twardosz A, et al. Microarrayed allergen molecules: diagnostic gatekeepers for allergy treatment. FASEB J. 2002;16:414–6.

12. https://www.futuremarketinsights.com/reports/ige-allergy-blood-tests-market. Visited on 15 Aug 2023.
13. Valenta R, Vrtala S, Laffer S, Steinberger P, Ball T, Ferreira F, Scheiner O, Kraft D. B-cell epitopes of allergens determined by recombinant techniques; use for diagnosis and therapy of type I allergy. Arb Paul Ehrlich Inst Bundesamt Sera Impfstoffe Frankf A M. 1994;87:235–46.
14. Van Ree R, Aalberse M. Pollen-vegetable food cross-reactivity: serological and clinical relevance of cross-reactive IgE. J Clin Immunoass. 1993;16:124–30.
15. Radauer C, Breiteneder H. Pollen allergens are restricted to few protein families and show distinct patterns of species distribution. J Allergy Clin Immunol. 2006;117:141–7.
16. Santos A, Van Ree R. Profilins: mimickers of allergy or relevant allergens? Int Arch Allergy Immunol. 2011;155:191–204.
17. Ebner C. Kreuzreagierende Allergene—Panallergene [Cross-reacting allergens—panallergens]. Wien Med Wochenschr. 1996;146:404–5.
18. Kazemi-Shirazi L, Niederberger V, Linhart B, Lidholm J, Kraft D, Valenta R. Recombinant marker allergens: diagnostic gatekeepers for the treatment of allergy. Int Arch Allergy Immunol. 2002;127:259–68.
19. Matricardi PM. Allergen-specific immunoprophylaxis: toward secondary prevention of allergic rhinitis? Pediatr Allergy Immunol. 2014;25:15–8.
20. Hatzler L, Panetta V, Lau S, Wagner P, Bergmann RL, Illi S, et al. Molecular spreading and predictive value of preclinical IgE response to Phleum pratense in children with hay fever. J Allergy Clin Immunol. 2012;130:894–901.e5.
21. Blands J, Lowenstein H, Weeke B. Characterization of extract of dog hair and dandruff from six different dog breeds by quantitative immunoelectrophoresis. Identification of allergens by crossed radioimmunoelectrophoresis (CRIE). Acta Allergol. 1977;32:147–69.
22. Christensen LH, Holm J, Lund G, Riise E, Lund K. Several distinct properties of the IgE repertoire determine effector cell degranulation in response to allergen challenge. J Allergy Clin Immunol. 2008;122:298–304.
23. Marrs T, Brough HA, Kwok M, Lack G, Santos AF. Basophil CD63 assay to peanut allergens accurately diagnoses peanut allergy in patient with negative skin prick test and very low specific IgE. Pediatr Allergy Immunol. 2022;33:e13739.
24. Matricardi PM. The very low IgE producer: allergology, genetics, immunodeficiencies, and oncology. Biomedicines. 2023;11:1378.
25. Aalberse RC, Aalberse JA. Molecular allergen-specific IgE assays as a complement to allergen extract-based sensitization assessment. J Allergy Clin Immunol Pract. 2015;3:863–9.
26. Harwanegg C, Laffer S, Hiller R, Mueller MW, Kraft D, Spitzauer S, et al. Microarrayed recombinant allergens for diagnosis of allergy. Clin Exp Allergy. 2003;33:7–13.
27. Sutton BJ, Gould HJ. The human IgE network. Nature. 1993;366:421–8.
28. Beavil AJ, Beavil RL, Chan CM, Cook JP, Gould HJ, Henry AJ, et al. Structural basis of the IgE-Fc epsilon RI interaction. Biochem Soc Trans. 1993;21:968–72.
29. Ishizaka T, Ishizaka K. Immunological events at the surface of basophil granulocytes and mast cells which induce degranulation. Scand J Respir Dis Suppl. 1977;98:13–22.
30. McDonnell JM, Dhaliwal B, Sutton BJ, Gould HJ. IgE, IgE receptors and anti-IgE biologics: protein structures and mechanisms of action. Annu Rev Immunol. 2023;41:255–75.
31. Metzger H, Goldstein B, Kent U, Mao SY, Pribluda C, Pribluda V, et al. Quantitative aspects of receptor aggregation. Adv Exp Med Biol. 1994;365:175–83.
32. MacGlashan D Jr, Lichtenstein LM. Studies of antigen binding on human basophils. I. Antigen binding and functional consequences. J Immunol. 1983;130:2330–6.
33. Flicker S, Valenta R. Renaissance of the blocking antibody concept in type I allergy. Int Arch Allergy Immunol. 2003;132(1):13–24.
34. Hamilton RG, Saito H. IgE antibody concentration, specific activity, clonality, and affinity measures from future diagnostic confirmatory tests. J Allergy Clin Immunol. 2008;122:305–6.
35. Wide L, Bennich H, Johansson SGO. Diagnosis of allergy by an in vitro test for allergen antibodies. Lancet. 1967;2:1105–7.
36. Dati F, Ringel EP. Reference values for serum IgE in healthy non-atopic children and adults. Clin Chem. 1982;28:1556.
37. Sacco C, Perna S, Vicari D, Alfò M, Bauer CP, Hoffman U, et al. Growth curves of "normal" serum total IgE levels throughout childhood: a quantile analysis in a birth cohort. Ped Allergy Immunol. 2017;28:525–34.
38. Hemmings O, Niazi U, Kwok M, James LK, Lack G, Santos AF. Peanut diversity and specific activity are the dominant IgE characteristics for effector cell activation in children. J Allergy Clin Immunol. 2021;148:495–505.
39. Hatzler L, Panetta V, Illi S, Hofmaier S, Rohrbach A, Hakimeh D, et al. Parental hay fever reinforces IgE to pollen as pre-clinical biomarker of hay fever in childhood. Pediatr Allergy Immunol. 2014;25:366–73.
40. Posa D, Hofmaier S, Arasi S, Matricardi PM. Natural evolution of IgE responses to mite allergens and relationship to progression of allergic disease: a review. Curr Allergy Asthma Rep. 2017;17:28.
41. Posa D, Perna S, Resch Y, Lupinek C, Panetta V, Hofmaier S, et al. Evolution and predictive value of IgE responses toward a comprehensive panel of house dust mite allergens during the first 2 decades of life. J Allergy Clin Immunol. 2017;2:541–9.
42. Asarnoj A, Hamsten C, Lupinek C, Melén E, Andersson N, Anto JM, et al. Prediction of peanut allergy in adolescence by early childhood storage

protein-specific IgE signatures: the BAMSE population-based birth cohort. J Allergy Clin Immunol. 2017;140:587–90.
43. Custovic A, Sonntag H-J, Buchan I, Belgrave D, Simpson A, Prosperi MCF. Evolution pathways to IgE responses to grass and mite allergens throughout childhood. J Allergy Clin Immunol. 2015;136:1645–52.
44. Huang X, Tsilochristou O, Perna S, Hofmaier S, Cappella A, Bauer CP, et al. Evolution of the IgE and IgG repertoire to a comprehensive array of allergen molecules in the first decade of life. Allergy. 2018;73:421–30.
45. Matricardi PM, Dramburg S, Potapova E, Skevaki C, Renz H. Molecular diagnosis for allergy immunotherapy. J Allergy Clin Immunol. 2019;143:831–43.
46. Brindisi G, Cipriani F, Potapova ES, Tripodi S, Panetta V, Bernardini R, et al. Inverse association between the molecular spreading of IgE to grass pollen and the IgE response to Dermatophagoides pteronyssinus among children with seasonal allergic rhinitis. World Allergy Organ J. 2024;17:100975.
47. Fontanella S, Frainay C, Murray CS, Simpson A, Custovic A. Machine learning to identify pairwise interactions between specific IgE antibodies and their association with asthma: a cross-sectional analysis within a population-based birth cohort. PLoS Med. 2018;15:e1002691.
48. Godfrey RC, Gradidge CF. Allergic sensitization of human lung fragments prevented by saturation of IgE binding sites. Nature. 1976;259:484–6.
49. Howard R, Belgrave D, Papastamoulis P, Simpson A, Rattray M, Custovic A. Evolution of IgE responses to multiple allergen components throughout childhood. J Allergy Clin Immunol. 2018;142:1322–30.
50. Potapova E, Panetta V, Grabenhenrich L, Icke K, Grübl A, Müller C, et al. A singleplex IgE test to a mixture of molecules from multiple airborne allergen sources: innovating in vitro screening of respiratory allergies. Pediatr Allergy Immunol. 2022;33:e13867.
51. Potapova E, Bauersachs D, Villella V, Meneguzzi G, Scala E, Sfika I, et al. Validation study of a new chemiluminescent singleplex IgE assay in a set of Italian allergic rhinitis patients. Clin Exp Allergy. 2021;51:604–13.
52. Bauersachs D, Potapova E, Renz H, Benes SH, Matricardi PM, Skevaki C. Validation of the analytical performance of the NOVEOS™ System, a system which improves upon the third-generation in vitro allergy testing technology. Clin Chem Lab Med. 2020;58:1865–74.
53. Mari A, Ballmer-Weber BK, Vieths S. The oral allergy syndrome: improved diagnostic and treatment methods. Curr Opin Allergy Clin Immunol. 2005;5:267–73.
54. Vieths S, Scheurer S, Ballmer-Weber B. Current understanding of cross-reactivity of food allergens and pollen. Ann N Y Acad Sci. 2002;964:47–68.
55. Mastrorilli C, Tripodi S, Caffarelli C, Perna S, Di Rienzo-Businco A, Sfika I, et al. Endotypes of pollen-food syndrome in children with seasonal allergic rhinoconjunctivitis: a molecular classification. Allergy. 2016;71:181–91.
56. Skypala IJ, Asero R, Barber D, Cecchi L, Diaz Perales A, Hoffmann-Sommergruber K, et al. Non-specific lipid-transfer proteins: allergen structure and function, cross-reactivity, sensitization, and epidemiology. Clin Transl Allergy. 2021;11:e12010.
57. Cipriani F, Mastrorilli C, Tripodi S, Ricci G, Perna S, Panetta V, et al. Diagnostic relevance of IgE sensitization profiles to eight recombinant Phleum pratense molecules. Allergy. 2018;73:673–82.
58. Weghofer M, Grote M, Resch Y, Casset A, Kneidinger M, Kopec J, et al. Identification of Der p 23, a peritrophin-like protein, as a new major Dermatophagoides pteronyssinus allergen associated with the peritrophic matrix of mite fecal pellets. J Immunol. 2013;190(7):3059–67.
59. Forchert L, Potapova E, Panetta V, Dramburg S, Perna S, Posa D, et al. Der p 23-specific IgE response throughout childhood and its association with allergic asthma: a birth cohort study. Pediatr Allergy Immunol. 2022;33:e13829.
60. Kleine-Tebbe J, Matricardi PM, Hamilton RG. Allergy work-up including component-resolved diagnosis: how to make allergen-specific immunotherapy more specific. Immunol Allergy Clin N Am. 2016;36:191–203.
61. Dramburg S, Grittner U, Potapova E, Travaglini A, Tripodi S, Arasi S, et al. Heterogeneity of sensitization profiles and clinical phenotypes among patients with seasonal allergic rhinitis in Southern European Countries—the @IT.2020 multicenter study. Allergy. 2024;79:908–23.
62. Sastre J, Rodriguez F, Campo P, Laffond E, Marin A, Alonso MD. Adverse reactions to immunotherapy are associated with different patterns of sensitization to grass allergens. Allergy. 2015;70:598–600.
63. Tuppo L, Alessandri C, Giangrieco I, Ciancamerla M, Rafaiani C, Tamburrini M, et al. Isolation of cypress gibberellin-regulated protein: analysis of its structural features and IgE binding competition with homologous allergens. Mol Immunol. 2019;114:189–95.
64. Shahali Y, Sutra J-P, Peltre G, Charpin D, Sénéchal H, Poncet P. IgE reactivity to common cypress (C. sempervirens) pollen extracts: evidence for novel allergens. World Allergy Organiz J. 2010;3:229–34.
65. Inomata N, Okazaki F, Moriyama T, Nomura Y, Yamaguchi Y, Honjoh T, et al. Identification of peamaclein as a marker allergen related to systemic reactions in peach allergy. Ann Allergy Asthma Immunol. 2014;112:175–177.e3.
66. Flückiger S, Fijten H, Whitley P, Blaser K, Crameri R. Cyclophilins, a new family of cross-reactive allergens. Eur J Immunol. 2002;32:10–7.

67. Kleine-Tebbe J, Ackermann-Simon J, Hanf G. Molecular allergy diagnosis using pollen marker allergens and pollen panallergens: five patterns seen in multiple test reactions to pollen extracts. Allergol Select. 2021;5:180–6.
68. Mattson L, Valcour A, Holmqvist M, Larsson H, Lidholm J. Cyclophilin—a novel cross-reactive determinant in peanut. Clin Exp Allergy. 2021;51:620–2.
69. Potapova ES, Tripodi S, Panetta V, Gattinger P, Bernardini R, Caffarelli C, et al. IgE to cross-reactive carbohydrate determinants (CCD) in childhood: biological and clinical correlates. Clin Exp Allergy. 2024;54:195–206.
70. Aalberse RC, Koshte V, Clemens JG. Immunoglobulin E antibodies that cross-react with vegetable foods, pollen, and Hymenoptera venom. J Allergy Clin Immunol. 1981;68:356–64.
71. Matricardi PM. IgE to cross-reactive carbohydrate determinants: origins, functions, and confounding role in nPhl p 4-IgE assays. J Allergy Clin Immunol. 2020;145:1554–5.
72. Tsakok T, Marrs T, Mohsin M, Baron S, du Toit G, Till S, et al. Does atopic dermatitis cause food allergy? A systematic review. J Allergy Clin Immunol. 2016;137:1071–8.
73. Osborne NJ, Koplin JJ, Martin PE, Gurrin LC, Lowe AJ, Matheson MC, et al. Prevalence of challenge-proven IgE-mediated food allergy using population-based sampling and predetermined challenge criteria in infants. J Allergy Clin Immunol. 2011;127:668–76.e1–2.
74. Nicolaou N, Poorafshar M, Murray C, Simpson A, Winell H, Kerry G, et al. Allergy or tolerance in children sensitized to peanut: prevalence and differentiation using component-resolved diagnostics. J Allergy Clin Immunol. 2010;125:191–7.e1–13.
75. Santos AF, Douiri A, Becares N, Wu SY, Stephens A, Radulovic S, et al. Basophil activation test discriminates between allergy and tolerance in peanut-sensitized children. J Allergy Clin Immunol. 2014;134:645–52.
76. Krawiec M, Radulovic S, Foong RX, Marques-Mejias A, Bartha I, Kwok M, et al. Diagnostic utility of allergy tests to predict baked egg and lightly cooked egg allergies compared to double-blind placebo-controlled food challenges. Allergy. 2023;78:2510–22.
77. Ji C, Huang Y, Yeung LH, Hemmings O, Jama Z, Kwok M, et al. Ara h 2-specific IgE presence rather than its function is the best predictor of mast cell activation in children. J Allergy Clin Immunol Pract. 2023;11:1154–61.e3.
78. Santos AF, Du Toit G, O'Rourke C, Becares N, Couto-Francisco N, Radulovic S, et al. Biomarkers of severity and threshold of allergic reactions during oral peanut challenges. J Allergy Clin Immunol. 2020;146:344–55.
79. Suarez-Farinas M, Suprun M, Bahnson HT, Raghunathan R, Getts R, duToit G, et al. Evolution of epitope-specific IgE and IgG(4) antibodies in children enrolled in the LEAP trial. J Allergy Clin Immunol. 2021;148:835–42.
80. du Toit G, Sayre PH, Roberts G, Lawson K, Sever ML, Bahnson HT, et al. Allergen specificity of early peanut consumption and effect on development of allergic disease in the Learning Early About Peanut Allergy study cohort. J Allergy Clin Immunol. 2018;141:1343–53.
81. Santos AF, Barbosa-Morais NL, Hurlburt BK, Ramaswamy S, Hemmings O, Kwok M, et al. IgE to epitopes of Ara h 2 enhance the diagnostic accuracy of Ara h 2-specific IgE. Allergy. 2020;75:2309–18.
82. van der Veen MJ, van Ree R, Aalberse RC, Akkerdaas J, Koppelman SJ, Jansen HM, et al. Poor biologic activity of cross-reactive IgE directed to carbohydrate determinants of glycoproteins. J Allergy Clin Immunol. 1997;100:327–34.
83. Zuidmeer-Jongejan L, Fernandez-Rivas M, Winter MG, Akkerdaas JH, Summers C, Lebens A, et al. Oil body-associated hazelnut allergens including oleosins are underrepresented in diagnostic extracts but associated with severe symptoms. Clin Transl Allergy. 2014;4:4.
84. Petersen A, Kull S, Rennert S, Becker WM, Krause S, Ernst M, et al. Peanut defensins: novel allergens isolated from lipophilic peanut extract. J Allergy Clin Immunol. 2015;136:1295–301.e1–5.
85. Schwager C, Kull S, Behrends J, Rockendorf N, Schocker F, Frey A, et al. Peanut oleosins associated with severe peanut allergy-importance of lipophilic allergens for comprehensive allergy diagnostics. J Allergy Clin Immunol. 2017;140:1331–8.e8.
86. Fernandez-Rivas M, van Ree R, Cuevas M. Allergy to Rosaceae fruits without related pollinosis. J Allergy Clin Immunol. 1997;100(6 Pt 1):728–33.
87. Fernandez-Rivas M, Bolhaar S, Gonzalez-Mancebo E, Asero R, van Leeuwen A, Bohle B, et al. Apple allergy across Europe: how allergen sensitization profiles determine the clinical expression of allergies to plant foods. J Allergy Clin Immunol. 2006;118:481–8.
88. Foong RX, Dantzer JA, Wood RA, Santos AF. Improving diagnostic accuracy in food allergy. J Allergy Clin Immunol Pract. 2021;9:71–80.
89. Riggioni C. Systematic review and meta-analyses on the accuracy of diagnostic tests for IgE-mediated food allergy. Allergy. 2023;79:324–52.
90. Foong RX, Santos AF. Biomarkers of diagnosis and resolution of food allergy. Pediatr Allergy Immunol. 2021;32(2):223–33.
91. McKendry RT, Kwok M, Hemmings O, James LK, Santos AF. Allergen-specific IgG show distinct patterns in persistent and transient food allergy. Pediatr Allergy Immunol. 2021;32:1508–18.

92. Qamar N, Fishbein AB, Erickson KA, Cai M, Szychlinski C, Bryce PJ, et al. Naturally occurring tolerance acquisition to foods in previously allergic children is characterized by antigen specificity and associated with increased subsets of regulatory T cells. Clin Exp Allergy. 2015;45:1663–72.
93. Santos AF, James LK, Bahnson HT, Shamji MH, Couto-Francisco NC, Islam S, et al. IgG4 inhibits peanut-induced basophil and mast cell activation in peanut-tolerant children sensitized to peanut major allergens. J Allergy Clin Immunol. 2015;135:1249–56.
94. Du Toit G, Roberts G, Sayre PH, Bahnson HT, Radulovic S, Santos AF, et al. Randomized trial of peanut consumption in infants at risk for peanut allergy. N Engl J Med. 2015;372:803–13.

24 Corticosteroids for Inflammation Control in the Allergic Child

Fabio Cardinale, Dora Alba Ciccarone, Valentina Tranchino, and Carla Mastrorilli

Abstract

Corticosteroids are powerful drugs with anti-inflammatory properties, commonly used in treating pediatric allergic diseases. The physiological and pharmacological functions of corticosteroids are mediated by different mechanisms, based on suppression of the genetic transcription of inflammatory cytokines (transrepression), or activation of inhibitory cytokine transcription (transactivation). The onset of action for these mechanisms taking place is usually 4–24 h. Other mechanisms mediated through non-genomic pathways have been studied. These effects are characterized by a rapid onset and short duration of action. Understanding the different mechanisms may help in the development of new and more selective anti-inflammatory drugs paving the way to new strategies in the management of allergic diseases. However, the decision whether or not to administer a corticosteroid for allergic diseases must be based on evidence of efficacy and according to guidelines. There are no convincing data supporting the use of corticosteroids to treat anaphylactic reactions. Oral corticosteroids may be beneficial in children with non-IgE-mediated food allergies, such as eosinophilic esophagitis and food protein-induced enterocolitis. Furthermore, the role of steroids in cutaneous atopic diseases including chronic urticaria and atopic dermatitis has been widely studied. In moderate-to-severe asthma exacerbations, clinical guidelines agree that oral corticosteroids should be promptly administered since they result in fewer and shorter hospitalizations. However, the efficacy in pre-school wheezing is debated. Finally, topical nasal corticosteroids are the treatment of choice for children with persistent allergic rhinoconjunctivitis. Although corticosteroids exert a beneficial effect on the course of several different allergic diseases in childhood, the type of corticosteroid to administer and the appropriate dosage should be carefully evaluated in order to minimize potential adverse effects.

Keywords

Allergy · Allergic rhinitis · Anaphylaxis · Asthma · Atopic dermatitis · Children · Chronic urticaria · Corticosteroids · Food allergy · Glucocorticoid receptor · Immune system · inflammation · Pediatric

F. Cardinale (✉) · D. A. Ciccarone · V. Tranchino
C. Mastrorilli
Department of Pediatrics, Pediatric Hospital Giovanni XXIII, University of Bari, Bari, Italy

C. Caffarelli, G. L. Marseglia (eds.), *Textbook of Pediatric Allergy*,
https://doi.org/10.1007/978-3-031-71283-8_24

Test your learning and check your understanding of this book's contents: use the "Springer Nature Flashcards" app to access questions using ▶ https://sn.pub/nspbjm. To use the app, please follow the instructions in Chap. 1.

24.1 Introduction

Corticosteroids represent the cornerstone for the treatment of many allergic diseases and inflammatory disorders. The meaning of the term "corticosteroid" arises from its glucocorticoid activity, although this term comprises two classes of steroids synthetized by the adrenal cortex (glucocorticoids and mineralocorticoids). The prototypical endogenous steroid with glucocorticoid activity is cortisol that is produced by the adrenal gland through cholesterol metabolism. Since other hormones, such as mineralocorticoid, aldosterone, and sex hormones, are produced through the same pathway, some side effects can be associated with this similarity. Cortisol levels change throughout the day since it is controlled by local and central circadian patterns (the hypothalamic-pituitary-adrenal axis) that regulate the endogenous anti-inflammatory responses, resulting in plasma concentration typically highest in the morning and lowest during the night. Under stress conditions, the hypothalamus secretes a corticotrophin-releasing hormone, stimulating the hypophysis gland, that in turn produces the adrenocorticotrophin hormone (ACTH). The latter acts on the cortex of the suprarenal gland that releases glucocorticoids into the blood. Glucocorticoids have a variety of effects on physiologic properties on carbohydrate, protein and lipid metabolism, bone mineralization, cardiovascular homeostasis, central nervous system function, fluid, and electrolyte balance. Moreover, they also determine upregulation of β_2-adrenergic receptor functions.

24.2 Mechanisms of Action

Corticosteroids are lipophilic substances with low molecular weight that can easily pass cellular membranes and bind to the glucocorticoid receptor in the cytosol, generating a hormone-receptor complex which moves into the cell nucleus and fixes to target DNA-binding sites (called glucocorticoid response elements), regulating gene expression [1] (Fig. 24.1). These agents are associated with genes that can suppress or stimulate transcription of target genes, which results in two effects called transrepression or transactivation, respectively. Likewise, corticosteroids weaken gene expression by a mechanism called cis-repression that implies binding to negative glucocorticoid response elements [2]. Moreover, corticosteroids also act by non-genomic mechanisms that are triggered by proteins released by the hormone-receptor complex and by interaction with cellular membranes, that involve the synthesis of nitric oxide, resulting in inhibition of vasodilatation. Since the action of corticosteroids is intracellular, the effect persists, even when they are no longer detected in the plasma.

The genomic effects on gene expression occur over hours to days and implicate the activation or repression of multiple genes [1]. Corticosteroids upregulate the transcription of several anti-inflammatory genes, such as annexin 1 (also named lipocortin-1), that blocks the synthesis of cytosolic phospholipase A2-α (which produces several inflammatory mediators) and inhibits the release of arachidonic acid from membrane phospholipids (Table 24.1). Moreover, they enhance genes encoding β_2-adrenergic receptors and the anti-inflammatory proteins secretory leukoprotease inhibitor and mitogen-activated protein kinase (MAPK) phosphatase 1, that inactivate the MAPK cascades, thus reversing the phosphorylation of GATA3 and inhibiting the transcription of T2 cytokines. From the other side, glucocorticoids, by activating histone deacetylase 2 (HDAC2), suppress the expression of several inflammatory genes which translates into switching off encoding cytokines, chemokines, adhesion molecules, inflammatory enzymes, receptors and proteins, such as

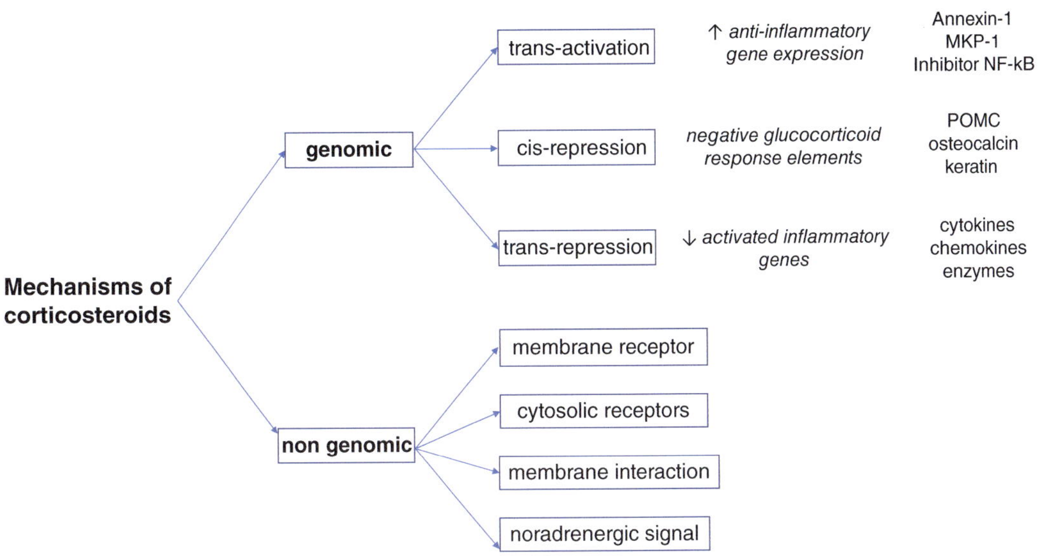

Fig. 24.1 Mechanisms of corticosteroids

Table 24.1 Effects of corticosteroids on gene transcription

Transactivation
Annexin-1
Inhibitor of nuclear factor-kB
β_2-adrenergic receptor
Secretory leukoprotease inhibitor
Phospholipase A_2 inhibitor
MKP-1 (inhibits MAP kinase pathways)
Anti-inflammatory cytokines (IL-10, IL-12, IL-1 receptor antagonist)
Glucocorticoid-inducible leucine zipper (GILZ)
Transrepression
Cytokines (IL-1 to IL-6, IL-9, IL-11 to IL-13, IL-16 to IL-18, TNF-α, GM-CSF, SCF)
Chemokines (CCL1, CCL5, CCL11, IL-8)
Adhesion molecules (ICAM-1, VCAM-1)
Inflammatory enzymes (iNOS, inducible COX-2, inducible phospholipase A_2)
Inflammatory receptors (neurokinin-1, bradykinin B_2 receptors)
Peptides (endothelin-1)

Modified from Barnes [1] and Barnes 2
IL interleukin, *GM-CSF* granulocyte-macrophage colony-stimulating factor, *SCF* stem cell factor, *CCL* C-C motif chemokine Ligand, *ICAM* intercellular adhesion molecule, *VCAM* vascular cell adhesion molecule, *iNOS* inducible nitric oxide synthase

nuclear factor-κb (NF-κb). This results in the switching off cyclooxygenase-2 (COX-2) that reduces neutrophil migration to inflammatory sites [2]. In addition, since NF-κB stimulates the expression of nitric oxide synthase, the production of nitric oxide is reduced, contributing to the reduction of inflammatory manifestations of asthma, such as vasodilatation and inflammatory cell recruitment. Furthermore, corticosteroids have post-genomic effects, mediated through a rapid degradation of mRNA, causing a reduction of inflammatory proteins, such as TNF-α. This action is dose-dependent and is characterized by a rapid onset (seconds to minutes) and a short duration (60–90 min). The interaction of corticosteroids with negative glucocorticoid response elements (cis-repression) is considered responsible for side effects, including suppression of gene regulating the hypothalamo-pituitary axis (corticotrophin-releasing factor), bone metabolism (osteocalcin), and skin structure (keratins) [1, 2]. Non-genomic actions have been classified into four categories according to the interaction of corticosteroids: (a) interaction with cell membrane, (b) membrane-bound receptors, (c) cytosolic receptors, and (d) inhibition of extra-neuronal monoamine transporter-mediated uptake of norepinephrine [3]. Finally, since corticosteroids enhance the transcription of the β_2-receptor gene, the expression of cell surface receptors increases, as well as the responses to β_2-agonists. This effect results in a rapid improvement of airway edema, explaining the beneficial effects of corticosteroids in asthma therapy [4].

Resistance to therapeutic effects of corticosteroids is a complex mechanism that can rarely occur, depending on genetic or acquired factors (Table 24.2) [5]. It has been shown, for example, that oxidative stress reduces the activity and expression of HDAC2, through the activation of phosphoinositide 3-kinase delta (PI3Kd), thus counteracting the activity of corticosteroids [6]. Genetic resistance factors have been also identified. Zein et al. demonstrated in a cohort of asthmatic adults that resistance to corticosteroids was linked to polymorphisms of the HSD3B1 gene encoding for 3β-hydroxysteroid dehydrogenase-1, responsible for the catabolism of dehydroepiandrosterone (DHEA) [7]. The adrenal restrictive genotype HSD3B1(1245) was associated with corticosteroid resistance as demonstrated by the fact that blood levels of DHEA were correlated with lower FEV1 [7]. Tantisira et al. also found a significant relationship between a polymorphism in glucocorticoid-induced transcript 1 gene (*GLCCI1*) and lung function response to inhaled corticosteroids [8]. Long-term complications of chronic steroid use have been widely studied, although serious adverse effects after short-term, high-dose therapy as those used in the treatment of allergic diseases, can rarely occur (Table 24.3). The

Table 24.2 Proposed molecular mechanisms of corticosteroid resistance

Genetic abnormalities in GRs
Reduced GR-α expression
Defective GC binding to GR-α
Reduced GR-α translocation due to increased phosphorylation by kinases such as p38 MAPK and JNK
Defective histone acetylation (↓ HDAC2 activity and ↑ oxidative stress)
Increased pro-inflammatory transcription factor activation (such as NF-κB and AP-1)
Increased GR-β expression

Modified from Henderson [5] and Barnes [6]
GR glucocorticoid receptor, *GC* glucocorticoid, *MAPK* mitogen-activated protein kinase, *JNK* c-Jun N-terminal kinase, *HDAC* histone deacetylase, *NF-κB* nuclear factor-κB, *AP1* activator protein-1

Table 24.3 Tissue-specific side effects of high-dose or prolonged corticosteroid treatment [9]

Tissue	Side effects
Adrenal gland	Adrenal atrophy, Cushing's syndrome
Cardiovascular system	Dyslipidemia, hypertension, thrombosis, vasculitis
Central nervous system	Changes in behavior, cognition, memory, and mood (i.e., glucocorticoid-induced psychoses), cerebral atrophy
Gastrointestinal tract	Gastrointestinal bleeding, pancreatitis, peptic ulcer
Immune system	Broad immunosuppression, activation of latent viruses
Skin	Atrophy, delayed wound healing, erythema, hypertrichosis, perioral dermatitis, petechiae, glucocorticoid-induced acne, striae rubrae distensae, telangiectasia
Musculoskeletal system	Bone necrosis, muscle atrophy, osteoporosis, retardation of longitudinal bone growth
Eyes	Cataracts, glaucoma
Kidney	Increased sodium retention and potassium excretion
Reproductive system	Delayed puberty, fetal growth retardation, hypogonadism

prevalence of psychiatric adverse effects is dose-dependent, with an incidence between 2% and 60% [10] mainly occurring within the first 7–14 days and ranging from mild depression and anxiety to psychosis with hallucinations [11]. A well-documented steroids' adverse effect is hyperglycemia that may occur within hours of administration [12]. No data are available on the incidence of clinically relevant hyperglycemia in patients using short-term corticosteroids; however, it should be considered among vulnerable subjects, including diabetic patients. Moreover, some reports exist of avascular necrosis after short-term use of corticosteroids [13, 14] (Table 24.3).

24.3 Corticosteroids in Medical Practice

Corticosteroids can be used systemically or topically (inhaled, nasal, cutaneous). Topical steroid treatment can be used for longer periods of time and is generally assumed as safe because of minimal systemic absorption. Chemical and structural modifications of different formulations significantly influence the pharmacokinetic and pharmacodynamic of steroids, with changes in efficacy and safety from individual to individual.

Systemically used corticosteroids are classified based on their anti-inflammatory potency, which is related to the duration of action and to the capability of inhibiting the hypothalamic-pituitary-adrenal (HPA) axis (Table 24.4). Each corticosteroid administered in clinical practice has an equivalent dose calculated on the peculiar anti-inflammatory potency when obtaining the same anti-inflammatory effect [9]. Since the genomic and non-genomic effects applied by different corticosteroids depend on their relative potencies, these features are used to describe the clinical efficacy of each molecule. For instance, betamethasone has a very low non-genomic potency and a higher genomic potency differently by prednisolone, meaning that the latter has a lower anti-inflammatory potency but a faster onset of action [9].

Since endogenous cortisol has its peak early in the morning, corticosteroids should be preferably given in single dose at morning. If twice daily dosing is required according to the type of molecule, two-thirds of the dose may be administered at morning and one-third in the afternoon, mimicking the circadian rhythm of adrenal secretion [15].

In light of the suppression of HPA axis, the use of corticosteroids is associated with various adverse events, particularly depending on dosage, type, route of administration, and duration of treatment (Table 24.4). In children, short-course oral corticosteroids can provoke vomiting, infections, behavioral changes, and sleep disorders, whereas prolonged treatment may trigger growth retardation, bone metabolism disorders or perturbation of adrenal function [16]. A longer biological half-life may result in a more prolonged and stronger suppression of HPA axis even after a single dose. In clinical practice, intermediate

Table 24.4 Classification and comparison of the most frequently used systemic corticosteroids [14]

Corticosteroid	Equivalent dose (mg)	Anti-inflammatory potency[a]	Salt retention[a]	Suppressive HPA potency[a]	Biological half-life (h)
Hydrocortisone	20	1	1	1	8–12 Short
Cortisone	25	0.8	0.8	2	8–12 Short
Prednisolone	5	4	0.8	1	12–36 Intermediate
Prednisone	5	4	0.8	1	12–36 Intermediate
Methylprednisolone	4	4–5	0.2–0.5	5	12–36 Intermediate
Triamcinolone	4	5–10	0	5	12–36 Intermediate
Dexamethasone	0.75	25	0	50	36–72 Long
Betamethasone	0.75	25	0	50	36–72 Long

PA hypothalamic–pituitary–adrenal axis
[a] Hydrocortisone as reference drug set equal to 1

half-life compounds, such as prednisolone or prednisone, should be preferred since they exert a little and transient suppression of HPA axis without negative feedback on pituitary gland or hypothalamus [17]. When a prolonged treatment is stopped abruptly, withdrawal syndrome may appear, clinically characterized by nausea/vomits, anorexia, asthenia/lethargy, headache, and arthromyalgia [9, 15]. This means that the drug dose should be progressively reduced. A treatment duration up to 3–10 days of compounds with short or intermediate biological half-life is not associated with withdrawal complications [18].

Strategies to reduce the risk of corticosteroids' adverse events avoiding the HPA suppression:

- Prefer an intermediate half-life analog (such as prednisolone or prednisone)
- Select the type for well-documented indications
- Apply the minimal effective dose for the shortest period possible
- When prolonged therapies are scheduled administer the drug in the morning in a single dose, or if possible, on alternate days and reduce the dose progressively.

24.4 Corticosteroids in Asthma

Corticosteroids are essential drugs in asthma treatment, being able to counteract all cellular elements and mediators involved in type 2 inflammation [19]. They inhibit phospholipase A2 and reduce the expression of COX-2 and the production and release of pro-inflammatory cytokines by macrophages and lymphocytes. Subsequently, they act on the adhesive molecules, such as intercellular adhesion molecule-1 (ICAM-1) and endothelial leukocyte adhesion molecule-1 (ELAM-1), inhibit the IgE-dependent release of histamine and leukotriene 4, promote apoptosis of eosinophils, and reduce mast cell density and fibroblast proliferation [14].

Furthermore, corticosteroids have the capacity to prevent the downregulation of beta-2 receptors by short-acting and long-acting beta agonists (SABA and LABA). In fact, there is a complex inter-relationship among beta-2 receptors, corticosteroid receptors, and LABA. Inhaled corticosteroids promote beta-2 receptor expression, coupling with their signal molecules. In turn, LABA exert an anti-inflammatory action as, acting on glucocorticoid receptors, stimulate the translocation within the nucleus and promote binding with the responsive sequences. As a result, LABA and inhaled corticosteroids are mutually reinforcing. The non-genomic effect especially concerns inhaled corticosteroids and their vasoconstrictor effect exerted at the level of vessels' smooth muscles of the respiratory tree; it depends on the ability of the inhaled corticosteroids to inhibit the re-uptake of norepinephrine by the sympathetic nerve endings and to concentrate its action on the α-receptors. This effect takes place within a few minutes, it is common to all inhaled corticosteroids, but is more evident for budesonide than fluticasone and beclomethasone [19].

Pharmacokinetic properties of different inhaled corticosteroids influence efficacy and safety of these drugs (Table 24.5) [19]. An ideal inhaled corticosteroid should be efficacious and safe. Efficacy is given by a strong link to the receptor (potency), a prolonged effect in the lung (lipophilia and lipid conjugation), and a high pulmonary deposition. Safety is conferred by negligible systemic effects (low oral bioavailability, high link to proteins, high systemic clearance) and minor oropharyngeal effects (low deposition, local activation).

Inhaled corticosteroids are offered as the first-line maintenance therapy in asthmatic children and adolescents with asthma-related symptoms more than twice a month. It is noteworthy that since 2018 asthma guidelines recommend their use also in mild asthma and whenever SABA are used instead that using SABA alone in children older than 5 years of age [20].

Table 24.5 Pharmacological features of inhaled corticosteroids

Corticosteroid—dose form	Relative glucocorticoid receptor binding affinity	Lipophilicity (log P)	Aqueous solubility (μg/mL)	Plasma protein binding (%)	Volume of distribution at steady state (L)	Plasma clearance (L/h)	Absolute bioavailability determined in healthy subjects (%)
Fluticasone furoate DPI	2989	4.17	0.03	99.7	608	65	15DPI 1oral
Mometasone furoate DPI	2100	4.73	<0.1	99.5	332	54	11DPI 1oral
Fluticasone propionate DPI	1775	3.89	0.14	99.3	318	69	16DPI 1oral
Beclomethasone dipropionate (BMP) MDI	53 (1345)	4.59 (3.27)	0.13 (15.5)	95.9	424	120	62CFC 82HFA 41oral
Ciclesonide (des-CIC) MDI	12 (1200)	3.2 (3.0)	<0.1 (7)	98.7	396	228	63HFA 1oral
Budesonide DPI	935	2.32	16	91.4	180	84	39DPI 11oral
Triamcinolone acetonide MDI	233	1.85	21	73.2	103	37	25CFC 23oral
Flunisolide MDI	190	1.36	140	61.2	96	58	33CFC 70HFA 20oral
Prednisolone oral	12	1.65	223	57.6	93	37	82oral

Modified from Daley-Yates [19]

For beclomethasone dipropionate (BDP) and ciclesonide (CIC), values in parenthesis are for the active metabolites—beclomethasone 17-monopropionate (BMP) and desisobutyryl ciclesonide (des-CIC). Glucocorticoid receptor binding affinity is relative to dexamethasone where dexamethasone affinity = 100

MDI metered-dose inhaler, *DPI* dry-powder inhaler

International guidelines focus on the early use of systemic corticosteroids in the treatment of asthma attacks [20–22]. Indeed, it has been demonstrated that a single dose of corticosteroids can improve lung function and reduce hospitalization rates and duration [23]. Based on half-life corticosteroids are divided into short, intermediate, and long half-life steroids. Higher anti-inflammatory power also corresponds to a more pronounced and prolonged inhibition of HPA axis. Long-lived molecules, such as dexamethasone and betamethasone, have the ability to inhibit the adrenal gland 50 times greater than intermediate half-life steroids (i.e., prednisone, prednisolone, and deflazacort), the latter having less potency, but also less interference with the adrenal gland function. Therefore, intermediate half-life steroids are the recommended corticosteroids in the acute attack of asthma. Regardless of the potency of the molecule, the action of corticosteroids is expressed over 2–4 h, so they should be introduced early in the treatment of acute asthma attack to optimize their effectiveness.

It has been shown that there are no substantial differences between oral or parenteral corticosteroid administration in acute asthma attacks [24, 25]. Oral route is indeed recommended since it is easier to administer, less expensive, and less invasive [21]. However, parenteral methylprednisolone represents the reference corticosteroid in severe asthma, due to increased affinity for lung tissue, as demonstrated in animal studies [26]. When choosing a corticosteroid molecule, side effects should also be considered [17]. In a milligram-to-milligram comparison, prednisolone approximatively has the capacity to suppress the blastulation of PBMC in vitro 11 times less than methylprednisolone and 13 times less than betamethasone [27]. Preliminary observations found deflazacort, a corticosteroid with an intermediate half-life to have similar efficacy to prednisolone in improving pulmonary function and clinical symptoms in children with moderate exacerbations of asthma [28]. Some studies found that deflazacort has less interference on bone metabolism and less effect on inhibition of GH production [29, 30]. The ratio of equipotency between deflazacort and prednisolone is 1.5:1 [9]. The recommended dosage for prednisone, prednisolone methylprednisolone, and deflazacort is 1–2 mg/kg/day in 2–3 sub-doses (maximum dose 80 mg). High-dose inhaled corticosteroids can also reduce emergency department visits and hospitalizations compared with placebo in asthma exacerbations. However, although no evidence of a difference between inhaled corticosteroids and systemic corticosteroids has been found in metanalysis or systematic reviews in terms of hospital admission rates, unscheduled visits, and need of additional course of steroids, their use is not recommended as an alternative or adjunctive therapy to systemic corticosteroids due to higher costs and feasibility [4, 31, 32].

- Systemic corticosteroids should be introduced early in the treatment of asthma attacks since they need 2–4 h to be efficacious.
- Although equal efficacy of the parental route compared to the oral route, oral corticosteroids are usually preferred, except from severe asthma or vomiting.
- There is no evidence of the superiority from one compound over another at equipollent doses. However, reference corticosteroids are prednisolone and methylprednisolone.

24.5 Corticosteroids in Anaphylaxis

Anaphylaxis is a systemic life-threatening acute immunological or non-immunological hypersensitivity reaction [33]. All healthcare personnel must be able to recognize and manage it. Anaphylaxis is potentially lethal, being characterized by a rapid onset of symptoms involving simultaneously the skin, the airways, the gastrointestinal or cardiovascular systems and requires immediate medical intervention. Despite the fact that mortality due to anaphylaxis remains low, hospitalization caused by food- and drug-induced anaphylaxis is still increasing. Most anaphylactic reactions are uniphasic [34]. Nevertheless, delayed onset, biphasic reactions, and protracted or persistent reactions have been described. Biphasic reactions are characterized by a symptom-free period followed by a second wave of symptoms, which may be more severe and refractory to therapy. The exact mechanism involved in each of these patterns is not yet fully understood.

Anaphylaxis characteristically occurs through an IgE-mediated mechanism and is usually triggered by foods, insect venom stings, or drugs, although pathophysiological events such as IgE-independent immunologic mechanisms and non-immunological mast cell activation can be also involved. Co-factors like exercise, stress, infection, or non-steroidal anti-inflammatory drugs may be aggravating factors [34].

Epinephrine is the single best therapy for anaphylaxis and is therefore universally recommended as first-line therapy in anaphylaxis guidelines and patient-centered emergency plans. In spite of this, data collected in the emergency departments show an underuse of epinephrine and a delayed administration during anaphylaxis worldwide [33]. Second-line drugs for the treatment of anaphylaxis include antihistamines (both anti-H1 and anti-H2) and corticosteroids. Disappointingly, although not life-saving, corticosteroids are frequently used worldwide in anaphylaxis, including in severe cases, leading often to underuse or delayed administration of epinephrine.

Considering the mechanism of action of corticosteroids, it may seem natural to use them during an anaphylaxis episode. However, due to their slow-onset action, corticosteroids are not first-line drugs in treatment anaphylaxis. The rationale of their use as an adjunctive therapy to epinephrine could be to prevent protracted symptoms and possibly biphasic reactions. So far no convincing evidence of their effectiveness in anaphylaxis still exists [34]. Actually, the use of glucocorticoid has been found to increase the risk for biphasic anaphylaxis in children, even if a confounding effect of severity may not be excluded [35]. Disappointingly, some studies found an increased risk of hospital or intensive care admission in patients treated at a home level with steroids for an episode of anaphylaxis [36]. A Cochrane review published in 2010 concluded that there is no evidence for the use of steroids in the emergency management of anaphylaxis [37]. Therefore, these drugs have been not incorporated in the last international anaphylaxis guidelines [38–40].

- No convincing evidence has been described on the effectiveness of corticosteroids in anaphylaxis.

24.6 Corticosteroids in Non-IgE-Mediated Food Allergy

Several adverse food reactions have been classified as non-IgE-mediated food allergies since the pathological immunologic response to food is mediated by the cell compartment of the immune system. These include food protein-induced enterocolitis syndrome (FPIES) that is distinguished into acute and chronic forms [41]. Acute FPIES is characterized by profuse and repetitive vomiting, often associated with pallor and/or lethargy, classically taking place 1–4 h after the ingestion of the culprit food. The pathophysiology of FPIES is not well understood; however, it has been assumed that food allergens may activate intestinal T cells, resulting in local inflammation, increased intestinal mucosa permeability, and fluid shift. The acute management of FPIES reactions requires rehydration and control of emesis. In mild reactions, oral rehydration at home may be suitable when fluids are tolerated. In case of severe emesis and lethargy, or in the event of hypotension, intravenous hydration in medical setting is needed. Corticosteroids should be administered in patients with a history of severe reactions attributable to FPIES, and this treatment could be considered also for patients with non-severe symptoms [42]. In particular, intravenous steroids should be considered in case of symptoms of acute FPIES during oral challenge. The role of the single dose of intravenous steroids is based on the presumed inflammatory pathophysiology of FPIES. However, there are no randomized studies demonstrating the usefulness of corticosteroids and, indeed, even of intravenous fluids [43].

Other diseases ascribable to non-IgE-mediated food allergy are represented by eosinophilic gastrointestinal disorders (EGD). EGD can be also successfully treated with steroids, both oral and topical [44]. In particular, oral steroids can treat eosinophilic esophagitis (EoE) inducing clinical and histological remission. Moreover, systemic corticosteroids should be administered for emergency cases, including severe dysphagia, hospitalization, and weight loss. Given the chronicity of this condition, steroids can carry significant adverse effects if used as long-term therapy. Currently, topical corticosteroid therapy can be considered in all children and adults affected by EoE for both starting and maintenance treatment since they are efficacious in inducing EoE remission [45]. However, steroid resistance (as demonstrated by the failure of histological responsiveness and the lack of variation from local esophageal gene expression) has been described [46].

- Intravenous corticosteroids should be administered in patients with a history of food protein-induced enterocolitis (FPIES) particularly in case of severe reactions and during oral challenge.
- Corticosteroids are efficacious in inducing clinical and histological remission of eosinophilic esophagitis (EoE).
- Topical steroid therapy can be considered in children affected by EoE as starting a maintenance treatment.
- Systemic corticosteroids can be useful in severe cases of EoE, such as dysphagia, weight loss, and hospitalization.

24.7 Corticosteroids in Cutaneous Atopic Diseases

Urticaria is defined as the development of wheals, angioedema, or both. According to the duration, it can be differentiated into acute or chronic (less or more than 6 weeks). Current guidelines of chronic urticaria in children suggest a stepwise approach for its treatment [47]. Generally, corticosteroids (prednisone or prednisolone up to 1 mg per kg per day) are used for short periods (3–10 days) for controlling flare-ups in chronic urticaria; long-term use is not suggested because of adverse effects. Delayed-pressure urticaria could benefit from topical corticosteroids [48]. Once the symptoms are adequately controlled, treatment should be tapered sequentially [49]. There are no studies confirming the use of corticosteroids in patients with chronic urticaria, even if they are valuable in clinical practice to control symptoms.

Atopic dermatitis represents the most frequent chronic inflammatory cutaneous disease in childhood with a prevalence among 16–20% worldwide. In severe forms, healthcare and social costs are relevant because of the strong impact of the disease on patients' and families' quality of life, sleep deprivation, attention disorders, and irritability [50]. Topical corticosteroids (TCS) have been the mainstay of atopic dermatitis therapy over the past 40 years. Effectiveness and good safety profile of TCS, even with long-term therapies contributed to the spread of their usage. Actually, TCS inhibit the transcription of several pro-inflammatory cytokines involved in skin diseases (e.g., IL-1, IL-2, IL-6, TNF-α, and INF-γ) and stimulate gene expression of anti-inflammatory cytokines, such as TGF-β and IL-10. Through this cytokine regulation, corticosteroids likely play an effective role in balancing the ratio of lymphocytes Th1 and Th2 at the skin lesions level [51]. Other anti-inflammatory effects include acceleration of eosinophils' and T lymphocytes' apoptosis, suppression of endothelial cells and lymphocyte activation, inhibition of edema at dermis, together with the dilatation of the capillaries, and the reduction of vascular per-

Table 24.6 Potency of topical corticosteroids

Low powerful	Moderately powerful	Powerful	Highly powerful
• Hydrocortisone • Hydrocortisone acetate	• Alclometasone dipropionate • Clobetasol butyrate • Dexamethasone sodium phosphate • Dexamethasone valerate • Desonide • Fluocortinbutylester • Hydrocortisone butyrate	• Beclomethasone dipropionate • Betamethasone benzoate, dipropionate and budesonide valerate • Budesonide • Desoximetasone • Diflucortolone valerate • Fluocinolone acetonide • Fluocinonide • Fluocortolone • Fluocortolone caproate • Fluticasone propionate • Methylprednisolone aceponate • Mometasone furoate • Prednicarbate	• Halcinonide • Clobetasol propionate
Group I	*Group II*	*Group III*	*Group IV*

From Galli et al. [50]

meability. Also, TCS showed antiproliferative effects on various cells, including T lymphocytes. Choosing the right TCS molecule should take account of different factors: the potency of the drug, the vehicle of the preparation, the age of the patient, and the site and body surface area to be treated. According to their potency in the European classification, TCS are classified into four groups, starting from group I, with low potency molecules, to the IV group with highly potent TCS (Table 24.6).

The choice of the TCS according to its potency, vehicle, and amount to be applied should be based on the patient's age and region of application. Different areas of the body surface show substantial differences (e.g., thickness of the stratum corneum and density of hair follicles) in TCS penetration and absorption [52]. TCS absorption may be also higher in infants and toddlers. Therefore, when TCS are applied to areas with the highest absorption, such as eyelids, genitals, face and skin folds, a careful monitoring of possible side effects is required. So, in these areas a prolonged use of corticosteroids should be avoided, especially those with moderate-high potency and with ointment vehicles. As discussed above, the risk of side effects, such as atrophy, telangiectasias, hypertrichosis, and striae rubrae, is very limited if the steroids are used appropriately.

As far as concerns systemic effects, a clinically significant suppression of the axis hypothalamic-pituitary-adrenal has never been reported in the routine treatment of pediatric patients with atopic eczema. As well, the expected prevalence of low bone mineral density in children treated with topical steroids is the same with respect to the general population.

Oral corticosteroids have a limited role in atopic dermatitis therapy without comorbidities [53]. They act in a short time on the acute symptoms of atopic dermatitis reducing inflammation, although few randomized controlled trials have been performed to confirm their real effectiveness compared to other drugs. Instead, they have a limited role in itching and pain. Despite their efficacy, rebound effect after discontinuation of therapy and side effects limit their use. Therefore, oral corticosteroids should be employed in exceptional cases such as major exacerbations in patients with severe atopic dermatitis, as a bridge therapy before starting other treatments with drugs with a better safety profile such as TCS and biologics (dupilumab).

- Short course of oral corticosteroids should be used for short periods (3–10 days) for controlling flare-ups in chronic urticaria.
- Topical corticosteroids can be beneficial in delayed-pressure urticaria.
- Topical corticosteroids represent the mainstay of atopic dermatitis treatment.
- Oral corticosteroids should be employed exceptional cases such as major exacerbations in patients with severe atopic dermatitis.

24.8 Corticosteroids in Allergic Rhinitis

Allergic rhinitis, with or without conjunctivitis, is the most prevalent allergic diseases resulting in a chronic, mostly eosinophilic, inflammation of the nasal mucosa and conjunctiva. Symptoms include itching, sneezing, watery nasal discharge, and nasal congestion. Commonly, there are associated ocular symptoms (watery, red, and/or itchy eyes). Symptoms may be described as seasonal and/or perennial; as intermittent or persistent; or mild, moderate, or severe according to their impact on the patient's quality of life [54].

Clinical manifestation of persistent forms is essentially characterized by obstructive symptomatology, compared with that of intermittent forms from seasonal allergens in which the irritative component prevails (rhinorrhea, sneezing, ocular involvement). The measures to be implemented for the care of the child with allergic rhinitis are based primarily on environmental prevention; the aim is to avoid as much as possible the exposure of the nasal mucosa with the sensitizing allergen. Secondarily, it is necessary to set up a correct and appropriate drug therapy. Intranasal corticosteroids (INC) are the mainstay of treatment for persistent moderate-to-severe allergic rhinitis. Indeed, numerous evidence have shown that topical nasal corticosteroids interact with mediators and cells involved in both early and late inflammatory reaction. INC indeed reduce the number of antigen-presenting cells and mast cells in the mucosa, inhibit the release of cytokines and chemokines, and are able to markedly decrease the inflammatory cell infiltrate. A reduction in neurogenic inflammation as well as a potent anti-permeabilizing and anti-oedematous effect has also been demonstrated [55]. The anti-inflammatory effect of INC improves nasal obstruction and indirectly also shows moderate efficacy on irritative syndromes: rhinorrhea, itching, and also sneezing [56]. Numerous studies have demonstrated the efficacy of INC in the treatment of both intermittent allergic rhinitis from seasonal allergens and persistent forms from perennial allergens. Their onset of action can be less than 30 min, although peak effect may take several hours to days, with maximum effectiveness usually is noted after 2–4 weeks of use; this emphasizes that INC are not drugs to be used on an as-needed basis, but continued use is recommended and prolonged according to clinical manifestations and periodicity of symptoms. The currently available molecules (mometasone furoate, fluticasone propionate, budesonide, flunisolide, beclomethasone dipropionate), which can be used in the pediatric age group, allow for maximum efficacy while minimizing potential systemic effects from absorption. So far, there is no evidence for the superiority of a INC. Corticosteroids used topically for allergic rhinitis are well tolerated. Most common adverse effects of intranasal corticosteroids are throat irritation, epistaxis, stinging, burning, and nasal dryness. Local side effects are almost always attributable to incorrect use of the nozzle when oriented toward the nasal septum and not the lateral wall. Although there has been concern about potential systemic adverse effects, including the suppression of the hypothalamic-pituitary axis, these effects have not been shown with currently available INC. Some data had previously shown significant growth retardation after prolonged use of endonasal beclomethasone, but no other ICN has shown systemic effects on growth [57]. However careful monitoring of height is required in children treated for long periods with both medium- and high-dose inhaled corticosteroid for asthma and INC for allergic rhinitis.

Usually, a combination of intranasal corticosteroid and a topical or oral antihistamine is enough to treat moderate-to-severe allergic rhinitis. Recent EAACI recommendations stated that pediatric allergic rhinitis should be treated with oral steroids only in particular cases with highly severe symptoms for a limited period of time. Systemic corticosteroids should never be considered as a first-line treatment for allergic rhinitis [58]. Therefore, it is always recommended a stepped-care approach according to disease severity [59, 60].

- Intranasal corticosteroids are recommended as first-line treatment of persistent allergic rhinitis.

24.9 Conclusions

Corticosteroids are a group of structurally related molecules that comprise natural hormones and synthetic drugs with anti-inflammatory activity. They play a crucial role in the treatment of allergic diseases since childhood. However, the decision of the type and the dosage of corticosteroid to be administered should be thoroughly assessed in order to reduce possible adverse reactions. Furthermore, administration of corticosteroids must be established on evidence of clinical benefits taking into account guidelines.

Take-Home Messages

- Corticosteroids prevent or suppress inflammation in response to immunological, radiant, mechanical, chemical, and infectious stimuli. Oral route of administration determines a good absorption and effectiveness.
- Corticosteroids have been correlated to various adverse effects, principally related to dosage, type, route of administration, and treatment duration. Prolonged corticosteroid treatment can be linked with suppression of HPA axis function and growth retardation.
- Administration of corticosteroids with intermediate biological half-life (e.g., prednisolone or prednisone) for 3–6 days is not associated with withdrawal symptoms.

Glossary

Allergic rhinitis Allergic reaction that causes inflammation of the nose that occurs when the immune system overreacts to inhaled allergens. Clinically, it is characterized by sneezing, congestion, itchy nose, and sore throat.

Anaphylaxis Acute life-threatening hypersensitivity disorder, defined as a generalized, rapidly evolving, multi-organ allergic reaction.

Asthma It is the most prevalent chronic respiratory disease in childhood, characterized by airway inflammation and hyperresponsiveness to various stimuli. Clinically, asthma is characterized by cough, wheezing, difficult breathing, and chest tightness.

Corticosteroids Group of steroid hormones produced in the adrenal cortex that are classified into glucocorticoids and mineralocorticoid. They have several metabolic functions and synthetic analogs of these hormones are used to treat inflammation.

Eosinophilic esophagitis (EoE) Chronic allergic/immune-mediated eosinophilic disease of the esophagus. Symptoms include swallowing difficulty, food impaction, vomiting, and heartburn.

Food protein-induced enterocolitis syndrome (FPIES) A non-IgE-mediated food allergy that affects mainly the gastrointestinal (GI) tract. Symptoms are delayed (2–4 h) and characterized by projectile vomiting, diarrhea and dehydration, lethargy, changes in blood pressure, and body temperature.

Glucocorticoid-responsive element Short sequences of DNA typically found in the promoter of glucocorticoid-responsive genes that are able to bind glucocorticoid receptor and regulate transcription of steroid-responsive genes.

Oxidative stress Disturbance in the balance between the production of reactive oxygen species (ROS) and antioxidants. ROS levels increase during environmental stress with the creation of cellular damage by reacting with intracellular constituents, such as DNA and membrane lipids.

Transactivation Stimulation of a gene transcription by a specific protein (i.e., transcription factor).

Transrepression Inhibition of a gene transcription by a specific protein (i.e., transcription factor).

References

1. Barnes PJ. Corticosteroid effects on cell signalling. Eur Respir J. 2006;27:413–26.
2. Barnes PJ. Glucocorticosteroids. Handb Exp Pharmacol. 2017;237:93–115.
3. Alangari AA. Genomic and non-genomic actions of glucocorticoids in asthma. Ann Thorac Med. 2010;5:133–9.
4. Beigelman A, Chipps BE, Bacharier LB. Update on the utility of corticosteroids in acute pediatric respiratory disorders. Allergy Asthma Proc. 2015;36:332–8.
5. Henderson I, Caiazzo E, McSharry C, Guzik TJ, Maffia P. Why do some asthma patients respond poorly to glucocorticoid therapy? Pharmacol Res. 2020;160:105189.
6. Barnes PJ. Corticosteroid resistance in patients with asthma and chronic obstructive pulmonary disease. J Allergy Clin Immunol. 2013;131:636–45.
7. Zein J, Gaston B, Bazeley P, DeBoer MD, Igo RP, Bleecker ER, et al. HSD3B1 genotype identifies glucocorticoid responsiveness in severe asthma. Proc Natl Acad Sci USA. 2020;117:2187–93.
8. Tantisira KG, Lasky-Su J, Harada M, Murphy A, Litonjua AA, Himes BE, et al. Genomewide association between GLCCI1 and response to glucocorticoid therapy in asthma. N Engl J Med. 2011;365:1173–83.
9. Cutrera R, Baraldi E, Indinnimeo L, Miraglia Del Giudice M, Piacentini G, Scaglione F, et al. Management of acute respiratory diseases in the pediatric population: the role of oral corticosteroids. Ital J Pediatr. 2017;43:31.
10. Warrington TP, Bostwick JM. Psychiatric adverse effects of corticosteroids. Mayo Clin Proc. 2006;81:1361–7.
11. Kenna HA, Poon AW, de los Angeles CP, Koran LM. Psychiatric complications of treatment with corticosteroids: review with case report. Psychiatry Clin Neurosci. 2011;65:549–60.
12. Poetker DM, Reh DD. A comprehensive review of the adverse effects of systemic corticosteroids. Otolaryngol Clin N Am. 2010;43:753–68.
13. Powell C, Chang C, Naguwa SM, Cheema G, Gershwin ME. Steroid induced osteonecrosis: an analysis of steroid dosing risk. Autoimmun Rev. 2010;9:721–43.
14. McKee MD, Waddell JP, Kudo PA, Schemitsch EH, Richards RR. Osteonecrosis of the femoral head in men following short-course corticosteroid therapy: a report of 15 cases. CMAJ. 2001;164:205–6.
15. Rhen T, Cidlowski JA. Antiinflammatory action of glucocorticoids—new mechanisms for old drugs. N Engl J Med. 2005;353:1711–23.
16. Fernandes RM, Oleszczuk M, Woods CR, Rowe BH, Cates CJ, Hartling L. The Cochrane library and safety of systemic corticosteroids for acute respiratory conditions in children: an overview of reviews. Evid Based Child Health. 2014;9:733–47.
17. Morimoto Y, Oishi T, Hanasaki N, Miyatake A, Noma K, Yamamura Y. Relative potency in acute and chronic suppressive effects of prednisolone and betamethasone on the hypothalamic-pituitary-adrenal axis in man. Endocrinol Jpn. 1980;27:659–66.
18. de Benedictis FM, Bush A. Corticosteroids in respiratory diseases in children. Am J Respir Crit Care Med. 2012;185:12–23.
19. Daley-Yates PT. Inhaled corticosteroids: potency, dose equivalence and therapeutic index. Br J Clin Pharmacol. 2015;80:372–80.
20. Levy ML, Bacharier LB, Bateman E, Boulet LP, Brightling C, Buhl R, et al. Key recommendations for primary care from the 2022 Global Initiative for Asthma (GINA) update. NPJ Prim Care Respir Med. 2023;33:7.
21. Krishnan JA, Cloutier MM, Schatz M. National Asthma Education and Prevention Program 2020 guideline update: where do we go from here? Am J Respir Crit Care Med. 2021;203:164–7.

22. British Thoracic Society. British guideline on the management of asthma.
23. Indinnimeo L, Chiappini E, Miraglia Del Giudice M, et al. Italian Panel for the management of acute asthma attack in children. Guideline on management of the acute asthma attack in children by Italian Society of Pediatrics. Ital J Pediatr. 2018;44:46.
24. Becker JM, Arora A, Scarfone RJ, Spector ND, Fontana-Penn ME, Gracely E, et al. Oral versus intravenous corticosteroids in children hospitalized with asthma. J Allergy Clin Immunol. 1999;103:586–90.
25. Kirkland SW, Cross E, Campbell S, Villa-Roel C, Rowe BH. Intramuscular versus oral corticosteroids to reduce relapses following discharge from the emergency department for acute asthma. Cochrane Database Syst Rev. 2018;6:CD012629.
26. Vichyanond P, Irvin CG, Larsen GL, Szefler SJ, Hill MR. Penetration of corticosteroids into the lung: evidence for a difference between methylprednisolone and prednisolone. J Allergy Clin Immunol. 1989;84:867–73.
27. Fiel SB, Vincken W. Systemic corticosteroid therapy for acute asthma exacerbations. J Asthma. 2006;43:321–31.
28. Parente L. Deflazacort: therapeutic index, relative potency and equivalent doses versus other corticosteroids. BMC Pharmacol Toxicol. 2017;18:1.
29. Ferraris JR, Fainstein Day P, Gutman R, Granillo E, Ramirez J, Ruiz S, et al. Effect of therapy with a new glucocorticoid, deflazacort, on linear growth and growth hormone secretion after renal transplantation. J Pediatr. 1992;121:809–13.
30. Balsan S, Stéru D, Bourdeau A, Grimberg R, Lenoir G. Effects of long-term maintenance therapy with a new glucocorticoid, deflazacort, on mineral metabolism and statural growth. Calcif Tissue Int. 1987;40:303–9.
31. Beckhaus AA, Riutort MC, Castro-Rodriguez JA. Inhaled versus systemic corticosteroids for acute asthma in children. A systematic review. Pediatr Pulmonol. 2014;49:326–34.
32. Su XM, Yu N, Kong LF, Kang J. Effectiveness of inhaled corticosteroids in the treatment of acute asthma in children in the emergency department: a meta-analysis. Ann Med. 2014;46:24–30.
33. Shaker MS, Wallace DV, Golden DBK, Oppenheimer J, Bernstein JA, Campbell RL, et al. Anaphylaxis—a 2020 practice parameter update, systematic review, and Grading of Recommendations, Assessment, Development and Evaluation (GRADE) analysis. J Allergy Clin Immunol. 2020;145:1082–123.
34. Muraro A, Worm M, Alviani C, Cardona V, DunnGalvin A, Garvey LH, et al. EAACI guidelines: anaphylaxis (2021 update). Allergy. 2022;77:357–77.
35. Ring J, Beyer K, Biedermann T, Bircher A, Duda D, Fischer J, et al. Guideline for acute therapy and management of anaphylaxis: S2 guideline of the German Society for Allergology and Clinical Immunology (DGAKI), the Association of German Allergologists (AeDA), the Society of Pediatric Allergy and Environmental Medicine (GPA), the German Academy of Allergology and Environmental Medicine (DAAU), the German Professional Association of Pediatricians (BVKJ), the Austrian Society for Allergology and Immunology (ÖGAI), the Swiss Society for Allergy and Immunology (SGAI), the German Society of Anaesthesiology and Intensive Care Medicine (DGAI), the German Society of Pharmacology (DGP), the German Society for Psychosomatic Medicine (DGPM), the German Working Group of Anaphylaxis Training and Education (AGATE) and the patient organization German Allergy and Asthma Association (DAAB). Allergol J Int. 2014;23:96–112.
36. Gabrielli S, Clarke A, Morris J, Eisman H, Gravel J, Enarson P, et al. Evaluation of prehospital management in a Canadian emergency department anaphylaxis cohort. J Allergy Clin Immunol Pract. 2019;7:2232–2238.e3.
37. Campbell RL, Li JT, Nicklas RA, Sadosty AT. Emergency department diagnosis and treatment of anaphylaxis: a practice parameter. Ann Allergy Asthma Immunol. 2014;113:599–608.
38. Choo KJL, Simons E, Sheikh A. Glucocorticoids for the treatment of anaphylaxis: Cochrane systematic review. Allergy. 2010;65:1205–11.
39. Cardona V, Ansotegui IJ, Ebisawa M, El-Gamal Y, Fernandez Rivas M, Fineman S, et al. World allergy organization anaphylaxis guidance 2020. World Allergy Organ J. 2020;13:100472.
40. Li X, Ma Q, Yin J, Zheng Y, Chen R, Chen Y, et al. A clinical practice guideline for the emergency management of anaphylaxis (2020). Front Pharmacol. 2022;13:845689.
41. Nowak-Węgrzyn A, Katz Y, Mehr SS, Koletzko S. Non-IgE-mediated gastrointestinal food allergy. J Allergy Clin Immunol. 2015;135:1114–24.
42. Leonard SA, Pecora V, Fiocchi AG, Nowak-Wegrzyn A. Food protein-induced enterocolitis syndrome: a review of the new guidelines. World Allergy Organ J. 2018;11:4.
43. Sicherer SH. Food protein-induced enterocolitis syndrome: case presentations and management lessons. J Allergy Clin Immunol. 2005;115:149–56.
44. Cianferoni A. Non-IgE mediated food allergy. Curr Pediatr Rev. 2020;16:95–105.
45. Licari A, Votto M, D'Auria E, Castagnoli R, Caimmi SME, Marseglia GL. Eosinophilic gastrointestinal diseases in children: a practical review. Curr Pediatr Rev. 2020;16:106–14.
46. Caldwell JM, Blanchard C, Collins MH, Putnam PE, Kaul A, Aceves SS, Bouska CA, Rothenberg ME. Glucocorticoid-regulated genes in eosinophilic esophagitis: a role for FKBP51. J Allergy Clin Immunol. 2010;125:879–888.e8.

47. Caffarelli C, Paravati F, El Hachem M, Duse M, Bergamini M, Simeone G, et al. Management of chronic urticaria in children: a clinical guideline. Ital J Pediatr. 2019;45:101.
48. Zuberbier T, Abdul Latiff AH, Abuzakouk M, Aquilina S, Asero R, Baker D, et al. The international EAACI/GA²LEN/EuroGuiDerm/APAAACI guideline for the definition, classification, diagnosis, and management of urticaria. Allergy. 2022;77:734–66.
49. Schaefer P. Acute and chronic urticaria: evaluation and treatment. Am Fam Physician. 2017;95:717–24.
50. Galli E, Neri I, Ricci G, Baldo E, Barone M, Belloni Fortina A, et al. Consensus conference on clinical management of pediatric atopic dermatitis. Ital J Pediatr. 2016;42:26.
51. Galli E, Fortina AB, Ricci G, Maiello N, Neri I, Baldo E, et al. Narrative review on the management of moderate-severe atopic dermatitis in pediatric age of the Italian Society of Pediatric Allergology and Immunology (SIAIP), of the Italian Society of Pediatric Dermatology (SIDerP) and of the Italian Society of Pediatrics (SIP). Ital J Pediatr. 2022;48:95.
52. Chiricozzi A, Comberiati P, D'Auria E, Zuccotti G, Peroni DG. Topical corticosteroids for pediatric atopic dermatitis: thoughtful tips for practice. Pharmacol Res. 2020;158:104878.
53. Drucker AM, Eyerich K, de Bruin-Weller MS, Thyssen JP, Spuls PI, Irvine AD, et al. Use of systemic corticosteroids for atopic dermatitis: International Eczema Council consensus statement. Br J Dermatol. 2018;178:768–75.
54. Roberts G, Pfaar O, Akdis CA, Ansotegui IJ, Durham SR, Gerth van Wijk R, et al. EAACI guidelines on allergen immunotherapy: allergic rhinoconjunctivitis. Allergy. 2018;73:765–98.
55. Daley-Yates PT, Larenas-Linnemann D, Bhargave C, Verma M. Intranasal corticosteroids: topical potency, systemic activity and therapeutic index. J Asthma Allergy. 2021;14:1093–104.
56. Scadding GK. Corticosteroids in the treatment of pediatric allergic rhinitis. J Allergy Clin Immunol. 2001;108:S59–64.
57. Bensch GW. Safety of intranasal corticosteroids. Ann Allergy Asthma Immunol. 2016;117:601–5.
58. Hox V, Lourijsen E, Jordens A, Aasbjerg K, Agache I, Alobid I, et al. Benefits and harm of systemic steroids for short- and long-term use in rhinitis and rhinosinusitis: an EAACI position paper. Clin Transl Allergy. 2020;10:1.
59. Brożek JL, Bousquet J, Agache I, Agarwal A, Bachert C, Bosnic-Anticevich S, et al. Allergic Rhinitis and its Impact on Asthma (ARIA) guidelines—2016 revision. J Allergy Clin Immunol. 2017;140:950–8.
60. Dykewicz MS, Wallace DV, Amrol DJ, Baroody FM, Bernstein JA, Craig TJ, et al. Rhinitis 2020: a practice parameter update. J Allergy Clin Immunol. 2020;146:721–67.

25 Monoclonal Antibodies in Pediatric Allergy Treatment

Riccardo Castagnoli, Maria De Filippo, Adelaide Corvaglia, Matea Jankovic, Martina Votto, Amelia Licari, and Gian Luigi Marseglia

Abstract

Remarkable therapeutic progress has been accomplished in pediatric allergology in recent decades, driven by the advances in molecular biology and immunopharmacology and the understanding of the inflammatory pathogenic mechanisms in primary allergic conditions. Notably, a shared feature among diseases with different clinical manifestations, such as atopic dermatitis (AD) and allergic asthma, is a "Type 2 helper T cell" (Th2) response. Biologically active proteins targeting specific therapeutic pathways exemplify the paradigm of tailored and precision medicine, yielding successful outcomes, particularly in the context of severe allergic skin and respiratory diseases. Monoclonal antibodies are humanized or chimeric immunoglobulins generated in vitro from a single immortalized clone of B lymphocytes. Currently, only a select few of these biologics are approved for clinical use as anti-IgE (omalizumab), anti-IL5 (mepolizumab), and anti-IL4/13 (dupilumab) for pediatric and adolescent populations, while others are still in the clinical trial phase.

The following sections outline the main and updated applications of biological drugs in various allergic diseases.

Keywords

Monoclonal antibodies · Dupilumab · Omalizumab · Mepolizumab · Benralizumab · Tezepelumab · Atopic dermatitis · Severe allergic asthma · Food allergy · Chronic spontaneous urticaria · Chronic rhinosinusitis with nasal polyps

Test your learning and check your understanding of this book's contents: use the "Springer Nature Flashcards" app to access questions using ▶ https://sn.pub/nspbjm. To use the app, please follow the instructions in Chap. 1.

R. Castagnoli · M. De Filippo · A. Corvaglia
M. Jankovic · M. Votto · A. Licari
G. L. Marseglia (✉)
Pediatric Unit, Department of Clinical, Surgical, Diagnostic and Pediatric Sciences, University of Pavia, Pavia, Italy

Pediatric Clinic, Fondazione IRCCS Policlinico San Matteo, Pavia, Italy
e-mail: gianluigi.marseglia@unipv.it

C. Caffarelli, G. L. Marseglia (eds.), *Textbook of Pediatric Allergy*,
https://doi.org/10.1007/978-3-031-71283-8_25

25.1 Atopic Dermatitis

Atopic dermatitis (AD) is a chronic, relapsing inflammatory skin disease typically characterized by skin xerosis, pruritus, and hyperreactivity. Pathogenesis is multifactorial, with an interplay between genetic predisposition and environmental factors, leading to abnormal immune response and skin barrier impairment with increased permeability to environmental allergens.

Prevalence in children is up to 20% and decreases with age. Nevertheless, one-third of adolescents with AD have moderate or severe disease, with a high impact on quality of life.

Current guidelines suggest an individualized, multidisciplinary, and step approach with increasing levels of treatment according to the AD severity, which is measured through various objective scales such as the Severity Scoring of Atopic Dermatitis (SCORAD) or Eczema Area and severity index EASI (EASI).

According to the latest Italian Intersocieties Consensus, **moderate-to-severe AD** is defined by one of the following criteria:

- EASI ≥24 or localization in visible or sensible areas (face, neck, hands, or genitalia)
- Numeric Rating Scale (NRS) itch ≥7
- Children Dermatology Life Quality Index (CDLQI) ≥10

Treating moderate-to-severe AD in adolescents is exceptionally challenging because it is poorly controlled by topical corticosteroids (TCSs), and limited treatment alternatives are available. Systemic immunosuppressive drugs, such as cyclosporine A, methotrexate, azathioprine, or mycophenolate mofetil, are off-label and are burdened by medium- and long-term adverse effects (AEs).

Understanding that the primary immunological mechanism that underlies AD is an excessive type 2 inflammatory response has laid the groundwork for the use of biological drugs that target specific critical cytokines involved in this type of inflammation [1].

25.1.1 Dupilumab in AD

Dupilumab is a human monoclonal IgG4 antibody targeting the alpha subunit of the interleukin 4 receptor (IL-4R), also shared by the interleukin 13 receptor (IL-13R). It exerts a dual inhibitory effect on the Th2 inflammatory cascade by targeting a common receptor subunit of these two cytokines.

Type I IL4R, expressed on hematopoietic cells, consists of the IL-4Rα subunit and the γc subunit and binds only IL-4. Conversely, type II IL-4R is expressed on cutaneous and bronchial epithelial cells, comprising the IL-4Rα subunit and the low-affinity receptor for IL-13 (IL-13Rα1). The binding of IL-4 and IL-13 to their respective receptors triggers transphosphorylation and activation of Janus family protein kinases (JAKs) associated with cytokine receptors, facilitating the recruitment of STAT6 (signal transducer and activator of transcription 6). This process initiates specific transcriptional and transduction programs, ultimately resulting in the activation of an adaptive pro-allergic immune response characterized by class switching to IgE production and the reprogramming of regulatory T cells (Tregs) into Th2 CD4+ cells and consequent alteration of immunotolerance.

The inflammatory pattern of eczematous skin lesions is characterized prominently by the expression of Th2 lymphocytes and innate type 2 lymphoid cells (ILC2).

Moreover, in AD, IL-4 and IL-13 inhibit the production of proteins involved in maintaining skin barrier integrity and contribute to the differentiation of keratinocytes while downregulating the production of filaggrin, loricrin, involucrin, adhesion molecules, antimicrobial peptides (such as beta-defensins and cathelicidin LL-37), and ceramides, which ultimately exacerbates the damage to the skin barrier. Additionally, IL-4, IL-13, IL-33, and thymic stromal lymphopoietin (TSLP) are implicated in itch, significantly impacting sleep quality and increasing the risk of bacterial and viral skin infections. The detection of IL-4Rα receptors on afferent neurons demonstrates the link.

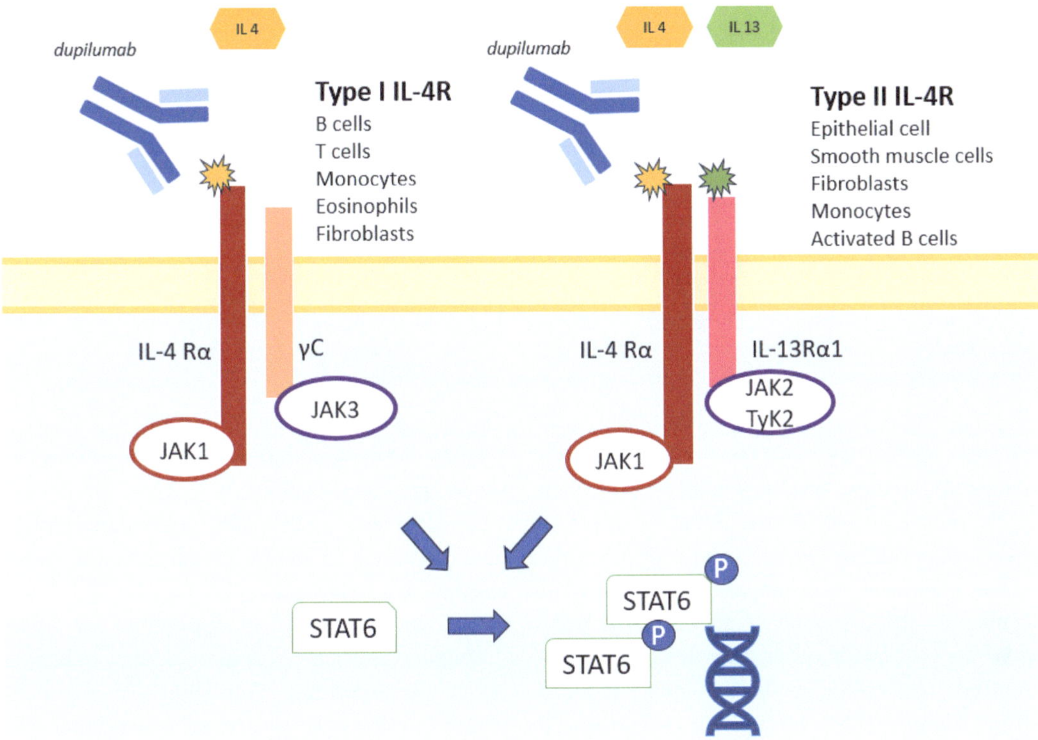

Fig. 25.1 Mechanism of action of dupilumab (anti-IL-4Rα). The binding of IL-4 and IL-13 to their respective receptors triggers the transphosphorylation and activation of receptor-associated kinases, the consequent recruitment of STAT6, and the activation of specific gene transcription programs. Dupilumab inhibits this pathway

Dupilumab exerts its mechanism of action by effectively inhibiting IL4R signaling upon binding both IL-4 and IL-13, leading to the downregulation of the Th2 inflammatory response (Fig. 25.1).

Dupilumab was the first biologic to gain regulatory approval for managing AD in 2017 for adults with moderate or severe forms of candidates for systemic therapy.

In 2019, the Food and Drug Administration (FDA) and European Medicine Agency (EMA) approved the use of dupilumab for the treatment of moderate-to-severe AD in adolescents (12–17 years) who have an inadequate response to standard-of-care therapies. Subsequently, the approval was extended by the FDA and EMA and, in 2022, by the Italian Medicines Agency (AIFA) for children aged >6 years with refractory AD. More recently, first by the FDA, followed by the EMA in March 2023, dupilumab has been approved for treating children aged 6 months to 5 years as an adjunctive treatment for moderate-to-severe forms of AD inadequately controlled.

Dupilumab is currently available in prefilled syringes or pens for injection (200 mg or 300 mg), formulated as a subcutaneous (sc) solution, for administration with dosage regimens that depend on the patient's age and weight, as indicated in Table 25.1.

Data regarding the utilization of dupilumab in children aged 6 months and above, as well as adolescents, are currently accessible. The numerous clinical trials evaluating the safety, pharmacokinetics, and efficacy of dupilumab in toddlers,

Table 25.1 Dupilumab dosage schedule in moderate-to-severe AD

		Starting dose	Subsequent doses
Adults >18 years		600 mg sc	300 mg sc every 2 weeks
Adolescents 12–17 years	>60 kg	600 mg sc	300 mg sc every 2 weeks
	<60 kg	400 mg sc	200 mg sc every 2 weeks
Children 6–11 years	15–60 kg	300 mg sc on day 1 + 300 mg sc on day 15	300 mg sc every 4 weeks[a]
	>60 kg	600 mg sc	300 mg sc every 2 weeks
Children 6 months–5 years	5–15 kg	–	200 mg sc every 4 weeks[b]
	15–30 kg	–	300 mg sc every 4 weeks[b]

[a] Starting 4 weeks after the second dose (day 15). The loading dose consists of two injections administered at two different sites

[b] In children aged 6 months to 5 years, the loading dose should not be administered

children, and adolescents have yielded results comparable to those observed in adults.

The most reported AEs are injection site reactions (pain, erythema, edema) and conjunctivitis.

The underlying mechanism of conjunctivitis is linked to the reduction of goblet cell activity and decreased mucin production, leading to conjunctival hyperemia, ocular itching, reduced visual acuity, or a foreign body sensation. It appears to be a characteristic AE explicitly observed in patients with AD undergoing treatment with this biologic. It is advisable to consider evaluating the potential presence of ophthalmic symptoms or prior episodes of conjunctivitis before initiating dupilumab treatment. Additionally, conducting a baseline ophthalmic assessment can be prudent in these cases.

Moreover, some studies highlight hypereosinophilia as a less common potential AE of using dupilumab. Approximately 20% of AD patients treated with dupilumab experienced increased eosinophil counts compared to their baseline levels, and this association could be explained by the mechanism of action of dupilumab, which blocks the IL-4 and IL-13 axis, thereby inhibiting the migration of eosinophils to the tissues without reducing their baseline production in the bone marrow. However, dupilumab-related hypereosinophilia is typically transient and not associated with clinical consequences.

Regarding efficacy, dupilumab therapy has shown an enhanced quality of life with relief from itching, as demonstrated by AD assessment scales and clinical improvement in comorbid conditions such as allergic rhinitis and asthma. Moreover, this therapy decreases allergen-specific IgE concentrations and reduces baseline blood eosinophil count.

If there is no observable improvement in the condition after 16 weeks, the physician may discontinue the treatment.

The increasing use of dupilumab for atopic dermatitis children has stimulated new questions about immunization. According to the most recent international consensus, coadministration of live and live attenuated vaccines with dupilumab is not recommended due to the lack of established safety and clinical efficacy data. It is recommended that patients receive appropriate immunizations with this type of vaccine before initiating dupilumab treatment. Instead, inactivated vaccines and COVID-19 vaccines are also recommended during biological therapy. Previous studies on patients undergoing dupilumab therapy who received tetanus toxoid vaccination and meningococcal polysaccharide vaccine have shown that the efficacy of immunization remained unaffected. Based on the most recent guidelines, it is recommended to schedule the COVID-19 vaccination between two dupilumab injections, with a 1-week interval between the vaccination and the biological treatment [2–6].

25.1.2 New Monoclonal Antibodies in AD Treatment

Lebrikizumab is an innovative humanized monoclonal antibody that targets soluble IL-13.

In phase 3 randomized trial including 211 adults and adolescents with moderate to severe AD, the administration of subcutaneous lebrikizumab in addition to topical corticosteroids resulted in a significant outcome: 41% of patients achieved an Investigator's Global Assessment (IGA) score indicating clear or almost clear skin after 16 weeks versus of 22% observed among patients who received placebo in conjunction with topical corticosteroids.

Also, **Tralokimumab**, anti-IL-13 as lebrikizumab, shows a good efficacy and tolerability profile in phase 2 clinical trials.

In treating mild to moderate AD, a highly promising appears to be **Brepocitinib**, a small-molecule tyrosine kinase 2 (TYK2)/JAK1 inhibitor that inhibits the IL-12 and IL-23 pathways.

However, none of these drugs are approved for pediatric patients with AD; more data on long-term efficacy and safety are needed [7–8].

25.2 Chronic Urticaria (CU)

Urticaria is characterized by developing wheals (hives) with or without angioedema. Hives are transient and usually last less than 24 h. Urticaria and angioedema are commonly classified as acute or chronic, depending on symptoms that occur or recur for less or more than 6 weeks. This distinction has significant clinical implications regarding the cause, disease course, and treatment. Chronic urticaria is less common in children than adults, and the overall prevalence estimate for children is about 0.5–5%. CU is defined as spontaneous or inducible if it occurs in response to specific triggers. Chronic spontaneous urticaria (CSU) is diagnosed when no eliciting triggers are found. Therefore, the time from symptom (CU) onset to proper diagnosis and correct management is usually long. CSU is the most common form of chronic urticaria. Wheels and angioedema can occur together (40% of cases) or alone in patients with CSU. Urticaria Activity Score (UAS7) is the most commonly used score to determine disease activity and how it interferes with a patient's daily exercise and sleep. No official score is validated for CU in children, but some authors proposed to use this one by adapting the body surface to a pediatric patient.

According to the European Academy of Allergology and Clinical Immunology (EAACI) and the World Allergy Organization (WAO), the standard therapy of CSU is based on using second-generation antihistamines once daily. If there is a poor response to the treatment or symptoms persist after 2–4 weeks, the daily antihistamine dosage can be increased up to four times daily. In the event of an inadequate response after 2–4 weeks, despite good adherence to the optimized maximal antihistamine therapy, the therapeutic approach can be augmented by introducing omalizumab.

25.2.1 Omalizumab in CSU

Omalizumab, a humanized monoclonal antibody of the IgG1 class, is a representative anti-IgE drug and operates through multiple mechanisms.

1. Omalizumab binds to free IgE molecules, preventing them from attaching to specific high-affinity receptors (FcεRI) on the mast and dendritic cells. This blocking action inhibits the activation of these cells and reduces the release of inflammatory mediators, thereby mitigating the allergic response.
2. Omalizumab also downregulates the expression of FcεRI receptors on mast cells and dendritic cells. By reducing the number of these receptors, omalizumab further limits the binding of IgE and subsequent cell activation, which helps to disrupt the inflammatory cascade involved in allergic reactions. Additionally, this downregulation of FcεRI expression helps to modulate the immune response and decrease the overall allergic response (Fig. 25.2).

By binding to IgE, omalizumab reduces the inflammatory response and relieves symptoms associated with CSU, such as itchy wheals and angioedema.

Omalizumab is the only monoclonal antibody currently approved for CSU and is recommended

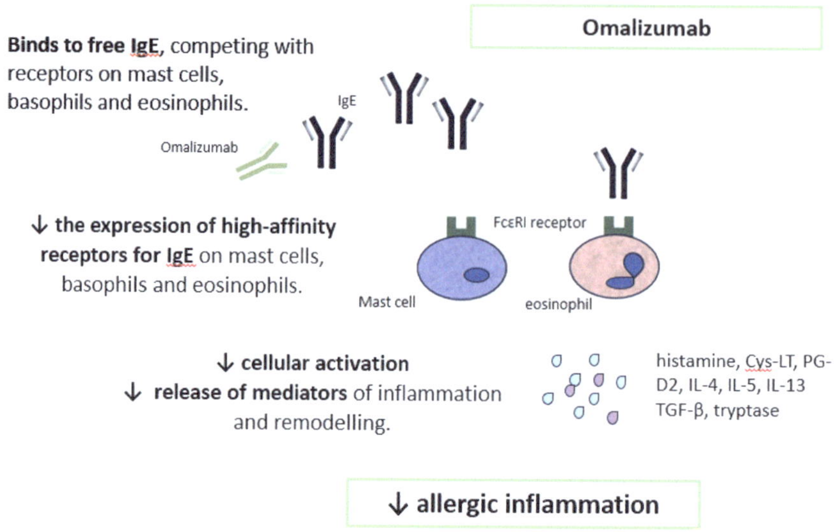

Fig. 25.2 Mechanism of omalizumab

as a third-line treatment for patients aged 12 and above. It is administered subcutaneously at the recommended 150 or 300 mg doses every 4 weeks. The dosage is not dependent on serum IgE (free or total) levels or body weight. However, if patients continue to experience symptoms before the 4-week mark, adjusting the dosage to 150 mg and administering it every 2 weeks may offer improved symptom management.

The most frequently observed side effects of omalizumab administration include local reactions at the injection site, such as bruising, burning sensation, and erythema. Additionally, mild headaches can occur as potential side effects.

The effectiveness of the treatment can be assessed after 6 months of therapy with omalizumab. If symptoms persist, the guidelines recommend considering the use of oral cyclosporine.

Several investigational biologics are being studied for the management of treatment-refractory CSU. These include ligelizumab, a monoclonal antibody with high affinity for IgE; dupilumab, a monoclonal antibody targeting IL-4 and IL-13, benralizumab, a monoclonal antibody against the IL-5 receptor alpha; and several promising novel drugs that are currently in the developmental phase.

25.3 Food Allergy

Food allergy (FA) is a pathological and potentially deadly immune response caused by exposure to specific food allergens. Epidemiological global data suggest that FA prevalence ranges from 0.45% to 10% among children younger than 5 years old. It has been estimated that approximately 40% of patients with FA have experienced a life-threatening allergic reaction and that 30% of children with FA show multiple FAs. Based on the underlying immune mechanism, FA is broadly classified into immunoglobulin (Ig) E-mediated (characterized by immediate reactions), non-IgE-mediated (characterized by delayed reactions), or mixed (represented by both IgE-dependent and IgE-independent mechanisms). IgE-mediated FA is the most common subtype affecting up to 10% of the pediatric population. Although the allergens triggering the FA vary with country and dietary habits, milk, egg, peanut, wheat, soy, and shellfish are currently the most common foods to induce IgE-mediated FA.

Following exposure to the allergenic substance, epitopes derived from food allergens bind to IgE antibodies and interact with the FcεRI receptors located on the surface of mast cells and basophils. This interaction initiates an IgE-mediated degranulation process, leading to the release of preformed histamine, leukotrienes (LTs), platelet-activating factor (PAF), and various cytokines such as IL-4, IL-5, and IL-13. These bioactive compounds are crucial in sustaining and amplifying the allergic immune response.

In the clinical setting, the initial manifestation of an allergic reaction can involve one or multiple organ systems, including the skin, respiratory, gastrointestinal, and cardiovascular systems. Anaphylaxis is a potentially life-threatening event that demands immediate and decisive intervention.

Currently, there is a lack of targeted treatments for food allergies (FAs), with the primary approach being avoidance of allergenic foods. However, there is growing optimism surrounding allergen-specific therapy, also known as immunotherapy, which has shown promising outcomes. Additionally, emerging therapeutic strategies are aimed at reinstating immune tolerance to the specific food epitopes that trigger allergic reactions.

Notably, the utilization of monoclonal antibodies as a therapeutic tool has recently yielded encouraging results in altering the progression of the disease, highlighting their significant importance in FA treatment [9–10].

25.3.1 Omalizumab in FA

IgE is crucial in FA, making it a potential therapy target. In a real-life study, omalizumab was used to treat 15 children with severe asthma who were also allergic to 37 foods. The treatment increased the threshold for cow's milk, hen's egg, wheat, and hazelnut, allowing the subjects to tolerate higher doses of these allergenic foods. After 4 months of omalizumab therapy, 70.4% of the participants could consume regular servings of these foods without requiring oral immunotherapy (OIT) procedures. The study suggests that omalizumab as a monotherapy has the potential to benefit a specific subset of patients with food allergies. Another explored approach is using omalizumab as a pretreatment or concomitant therapy alongside OIT. A multicenter, randomized clinical trial is currently underway, evaluating the effectiveness of omalizumab as a monotherapy or in combination with multifood OIT in individuals allergic to peanuts and at least two other foods. Overall, these findings highlight the potential of omalizumab as a viable therapeutic option in food allergy patients by increasing the tolerance threshold, thereby reducing the risk of severe AEs in cases of accidental ingestion. The FDA has yet to approve omalizumab as a treatment for food allergies, and the optimal dosage has yet to be established. Ongoing trials are investigating the role of omalizumab as a monotherapy or in combination with OIT.

25.3.2 Etokimab in FA

Etokimab, also known as ANB020 (AnaptysBio), is a monoclonal antibody designed to target IL-33, a cytokine that promotes the production of IgE antibodies and contributes to inflammation. It has a long half-life of approximately 372 h. In a 6-week clinical placebo-controlled phase II trial involving 15 adult participants (aged 19–54 years) with food allergies, cetuximab was found to be safe and well-tolerated compared to a placebo. Notably, a single dose of cetuximab administered as a standalone treatment demonstrated the ability to induce immune tolerance to peanuts and reduce allergic reactions related to atopy in the enrolled patients.

In food allergy, promising results have been obtained regarding the role of downregulating the allergic immune response using monoclonal antibodies. Further studies are needed to bolster and reinforce these data.

25.4 Chronic Rhinosinusitis (CRS)

CRS is a persistent nasal mucous and sinuses inflammation lasting over 12 weeks. It can occur with or without nasal polyps and is characterized by symptoms like nasal obstruction, facial pain, and a reduced sense of smell. Chronic rhinosinusitis with nasal polyps (CRSwNP) can be challenging to treat and can be associated with comorbidities such as asthma.

Recently (June 2019), the FDA-approved dupilumab to treat adults with inadequately controlled CRSwNP. Several clinical trials have demonstrated its efficacy in reducing nasal polyp size and nasal congestion, improving the sense of smell, and reducing the need for nasal polyp surgery and oral steroids. Data on the pediatric population is currently not available.

Results from three Phase III trials (NCT03280537, NCT03280550, and NCT03478930) have shown the efficacy of omalizumab, now approved for treating adult patients (18 years and older). It has demonstrated that patients treated with omalizumab experience a significant reduction in respiratory symptoms and nasal polyp size (measured by the Nasal Congestion Score) as early as 4 weeks into treatment.

In addition, the effectiveness of IL-5 inhibitors in treating CRSwNP is currently being studied. Gavaert et al. demonstrated the efficacy of mepolizumab in reducing symptoms and polyp size in adults with treatment-resistant CRSwNP. Two Phase III trials (NCT03085797, NCT03401229) have shown that mepolizumab and reslizumab are effective and safe adjunctive therapies for bilateral CRSwNP [11].

25.5 Asthma

Asthma is a chronic inflammatory disease of the airways characterized by recurrent shortness of breath, chest tightness, and cough associated with airway hyperresponsiveness and reversible bronchoconstriction. Asthma is a heterogeneous clinical condition, and its inflammatory substrate emerges due to complex genetic and environmental interactions. The therapeutic strategies are organized in multiple-step levels according to the clinical severity. Approximately up to 2.5% of children with asthma have **severe asthma**.

It is crucial to distinguish between difficult-to-treat asthma, where effective symptom control can be achieved by identifying and managing specific treatable characteristics, and severe asthma. These patients show chronic respiratory symptoms and recurrent life-threatening asthma attacks requiring hospitalization, despite high-dose treatment and resolution of treatable traits. This leads to a reduced QoL and the exposition of medication side effects.

The clinical definition of severe asthma for patients aged >6 years was established in 2014 through a collaborative effort between the American Thoracic Society (ATS) and the European Respiratory Society (ERS). According to this definition, asthma is classified as "severe" when the patient requires continuous treatment at steps 4–5 of the Global Initiative for Asthma (GINA) Guidelines throughout the previous year or when they have received systemic steroid treatment for a duration exceeding 6 months within the last year, with persistent uncontrolled symptoms or worsening despite escalated therapy.

Severe asthma requires additional therapies with biologics to mitigate the overall disease burden (step 5).

Before starting biological therapy, it is essential to validate the diagnosis of severe asthma by considering differential diagnoses, ruling out mimicking conditions, and assessing patient adherence. Furthermore, eventual coexisting needs should be identified and treated, and persistent triggers, such as allergens, should be minimized or eliminated where possible.

The choice of the appropriate biological treatment should consider the biological heterogeneity of severe asthma and the patient's age.

It is essential to differentiate the inflammatory phenotype of asthma into type 2 or nontype 2 and recognize the predominant endotype (type 2-high or type 2-low) based on the underlying pathogenic mechanisms. In childhood, the most common inflammatory phenotype is type 2, precisely type 2-high, characterized by eosinophilic airway inflammation characterized and mostly driven by allergic mechanisms. The inflammatory subset of the type 2-high endotype is supported by specific cytokines such as IL-4, IL-5, and IL-13, mainly produced by Th2 lymphocytes, type 2 innate lymphoid cells, and mast cells. It is associated with increased eosinophil count in peripheral blood, elevated serum IgE levels, and fractional exhaled nitric oxide values (FeNO). Conversely, type 2-low asthma, less common in pediatric age, is distinguished by neutrophilic or paucigranulocytic airway inflammation and is driven by different cytokines such as IL-8, IL-17, IL-22, and other T cell-related cytokines.

Currently, for managing severe asthma, various biologics are available, targeting circulating IgE and specific cytokines of type 2 inflammation, although the landscape of these therapies is continuously expanding [12–22].

25.5.1 Omalizumab

Omalizumab was the first monoclonal antibody used in allergology. Initially, it was approved by the FDA in 2003 for treating moderate-severe allergic asthma in adults and adolescents ≥12 years. Since 2009, EMA extended its use to children aged 6 years and above; since 2016, also in the United States.

It is suggested as first-line adjunctive therapy for managing severe allergic asthma in children with elevated IgE levels and positive-specific IgE for at least one aeroallergen.

It exerts its anti-IgE action by targeting the Fc fragment of circulating IgE, with consequent reduction of free IgE levels, and preventing interaction of IgE with its high-affinity IgE receptor (FcεRI) on mast cells, basophils, and low-affinity IgE receptor (FcεRII) on dendritic cells and eosinophils, thereby interrupting the release of inflammatory mediators.

Moreover, omalizumab enhances the inhibition of allergic cascade, downregulating the expression of FcεRI and decreasing cellular activation and the release of soluble mediators by mast cells and basophils. Recent evidence has shown the potential role of omalizumab in reducing the expression of mediators of bronchial tissue remodeling.

Omalizumab is administered via subcutaneous injection every 2–4 weeks. The dosage range is between 75 and 375 mg sc and is based on the patient's body weight and baseline total serum IgE levels.

Insufficient data on validated biomarkers that predict the response to omalizumab therapy in children is currently available.

Recent studies demonstrated that patients with more likely to benefit from omalizumab treatment show:

- Pretreatment serum total IgE between 30 and 1500 IU/mL
- Multiple allergic comorbidities
- Positive skin prick test or specific IgE to a perennial aeroallergen
- High pretreatment peripheral eosinophil counts (>260 cells/mL)
- High pretreatment fractional exhaled nitric oxide (FeNO >20 ppb)
- Low FEV_1 (Forced Expiratory Volume in the first second) at baseline (<80%) in adolescents ≥12 years

An emerging approach for identifying predictive biomarkers of response to omalizumab involves the field of metabolomics. In a recent multicenter prospective study in children with severe asthma treated with omalizumab, Carraro et al. identified a specific metabolic signature enriched in amino acids, specifically L-Histidine and L-Kynurenine, which showed a strong association with a positive response to omalizumab therapy. Therefore, further research and investigation are required.

Various randomized controlled trials have demonstrated omalizumab's efficacy and safety in pediatric patients. Omalizumab is generally well tolerated in children and adolescents. Regarding safety, the main AEs reported were injection site reactions or headaches, with a good prognosis and short resolution. Severe hypersensitivity reactions such as anaphylaxis are observed in 0.1–0.2% of adult or adolescent patients treated with omalizumab. The incidence is like that observed with other drugs such as oral penicillin, aspirin, and nonsteroidal anti-inflammatory drugs, as well as the incidence of anaphylaxis in the general population. Moreover, a recent analysis emphasizes no documented evidence of an elevated risk of malignant neoplasia in patients receiving long-term treatment with omalizumab.

Once treatment is initiated, evaluating the treatment response after 4–6 months is advised. The valuation of efficacy should consider the following parameters:

- Number of exacerbations and/or hospitalizations
- Reduction in daily oral corticosteroid usage
- General improvement in symptoms (daytime and nighttime) and QoL
- Respiratory function tests (FEV1)

Although a universally accepted definition of treatment response for biologic therapy in the pediatric population is currently lacking, if there is a suboptimal response, such as a reduction of exacerbations by less than 50% or a lack of improvement in lung function, it is recommended to propose a therapeutic switch to an alternative biologic.

The duration of therapy should be at least 2 years. In the case of inactive bronchial asthma, the possibility of discontinuation can be evaluated by continuing the follow-up. Long-term studies have documented that omalizumab effectively reduces circulating IgE levels even following therapy discontinuation.

25.5.2 Antibodies Against Interleukin-5 and Interleukin-5R

Mepolizumab is a humanized monoclonal antibody that exerts its therapeutic effect by binding to and inhibiting circulating IL-5, a crucial cytokine involved in the recruitment of eosinophils and enhancement of their survival, proliferation, and activation within peripheral tissues. It inhibits the interaction between IL-5 and its receptor's α chain (IL-5Ralpha).

It has obtained regulatory approval as add-on therapy by FDA and EMA for asthmatic patients aged 6 years and above, who exhibit refractory disease and an eosinophilic phenotype, alongside a documented history of asthma exacerbations.

Mepolizumab is administered via the subcutaneous route, with a recommended dosage of 100 mg for adolescents aged 12 years and above (or patients with body weight >40 kg) and 40 mg for children aged 6–11 years (or patients with body weight <40 kg). The administration is performed once every 4 weeks.

Although standardized response criteria are currently unavailable, in various studies it was observed that blood eosinophilia could represent an accurate indicator for predicting a positive response to anti-interleukin-5 antibodies and, in particular a blood eosinophil count of ≥300 cells/μL or ≥150 cells/μL in patients with well-characterized eosinophilic asthma. Other clinical and laboratory parameters have been proposed as predictive tools for assessing therapy efficacy for patients requiring multiple cycles of OCS. Additionally, recent research has highlighted the importance of improvements in FEV_1 as an indicator of response to mepolizumab therapy.

Headache, injection site reactions, and back pain were the most observed AEs in safety studies of mepolizumab.

Another monoclonal Ab anti-IL-5 is **reslizumab**, currently approved only for treating patients aged ≥18 years with severe eosinophilic asthma. The NICE Appraisal Committee strongly recommends considering reslizumab as a treatment option for individuals with severe asthma who remain uncontrolled despite receiving high-dose inhaled corticosteroids (ICS) and other therapy. This recommendation applies to patients meeting the following criteria: peripheral eosinophil count ≥400 cells/μL, experiencing at least three asthma exacerbations within a year, and with the availability of the monoclonal antibody at the agreed discounted price. It is administered intravenously, and the dosage is based on the patient's weight (3 mg/kg every 4 weeks IV). Although multiple studies demonstrate its effectiveness and safety in adults, there is currently a lack of evidence in the population of children and adolescent patients. Moreover, intravenous administration may impact therapeutic compliance.

Benralizumab is a humanized monoclonal antibody that specifically targets the alpha subunit of the interleukin-5 receptor on eosinophils. It triggers apoptosis through antibody-dependent cell-mediated cytotoxicity. FDA approved benralizumab as an add-on maintenance treatment in patients with ≥12 years and adults with severe eosinophilic asthma. It has demonstrated efficacy in reducing asthma exacerbations and symptoms while having a modest to moderate impact on FEV1. Moreover, for patients with blood eosinophils exceeding 150/μL, it may allow for a reduction or discontinuation of oral glucocorticoids. Notably, treatment with this medication has also been associated with improved quality of life.

Benralizumab is subcutaneously administered 30 mg every 4 weeks for the first three doses, then 30 mg every 8 weeks.

25.5.3 Dupilumab

Dupilumab, a fully human monoclonal antibody, blocks the receptors for IL-4 and IL-13.

According to EMA, it is indicated as an adjunctive maintenance therapy for patients with type 2 asthma characterized by high blood eosinophils and/or elevated FeNO levels. According to FDA, it is approved for patients with severe eosinophilic asthma and glucocorticoid-dependent patients who have insufficient control with high-dose ICS and additional medication.

It is approved for patients aged 6 years and older. The dosage of dupilumab depends on the patient's weight and age (see Fig. 25.3).

Regarding its efficacy, dupilumab has exhibited substantial improvement in lung function and a significant decrease in the rate of asthma exacer-

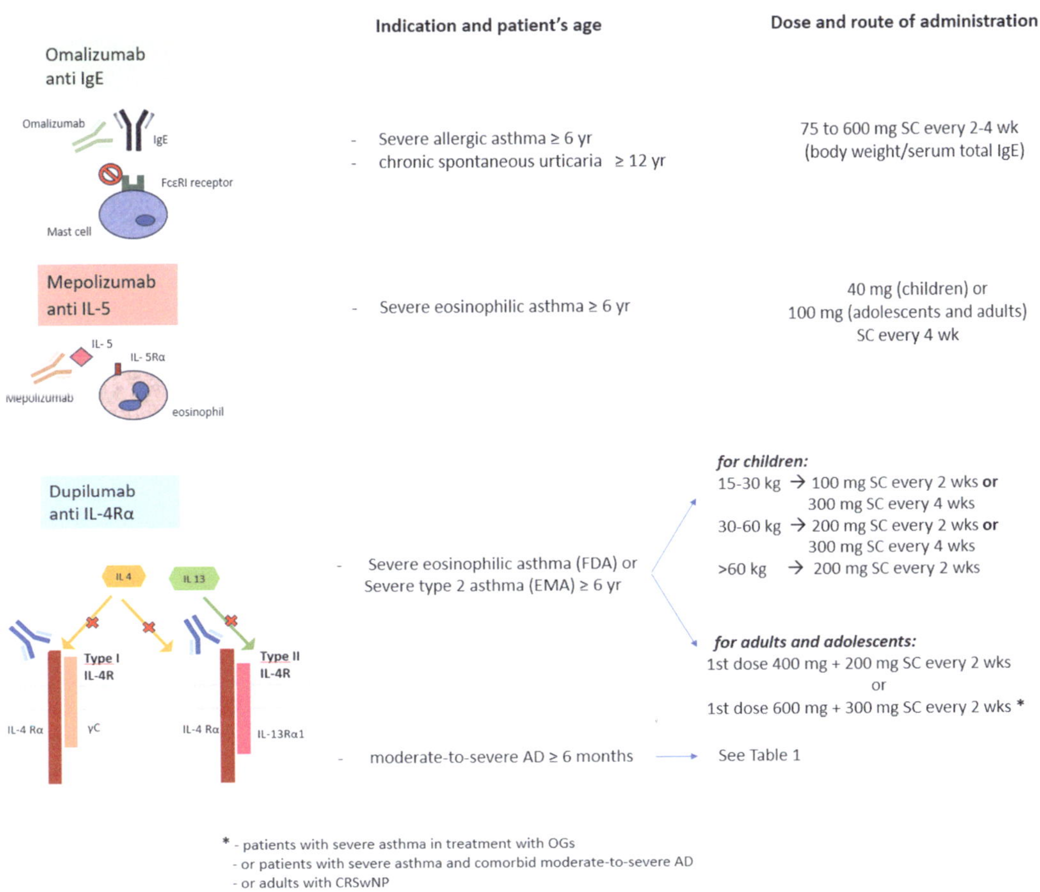

Fig. 25.3 Main indications of omalizumab, dupilumab, and mepolizumab

bations, especially among patients with either a baseline blood eosinophil level ≥150 cells/mcL and/or baseline FeNO level ≥25 ppb. Furthermore, patients treated with dupilumab have demonstrated reduction or discontinuation of oral glucocorticoids (OGs) and improved quality of life.

Treatment is generally well-tolerated by patients, with the most commonly observed AEs being localized reactions at the injection site, including pruritus, pain, and edema. Other AEs described include conjunctivitis, blepharitis, and oral herpes.

25.5.4 Tezepelumab

Tezepelumab is a human monoclonal antibody designed to specifically target and inhibit epithelial alarmin known as thymic stromal lymphopoietin (TSLP). This airway epithelial-derived cytokine is involved in activating the type 2 inflammatory pathways. In 2021, tezepelumab received approval for treating severe asthma in adolescents (12 years and older) and adults, regardless of their specific endotype or phenotype. Tezepelumab exhibited simultaneous reductions in blood eosinophil count, Feno levels, and IgE levels, suggesting its ability to suppress multiple inflammatory pathways. These effects are likely attributed to decreased levels of interleukin-5 and interleukin-13. Moreover, the observed decrease in total IgE levels can be attributed to reduced levels of interleukin-4 and interleukin-13, resulting in a gradual shift in B-cell switching from IgM to IgE production.

The recommended dosage of tezepelumab is administered subcutaneously at a dose of 210 mg once every 4 weeks.

Significant reductions in exacerbations were observed with tezepelumab in adults and adolescents with severe, uncontrolled asthma, including those with low blood eosinophil counts. Additionally, improvements were noted in lung function, asthma control, and QoL.

The most frequently reported AEs of tezepelumab included arthralgias, back pain, and pharyngitis. Overall, the medication was well tolerated in terms of safety.

25.6 Summary

Monoclonal antibody therapy shows promise in treating various conditions, including atopic dermatitis, chronic spontaneous urticaria, asthma, chronic rhinosinusitis with nasal polyps, and food allergies. Two notable examples are dupilumab, which targets IL-4R and IL-13R, thereby inhibiting the Th2 inflammatory cascade, and omalizumab, which blocks circulating IgE and reduces its binding to receptors on mast cells and dendritic cells, effectively reducing the allergic response. Other monoclonal antibodies include mepolizumab, which inhibits IL-5 crucial for eosinophil activity, and benralizumab, which induces eosinophil apoptosis. Ongoing clinical trials aim further to explore the potential of these additional drugs and establish long-term safety profiles.

References

1. Galli E, Fortina AB, Ricci G, Maiello N, Neri I, Baldo E, Berti I, Bonamonte D, Capra L, Carboni E, Carello R, Caroppo F, Cavagni G, Chinellato I, Cipriani F, Comberiati P, Diociaiuti A, Di Lernia V, Duse M, Filippeschi C, Giannetti A, Giovannini M, Licari A, Marseglia GL, Pace M, Patrizi A, Pajno GB, Peroni D, Villani A, Eichenfield L. Narrative review on the management of moderate-severe atopic dermatitis in pediatric age of the Italian Society of Pediatric Allergology and Immunology (SIAIP), of the Italian Society of Pediatric Dermatology (SIDerP) and of the Italian Society of Pediatrics (SIP). Ital J Pediatr. 2022;48(1):95. https://doi.org/10.1186/s13052-022-01278-7.
2. Licari A, Castagnoli R, Marseglia A, Olivero F, Votto M, Ciprandi G, Marseglia GL. Dupilumab to treat type 2 inflammatory diseases in children and adolescents. Paediatr Drugs. 2020;22(3):295–310. https://doi.org/10.1007/s40272-020-00387-2.
3. Votto M, Delle Cave F, De Filippo M, Marseglia A, Marseglia GL, Brazzelli V, Licari A. Rapid response to dupilumab treatment in children with moderate-to-severe atopic dermatitis: a case series. Pediatr Allergy Immunol. 2022;33(Suppl 27):31–3. https://doi.org/10.1111/pai.13623.
4. Stingeni L, Bianchi L, Antonelli E, Caroppo ES, Ferrucci SM, Ortoncelli M, Fabbrocini G, Nettis E, Schena D, Napolitano M, Gola M, Bonzano L, Rossi M, Belloni Fortina A, Balato A, Peris K, Foti C, Guarneri F, Romanelli M, Patruno C, Savoia P, Fargnoli MC, Russo F, Errichetti E, Bianchelli

T, Bianchi L, Pellacani G, Feliciani C, Offidani A, Corazza M, Micali G, Milanesi N, Malara G, Chiricozzi A, Tramontana M, Hansel K, DADA—Dupilumab for Atopic Dermatitis of the Adolescence Study Group. Moderate-to-severe atopic dermatitis in adolescents treated with dupilumab: a multicentre Italian real-world experience. J Eur Acad Dermatol Venereol. 2022;36(8):1292–9. https://doi.org/10.1111/jdv.18141. Epub 2022 Apr 22.

5. Zhang S, Lu L, Feng J, Hu Z, Song H, Yang L, Liu Y, Chen D, Wang T. Uveitis and hypereosinophilia associated with dupilumab in an atopic dermatitis patient. J Dermatolog Treat. 2023;34(1):2229466. https://doi.org/10.1080/09546634.2023.2229466.
6. Pfaar O, Klimek L, Hamelmann E, et al. COVID-19 vaccination of patients with allergies and type-2 inflammation with concurrent antibody therapy (biologicals)—a position paper of the German Society of Allergology and Clinical Immunology (DGAKI) and the German Society for Applied Allergology. Allergol Select. 2021;5:140–7. https://doi.org/10.5414/ALX02241E.
7. Simpson EL, Gooderham M, Wollenberg A, Weidinger S, Armstrong A, Soung J, Ferrucci S, Lima RG, Witte MM, Xu W, ElMaraghy H, Natalie CR, Pierce E, Blauvelt A, ADhere Investigators. Efficacy and safety of lebrikizumab in combination with topical corticosteroids in adolescents and adults with moderate-to-severe atopic dermatitis: a randomized clinical trial (ADhere). JAMA Dermatol. 2023;159(2):182–91. https://doi.org/10.1001/jamadermatol.2022.5534.
8. Landis MN, Arya M, Smith S, Draelos Z, Usdan L, Tarabar S, Pradhan V, Aggarwal S, Banfield C, Peeva E, Vincent MS, Sikirica V, Xenakis J, Beebe JS. Efficacy and safety of topical brepocitinib for the treatment of mild-to-moderate atopic dermatitis: a phase IIb, randomized, double-blind, vehicle-controlled, dose-ranging and parallel-group study. Br J Dermatol. 2022;187(6):878–87. https://doi.org/10.1111/bjd.21826. Epub 2022 Oct 23
9. Manti S, Pecora G, Patanè F, Giallongo A, Parisi GF, Papale M, Licari A, Marseglia GL, Leonardi S. Monoclonal antibodies in treating food allergy: a new therapeutic horizon. Nutrients. 2021;13(7):2314. https://doi.org/10.3390/nu13072314.
10. Fiocchi A, Artesani MC, Riccardi C, Mennini M, Pecora V, Fierro V, Calandrelli V, Dahdah L, Valluzzi RL. Impact of omalizumab on food allergy in patients treated for asthma: a real-life study. J Allergy Clin Immunol Pract. 2019;7(6):1901–1909.e5. https://doi.org/10.1016/j.jaip.2019.01.023. Epub 2019 Feb 20.
11. Licari A, Castagnoli R, De Filippo M, Foiadelli T, Tosca MA, Marseglia GL, Ciprandi G. Current and emerging biologic therapies for allergic rhinitis and chronic rhinosinusitis. Expert Opin Biol Ther. 2020;20(6):609–19. https://doi.org/10.1080/14712598.2020.1729350. Epub 2020 Feb 19.
12. Castagnoli R, De Filippo M, Votto M, Marseglia A, Montagna L, Marseglia GL, Licari A. An update on biological therapies for pediatric allergic diseases. Minerva Pediatr. 2020;72(5):364–71. https://doi.org/10.23736/S0026-4946.20.05993-9. Epub 2020 Jul 20.
13. 2022 GINA Report. Global strategy for asthma management and prevention. https://ginasthma.org/gina-reports/. Accessed 11 Jun 2023.
14. Castagnoli R, Brambilla I, Giudice MMD, Marseglia GL, Licari A. Applying the new guidelines to asthma management in children. Curr Opin Allergy Clin Immunol. 2023;23(2):132–6. https://doi.org/10.1097/ACI.0000000000000892. Epub 2023 Jan 12.
15. Brusselle GG, Koppelman GH. Biologic therapies for severe asthma. N Engl J Med. 2022;386(2):157–71. https://doi.org/10.1056/NEJMra2032506.
16. Votto M, De Filippo M, Licari A, Marseglia A, De Amici M, Marseglia GL. Biological therapies in children and adolescents with severe uncontrolled asthma: a practical review. Biologics. 2021;15:133–42. https://doi.org/10.2147/BTT.S252574.
17. Marseglia GL, Licari A, Tosca MA, Ciprandi G. Biologics to treat severe asthma in children and adolescents: a practical update. Pediatr Allergy Immunol Pulmonol. 2020;33(4):168–76. https://doi.org/10.1089/ped.2020.1212. Epub 2020 Nov 13.
18. Castagnoli R, Licari A, Manti S, Chiappini E, Marseglia GL. Type-2 inflammatory mediators as targets for precision medicine in children. Pediatr Allergy Immunol. 2020;31(Suppl 26):17–9. https://doi.org/10.1111/pai.13340.
19. Pajno GB, Castagnoli R, Arasi S, Licari A, Caminiti L, Marseglia GL. Pediatric use of omalizumab for allergic asthma. Expert Opin Biol Ther. 2020;20(7):695–703. https://doi.org/10.1080/14712598.2020.1751115. Epub 2020 Apr 13.
20. De Filippo M, Votto M, Caminiti L, Carella F, Castro G, Landi M, Olcese R, Panasiti I, Vernich M, Barberi S, Ciprandi G, Marseglia GL. Omalizumab and allergen immunotherapy for respiratory allergies: a mini-review from the Allergen-Immunotherapy Committee of the Italian Society of Pediatric Allergy and Immunology (SIAIP). Allergol Immunopathol (Madr). 2022;50(6):47–52. https://doi.org/10.15586/aei.v50i6.495.
21. Bagnasco D, Canevari RF, Del Giacco S, Ferrucci S, Pigatto P, Castelnuovo P, Marseglia GL, Yalcin AD, Pelaia G, Canonica GW. Omalizumab and cancer risk: current evidence in allergic asthma, chronic urticaria, and chronic rhinosinusitis with nasal polyps. World Allergy Organ J. 2022;15(12):100721. https://doi.org/10.1016/j.waojou.2022.100721.
22. De Filippo M, Votto M, Licari A, Pagella F, Benazzo M, Ciprandi G, Marseglia GL. Novel therapeutic approaches targeting endotypes of severe airway disease. Expert Rev Respir Med. 2021;15(10):1303–16. https://doi.org/10.1080/17476348.2021.1937132.

26 Allergen-Specific Immunotherapy

Carlo Caffarelli, Salvatore Barberi, and Giovanni Traina

Abstract

Allergen immunotherapy (AIT) has been used as a desensitizing therapy for allergic diseases for over 100 years and represents the only potentially curative treatment. There have been major progresses in understanding the complex regulatory mechanisms of immune-mediated diseases and this has led to increasingly targeted therapeutic approaches. The mechanisms of AIT include the desensitization effects, modulation of T and B cell responses, inhibition of migration into tissues, and mediator releasing of eosinophils, basophils, and mast cells. AIT acts on dendritic cells and on regulatory T (Treg) cells that have a key role in the immunological processes for achieving allergen tolerance. The efficacy of AIT has been shown in allergen-driven diseases. Subcutaneous immunotherapy is recommended in children with allergic rhinitis, allergic asthma, and hymenoptera venom allergy. Oral immunotherapy has been used for food allergies. Sublingual immunotherapy is recommended for allergic rhinitis, and allergic asthma particularly due to house dust mites associated with allergic rhinitis. Other indications are debated because of the heterogeneity of products and drawbacks of studies.

Keywords

Allergen-specific immunotherapy · Regulatory T cells · IgE · IgG4 · Mast cell · Sublingual allergen immunotherapy · Subcutaneous allergen immunotherapy · Allergic rhinitis · Asthma · Food allergy

Test your learning and check your understanding of this book's contents: use the "Springer Nature Flashcards" app to access questions using ▶ https://sn.pub/nspbjm. To use the app, please follow the instructions in Chap. 1.

26.1 Introduction

The complexity and uniqueness of the immune system determine a network of interactivity with the tissues that protect the host from different

C. Caffarelli
Clinica Pediatrica, Azienda Ospedaliero-Universitaria, Dipartimento di Medicina e Chirurgia, Università di Parma, Parma, Italy
e-mail: carlo.caffarelli@unipr.it

S. Barberi
Dipartimento Materno Infantile, ASST Rhodense, Milan, Italy
e-mail: salvatore.barberi@unikore.it

G. Traina (✉)
Dipartimento Materno Infantile, ASST Melegnano-Martesana, Milan, Italy

C. Caffarelli, G. L. Marseglia (eds.), *Textbook of Pediatric Allergy*,
https://doi.org/10.1007/978-3-031-71283-8_26

pathogens, while a certain degree of tolerance toward self and nonself-antigens considered harmless is maintained. In allergic diseases, there is an immune dysregulation that is directly linked with the loss of immune tolerance. Allergen immunotherapy (AIT) is the only therapeutic approach that at variance from drugs, can change the immune response to allergens making it possible to modify the disease course and to prevent or reduce the onset of symptoms in sensitized patients who are exposed to the allergens. AIT is indicated in patients with IgE-mediated allergic symptoms. It involves the administration of the allergen, to which the person is allergic. AIT is recommended for treating allergic rhinitis, allergic asthma due to inhalant allergens, hymenoptera venom allergy, and food allergy. Generally, increasing doses followed by years of maintenance treatment are necessary for achieving immune tolerance [1–13].

26.2 Mechanisms of AIT

The immunological basis of allergic diseases has two phases: sensitization and activation of T and B cell and IgE responses (initial phase) and effector functions related to inflammation and tissue damage (late phase) [14]. Differentiation of allergen-specific Th2 CD4+ producing IL-4 and IL-3 is necessary for inducing class-shifting to a heavy chain of IgE antibodies in B cells and the production of allergen-specific IgE during the sensitization phase. Allergen-specific IgE antibodies bind high-affinity receptor FcεRI on the surface of mast cells and basophils. Subsequently, when the subject is exposed to the allergen, a crosslinking of FcεRI IgE complexes on sensitized basophils and mast cells takes place. This activates basophils and mast cells that release inflammatory and anaphylactogenic mediators responsible for the immediate symptoms of type 1 hypersensitivity. Innate immune response of substances co-exposed with the antigen and co-signals for cell differentiation can differentiate T CD4+ naive into several lineages including Th1, Th2, Th9, Th17, Th22, and memory cells promoting different pathways of inflammatory responses. Th2 cells produce IL-4, IL-5, IL-9, IL-13, epithelial cells, and dendritic cells IL-25, IL-31, IL-33 [15–25]. These cytokines play a key role in producing allergen-specific IgE antibodies, eosinophilia, the permeability of vessels, recruiting of inflammatory cells, mucus production, smooth muscle hypertrophy, and reduced threshold of contraction [26–28]. Th1 cells contribute to the development of allergic diseases, with their role in epithelial apoptosis in asthma and atopic dermatitis and smooth muscle cell apoptosis in fatal asthma [8, 25, 29]. Th17 cells are characterized by the expression of IL-17, IL-17F, IL-6, IL-8. TNF-y, IL-22, and IL-26 [27, 28, 30]. Inhibition of IL-17 and Th17 resolves tissue pathology in autoimmunity models, reduces joint damage in experimental arthritis, and reduces neutrophil infiltration in experimental models of asthma, while increasing eosinophil infiltration [31–34]. In atopic dermatitis, T cells independently express IL-22 with low levels of IL-17. T cell subpopulations and their cytokines represent targets in the treatment of allergic diseases. The induction of Treg cells counteracts the excessive activation of Th2 cells that results in a progressive immune tolerance of the allergen [35]. It has been shown that both subcutaneous and sublingual AIT induce the differentiation of allergen-specific Treg cells that may explain why AIT is an effective treatment.

26.2.1 AIT and the Immune System

AIT induces a long-term tolerance to allergens by inhibiting allergen-specific TH2 cell responses, by an immune deviation toward a TH1 cell response (and by increasing activation threshold of mast cells and basophils). AIT rapidly induces peripheral T cell tolerance, but not B cell [36]. Despite decreasing IgE antibody levels and IgE-mediated skin sensitivity requires at least 3 years of treatment with AIT, most patients are protected from bee stings or pass a challenge to hymenoptera venom or grasses from the first months of AIT treatment [37, 38]. A key factor for the success of AIT is that both subcutaneous allergen immunotherapy (SCIT) and sublingual allergen immunotherapy (SLIT) induce tolerogenic dendritic cells that predispose to the production of regulatory T (Treg) and regulatory B (Breg) cells that determine tolerance [38]. The sublingual route is considered effective to induce allergen tolerance in animal models especially because oral mucosa contains many dendritic cells and few mast cells [39]. Allergen-specific Tregs produce thymus-derived FOXP3+ Treg cells (Foxp3+ CD25+ CD3+) that are increased in the circulation and at the nasal mucosa following pollen AIT and associated with clinical efficacy and inhibition of seasonal allergic inflammation [40, 41]. Treg cells suppress Th2 differentiation [42]. Furthermore, Treg cells express IL-10 that induces B cells to switch to allergen-specific IgG1 and IgG4, transforming growth factor-β (TGFβ) that switches B cells to IgA synthesis, IL-35 [43]. At the beginning of AIT, serum-specific IgE concentration increases, then progressively diminishes over the treatment period and it is persistently suppressed following discontinuation of treatment [44]. Following AIT, Treg differentiates B cells to produce allergen-specific IgG4 and IgA whose circulant levels increase 10–100 times blocking the allergic reaction [45, 46]. Allergen-specific blocking antibodies bound allergens before they link to IgE on the surface of mast cells inhibiting cell degranulation of mast cells and basophils. Blocking antibodies are present in serum and nasal fluid. In SCIT, they are mainly IgG4, while in SLIT, they are largely IgA1 and/or IgA2 [47]. Consequently, it has been shown that serum from individuals treated with AIT for hay fever to ragweed injected intradermally blocked skin response to ragweed in sensitized patients [40]. The IgG4 hinge has unique structural characteristics that determine a lower affinity for some Fcγ receptors and the ability to separate and repair through the dynamic exchange of the Fab arm. This leads to bi-specific antibodies that are functionally monomeric [41, 48]. Furthermore, IgG4 does not activate complement and inhibits the formation of immunocomplexes by other isotypes, giving this specific isotype anti-inflammatory characteristics. One of the main soluble factors released by mast cells following allergenic stimulation is histamine. There are four histamine receptors [39, 42, 43]. H1 receptor has pro-inflammatory and cell activation properties. H2 receptor is coupled to the adenylate cyclase and second messenger phosphoinositide systems and it is thought to be involved in tolerogenic immune responses [44]. AIT suppression of mast cells and basophils mast cells and basophils appear to be affected by the generation of allergen-specific Treg cells and the decrease of specific IgE levels [45, 46]. Regarding other immune pathways, Breg cells promote allergen immune tolerance, particularly by producing IL-10 and IgG4. They also release TGF-β. The activation of type2 innate lymphoid cells (ILC2) by cytokines released by epithelial cells is decreased following grass pollen AIT while ILC2s releasing IL-10 are increased [49, 50].

Effects related to AIT adjuvant have been shown. Aluminum hydroxide is a safe commonly used adjuvant in AIT with good results. Novel adjuvants activating TLR that controls the overexpression of Th2 cytokines by polarizing the Th1–Th2 balance toward a Th1 and Treg profile were effective in vivo models. A few applications of allergens by means of skin patches for a few weeks seem to obtain a lasting improvement of symptoms. So, the epicutaneous AIT that acts on the high number of Langerhans cells in the epidermis layer has been recently proposed as a therapeutic option [47]. Finally, in oral food immunotherapy, it has also been shown an increase in peripheral IL-10, an increase of Treg cells and IgG4, a suppression of TH2 cells, and a decrease in basophil activation [51–53].

26.3 Respiratory Allergy

Both SLIT and SCIT should be offered by a doctor expert in allergy, for the treatment of IgE-mediated allergic rhinitis and/or allergic asthma with worsening symptoms following exposure to aeroallergens, such as pollens, house dust mites, molds, and animal epithelia [11]. AIT is recommended when the allergen is difficult to avoid, such as grass pollen, or interventions for reducing allergen exposure have been unsuccessful. AIT should be considered when the medications do not well control symptoms or adverse reactions to drugs occur. It can be helpful for people who would like to reduce the long-term medication burden. In children, SCIT and SLIT are recommended for both intermittent and persistent moderate-severe allergic rhinitis. SCIT is recommended in children >5 years of age with mild to moderate controlled allergic asthma with acute symptoms (e.g., allergy to pets), seasonal symptoms (e.g., allergy to grass pollen), or perennial symptoms (e.g., allergy to house dust mites) [54]. The use of SLIT is particularly recommended in controlled asthmatics with allergic rhinitis to house dust mites and FEV1 ≥70% [55]. SLIT can be given at any age. However, in preschool children, evidence is scarce [56]. SLIT drops should be preferred in children <5 years of age.

Another issue is that most children with respiratory allergy are sensitized to many pollens that have the same seasonality. These multiple sensitizations are often due to cross-reactive panallergens. To use AIT only in children sensitized to genuine allergens would probably improve the efficacy of the treatment [57]. Improvement with both SCIT and SLIT does not quickly occur. It typically needs at least 3–5 months of administration. So, SLIT efficacy should be assessed after at least 6 months of preco-seasonal SLIT for pollens or at least 12 months for chronic symptoms. SLIT can be interrupted when symptoms do not improve. Both SCIT and SLIT should be taken for at least 3 years [58] to 5 years [59] to maintain benefits over time. Medications should be continued during AIT, which should be considered an add-on treatment.

There is evidence that both SCIT and SLIT are effective in improving symptoms of rhinoconjunctivitis and asthma. They reduce severity and frequency of symptoms, lung function, and drug consumption, in the short- and long-term follow-up [60–66]. In children, the efficacy of AIT following discontinuation of treatment has been documented for SCIT and SLIT after 2 years [67]. Both SCIT and SLIT for seasonal allergic rhinitis prevent the development of asthma in children [18, 68–70]. Research studies on primary prevention of allergic diseases to inhalants with SLIT drops to house dust mites are promising [71]. There is availability of products for AIT with distinct characteristics and effectiveness. It would be necessary to consider each product to prevent misperception and calculate advantages since there are no data of studies comparing existing products. For example, allergoids are chemically modified allergens for reducing side effects. They have been shown to be effective and safe but a comparison with traditional extracts is lacking [72, 73].

26.3.1 Subcutaneous and Sublingual Immunotherapy

There is no evidence that there are differences in efficacy between SLIT and SCIT. Consideration should be given to the preferences of patients and caregivers, patient convenience, likely compliance, product availability, and costs when prescribing SLIT or SCIT. Administration schedule of SCIT with depot extract consists of a build-up phase with increasing weekly doses for 1–3 months, followed by a monthly maintenance phase over 3–5 years. Preseasonal or preco-seasonal treatments or all year for pollens are available. SCIT may trigger allergic reactions including anaphylaxis. They are uncommon but unpredictable. So, patients should receive SCIT in a setting with personnel trained and equipment for managing life-threatening reactions. Patients should remain under doctor surveillance for at least 30 min after injection and avoid exercising for at least 3–24 h. Many patients develop swelling at the site of injection in the deltoid region. It is advisable to apply steroid cream and avoid scratching. The next dose should not be increased if the circumference of wheal is >5 cm and reduced if >10 cm. Overall, SCIT use is hampered by frequent injections at the office of the doctor and the possible onset of systemic reactions. SLIT for inhalants allergens has been recently developed to improve safety and accessibility in young children and in patients who are afraid of getting struck with a needle. SLIT is given as liquid drops or tablets that are taken under the tongue or in the mouth for 60′–120′ or until dissolution and then swallowed. So far,

SLIT tablets for grass pollen, timothy, birch, ragweed, cedar pollen, and house dust mites have been licensed by regulatory Agencies of different regions. SLIT aqueous solutions and some tablets are commercialized as "named patient products" (NPP), that are prepared according to Good Manufacturing Practice, without approval by Health Authority. The SLIT build-up phase that is often not mandatory can last from a few days to 3 weeks. The duration of SLIT is 3–5 years. There are preseasonal and preco-seasonal schemes for pollens. The adherence to SLIT is low since in the maintenance phase, SLIT requires to be taken 2–7 days a week. On the other hand, SLIT is safer than SCIT, therefore, it is self-administered at home. Adverse events are rare and mild, such as swelling and itching in lips, oral cavity, pharynx, esophageal/stomach burning, nausea, and vomiting in the first weeks. Systemic allergic adverse reactions are only anecdotally reported [74]. They can be controlled by provisionally decreasing and individualizing the dose or premedication with an oral antiH1 antihistamine. It is not usually necessary to interrupt the treatment since adverse events usually resolve in a short time. AIT is contraindicated in patients with severe immune-associated disorders (e.g., severe immunodeficiencies), tumors, severe chronic diseases (e.g., organ insufficiency, chronic infections, psychiatric diseases), and uncontrolled asthma [75]. Beta-blocker treatment is not an absolute contraindication. The AIT administration should be postponed in children with acute asthma and fever. SLIT should not be given to children with lesions at the mouth.

26.4 Other Allergies

SCIT is mandatory for children at risk of anaphylactic reaction to hymenoptera venom, bee and wasp in Europe. Therefore, SCIT should be performed in children with previous systemic reactions to hymenoptera venom. Moreover, SCIT could be considered in children who have had general urticaria and large local reactions >10 cm when they are at risk of frequent insect stings, or a quick rescue is not possible. The efficacy of SCIT in hymenoptera venom has been in more than 90% of treated patients. It is higher for wasp than for bee venom. Oral immunotherapy for IgE-mediated food allergy seems promising [76]. It has been suggested particularly for milk, egg, and peanuts [77]. An oral peanut immunotherapy product has been approved for use in clinical practice by regulatory agencies. It has been shown to be effective in desensitizing children in about 71% of patients after 134 weeks of treatment [78]. However, sustained remission was observed in approximately 15–20% after discontinuation of immunotherapy. AIT to peanut elicited several allergic reactions, including anaphylaxis both in the build-up phase at the hospital and in the maintenance period at home [78–80]. Partial efficacy, side effects, and the need of increasing the dose at the doctor's office several times hamper the use of oral immunotherapy for food allergies. Epicutaneous AIT for peanuts achieved long-term desensitization in about 35% of the children. Side effects were less frequent than with oral AIT and they mostly occurred at the application site [81]. AIT, particularly to house dust mites, for atopic eczema should be considered an experimental approach that is only occasionally recommended as there is limited evidence.

26.5 Future Developments

Novel approaches have been proposed to improve efficacy, safety, tolerability, duration, and adherence [14, 82–90]. Among them, there are new compounds, including natural and hypoallergenic recombinant allergens, combined recombinant peptides of grass pollen allergens and Pre-S protein derived from hepatitis B virus, cat peptides, a mixture of T cells epitope peptides, mRNA, DNA or alternative route of administration, such as needle-free, epicutaneous, and intralymphatic [15, 16, 91].

The development in understanding the molecular mechanism of allergic diseases will provide new therapeutic targets such as micro-RNAs that together with partner proteins induce gene silencing through the degradation of mRNA target inhibition of translation to a functional protein [36]. The role of adding bacterial extracts to allergen extracts for SLIT is unclear. The efficacy of the combination of AIT with biologics targeting T2 cytokines is currently being investigated.

Serum IgG4 levels may potentially support the clinical assessment of the AIT response. However, the relationship between the effectiveness of AIT and the induction of allergen-specific IgG4 is controversial and further studies are warranted [11, 54].

26.6 Conclusions

AIT has multiple mechanisms of action with the involvement of several cell subsets [58]. AIT induces tolerance of dendritic cells and allergen-specific T cells and regulates B cells' production of IgE, IgA, and IgG4. The immunosuppressive functions of IL-10 play a key role. So far AIT should be considered an excellent model of personalized medicine in clinical allergy. AIT is an important therapeutic option, especially in childhood, to mitigate and modify the natural history of allergic asthma and allergic rhinitis, to prevent allergic reactions to hymenoptera venom and it may help to control food allergy.

References

1. Akdis CA. Allergy and hypersensitivity: mechanisms of allergic disease. Curr Opin Immunol. 2006;18:718–26.
2. Akdis M, Akdis CA. Therapeutic manipulation of immune tolerance in allergic disease. Nat Rev Drug Discov. 2009;8:645–60.
3. Akdis M,Burgler S, Crameri R, Eiwegger T, Fujita H, Gomez E, et al. Interleukins, from 1 to 37, and interferon-gamma: Receptors, functions, and roles in diseases. J Allergy Clin Immunol. 2011;127(3):701–21.e70.
4. Soyer OU, Akdis M, Akdis CA. Mechanisms of subcutaneous allergen immunotherapy. Immunol Allergy Clin North Am. 2011;31:175–90.
5. Knol EF. Requirements for effective IgE cross-linking on mast cells and basophils. Mol Nutr Food Res. 2006;50:620–4.
6. Akdis M, Akdis CA. Mechanisms of allergen-specific immunotherapy: multiple suppressor factors at work in immune tolerance to allergens. J Allergy Clin Immunol. 2014;133:621–31.
7. Akdis CA. Therapies for allergic inflammation: refining strategies to induce tolerance. Nat Med. 2012;18:736–49.
8. Akdis M, Akdis AC. Immune tolerance. In: Franklin Adkinson Jr BSBN, Wesley B, Busse WW, Holgate ST, Lemanske Jr RF, O'Hehir RE, editors. Middleton's allergy. 8th ed. Elsevier; 2013.
9. Akdis C, Papadopoulos N, Cardona V. Fighting allergies beyond symptoms: the European declaration on immunotherapy. Eur J Immunol. 2011;41:2802–4.
10. Akkoc T, Akdis M, Akdis CA. Update in the mechanisms of allergen-specific immunotheraphy. Allergy Asthma Immunol Res. 2011;3:11–20.
11. Pajno GB, Bernardini R, Peroni D, Arasi S, Martelli A, Landi M, et al. Clinical practice recommendations for allergen-specific immunotherapy in children: the Italian consensus report. Ital J Pediatr. 2017;43:13.
12. Bousquet J, Khaltaev N, Cruz AA, Denburg J, Fokkens WJ, Togias A, et al. Allergic rhinitis and its impact on asthma (ARIA) 2008 update (in collaboration with the World Health Organization, GA(2)LEN and AllerGen). Allergy. 2008;63:8–160.
13. Canonica GW, Cox L, Pawankar R, Baena-Cagnani CE, Blaiss M, Bonini S, et al. Sublingual immunotherapy: World Allergy Organization position paper 2013 update. World Allergy Organ J. 2014;7:6.
14. Focke-Tejkl M, Weber M, Niespodziana K, Neubauer A, Huber H, Henning R, et al. Development and characterization of a recombinant, hypoallergenic, peptide-based vaccine for grass pollen allergy. J Allergy Clin Immunol. 2014.
15. von Moos S, Johansen P, Tay F, Graf N, Kundig TM, Senti G. Comparing safety of abrasion and tape-stripping as skin preparation in allergen-specific epicutaneous immunotherapy. J Allergy Clin Immunol. 2014;134:965–7.
16. Spertini F, Perrin Y, Audran R, Pellaton C, Boudousquié C, Barbier N, et al. Safety and immunogenicity of immunotherapy with Bet v 1-derived contiguous overlapping peptides. J Allergy Clin Immunol. 2014;134:239–40.
17. Alviani C,Roberts G, Mitchell F, Martin J, Zolkipli Z, Michaelis LJ, et al. Primary prevention of asthma in high-risk children using HDM SLIT: assessment at age 6 years. J Allergy Clin Immunol. 2020;45:1711–3.
18. Larche M, Akdis CA, Valenta R. Immunological mechanisms of allergen-specific immunotherapy. Nat Rev Immunol. 2006;6:761–71.
19. Chatila TA, Li N, Garcia-Lloret M, Kim HJ, Nel AE. T-cell effector pathways in allergic diseases: transcriptional mechanisms and therapeutic targets. J Allergy Clin Immunol. 2008;121:812–23; quiz 24–5.
20. Kang CM, Jang AS, Ahn MH, Shin JA, Kim JH, Choi YS, et al. Interleukin-25 and interleukin-13 production by alveolar macrophages in response to particles. Am J Respir Cell Mol Biol. 2005;33:290–6.
21. Wang YH, Angkasekwinai P, Lu N, Voo KS, Arima K, Hanabuchi S, et al. IL-25 augments type 2 immune responses by enhancing the expansion and functions of TSLP-DC-activated Th2 memory cells. J Exp Med. 2007;204:1837–47.

22. Dillon SR, Sprecher C, Hammond A, Bilsborough J, Rosenfeld-Franklin M, Presnell SR, et al. Interleukin 31, a cytokine produced by activated T cells, induces dermatitis in mice. Nat Immunol. 2004;5:752–60.
23. Bilsborough J, Leung DY, Maurer M, Howell M, Boguniewicz M, Yao L, et al. IL-31 is associated with cutaneous lymphocyte antigen-positive skin homing T cells in patients with atopic dermatitis. J Allergy Clin Immunol. 2006;117:418–25.
24. Kakkar R, Lee RT. The IL-33/ST2 pathway: therapeutic target and novel biomarker. Nat Rev Drug Discov. 2008;7:827–40.
25. Rank MA, Kobayashi T, Kozaki H, Bartemes KR, Squillace DL, Kita H. IL-33-activated dendritic cells induce an atypical TH2-type response. J Allergy Clin Immunol. 2009;123:1047–54.
26. Romagnani S. Immunologic influences on allergy and the TH1/TH2 balance. J Allergy Clin Immunol. 2004;113:395–400.
27. Akkoc T, de Koning PJ, Ruckert B, Barlan I, Akdis M, Akdis CA. Increased activation-induced cell death of high IFN-gamma-producing T(H)1 cells as a mechanism of T(H)2 predominance in atopic diseases. J Allergy Clin Immunol. 2008;121:652–8.
28. Trautmann A, Akdis M, Kleemann D, Altznauer F, Simon HU, Graeve T, et al. T cell-mediated Fas-induced keratinocyte apoptosis plays a key pathogenetic role in eczematous dermatitis. J Clin Invest. 2000;106:25–35.
29. Prefontaine D, Nadigel J, Chouiali F, Audusseau S, Semlali A, Chakir J, et al. Increased IL-33 expression by epithelial cells in bronchial asthma. J Allergy Clin Immunol. 2010;125:752–4.
30. Meyer N, Zimmermann M, Bürgler S, Bassin C, Woehrl S, Moritz K, et al. IL-32 is expressed by human primary keratinocytes and modulates keratinocyte apoptosis in atopic dermatitis. J Allergy Clin Immunol. 2010;125:858–65.
31. Solarewicz-Madejek K, Basinski TM, Crameri R, Akdis M, Akkaya A, Blaser K, et al. T cells and eosinophils in bronchial smooth muscle cell death in asthma. Clin Exp Allergy. 2009;39:845–55.
32. Burgler S, Ouaked N, Bassin C, Basinski TM, Mantel PY, Siegmund K, et al. Differentiation and functional analysis of human T(H)17 cells. J Allergy Clin Immunol. 2009;123:588–95; 595.e1.
33. Zheng Y, Danilenko DM, Valdez P, Kasman I, Eastham-Anderson J, Wu J, et al. Interleukin-22, a T(H)17 cytokine, mediates IL-23-induced dermal inflammation and acanthosis. Nature. 2007;445:648–51.
34. Martin P, Gomez M, Lamana A, Matesanz Marín A, Cortés JR, Ramírez Huesca M, et al. The leukocyte activation antigen CD69 limits allergic asthma and skin contact hypersensitivity. J Allergy Clin Immunol. 2010;126:355–65; 65.e1–3.
35. Sergejeva S, Ivanov S, Lotvall J, Linden A. Interleukin-17 as a recruitment and survival factor for airway macrophages in allergic airway inflammation. Am J Respir Cell Mol Biol. 2005;33:248–53.
36. Renand A, Shamji MH, Harris KM, Qin T, Wambre E, Scadding GW, et al. Synchronous immune alterations mirror clinical response during allergen immunotherapy. J Allergy Clin Immunol. 2018;141:1750–1760.
37. Rangachari M, Mauermann N, Marty RR, Dirnhofer S, Kurrer MO, Komnenovic V, et al. T-bet negatively regulates autoimmune myocarditis by suppressing local production of interleukin 17. J Exp Med. 2006;203:2009–19.
38. Gueguen C, Bouley J, Moussu H, Luce S, Duchateau M, Chamot-Rooke J, et al. Changes in markers associated with dendritic cells driving the differentiation of either TH2 cells or regulatory T cells correlate with clinical benefit during allergen immunotherapy. J Allergy Clin Immunol. 2016;137:545–58.
39. Allam JP, Stojanovski G, Friedrichs N, Peng W, Bieber T, Wenzel J, Novak N. Distribution of Langerhans cells and mast cells within the human oral mucosa: new application sites of allergens in sublingual immunotherapy? Allergy. 2008;63:720–7.
40. Cooke RA, Barnard JH, Hebald S, Stull A. Serological evidence of immunity with coexisting sensitization in a type of human allergy (hay fever). J Exp Med. 1935;62:733–50.
41. Veldhoen M, Uyttenhove C, van Snick J, Helmby H, Westendorf A, Buer J, et al. Transforming growth factor-beta 'reprograms' the differentiation of T helper 2 cells and promotes an interleukin 9-producing subset. Nat Immunol. 2008;9:1341–6.
42. Ling EM, Smith T, Nguyen XD, Pridgeon C, Dallman M, Arbery J, Carr VA, et al. Relation of CD4+CD25+ regulatory T-cell suppression of allergen-driven T-cell activation to atopic status and expression of allergic disease. Lancet. 2004;363:608–15.
43. Durham SR, Shamji MH. Allergen immunotherapy: past, present and future. Nat Rev Immunol. 2023;23:317–28.
44. Varga EM, Francis JN, Zach MS, Klunker S, Aberer W, Durham SR. Time course of serum inhibitory activity for facilitated allergen–IgE binding during bee venom immunotherapy in in children. Clin Exp Allergy. 2009;39:1353–7.
45. Schmid JM, Wurtzen PA, Dahl R, Hoffmann HJ. Early improvement in basophil sensitivity predicts symptom relief with grass pollen immunotherapy. J Allergy Clin Immunol. 2014;134:741–4.
46. Senti G, Graf N, Haug S, Rüedi N, von Moos S, Sonderegger T, et al. Epicutaneous allergen administration as a novel method of allergen-specific immunotherapy. J Allergy Clin Immunol. 2009;124:997–1002.
47. Shamji MH, Larson D, Eifan A, Scadding GW, Qin T, Lawson K,et al. Differential induction of allergen-specific IgA responses following timothy grass subcutaneous and sublingual immunotherapy. J Allergy Clin Immunol. 2021;148:1061–1071.e1.
48. Akdis CA, Akdis M. Mechanisms and treatment of allergic disease in the big picture of regulatory T cells. J Allergy Clin Immunol. 2009;123:735–46; quiz 47–8.

49. Lao-Araya M, Steveling E, Scadding GW, Durham SR, Shamji MH. Seasonal increases in peripheral innate lymphoid type 2 cells are inhibited by subcutaneous grass pollen immunotherapy. J Allergy Clin Immunol. 2014;134:1193–1195.e4.
50. Golebski K, Layhadi JA, Sahiner U, Steveling-Klein EH, Lenormand MM, Li RCY, et al. Induction of IL-10-producing type 2 innate lymphoid cells by allergen immunotherapy is associated with clinical response. Immunity. 2021;54:291–307.
51. Wambre E, Bajzik V, DeLong JH, O'Brien K, Nguyen QA, Speake C, et al. A phenotypically and functionally distinct human TH2 cell subpopulation is associated with allergic disorders. Sci Transl Med. 2017;9:eaam9171.
52. Bajzik V, DeBerg HA, Garabatos N, Rust BJ, Obrien KK, Nguyen QA, et al. Oral desensitization therapy for peanut allergy induces dynamic changes in peanut-specific immune responses. Allergy. 2022;77:2534–48.
53. Vickery BP, Scurlock AM, Kulis M, Steele PH, Kamilaris J, Berglund JP, et al. Sustained unresponsiveness to peanut in subjects who have completed peanut oral immunotherapy. J Allergy Clin Immunol. 2014;133:468–75.
54. Expert Panel Working Group of the National Heart, Lung, and Blood Institute (NHLBI) administered and coordinated National Asthma Education and Prevention Program Coordinating Committee (NAEPPCC), et al. Focused updates to the asthma management guidelines: a report from the National Asthma Education and Prevention Program Coordinating Committee Expert Panel Working Group. J Allergy Clin Immunol. 2020;2020:1217–70.
55. Global strategy for asthma management and prevention. 2023. https://ginasthma.org/reports/.
56. Caffarelli C, Mastrorilli C, Procaccianti M, Santoro A. Use of sublingual immunotherapy for aeroallergens in children with asthma. J Clin Med. 2020;9:3381.
57. Stringari G, Tripodi S, Caffarelli C, Dondi A, Asero R, Di Rienzo Businco A, et al. The effect of component-resolved diagnosis on specific immunotherapy prescription in children with hay fever. J Allergy Clin Immunol. 2014;134:75–81.
58. Scadding GW, Calderon MA, Shamji MH, Eifan AO, Penagos M, Dumitru F, et al. Effect of 2 years of treatment with sublingual grass pollen immunotherapy on nasal response to allergen challenge at 3 years among patients with moderate to severe seasonal allergic rhinitis: the GRASS randomized clinical trial. JAMA. 2017;317:615–25.
59. Marogna M, Spadolini I, Massolo A, Canonica GW, Passalacqua G. Long-lasting effects of sublingual immunotherapy according to its duration: a 15-year prospective study. J Allergy Clin Immunol. 2010;126:969–75.
60. Cox L,Nelson H, Lockey R, Calabria C, Chacko T, Finegold I, et al. Allergen immunotherapy: a practice parameter third update. J Allergy Clin Immunol. 2011;12:S1–S55.
61. Bousquet J, Anto J, Auffray C, Akdis M, Cambon-Thomsen A, Keil T, et al. MeDALL (Mechanisms of the Development of ALLergy): an integrated approach from phenotypes to systems medicine. Allergy. 2011;66:596–604.
62. Casale TB, Stokes JR. Immunotherapy: what lies beyond. J Allergy Clin Immunol. 2014;133:612–9; quiz 20.
63. Soyka MB, van de Veen W, Holzmann D, Akdis M, Akdis CA. Scientific foundations of allergen-specific immunotherapy for allergic disease. Chest. 2014;146:1347–57.
64. Jutel M, Akdis CA. Novel immunotherapy vaccine development. Curr Opin Allergy Clin Immunol. 2014;14:557–63.
65. Cavkaytar O, Akdis CA, Akdis M. Modulation of immune responses by immunotherapy in allergic diseases. Curr Opin Pharmacol. 2014;17:30–7.
66. Akdis M, Akdis CA. Mechanisms of allergen-specific immunotherapy. J Allergy Clin Immunol. 2007;119:780–91.
67. Valovirta E, Petersen TH, Piotrowska T, Laursen MK, Andersen JS, Sørensen HF, et al. Results from the 5-year SQ grass sublingual immunotherapy tablet asthma prevention (GAP) trial in children with grass pollen allergy. J Allergy Clin Immunol. 2018;141:529–538.e13.
68. Akdis M. Healthy immune response to allergens: T regulatory cells and more. Curr Opin Immunol. 2006;18:738–44.
69. Durham SR, Walker SM, Varga E-V, Jacobson MR, O'Brien F, Noble W, et al. Long-term clinical efficacy of grass-pollen immunotherapy. N Engl J Med. 1999;341:468–75.
70. Ozdemir C, Kucuksezer UC, Akdis M, Akdis CA. Mechanisms of immunotherapy to wasp and bee venom. Clin Exp Allergy. 2011;41:1226–34.
71. Traina G, Martelli AG, Fiocchi AG, Franco V, Ronchi B, Betti F. Allergy… No more fear of neeedle! Eur J Allergy Clin Immunol. 2019;74:2277–9.
72. Caffarelli C, Sensi LG, Marcucci F, Cavagni G. Preseasonal local allergoid immunotherapy to grass pollen in children: a double-blind, placebo-controlled, randomized trial. Allergy. 2000;55:1142–7.
73. Worm M, Rak S, Samoliński B, Antila J, Höiby AS, Kruse B, et al. Efficacy and safety of birch pollen allergoid subcutaneous immunotherapy: a 2-year double-blind, placebo-controlled, randomized trial plus 1-year open-label extension. Clin Exp Allergy. 2019;49:516–25.
74. James C, Bernstein DI. Allergen immunotherapy: an updated review of safety. Curr Opin Allergy Clin Immunol. 2017;17:55–9.
75. Calderon MA, Simons FER, Malling HJ, Lockey RF, Moingeon P, Demoly P. Sublingual allergen immunotherapy: mode of action and its relationship with the safety profile. Allergy. 2012;67:302–11.
76. Bégin P, Chan ES, Kim H, Cellier MS, Favron-Godbout C, et al. CSACI guidelines for the ethical, evidence-based and patient-oriented clinical practice

of oral immunotherapy in IgE-mediated food allergy. Allergy Asthma Clin Immunol. 2020;16:20.
77. Pajno GB,Fernandez-Rivas M, Arasi S, Roberts G, Akdis CA, Alvaro-Lozano M, et al. EAACI guidelines on allergen immunotherapy: IgE-mediated food allergy. Allergy. 2018;73:799–815.
78. Chu DK,Wood RA, French S, Fiocchi A, Jordana M, Waserman S, et al. Oral immunotherapy for peanut allergy (PACE): a systematic review and meta-analysis of efficacy and safety. Lancet. 2019;393:2222–32.
79. Chinthrajah RS,Purington N, Andorf S, Long A, O'Laughlin KL, Lyu SC, et al. Sustained outcomes in oral immunotherapy for peanut allergy (POISED study): a large, randomised, double-blind, placebo-controlled, phase 2 study. Lancet. 2019;394:1437–49.
80. Jones SM, Kim EH, Nadeau KC, Nowak-Wegrzyn A, Wood RA, Sampson HA, et al. Efficacy and safety of oral immunotherapy in children aged 1–3 years with peanut allergy (the Immune Tolerance Network IMPACT trial): a randomised placebo-controlled study. Lancet. 2022;399:359–71.
81. Scurlock AM, Burks AW, Sicherer SH, Leung DYM, Kim EH, Henning AK, et al. Epicutaneous immunotherapy for treatment of peanut allergy: Follow-up from the Consortium for Food Allergy Research. J Allergy Clin Immunol. 2021;147:992–1003.
82. Pajno GB, Barberio G, De Luca F, Morabito L, Parmiani S. Prevention of new sensitizations in asthmatic children monosensitized to house dust mite by specific immunotherapy. A six-year follow-up study. Clin Exp Allergy. 2001;31:1392–7.
83. Moller C, Dreborg S, Ferdousi HA, Halken S, Høst A, Jacobsen L, et al. Pollen immunotherapy reduces the development of asthma in children with seasonal rhinoconjunctivitis (the PAT-study). J Allergy Clin Immunol. 2002;109:251–6.
84. Burks AW, Calderon MA, Casale T, Cox L, Demoly P, Jutel M, et al. Update on allergy immunotherapy: American Academy of Allergy, Asthma & Immunology/European Academy of Allergy and Clinical Immunology/PRACTALL consensus report. J Allergy Clin Immunol. 2013;131:1288–96.
85. Creticos PS, Maloney J, Bernstein DI, Casale T, Kaur A, Fisher R, et al. Randomized controlled trial of a ragweed allergy immunotherapy tablet in North American and European adults. J Allergy Clin Immunol. 2013;131:1342–9.
86. Witten M, Malling HJ, Blom L, Poulsen BC, Poulsen LK. Is intralymphatic immunotherapy ready for clinical use in patients with grass pollen allergy? J Allergy Clin Immunol. 2013;132:1248–52.
87. Tam H, Calderon MA, Boyle RJ. Efficacy of allergen-specific immunotherapy for patients with atopic dermatitis. J Allergy Clin Immunol. 2013;132:1012–3.
88. Patel P, Holdich T, von Weikersthal-Drachenberg KJF, Huber B. Efficacy of a short course of specific immunotherapy in patients with allergic rhinoconjunctivitis to ragweed pollen. J Allergy Clin Immunol. 2014;133:121–9.e1–2.
89. Swoboda I, Balic N, Klug C, Focke M, Weber M, Spitzauer S, et al. A general strategy for the generation of hypoallergenic molecules for the immunotherapy of fish allergy. J Allergy Clin Immunol. 2013;132:979–81.
90. Kiel MA, Roder E, Gerth van Wijk R, Al MJ, Hop WC, Rutten-van Molken MP. Real-life compliance and persistence among users of subcutaneous and sublingual allergen immunotherapy. J Allergy Clin Immunol. 2013;132:353–60.e2.
91. Kundig TM, Johansen P, Bachmann MF, Cardell LO, Senti G. Intralymphatic immunotherapy: time interval between injections is essential. J Allergy Clin Immunol. 2014;133:930–1.

Pollution, Climate Change, and Environmental Allergy

27

Amelia Licari, Stefano Forestieri, Giulia Milano, and Stefania La Grutta

Abstract

Climate change and air pollution are topics of current interest due to their impact on adults' and children's health: according to WHO, in most countries, more than 90% of people breathe polluted air. Due to climate change and global warming, extreme weather events such as floods, hurricanes, typhoons, droughts, and sandstorms have become increasingly frequent in recent years, arousing concern. Global and regional climate change causes a variation in airborne allergen amounts and distribution, affecting allergic diseases such as rhinoconjunctivitis and asthma. For physiological reasons, infants and children are particularly vulnerable to climate change and air pollution. In addition, exposure to extreme weather events and air pollution in childhood increases the risk of wheezing, asthma development or exacerbations, and lung function impairment. As many diseases linked to pollution and climate change have no curative treatments yet, it is important to engage today through environmental policies and interventions to reduce this serious problem.

Keywords

Asthma · Air pollution · Climate change · Global warming · Pollen seasons · Thunderstorm asthma · Cigarette smoke · Wildfire smoke · Particulate matter · Traffic-related air pollution

Test your learning and check your understanding of this book's contents: use the "Springer Nature Flashcards" app to access questions using ▶ https://sn.pub/nspbjm. To use the app, please follow the instructions in Chap. 1.

A. Licari (✉)
Pediatric Unit, Department of Clinical, Surgical, Diagnostic and Pediatric Sciences, University of Pavia, Pavia, Italy

Pediatric Clinic, Fondazione IRCCS Policlinico San Matteo, Pavia, Italy

Institute of Translational Pharmacology (IFT), National Research Council of Italy (CNR), Palermo, Italy
e-mail: amelia.licari@unipv.it

S. Forestieri
School of Pediatrics, University of Cagliari, Cagliari, Italy

G. Milano
Division of Pediatrics, Department of Health Sciences, University of Piemonte Orientale, Novara, Italy

S. La Grutta
Institute of Translational Pharmacology (IFT), National Research Council of Italy (CNR), Palermo, Italy

C. Caffarelli, G. L. Marseglia (eds.), *Textbook of Pediatric Allergy*,
https://doi.org/10.1007/978-3-031-71283-8_27

27.1 Introduction: Climate Change and Air Pollution

Climate change and air pollution are topics of current interest due to their impact on adults' and children's health. The first one acts directly intensifying extreme weather events such as heatwaves, wildfires, droughts, storms, hurricanes, and floods but also indirectly influencing air pollution and pollen seasons [1]; the second one, instead, is mainly due to the burning of fossil fuels, which is constantly increasing in the last years (Fig. 27.1).

Air pollutants can be classified as primary ones, directly emitted by sources such as carbon monoxide (CO), sulfur dioxide (SO_2), and particulate matter (PM), and secondary ones, due to chemical and physical reactions (nitrogen dioxide (NO_2), ozone (O_3), sulfates, and ultrafine particulates) [2].

Pollutants are present outdoors and indoors, mainly due to tobacco smoke and burning solid fuels (SF) as biomass and coal for healing, cooking, and lighting houses, especially in low-income countries [3].

According to the World Health Organization (WHO), more than 90% of people in most countries breathe polluted air, with many air pollutants exceeding the established safe threshold [4]. For this reason, pollution reduction is one of the

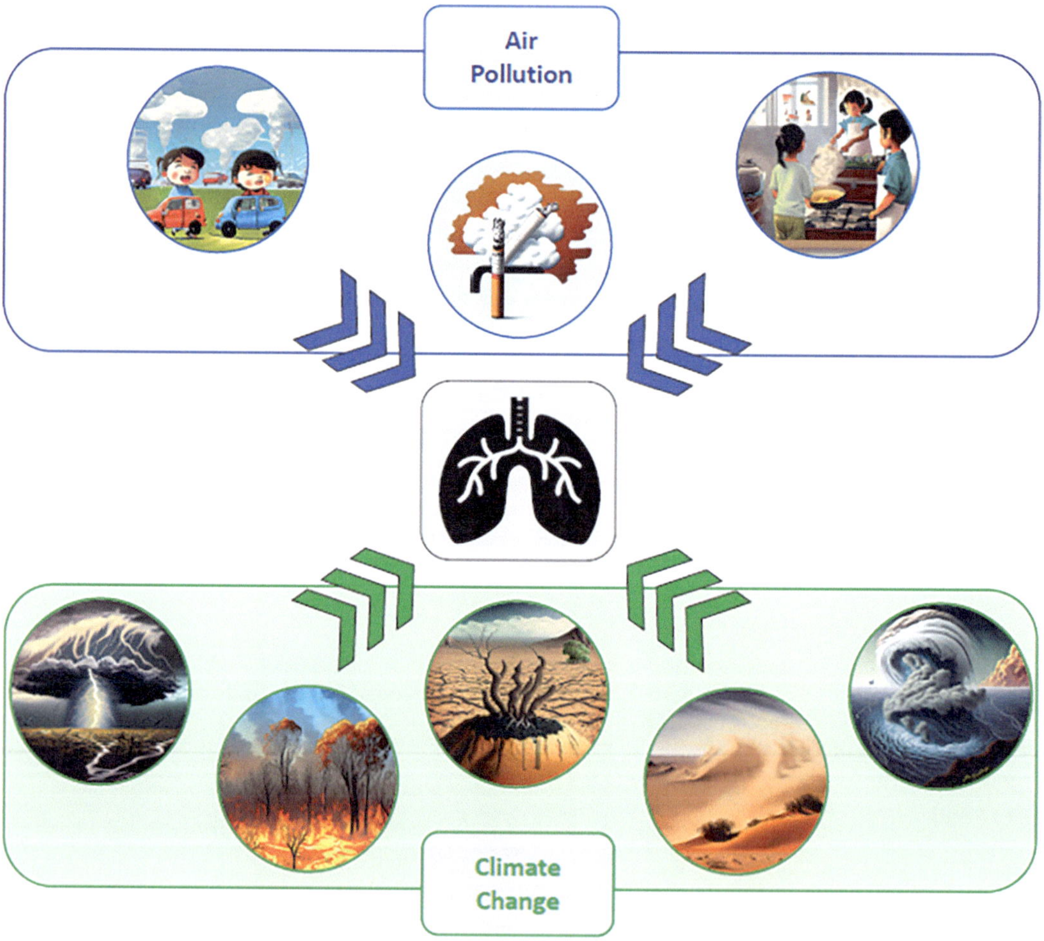

Fig. 27.1 How climate change and air pollution affect respiratory health

biggest challenges of our time. Actions of individual citizens can only mitigate air pollution, while the most important results can be reached from targeted policy interventions [3].

27.2 Children's Susceptibility

Children are affected by ambient air pollutants from the womb to adulthood. Infants and children are particularly vulnerable to the effects of climate change and air pollution due to physiological factors (Table 27.1): being at a developmental age, their respiratory, immune, and detoxifying systems are still immature, conferring their higher sensitivity to toxic chemicals and other stressors [3, 5].

Because of their lower height, children breathe air closer to the ground, where many pollutants (especially traffic-related ones) are concentrated. Infants' and children's respiratory rate is higher than adults, making them breathe more air relative to their body weight. Moreover, children usually have increased oral breathing, allowing pollutants to reach the lower parts of the respiratory tract [6]. Also, children spend much time playing outdoors, potentially increasing their exposure to environmental pollutants, which can trigger bronchoconstriction, also favored by their narrower airways. It should also be considered that children have a long residual life span and consequently a longer exposure to air pollutants, which may have potentially more time to cause respiratory diseases. Moreover, getting sick in childhood means living many years as a chronic patient, negatively affecting the quality of life [5].

Table 27.1 Children's vulnerability factors

Physiological immaturity of respiratory, immune, and detoxifying systems
Higher respiratory rate
Oral breathing
Lower height
More time spent outdoors with increased pollutant exposure
Narrower airways
Longer residual life span

27.3 Effects of Climate Change on Asthma

Asthma is the most common chronic lung disease in children and adolescents and is characterized by a history of respiratory symptoms such as shortness of breath, cough, chest tightness, and wheezing [7].

Allergic diseases such as rhinoconjunctivitis and asthma are affected by global and regional climate change as they cause airborne allergen amounts and distribution variation. Air pollutants and global warming affect not only pollen and mold allergenicity, but also the onset and length of pollen seasons; also, climate change promotes the growth of subtropical plants, changing the local pollen calendar. Finally, the increasing concentration of CO_2 in the atmosphere induces a faster and larger growth of plants, increasing the intensity and the flowering time [8, 9].

In addition to pollen, the growth of house dust mites (HDM) and molds is also affected by climate change. The HDM growth strongly depends on climate and seasons. The HDM ideal growing conditions are warm and humid environments (25–30 °C and relative humidity of 70%), as in tropical regions. The rise in temperature has also changed human lifestyles, increasing the time spent indoors, with more frequent use of air conditioning, which can affect exposure to HDM. Exposure to high amounts of HDM in childhood is considered a risk factor for developing allergic diseases later in life [10, 11].

The rising number of storms, rainfalls, and floods are related to mold infestation and damp problems inside houses and buildings [9]. Many studies have demonstrated an association between asthma exacerbations and increased atmospheric fungal spore counts, particularly *Alternaria alternata*. Moreover, *Alternaria alternata* sensitivity is associated with more severe phenotypes of asthma [12, 13].

The increasing concentration of greenhouse gases also contributes to the global surface temperature increase. As temperature rises, environmental dampness rises too, accentuating extreme rainfall, flooding, and devasting storms.

Another consequence of global warming is the increase of ocean surface water temperature, affecting the frequency and the extent of tropical storms, cyclones, hurricanes, and typhoons. Climate change also affects the availability of water resources in many geographical areas. As a result, drought can cause devasting sandstorms that can move large amounts of sand from one continent to another, favoring desertification with important consequences for the agricultural sector, and affecting the food supply. Because of climate change, extreme weather events are becoming more and more frequent in recent years, arousing growing concern [14].

Extreme weather events can aggravate preexisting respiratory conditions and increase the likelihood of asthma-related events. Many studies describe a significant association between extreme weather events and asthma symptoms in children. For example, during local thunderstorms, an increase in acute asthma exacerbation is well documented, and this phenomenon is known as thunderstorm asthma. Investigators suggest thunderstorm asthma results from a complex interaction between environmental and individual susceptibility factors as sensitization to seasonal aeroallergens. Thunderstorms favor the pollen's breakdown into smaller parts, allowing them to reach the deeper part of the lungs, and bring respirable allergen particles down to ground level, making them easier to be inhaled. Wind gusts generated during thunderstorms can carry pollen and pollutants over longer distances, reaching more people and amplifying this event [15]. It should be considered that, among asthma thunderstorm risk factors, there is also the sensitization to *Alternaria alternata* [13].

According to the European Respiratory Society (ERS), extreme weather events increase the risk ratio of asthma exacerbations in children by 1.19-fold and of asthma. Emergency Department (ED) visits by 1.52-fold with a subsequent increase in children's hospitalization [16].

27.4 Effects of Pollution on Asthma

The exposome, defined as the whole external environmental exposures with which an individual gets in touch starting from intrauterine life, interacts with the genome. In fact, genetic predisposition combined with environmental exposure to inhaled air pollutants is an important risk factor for developing allergic diseases.

Among external factors, climate, allergens, foods, and pollutants are involved in developing atopic dermatitis, allergic conjunctivitis, rhinitis, and asthma [3, 8, 9, 17, 18].

Air pollution is defined as any agent's contamination of indoor or outdoor air that modifies its natural characteristics [4, 6].

It has been recently established that air pollution not only affects patients with preexisting asthma but can also act to initiate it, modulating the airway epithelium function, disrupting its integrity facilitating the allergens penetration into mucous membrane, and playing a central role in inflammation by increasing oxidative stress with subsequent pro-inflammatory cytokine production [9, 19]. Air pollution exposure increases Th2 and Th17 lymphocyte response, as in some respiratory diseases such as asthma [20].

Oxidative stress and DNA damage are plausible mechanisms to explain how air pollution can affect respiratory health. Outdoor and indoor pollutants can cause lung injury due to oxidative stress, inducing inflammation and increasing reactive oxygen species (ROS) production. ROS contribute to epithelial cell inflammation, airway hyperreactivity, increased tight junction barrier permeability, and lung injury.

Oxidative stress is the result of an imbalance between ROS production and antioxidant defense systems. High oxidative stress levels sustain the pathophysiology of many diseases, including asthma. In fact, in asthmatic patients, ROS production and consequent oxidative stress levels are higher than in healthy people. In these patients, a vicious cycle of events supports the increase of oxidative stress: external insults such as allergens, pollution, and smoke can trigger oxidative stress events that, in turn, promote pro-inflammatory events, including the recruitment of activated inflammatory cells (eosinophils, neutrophils, and macrophages) that are the primary source of ROS. If not balanced by antioxidant molecules, an excess in ROS levels leads to oxidative stress and structural and functional damages, remodeling processes, and a worsened corticosteroid response. In conclusion, all these events promote asthma evolution toward the more severe forms [21].

Among the major air pollutants PM, NO_2, CO, SO_2, and O_3 are sources of particular concern (Table 27.2).

Table 27.2 Sources and effects of principal pollutants [3, 20]

Pollutant type	Pollutant source	Effect on children's health
Particulate matter (PM) • PM_{10} • $PM_{2.5}$ • $PM_{0.1}$	Fuel burning: motor vehicles, ships, airplanes, domestic heating, energy production, other industrial burning such as waste incineration, wood-burning stoves, and fireplaces Surface tire abrasion Traffic-related air pollution Construction work Chemical reaction products Pollens and other bioaerosols Wind-dispersed dust particles	Irritative rhinoconjunctivitis Worsening asthma and lung diseases Reduced lung function Reduces mucociliary activity Increase oxidative stress Pulmonary and systemic inflammation Promote disease progression as asthma and chronic obstructive pulmonary disease (COPD) Reduce life expectancy Possible carcinogenic effects Airway remodeling
Ozone (O_3)	Chemical reactions of volatile organic compounds in the atmospheric presence of sunlight	Irritation of lower airways: coughing, sore, and scratchy throat Increased susceptibility to respiratory infections Irritative rhinoconjunctivitis Reduced lung function Exacerbation of asthma and COPD
Nitrogen dioxide (NO_2)	Motor vehicle emission Transportation (airplanes, railways, ships) Ice resurfacing equipment Cooking with gas stoves Chemical reaction products Cigarette smoking	Airway inflammation in healthy people Increased susceptibility to lung infections in asthmatic patients Increased susceptibility to asthma triggers like pollen and exercise Increase asthma exacerbations with worsened symptoms
Carbon monoxide (CO)	Wood-burning stoves and malfunctioning or poorly ventilated heating ovens Outdoor heaters and home heating systems Gas lanterns Tools with gasoline engines	Cell hypoxia Loss of consciousness Death and fetal death
Sulfur dioxide (SO_2)	Burning fuels containing sulfur (diesel) Fossil fuel combustion at power plants and other industrial facilities Transportation (which burns residual fuel oil) Natural processes that release sulfur gases include the decomposition and combustion of organic matter, spray from the sea, and volcanic eruptions	Irritates the mucosa of the nose, throat, and lungs Susceptibility to infections Worsen existing respiratory diseases such as asthma Narrowing of the airways leads to wheezing, chest tightness, and shortness of breath More frequent asthma attacks in asthmatic patients

27.4.1 Particulate Matter

PM is microscopic solid particles and liquid droplets suspended in the air resulting from fuel burning (motor vehicles, energy production, heating, and cooking), natural fragments of pollens or spores, and wind-dispersed dust. Short-term exposure to PM exacerbates preexisting diseases such as asthma, while long-term exposure is associated with the onset of new diseases and their progression [22].

According to aerodynamic diameter, they are classified into PM 10 (<10 μm), PM 2.5 (<2.5 μm), and PM 0.1 (ultra-fine particulates, <0.1 μm). Depending on the size, they reach different respiratory airway levels: PM 10 reaches the nasal cavity and central airways (trachea, bronchi, and bronchioles), PM 2.5 arrives in alveoli, and PM 0.1 to alveoli, lung tissue, and blood. PM also reduces mucociliary activity, causes upper airway irritation, increases oxidative stress favoring pulmonary and systemic inflammation, promotes pulmonary remodeling, and can also have carcinogenic effects [3, 22].

Early-life exposure to PM has been associated with impaired lung function and eosinophilic inflammation, suggesting that it may contribute to airway inflammation and remodeling, with consequent asthma development. Also, a decrease in peak expiratory flow (PEF) rates and forced expiratory volume in the first second (FEV_1) has been documented, especially among asthmatic children, with an increased number of asthma exacerbations, visits to ED, hospitalizations, and deaths.

27.4.2 Ozone

Ozone is a highly reactive and unstable gas in the upper atmosphere and ground level. In the upper atmosphere, ozone has a protective effect by filtering out damaging ultraviolet radiation from the sun. Ozone at ground level, instead, is dangerous for health [23]. Ground-level ozone is the main component of smog and derives from the interaction between sunlight, motor vehicles, and industrial emissions. Ground-level ozone can be harmful to our health, even at low levels. Moreover, ozone can reach long distances and accumulate far away from the sources of the original pollutants. The potentially harmful effects are listed in Table 27.2 [19].

27.4.3 Nitrogen Dioxide

Nitrogen dioxide is a highly reactive gas that can be present outdoors, especially near busy roads and inside, resulting from cigarette smoke and cooking with gas stoves. In outdoors, nitrogen dioxide contributes to ground-level ozone production and PM pollution. Nitrogen dioxide is considered a major irritant for respiratory airways [24].

27.4.4 Carbon Monoxide

Carbon monoxide is a poisonous, colorless, odorless, and tasteless gas. It originated from burning fuels like gas, wood, and charcoal in closed spaces without enough airflow. For this reason, all the devices that produce carbon monoxide, including outdoor heaters and barbeques, tools with gasoline, and vehicle engines, should never be used indoors. Common symptoms of carbon monoxide poisoning are headache, nausea, vomiting, dizziness, and weakness, up to more severe conditions such as loss of consciousness and death [24].

27.4.5 Sulfur Dioxide

Sulfur dioxide is a highly reactive gas with a pungent irritating smell. Natural processes that release sulfur gases include the decomposition and combustion of organic matter and volcanic eruptions; fossil fuel combustion can also be produced at industrial facilities. Sulfur dioxide exposure is associated with wheezing, chest tightness, and shortness of breath [24].

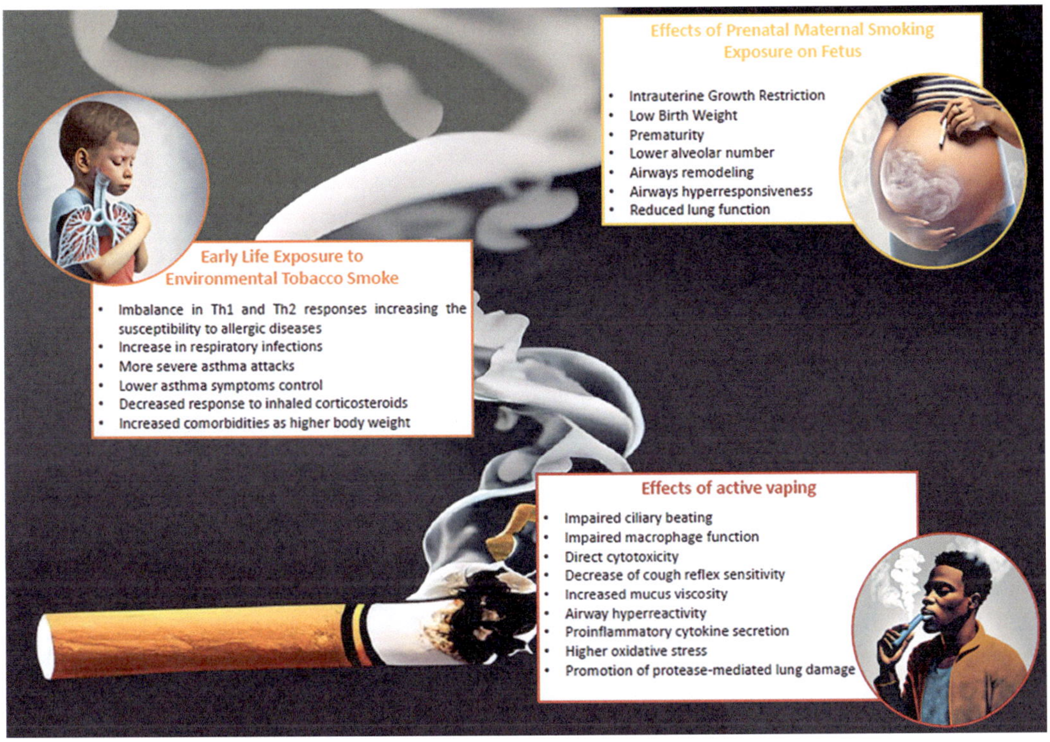

Fig. 27.2 Smoking and vaping effects at different ages

27.4.6 Cigarette and e-Cigarette Smoke

Cigarette smoke and vaping also contribute to air pollution, to which adults and children are exposed (Fig. 27.2). Cigarette smoking is widespread worldwide, and tobacco use is the major cause of preventable death. Environmental tobacco smoke (ETS) exposure is a recognized risk factor for both acute and chronic respiratory diseases. Both prenatal and early-life ETS exposure may impact the infant's susceptibility to developing respiratory diseases and impaired lung development [25]. It is also important to underline that there is no safe level of ETS exposure. ETS interferes with infant lung development and is associated with childhood upper and lower respiratory tract infections, wheezing, and asthma [26]. Further, exposure to ETS reduces lung function early in life, determining an increased lifelong risk of severe respiratory disease. Potential mechanisms for ETS-induced damage include impaired lung growth in the fetus and direct genotoxicity [26].

Further, there is evidence linking the effects of tobacco smoke exposure to impaired early-life immune function resulting in an imbalance in Th1 and Th2 responses, increasing the susceptibility to allergic diseases and childhood respiratory infections. ETS exposure has also been associated with more severe asthma attacks, lower asthma symptoms control with decreased response to inhaled corticosteroids (ICS), contributing to reduce efficacy in asthmatic children. Children with asthma and ETS exposure are twice as likely to be hospitalized for asthma and have more ED visits than unexposed asthmatics. Finally, ETS-exposed children have increased comorbid conditions with significantly higher body mass index (BMI) percentiles and are more likely to have more severe asthma than nonexposed controls [25].

Many policies have been implemented to limit exposure to passive smoke in public places, but no ban prevents exposure to indoor smoke in private locations yet [27]. Many children experience exposure to the ETS because of a smoking family member inside the houses with a degree of exposure closely related to smoking habits. A direct correlation has been demonstrated between the family's socioeconomic status and the children's ETS [28]. Nowadays, it is estimated that up to 40% of children are still exposed to tobacco smoke [6].

Tobacco smoke includes several chemicals and carcinogens that may affect the developing respiratory system. Smoke exposure is associated with anatomical airway changes that can lead to decreased airflow and increased resistance, resulting in decreased pulmonary function. It has been shown that enforcement of smoke-free policies was significantly associated with a reduction in hospital admissions (−9.8%) and lower respiratory tract infections (−18.5%), indicating that stringent smoke-free policies are necessary to gain maximum health benefits [3].

The use of electronic cigarettes is widespread, especially among adolescents. Although an increasing number of studies support the evidence of vaping-related damage to the respiratory tract, electronic nicotine delivery systems (ENDS) such as e-cigarettes are still considered less harmful than traditional cigarettes by the general population [29]. E-liquids and vaping contain many toxicants, and the health-related adverse effects depend on vaping habits, physical device factors, e-liquid components, heat-related chemical changes, and the e-cigarette user's health (e.g., asthma) [30].

The main effects of vaping on the airway mucosa are the recruitment of immune cells to the site of exposure, impaired ciliary beating and macrophage function, direct cytotoxicity, a decrease of cough reflex sensitivity, promotion of protease-mediated lung tissue damage, and increase of mucus viscosity, airway hyperreactivity, airflow resistance, pro-inflammatory cytokine secretion, and oxidative stress. The use of ENDS is increasing worldwide, especially among adolescents and young adults. Despite the growing spread of their use, evidence of their effects on asthma is limited. It is expected that vaping may be detrimental to asthmatic patients due to its pro-inflammatory and bronchoconstriction effects. Indeed, vape exposure among adolescents and young adults appears to be associated with acute respiratory symptoms. Moreover, there is insufficient evidence about the long-term effects on users' health and second- and third-hand vape exposure [29].

27.4.7 Wildfire Smoke

Due to droughts and heat waves due to climate change, an increase in wildfires was observed in the last years [31]. The rise of forest fires exposes the population to wildfire smoke and enhanced fine particulate levels, promoting wheezing, asthma exacerbations, pneumonia, and bronchitis, especially in children [5]. Researchers demonstrated an increase in the odds of ED visits on days with wildfire smoke exposure versus non-wildfire smoke exposure days, with peak odds on the first day of exposure [32].

27.4.8 Traffic-Related Air Pollution

Also, traffic-related air pollution (TRAP) is important in environmental pollution. Many studies have shown higher respiratory infection rates, wheezing, and asthma incidence in children living near busy roads [32]. An infant's early-life exposure to TRAP increases the risk of respiratory infection as bronchiolitis, increasing the risk of asthma development. TRAP also directly decreases lung function and is associated with developing respiratory symptoms and asthma, even if the exact pathogenetic mechanism is unclear [33–35].

27.4.9 Prenatal Exposure to Air Pollutants

The developing fetus is highly vulnerable to oxidative stress injury, as the immune system is still immature during the prenatal period. Maternal smoking exposure (MSE) and PM exposure are associated with asthma susceptibility later in life. Free radicals and chemicals inhaled during pregnancy can pass the blood-placental barrier, increasing the level of oxidative stress in the offspring and modifying the placental structure, which reduces nutrient delivery. Intrauterine nutrient deficiency may lead to intrauterine growth restriction (IUGR), low birth weight (LBW), and prematurity, with possible lung development impairment. The sequelae of these early-life events are airway remodeling, airway hyperresponsiveness, and inflammation, which are distinctive features of asthma.

Moreover, IUGR, LBW, and prematurity can result in lower alveolar numbers and reduced lung function, with an increased risk of childhood asthma in an MSE dose-dependent way. A direct correlation between the number of maternal cigarettes smoked and the prevalence of asthma symptoms has been reported. Overall, the oxidants inhaled by the mother can cause an increase in oxidative stress in the fetus that may result in persistent changes to both the fetal epigenome and lung structure [4, 36].

27.5 Conclusions

Climate change is now a reality we live with every day. However, its impact on future generations is impossible to predict [3]. Climate change is closely related to environmental pollution, whose deleterious effects on human health are already well known, particularly respiratory diseases like asthma. As available asthma therapies are still not curative, it is important to develop preventive strategies through environmental policies aimed at reducing pollution and environment preservation [18, 35].

Key Points

- Climate is changing: extreme weather events and air pollution are increasing.
- Asthma is affected by climate change and air pollution.
- Prenatal exposure and early-life exposure to pollutants can cause structural and functional damage favoring inflammation and pulmonary remodeling processes.
- Extreme weather events can aggravate preexisting respiratory conditions and increase asthma-related events such as thunderstorm asthma.
- The imbalance between ROS production and antioxidant defense systems plays an important role in lung inflammatory conditions such as asthma.
- Asthma can be worsened by oxidative stress, smoking exposure, and traffic-related air pollution.

Take-Home Messages

- Climate change and air pollution have a significant impact on adults' and children's health.
- Infants and children are more vulnerable than adults because of their physiological immaturity, higher respiratory rate, and different lifestyles.
- Climate change influences extreme weather events, pollen seasons, allergen amounts and distribution, house dust mites, and mold growth affecting allergic diseases such as rhinoconjunctivitis and asthma.
- Air pollution can cause lung injury due to oxidative stress-inducing inflammation and increasing ROS production, leading to structural and functional damage promoting wheezing and asthma.

(continued)

- Prenatal exposure to oxidative stress may lead to IUGR, LBW, and prematurity with possible lung development impairment and subsequent increased risk of childhood asthma.
- Smoking tobacco exposure is still a concerning problem: prenatal and infancy exposure can affect the developing respiratory system resulting in decreased pulmonary function.
- Climate change has deleterious effects on children's health: it is crucial to adopt preventive strategies to reduce pollution and preserve the environment.

References

1. Biagioni B, Cecchi L, D'Amato G, Annesi-Maesano I. Environmental influences on childhood asthma: climate change. Pediatr Allergy Immunol. 2023;34:e13961.
2. Goossens J, Jonckheere AC, Dupont LJ, Bullens DMA. Air pollution and the airways: lessons from a century of human urbanization. Atmosphere. 2021;12:898.
3. Urrutia-Pereira M, Guidos-Fogelbach G, Solé D. Climate changes, air pollution and allergic diseases in childhood and adolescence. J Pediatr. 2022;98(Suppl 1):S47–54.
4. Hoffmann B, Boogaard H, de Nazelle A, Andersen ZJ, Abramson M, Brauer M, et al. WHO Air Quality Guidelines 2021—aiming for healthier air for all: a joint statement by Medical, Public Health, Scientific Societies and Patient Representative Organisations. Int J Public Health. 2021;66:1604465.
5. Perera F, Nadeau K. Climate change, fossil-fuel pollution, and children's health. N Engl J Med. 2022;386:2303–14.
6. European Environmental Agency (EEA). Air pollution and children's health. 2023. https://www.eea.europa.eu/publications/air-pollution-and-childrens-health.
7. Global Initiative for Asthma. Global strategy for asthma management and prevention. 2023. www.ginasthma.org.
8. European Academy of Allergy and Clinical Immunology. Global atlas of asthma. EAACI. 2nd ed. European Academy of Allergy and Clinical Immunology; 2021. www.eaaci.org.
9. D'Amato G, Chong-Neto HJ, Monge Ortega OP, Vitale C, Ansotegui I, Rosario N, et al. The effects of climate change on respiratory allergy and asthma induced by pollen and mold allergens. Allergy. 2020;75:2219–28.
10. Acevedo N, Zakzuk J, Caraballo L. House dust mite allergy under changing environments. Allergy Asthma Immunol Res. 2019;11:450.
11. Di Cicco M, Del Tufo E, Fasola S, Gracci S, Marchi MG, Fibbi L, et al. The effect of outdoor aeroallergens on asthma hospitalizations in children in North-Western Tuscany, Italy. Int J Environ Res Public Health. 2022;19:3586.
12. O'Hollaren MT, Yunginger JW, Offord KP, Somers MJ, O'Connell EJ, Ballard DJ, et al. Exposure to an aeroallergen as a possible precipitating factor in respiratory arrest in young patients with asthma. N Engl J Med. 1991;324:359–63.
13. Pulimood TB, Corden JM, Bryden C, Sharples L, Nasser SM. Epidemic asthma and the role of the fungal mold Alternaria alternata. J Allergy Clin Immunol. 2007;120:610–7.
14. Centro Regionale di Informazione delle Nazioni Unite. Effetti del cambiamento climatico. Nazioni Unite. 2023. www.unric.org.
15. Thien F, Beggs PJ, Csutoros D, Darvall J, Hew M, Davies JM, et al. The Melbourne epidemic thunderstorm asthma event 2016: an investigation of environmental triggers, effect on health services, and patient risk factors. Lancet Planet Health. 2018;2:e255–63.
16. Makrufardi F, Manullang A, Rusmawatiningtyas D, Chung KF, Lin SC, Chuang HC. Extreme weather and asthma: a systematic review and meta-analysis. Eur Respir Rev. 2023;32:230019.
17. Ferrante G, Fasola S, Cilluffo G, Piacentini G, Viegi G, La Grutta S. Addressing exposome: an innovative approach to environmental determinants in pediatric respiratory health. Front Public Health. 2022;10:871140.
18. Wang J, Janson C, Malinovschi A, Holm M, Franklin KA, Modig L, et al. Asthma, allergic rhinitis and atopic dermatitis in association with home environment—the RHINE study. Sci Total Environ. 2022;853:158609.
19. Bontinck A, Maes T, Joos G. Asthma and air pollution. Curr Opin Pulm Med. 2020;26:10–9.
20. Glencross DA, Ho TR, Camiña N, Hawrylowicz CM, Pfeffer PE. Air pollution and its effects on the immune system. Free Radic Biol Med. 2020;151:56–68.
21. Vincenzo SD, Ferrante G, Ferraro M, Cascio C, Malizia V, Licari A, et al. Oxidative stress, environmental pollution, and lifestyle as determinants of asthma in children. Biology. 2023;12:133.
22. Akdis CA. Does the epithelial barrier hypothesis explain the increase in allergy, autoimmunity and other chronic conditions? Nat Rev Immunol. 2021;21:739–51.
23. Atkinson CE, Kesic MJ, Hernandez ML. Ozone in the development of pediatric asthma and atopic disease. Immunol Allergy Clin N Am. 2022;42:701–13.

24. New South Wales Health (NSW). https://www.health.nsw.gov.au/environment/air/Pages/common-air-pollutants.aspx.
25. Vanker A, Gie RP, Zar HJ. The association between environmental tobacco smoke exposure and childhood respiratory disease: a review. Expert Rev Respir Med. 2017;11:661–73.
26. Mescolo F, Ferrante G, La Grutta S. Effects of E-cigarette exposure on prenatal life and childhood respiratory health: a review of current evidence. Front Pediatr. 2021;9:711573.
27. Cilluffo G, Ferrante G, Cutrera R, Piacentini G, Bignamini E, Landi M, et al. Barriers and incentives for Italian paediatricians to become smoking cessation promoters: a GARD-Italy Demonstration Project. J Thorac Dis. 2020;12:6868–79.
28. Rocco I, Cilluffo G, Ferrante G, Cibella F, Marcon A, Marchetti P, et al. Investigating the relationship between parental education, asthma and rhinitis in children using path analysis. Int J Environ Res Public Health. 2022;19:14551.
29. Di Cicco M, Sepich M, Beni A, Comberiati P, Peroni DG. How E-cigarettes and vaping can affect asthma in children and adolescents. Curr Opin Allergy Clin Immunol. 2022;22:86–94.
30. Gordon T, Karey E, Rebuli ME, Escobar YNH, Jaspers I, Chen LC. E-cigarette toxicology. Annu Rev Pharmacol Toxicol. 2022;62:301–22.
31. Abatzoglou JT, Williams AP. Impact of anthropogenic climate change on wildfire across western US forests. Proc Natl Acad Sci USA. 2016;113:11770–5.
32. Doubleday A, Sheppard L, Austin E, Isaksen TB. Wildfire smoke exposure and emergency department visits in Washington state. Environ Res Health. 2023;1:025006.
33. Morgenstern V, Zutavern A, Cyrys J, Brockow I, Koletzko S, Krämer U, et al. Atopic diseases, allergic sensitization, and exposure to traffic-related air pollution in children. Am J Respir Crit Care Med. 2008;177:1331–7.
34. Lee JY, Leem JH, Kim HC, Lamichhane DK, Hwang SS, Kim JH, et al. Effects of traffic-related air pollution on susceptibility to infantile bronchiolitis and childhood asthma: a cohort study in Korea. J Asthma. 2018;55:223–30.
35. HEI Panel on the Health Effects of Long-Term Exposure to Traffic-Related Air Pollution. Systematic review and meta-analysis of selected health effects of long-term exposure to traffic-related air pollution. Special Report 23. Boston, MA: Health Effects Institute; 2022.
36. Wang B, Chen H, Chan YL, Wang G, Oliver BG. Why do intrauterine exposure to air pollution and cigarette smoke increase the risk of asthma? Front Cell Dev Biol. 2020;8:38.

Daily Life of Allergic Children 28

Giovanni Cavagni and Monica De Simone

Abstract

The management of a child or adolescent suffering from one or more allergic diseases cannot be separated from the appropriate consideration of the good rules to follow in everyday life. The chapter will first address the importance of virtuous relationships among the pediatrician, the specialist, and the family. It will continue with the analysis of the management of children suffering from atopic dermatitis, food allergy, respiratory allergy, severe asthma, and rhinitis in his/her daily life. The most important moments of the child's life will be taken into consideration, whether at home, at school, during sport activities, and in canteens. The article will distinguish the case of children and adolescents. The chapter ends with an analysis of socialization, outlining the rules to follow in order to overcome difficulties and dangers outside the domestic environment. The aim is to encourage normal socialization and avoid parents' fears leading to excessive protectionism.

Keywords

Allergic children · Atopic dermatitis · TEWL · Urticaria · Food allergy · Elimination diet · Bronchial asthma · Allergic rhinitis · Anaphylaxis · Salbutamol · Epinephrine · Local corticosteroids · School · Socialization · Self-management

Test your learning and check your understanding of this book's contents: use the "Springer Nature Flashcards" app to access questions using ▶ https://sn.pub/nspbjm. To use the app, please follow the instructions in Chap. 1.

Key Points

- Daily life of children with atopic dermatitis, food allergy, bronchial asthma, allergic rhinitis.
- Psychosocial problems in children with allergic diseases.
- How to deal with allergic emergencies at school and on school trips.
- Sport activities for allergic children.
- How to prevent relapses of food and respiratory allergies.
- The influence of complications on the behavior of allergic children.

G. Cavagni (✉)
Centro Diagnostico Europeo Dalla Rosa Prati, Parma, Italy

M. De Simone
University of Palermo and Representative for Relations with the Institutions of ARI-AAA3 ODV, Association for Research on Allergy, Asthma and the Environment, Palermo, Italy

C. Caffarelli, G. L. Marseglia (eds.), *Textbook of Pediatric Allergy*,
https://doi.org/10.1007/978-3-031-71283-8_28

28.1 Introduction

From earlier chapters, it is clear that the diagnostic process and the ensuing therapeutic approach are effective for treating the particular disorder known as allergic children (AC).

We use the term "specific" allergic disease because the multifactorial nature of allergies may be influenced by environmental and epigenetic factors, causing the disease to manifest itself in a variety of ways and affect various organs and bodily parts.

The fact is that AC can be affected by diseases like atopic dermatitis (AD), food allergies (FA), allergic rhinitis (AR), and asthma (BA). "Atopia"—ἀτοπία—is the body's sensitivity to certain environmental substances, which are normally innocuous to most people. However, in some cases, these substances can lead to excessive immune responses and organ manifestations.

The "Atopic March," which is now regarded as a combination of underlying immunologic mechanisms, describes the temporal progression of a variety of allergic conditions, from AD and food allergies in early childhood to the development of asthma and AR, to which the eosinophilic esophagitis most recently was added [1].

Therefore, one can understand the complexity of the subject matter that will be covered in this chapter, which is devoted to the daily struggles of children who have one or more allergic diseases or who have "Atopic March" [1].

This analysis will cover all interactions with doctors. A list of everyday behaviors at home, at school, during meals, at the grocery store, and during sports activities, will follow. The chapter will end with psychological aspects of adolescent and child desocialization as well as issues related to the self-regulation of the disease.

28.2 The Physician and the Specialist

The general practitioner (GP) or specialist (preferably a pediatrician) should take into consideration not only his or her own expertise and professional qualifications, but also children and parents' emotional intelligence. The proper course of treating a child suspected of having an allergy requires the Pediatrician to refer the child to the hospital's Allergologist. According to medical ethics, Allergologist is required to draft a specific report with diagnoses and instructions on how to manage AC at home.

The final task for the GP is to confirm the specialists' proposals and verify that parents are aware and ready to manage AC. They have to ensure that both AC and families maintain their quality of life on a daily basis and oversee the formal relationships required with local healthcare facilities, schools, and other socializing venues such as school gyms. If the tenure of the AC's support network falters, for example, due to the inability of some of the actors and bureaucratic shortcomings, it is likely that the young child's allergy condition will worsen [2].

28.3 Daily Life with Atopic Dermatitis

It is not difficult for a pediatrician or dermatologist to identify AD (refer to Chap. 6) when painful erythema develops on the face and spreads to the folds of the limbs as early as the first few months of life [3]. The chronic inflammatory condition, which may be the first sign of the "Atopic March," can be linked to food allergies, milk and eggs as early as the first year of life. Families are concerned about the potential chronicity of the sickness and the bothersome itching. They need to have patience and follow the daily therapies recommended by the pediatric specialist [3].

Transepidermal water loss (TEWL) is a prominent skin defect in children with AD. As a result, the skin needs to be maintained hydrated on a regular basis [4]. Daily skin care is also necessary to reduce itching and avoid skin flare-ups or infections (impetigo) [5, 6].

Medicinal baths or sterile compresses soaked in an antiseptic and decongestant solution are advised for the acute serous phase [7]. The itching gets worse after scratching, as the skin's nerve fibers get activated, making the itching even worse. In addition to moisturizers, the chronic treatment of dry erythema must include the corticosteroids cremes. These are the most effective anti-inflammatory medications that can reduce itching. Scratches can cause open sores and skin infections by infectious organisms [6, 8].

The itching caused by AD can interfere with sleeping rhythms because parents try to prevent children from scratching, resulting in a lack of sleep [9, 10].

Here are some helpful tips for families to avoid AD flare-ups:

1. Use mild, oil-free cleansers for about 10 min on a daily basis to reduce the dehydrating effects of bathing. Be sure to pat the skin dry with a soft towel, and apply moisturizers while the skin is still moist (within 3 min); fabrics in contact with the skin must be white and smooth, like cotton or silk.
2. Avoid scratchy garments like wool and colored fabrics next to the skin (warm clothes cause sweating, which is harmful); shower gels or detergents containing dyes, alcohol, or scents; food proteins coming in touch with the skin, such as creams or oils containing peanuts, almonds, or other food that may cause sensitization and food allergies [11–14].

28.4 Daily Life with Food Allergy

Parents may become alarmed when their infant develops anaphylactic symptoms due to a FA for the first time (refer to Chap. 10). These symptoms appear most frequently during breastfeeding or typically with weaning, after eating for a short period of time cow's milk and/or eggs [15]. Children's sensitivity to other foods, including fish and fruit (fresh and dried, such as hazelnuts, peaches, etc.) may increase as the diet is expanded [16, 17].

It should be underlined that a youngster with FA is often healthy unless exposed to the allergen in question. For this kind of allergy, it's important to follow at all times a strict diet plan and carry the epinephrine auto-injectors that the doctor has prescribed [18].

The intense focus on nutrition in children and adolescents has a significant impact on their development and behavior. Children who have had severe allergic reactions develop high levels of mistrust and anxiety about dangers they may encounter. Sudden changes in AC's daily routine and diet might disrupt the balance and social and emotional meanings associated with feeding.

The FA impairs the quality of life for both AC and their families; anxiety in children is frequently transmitted by parents who use it as a coping mechanism to feel more at ease; as a result, medical and psychological interventions are essential [19].

At Home: The best way to prevent accidental ingestion is to read the labels of all food ingredients. It is also important to take care when preparing meals, making sure they are free of any potential contaminants, and keeping a variety of kitchen utensils available only for "safe" foods. Foods containing the allergen in question must be eliminated or kept out of AC's reach. It is important to instruct family members, babysitters, and domestic workers on the risks that AC's encounter in contact with food or its contamination [20].

At School: From daycare on any child who is food allergic must notify the school administration with a medical certificate at the time of enrollment. Schools are in charge of children's health and must provide the following for the family: "safe" meals in the cafeteria avoiding cross-contamination with other children's meals; trained staff members in the injection of epinephrine in the event of accidental anaphylaxis must notify the family and emergency services. The same care, if not more, must be provided during school trips. Ideally, classmates' parents are also involved and asked not to bring lunches that may potentially contain dangerous foods for AC [21].

At the Restaurant: The regulation (EU) 1169/2011, in effect since December 13, 2014 [22], prescribes the obligation to single out ingredients on the label that may cause allergies (for e.g., using graphic aids like bold, a different color, underlining). The top 14 allergens that must be listed are: (1) gluten-containing grains, (2) shellfish, (3) eggs, (4) fish, (5) peanuts, (6) soy beans (7) cow's milk and dairy products (including lactose), (8) nuts, (9) celery, (10) mustard, (11) sesame seeds, (12) concentrations of sulfur dioxide and sulfites larger than 10 mg/kg or 10 mg/L in terms of total SO, (13) lupins, and (14) mollusk. Catering businesses providing ready-to-eat food are required to inform the ultimate consumer of the ingredients or products that can cause allergies or intolerances in accordance with Annex II of Regulation (EU) No. 1169/2011. The consumer must have easy access to this information, thus it must be kept in plain sight [23].

At the Supermarket: Avoid buying packaged goods that have an allergic item listed on the label. Parents should be alerted when coming across sentences such as "it could contain traces of…." For instance, a product that does not intentionally contain the allergen (for e.g., hazelnuts) in the recipe could still be contaminated by other products produced in the same factory [24]. The phrase "may contain traces of…" should be solely understood as valuable information for the consumer and not as a blanket discharge from all obligations for the food producer. Food that has been contaminated by allergens not disclosed on the label or placard is considered to be "at risk" [3], needing the prompt implementation of the corrective measures outlined in the "General Food Law" [25].

28.5 Daily Life with Respiratory Allergy

28.5.1 Children

Daycare attendance increases the risk of respiratory tract infections, which frequently cause breath wheezing due to the small size and mucus-clogged bronchi. However, in children who continue to suffer from bronchial obstruction as they age, this is a sign that they have bronchial asthma, one of the most common childhood diseases. Children of parents with AD have a very high probability of developing allergies. The first episodes of BA (refer to Chap. 4) are often confused with respiratory infections [26] and treated improperly with antibiotics or, even worse, with cough suppressants that are always ineffective [27]. After formulating a diagnosis based on symptoms, family history, and the results of allergy diagnostic tests (skin prick test), the specialist will explain to parents (often anxious when they witness a sudden acute asthma attack) the most effective drug treatment for acute attack and long-term control of your child's asthma. The therapy will initially consist of inhaled anti-inflammatories and bronchodilators. Experienced in both routine care and acute attack therapy, parents must appear confident and determined when administering medications because apprehension, or worst, fear, have an adverse effect on the child's response.

Parents must be aware of the impact and results of treatment:

- Identify the risk factors, and learn to eliminate or reduce them (e.g., keep the windows closed, if the child is sensitive to pollen or air in the bedroom and vacuum the mattress often, if allergic to dust mites, avoid passive smoking or perfumes intensely).
- The correct use of a spacer suitable for the child's age (with mask up to 5 years, with the mouthpiece in later ages) connected to a fast-acting bronchodilator delivered via a metered-dose inhaler.
- Learn to recognize a worsening or an imminent crisis of air hunger (e.g., shortness of breath, irritability, cough after playing, unexplained tiredness, purplish skin, disturbed sleep).
- Keep an asthma diary, in which the child's symptoms are recorded.
- Even the child himself can gradually learn to understand his/her condition and independently adhere to the recommended course of

treatment with cortisone and inhaled bronchodilators, yet always under the parent's watchful eye.
- In conclusion, an asthmatic child can maintain a normal life without giving up sports and school activities, as long as adequate care is given [28].

28.5.2 Adolescents

Allergic sensitization tends to evolve up to the developmental age. Then it tends to cool down but this phenomenon is not always accompanied by the control of asthmatic symptoms. Asthma can continue during adolescence, but crises may appear more distant from each other, leading the adolescent to underestimate and neglect it. Wheezing forces are sometimes caused by smoking, which is often a way to socialize for teenagers.

In the Italian context, the transition from the pediatrician to the GP, happening around the age of 14 years old, is another reason that tends to decrease attention to the problem. While during childhood, the frequency of the crises forced to maintain a constant relationship between families and specialists, in adolescence often the attacks tend to reduce, the presumed feeling of well-being and the transition phase, tend to neglect the disorder.

It has been demonstrated in adolescents between 12 and 15 years old, in 30% symptomatic, you can receive an incorrect diagnosis and therefore not be treated due to:

- Compromised family situations (complexity, economic hardship, low levels of education)
- A high body mass index
- Passive smoking
- Lack of physical activity
- The absence of concomitant allergic rhinitis

Conditions which, on the other hand, should induce the family and the GP to subject the adolescent to the specialist.

In essence, it is certain that asthma does not in any way preclude the possibility of carrying out a healthy physical activity. On the contrary, it can promote lung function thanks to the enhancement of musculature which, with training, tends to require less stress on the respiratory apparatus [29].

As already noted, it is important to encourage young people to pay closer attention to their bodies and, in the case of bronchial asthma diagnosed in childhood, make them responsible for their health in the face of risk factors and familiarity with asthma and allergy.

When adolescents with allergies cough while playing sports, they must correctly inhale the fast-acting bronchodilator (using a spacer) before the start of physical exertion. If the adolescent coughs when waking up, he must be cautious of the invisible dust mites present in his bed, to which he is allergic.

In order for adolescents to learn the importance of keeping healthy, parents must remind them of the fundamental therapy, clinical tests, and the spirometry (useful about every 3 months) [30].

28.6 Daily Life with Severe Asthma

Neglected or concomitant asthma can progress into severe asthma (refer to Chap. 5), a kind of asthma that requires high doses of corticosteroid and bronchodilator therapy to control or that does not respond to this medication. Comorbidities include diseases that share a common mechanism of action with asthma, such as rhinosinusitis or nasal polyposis, as well as chronic illnesses brought on by long-term use of systemic corticosteroids (such as obesity, diabetes, and high blood pressure), or made worse by psychological conditions like anxiety and depression.

These adolescents ought to adhere to a multidisciplinary treatment that can identify the instruments necessary for an accurate diagnosis and proper treatment of the illness.

A "value-based healthcare" vision calls for:

- Early detection.
- An optimization of the therapy that can also be tailored to the patient's particular conditions.
- An adequate follow-up process that can develop in a synergistic way between all the players involved in the complex approach to this pathology [30].

28.7 Daily Life with Allergic Rhinitis

Children and adolescents with rhinitis or rhinoconjunctivitis (refer to Chaps. 7 and 8) are disturbed by annoying typical symptoms such as rhinorrhea, nasal congestion, sneezing, and itchy nose and eyes, often edematous; the nasal obstruction can be such as to force them to sleep with an open mouth at night or, worse, to suffer from sleep apnea and consequently feeling tired throughout the day, resulting in poor concentration at school; frontal headache is a sign of subsequent sinusitis; adolescents also have practical problems, such as having to blow the nose often and therefore having pockets full of tissues, sometimes feeling embarrassed [31]. This greatly limits his daily activities and social relationships with a possible state of frustration and irritability. Both children and adolescents may experience school problems due to easy loss of concentration, tiredness, or easy irritability, as well as frequent absences. Younger children (6–12 years) are paradoxically more concerned about their symptoms and use handkerchiefs, take medicines, limit sports, contact with animals, and recreational activities. Adolescents suffering from RA are more likely to experience more lack of sleep, activity limitations, and dissatisfaction than asymptomatic peers. They may also experience another problem: continuous rhinorrhea and frequent sneezing can disturb their classmates and mock them, causing embarrassment and shame [32].

Prevention measures against allergens, such as pollen, aimed at reducing symptoms, can also limit the child's outdoor activities, who are often forced to stay indoors to avoid pollen and mold, thus reducing opportunities for interaction with peers. RA can also negatively impact the quality of the child's family life. Parents may become anxious and overprotective or feel guilty about their children. Lack of RA therapeutic treatment can lead to comorbid conditions including asthma, sinusitis, otitis media, recurrent respiratory infections, orthodontic malocclusions, OSAS, and all conditions which can have an additional negative impact [33]. The sanitizing and preventive action of nasal showers with physiological or hypertonic solutions, certainly effective, such as the toothbrush for dental care, should not be overlooked; this practice is the most effective remedy for the child with RA, provided that is kept constant over time associated with oral antihistamine and nasal anti-inflammatory treatment in the symptomatic phase if conjunctivitis is associated with rheumatoid arthritis, anti-inflammatory eye drops should not be forgotten. Allergen immunotherapy (AIT) may be the definitive treatment for asthma, rhinitis, and conjunctivitis when they are caused by the same allergen [34].

28.8 Cigarette Smoke

Smoke (refer to Chap. 27) is the biggest contaminant in enclosed spaces. At least one-third of the population is exposed to this domestic pollutant.

The phrase "*passive smoke*"or "*secondhand smoke*"refers to the inadvertent inhalation of smoke by individuals who do not smoke but who do so around others [35].

Active smokers exhale a combination of smoke (a complex of over 4000 chemicals in the form of particles and gases) from their cigarettes, pipes, or cigars. This mixture of smoke contains many of the harmful substances found in smoke, such as nicotine and carbon monoxide which are rapidly dispersed as they exit the cigarette, nicotine, and carbon monoxide spread quickly to damage the surroundings.

The term *thirdhand smoke*, on the other hand, considers the toxic residues of nicotine and other chemical substances which, after the combustion of the cigarette, are deposited in the environment. These can be detected on surfaces, on clothes, upholstery, objects, furniture, and even on the skin. Some of these components can be absorbed through the skin, ingested or inhaled with the powder.

Many studies have unequivocally shown that breathing secondhand smoke from people who smoke at home can cause health problems in children, such as bronchial asthma. These problems increase if both parents smoke [36, 37].

28.9 Socialization in Children and Teenagers with Allergic Diseases

Parental fear can lead to excessive protectionism. This can be avoided by taking the necessary precautions that do not limit but rather encourage normal socialization.

The risk of severe allergic reaction leading to anaphylaxis, air hunger leading to an asthmatic crisis, and extreme nasal obstruction are among the dangers that must be avoided in order to ensure the child and adolescent's successful socialization.

Schools are the most significant setting for children's initial socialization.

The management of AC at school can only be successful if all various players cooperate with each other and are accountable to ensure safety and the child's integration.

The AC's parents, family, friends, pediatrician, school administration, teachers, and support staff need to include the allergic child through the respect of some simple common rules, that ensure a clean environment, as free of allergens as possible, and that prevent the risk of contamination.

The first step for parents to safeguard their child's health is to issue an official and detailed certification. Thereafter schools will have the obligation to put all safety measure at place, such as a risk-prevention protocol in every circumstance of school life. The goal of such a document is to respect the AC's areas and possessions and reduce the possibility of an exacerbation of the disease: in the classroom, in any area courtyard, during the break, in the playground, in the gym, on a school trip, in the vehicles used in trips intended for educational activities, and in the canteen. For a student with an FA, canteens pose the biggest risk, particularly of anaphylaxis. In such a space, it is essential that the school adheres to preestablished protocols that eliminate the possibility of contamination throughout all processes, from food processing, packaging, and delivery, to the canteen preparation, meal handling, distribution, administration, and consumption. By adhering to these safety practices, ACs are safe to attend the canteen with classmates rather than being left alone.

Sports, both at school and in gyms for extracurricular activities, require the most attention for a kid or adolescent with respiratory allergies or AR. The child will be able to engage in physical activity if the practicing area is made as healthy as possible, and if the child is well guided through the administration of drugs that control the disease, and have those available to deal with any acute reaction.

The administration of medications at school, especially in the event of a severe asthmatic or anaphylactic crisis, is a very challenging component of managing the AC.

Unfortunately, the lack of legislation that specifies the procedures to be followed and lack of working staff in charge of administering first aid or life-saving drugs (self-injectable adrenaline, salbutamol inhaler) forces families, schools, pediatricians, and healthcare organizations to be actors who move extremely slowly in order to create a network of rescue. The therapeutic plan, which was created by the pediatrician in conjunction with the specialist, must include precise operational indications for the administration of the medications, and must be given to the school along with the aforementioned certified individual. The protocol must also include the name of the working staff in charge of overviewing the safety of the child. Unfortunately, Italy has not yet addressed these procedures, making it hard to guarantee widespread acceptability and uniformity.

Organizing children's parties is another crucial event that parents must learn to manage under the advice of a pediatrician, even with the help of his classmates and parents who have been made aware of the guidelines to prevent the risk of infection.

The catering establishments are yet another crucial location for the socialization of children, especially adolescents. The 2011 European directive represented a significant improvement in the safety of allergy patients. However, certain problems remain unresolved: the effective implementation of this legislation, which goes beyond generic and merely formal indications of allergen presence in the menu to indicate such presence in a specific manner and for each course; the training of all staff, including in the dining room, who is knowledgeable about food allergies and knows how to welcome the child and family or the now independent adolescent; the ongoing supervision of suppliers, who have the responsibility like restaurateur to follow the same legislation. We must not ignore the fact that anaphylactic shock deaths in restaurants occur in Italy on a yearly basis [38].

Identifying allergens is a similar issue with packaged goods. A very essential type of protection for allergy patients is undoubtedly the labeling regulation, which mandates listing all ingredients, including allergens, now specified in forms that highlight them in comparison to the others. Parents anxiously analyzing each product are frequently stressed out by the phrases "may contain traces" or "produced in an establishment where the allergen is present."

The phrase "without…" is still the best labeling for someone who has allergies.

Last but not least, a delicate subject concerns teenagers who have asthma, respiratory allergies, or food allergies, especially if they are severe. These teenagers need support in their development of self-management of their health condition through self-management of medications, both daily and acutely, to deal with respiratory or reaction crises to food allergens. It is common for people to let their guard down, disregard daily therapy, skip checkups, be careless, and refuse to carry emergency drugs, particularly adrenaline, out of a desire to fit in and not feel different. Certainly, avoiding such hazards can be facilitated by the pediatrician's and the practitioner's ongoing support along the adolescent route [39].

Take-Home Messages

- A virtuous relationship among the pediatrician, the specialist, and the family must be established.
- Pediatricians must guide parents and children in the daily management when they are suffering from atopic dermatitis, food allergy, respiratory allergy, severe asthma, and rhinitis.
- Particular attention must be paid to the life of allergic children, at home, at school, during sports activities, and in catering, appropriately considering the different types of allergies they suffer from and distinguishing the differences between children and adolescents.
- Pediatricians need to promote normal socialization and avoid the excessive protectionism that parental fear can cause.
- The best way to prevent accidental ingestion, in children with specific food allergy, is to read the labels of all ingredients.
- Avoiding second-hand and third-hand smoke from people who smoke at home because it can cause health problems in children, such as bronchial asthma and other allergic diseases. These problems increase if both parents smoke.

References

1. Hill DA, Grundmeier RW, Ramos M, Spergel JM. Eosinophilic esophagitis is a late manifestation of the allergic march. J Allergy Clin Immunol Pract. 2018;6:1528–33.
2. Stille CJ, Primack WA, McLaughlin TJ, Wasserman RC. Parents as information intermediaries between primary care and specialty physicians. Pediatrics. 2007;120:1238–46.

3. Page SS, Weston S, Loh R. Atopic dermatitis in children. Aust Fam Physician. 2016;45:293–6.
4. Rehbinder EM, Advocaat Endre KM, Lødrup Carlsen KC, Asarnoj A, Stensby Bains KE, et al. Predicting skin barrier dysfunction and atopic dermatitis in early infancy. J Allergy Clin Immunol Pract. 2020;8:664–73.
5. Mannschreck D, Feig J, Selph J, Cohen B. Disseminated bullous impetigo and atopic dermatitis: case series and literature review. Pediatr Dermatol. 2020;37:103–8.
6. Whalen-Browne A, Williams HC, Chu DK. Managing atopic dermatitis in infants. CMAJ. 2022;07:194.
7. Sabin BR, Peters N, Peters AT. Chapter 20: Atopic dermatitis. Allergy Asthma Proc. 2012;33(Suppl 1):67–9.
8. Kulthanan K, Tuchinda P, Nitiyarom R, Chunharas A, Chantaphakul H, Aunhachoke K, et al. Clinical practice guidelines for the diagnosis and management of atopic dermatitis. Asian Pac J Allergy Immunol. 2021;39:145–55.
9. Blume-Peytavi U, Metz M. Atopic dermatitis in children: management of pruritus. J Eur Acad Dermatol Venereol. 2012;26(Suppl 6):2–8.
10. Ramirez FD, Chen S, Langan SM, Prather AA, McCulloch CE, Kidd SA, et al. Association of atopic dermatitis with sleep quality in children. JAMA Pediatr. 2019;173:e190025.
11. Djurović MR,Janković J, Ćirković A, Spirić VT, Maksimović N, Timotijević ZS, et al. Quality of life in infants with atopic dermatitis and their families. Postepy Dermatol Alergol. 2020;37:66–72.
12. Williams HC, Chalmers J. Prevention of atopic dermatitis. Acta Derm Venereol. 2020;100:5771.
13. Caffarelli C, Giannetti A, Giannì G, Ricci G. Anti-inflammatory and biologic drugs for atopic dermatitis: a therapeutic approach in children and adolescents. Front Med (Lausanne). 2023;10:1214963.
14. Khan A, Adalsteinsson J, Whitaker-Worth DL. Atopic dermatitis and nutrition. Clin Dermatol. 2022;40:135–44.
15. Domínguez O, Plaza AM, Alvaro M. Relationship between atopic dermatitis and food allergy. Curr Pediatr Rev. 2020;16:115–22.
16. Bettcher CM, Rockwell PG, Ravikumar R. Managing food allergy in children: an evidence-based update. J Fam Pract. 2020;69:336;338.
17. Tedner SG, Asarnoj A, Thulin H, Westman M, Konradsen JR, Nilsson C. Food allergy and hypersensitivity reactions in children and adults—a review. J Intern Med. 2022;29:283–302.
18. Mendonca CE, Andreae DA. Food allergy. Prim Care. 2023;50:205–20.
19. Poowuttikul P, Seth D. Anaphylaxis in children and adolescents. Immunol Allergy Clin N Am. 2021;41:627–38.
20. Skypala IJ, McKenzie R. Nutritional issues in food allergy. Clin Rev Allergy Immunol. 2029;57:166–78.
21. Hui JW, Copeland M, Lanser BJ. Food allergy management at school in the era of immunotherapy. Curr Allergy Asthma Rep. 2020;20:32.
22. Regulation (EU) No 1169/2011 of the European Parliament and of the Council of 25 October 2011 on the provision of food information to consumers, amending Regulations (EC) No 1924/2006 and (EC) No 1925/2006 of the European Parliament and of the Council, and repealing Commission Directive 87/250/EEC, Council Directive 90/496/EEC, Commission Directive 1999/10/EC, Directive 2000/13/EC of the European Parliament and of the Council, Commission Directives 2002/67/EC and 2008/5/EC and Commission Regulation (EC) No 608/2004 (OJ L 304, 22.11.2011, p. 18).
23. Carter CA, Pistiner M, Wang J, Sharma HP. Food allergy in restaurants work group report. J Allergy Clin Immunol Pract. 2018;8:70–4.
24. Chafei H, El Harake MD, Toufeili I, Kharroubi SA. Knowledge, attitudes, and practices of consumers on food allergy and food allergen labeling: a case of Lebanon. Foods. 2023;12:933.
25. Zuberbier T, Dörr T, Aberer W, Alvaro M, Angier E, Arasi S, et al. Proposal of 0.5 mg of protein/100 g of processed food as threshold for voluntary declaration of food allergen traces in processed food—a first step in an initiative to better inform patients and avoid fatal allergic reactions: a GA^{2}LEN position paper. Allergy. 2022;77:1736–50.
26. Reddel HK, Bacharier LB, Bateman ED, Brightling CE, Brusselle GG, Buhl R, et al. Global Initiative for Asthma Strategy 2021: executive summary and rationale for key changes. Am J Respir Crit Care Med. 2022;205:17–35.
27. Morice AH, Millqvist E, Bieksiene K, Birring SS, Dicpinigaitis P, Domingo Ribas C, et al. ERS guidelines on the diagnosis and treatment of chronic cough in adults and children. Eur Respir J. 2020;55:1901136.
28. Bellin MH, Land C, Newsome A, Kub J, Mudd SS, Bollinger ME, et al. Caregiver perception of asthma management of children in the context of poverty. J Asthma. 2017;54:162–72.
29. Nish WA, Schwietz LA. Underdiagnosis of asthma in young adults presenting for USAF basic training. Ann Allergy. 1992;69:239–42.
30. Cloutier MM, Dixon AE, Krishnan JA, Lemanske RF Jr, Pace W, Schatz M. Managing asthma in adolescents and adults: 2020 asthma guideline update from the National Asthma Education and Prevention Program. JAMA. 2020;324:2301–17.
31. Schuler CF IV, Montejo JM. Allergic rhinitis in children and adolescents. Immunol Allergy Clin North Am. 2019;41:613–25.
32. D'Elia C, Gozal D, Bruni O, Goudouris E, Meira E, Cruz M. Allergic rhinitis and sleep disorders in children—coexistence and reciprocal interactions. J Pediatr. 2022;98:444–54.
33. Miraglia Del Giudice M, Marseglia A, Leonardi S, La Rosa M, Salpietro C, Brunese FP, et al. Allergic rhinitis and quality of life in children. Int J Immunopathol Pharmacol. 2011;24:25–8.

34. Dierick BJH, van der Molen T, Flokstra-de Blok BMJ, Muraro A, Postma MJ, Kocks JWH, et al. Burden and socioeconomics of asthma, allergic rhinitis, atopic dermatitis and food allergy. Expert Rev Pharmacoecon Outcomes Res. 2020;20:437–53.
35. Eisner MD, Klein J, Hammond SK, Koren G, Lactao G, Iribarren C. Directly measured second hand smoke exposure and asthma health outcomes. Thorax. 2005;60:814–21.
36. Di Cicco M, Sepich M, Beni A, Comberiati P, Peroni DG. How E-cigarettes and vaping can affect asthma in children and adolescents. Curr Opin Allergy Clin Immunol. 2022;22:86–94.
37. Allen Merritt T, Mazela J, Adamczak A, Merritt T. The impact of second-hand tobacco smoke exposure on pregnancy outcomes, infant health, and the threat of third-hand smoke exposure to our environment and to our children. Przegl Lek. 2012;69:717–20.
38. Morou Z, Tatsioni A, Dimoliatis ID, Papadopoulos NG. Health-related quality of life in children with food allergy and their parents: a systematic review of the literature. J Investig Allergol Clin Immunol. 2014;24:382–95.
39. Wu WC, Chang HY, Kuo KN, Chen CY, Tu YC, Yang YH. Psychosocial problems in children with allergic diseases: a population study in Taiwan. Child Care Health Dev. 2011;37:662–70.

29 Allergy Prevention

Alessandra Carmignani, Alice Bedini,
Diego Peroni, and Pasquale Comberiati

Abstract

Atopic diseases have become a public health concern in the last few decades. The recent increase in the prevalence of atopic diseases comes with high socioeconomic costs and underlines the need for effective prevention. Prevention can be directed to reduce the incidence of allergic diseases, in "high-risk" patients, as well as reducing the severity and impact on the quality of life of allergic patients.

The occurrence of atopic diseases depends on a complex interplay between genetic predisposition, environmental and allergen exposures, microbial imbalance, and immune dysfunction. Current preventive strategies for atopic diseases in children target mainly environmental and allergen exposures, both in pregnant women and in children during early infancy. Over the last decade, there has been an increasing interest in microbiome composition, development, and modulation as a possible preventive strategy for immune-mediated diseases such as allergic diseases.

This chapter focuses on available high-quality evidence on the role of prenatal and perinatal interventions for the prevention of allergic diseases in children and addresses the current preventive strategies recommended by international guidelines as well as unmet areas for future research.

Keywords

Allergy prevention · Allergen exposure · Genetic predisposition · Environmental exposures · Skin barrier dysfunction · Microbial diversity

Test your learning and check your understanding of this book's contents: use the "Springer Nature Flashcards" app to access questions using ▶ https://sn.pub/nspbjm. To use the app, please follow the instructions in Chap. 1.

Alessandra Carmignani and Alice Bedini contributed equally with all other contributors.

A. Carmignani · A. Bedini · D. Peroni (✉)
P. Comberiati (✉)
Department of Clinical and Experimental Medicine, Section of Paediatrics, University of Pisa, Pisa, Italy
e-mail: diego.peroni@unipi.it; pasquale.comberiati@unipi.it

C. Caffarelli, G. L. Marseglia (eds.), *Textbook of Pediatric Allergy*,
https://doi.org/10.1007/978-3-031-71283-8_29

Key Points

- There is no evidence to support the restriction of allergenic foods during pregnancy or breastfeeding to prevent allergies in the offspring.
- There is no recommendation for or against using breastfeeding to prevent food allergy in infants and young children, but breastfeeding has many benefits for infants and mothers and should be encouraged wherever possible.
- Do not routinely prescribe or recommend the use of any milk formula for the specific prevention of allergic diseases.
- The best timing for introducing allergenic food for the prevention of food allergy is still debated, besides the introduction of peanuts between 4 and 11 months in infants living in areas with a high prevalence of peanut allergy and at high risk for peanut allergy and cooked egg between 6 and 8 months.
- Current guidelines do not recommend the use of probiotics or vitamins for allergy prevention.

29.1 Introduction

Atopic diseases represent an increasing health problem in developed countries, affecting up to 20% of the population. The most frequent atopic disorders include atopic dermatitis (AD), asthma, allergic rhinoconjunctivitis, food allergy, venom allergy, drug allergy, and eosinophilic esophagitis [1]. The development and phenotypic expression of atopic diseases depend on a complex interplay between genetic predisposition, environmental and allergen exposures, microbial imbalance, and immune dysfunction (Fig. 29.1).

The increase in atopic diseases has been recognized as a modern pandemic. The burden they give rise to, healthcare needs, disability, and costs, have cumulated in the highly urbanized countries, thus emphasizing the need for effective allergy prevention [2].

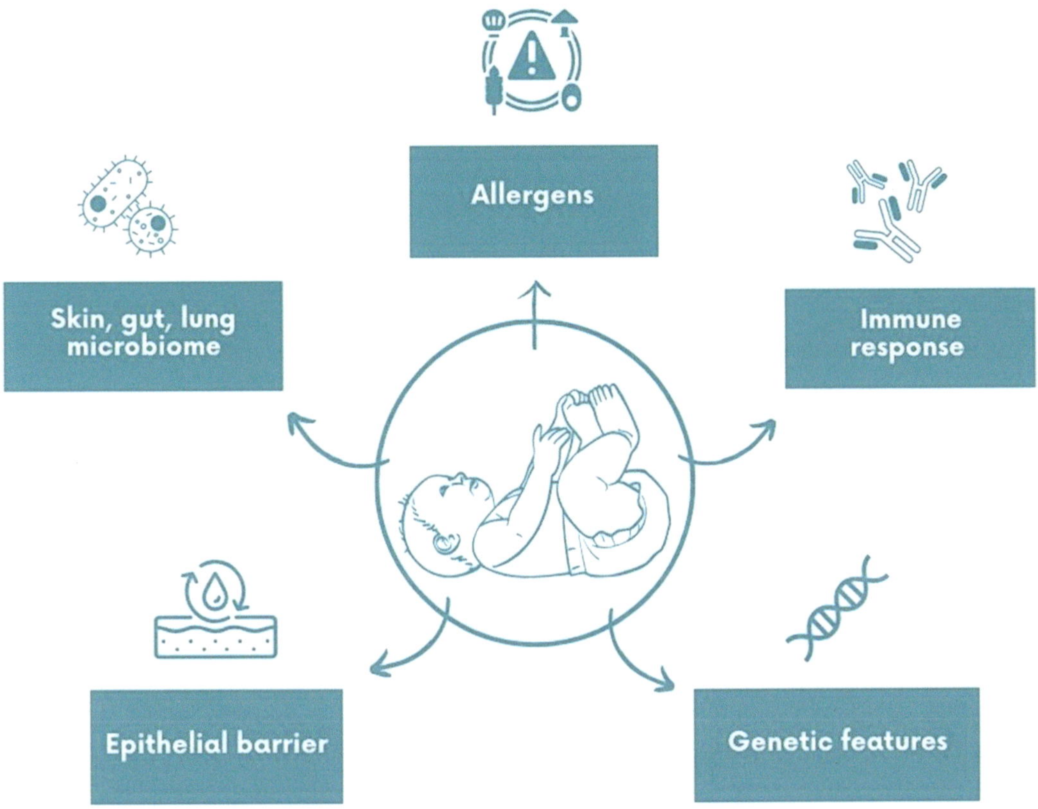

Fig. 29.1 Predisposing factors for the development of atopic diseases

29.2 Prevention of Allergic Diseases

Overall, the aims of allergy prevention include:

- Reducing the incidence of allergic diseases.
- Reducing the risk of the development of new atopic manifestations in allergic patients.
- Reducing the severity of the disease and the proportion of patients with severe symptoms.
- Increasing the possibility of remission.
- Increasing the quality of life in the patients.

Prevention may consist of a variety of prophylactic measures. There are three levels of allergy prevention in children [3]:

- *Primary prevention* aims to prevent allergic sensitization and the development of allergic diseases. It also includes any prophylactic measure undertaken by pregnant mothers.
- *Secondary prevention*: addresses children who already developed an allergic disease and, aims to reduce the development of additional diseases and prevent symptoms.
- *Tertiary prevention*: addresses patients with chronic diseases, reducing symptoms after disease expression and preventing further progression and deterioration.

29.3 Maternal Avoidance Diet During Pregnancy and Lactation

The available studies suggest that maternal avoidance of allergenic foods during pregnancy and lactation does not reduce the risk of allergic disease in the offspring, regardless of whether the infant is high-risk or not.

Specifically, the definition of "high-risk" infant as regards developing allergic diseases is given based upon a consensus among several committees representing the American Academy of Pediatrics (AAP), the joint guidelines of the European Society for Pediatric Allergology and Clinical Immunology (ESPACI), and the European Society for Pediatric Gastroenterology, Hepatology, and Nutrition (ESPGHAN) [4, 5], and is defined by the presence of at least one first-degree relative with a documented atopic condition, including AD, asthma, allergic rhinitis (AR), or food allergy [6].

The AAP, ESPACI, ESPGHAN, and EAACI guidelines on the prevention of food allergies advise against maternal dietary restrictions (i.e., avoidance of potent food allergens) during pregnancy or breastfeeding for allergy prevention in infants (Table 29.1) [5, 7, 10].

Also, current evidence does not provide enough support for prescribing specific recommendations regarding the targeted consumption of particular foods. However, all guidelines emphasize the importance of following a healthy, diverse, and well-balanced diet during pregnancy. This includes the incorporation of vegetables, milk, dairy products (such as yogurt), fruits, nuts, eggs, and fish [9].

Emerging studies indicate that the quality and diversity of maternal diets can impact allergy outcomes in infants. In this regard, clinical predictive scores, such as the Maternal allergy-preventive Diet Index (MDI), have been developed. The MDI index evaluates the intake of diverse food items, including vegetables, yogurt, fried potatoes, rice/grains, red meats, 100% fruit juice, and cold cereals, assigning them different weights [11]. The study assessing the clinical usefulness of the MDI index, which evaluated the development of allergic diseases in offspring at the age of 4, revealed that consumption of vegetables and yogurt was associated with a decreased likelihood of offspring developing

Table 29.1 Comparison of the latest international guidelines on allergy prevention strategies

	EAACI Guidelines [7]	AAAAI/ACAAI/CSACI Consensus Statement [8]	S3 German Guidelines [9]
Maternal nutrition during pregnancy and breastfeeding	There is no evidence to support the restriction of allergenic foods during pregnancy or breastfeeding to prevent allergies in the offspring Pregnant women should follow a balanced and healthy diet	Not recommend maternal exclusion of common allergens during pregnancy and lactation as a means to prevent food allergy Not recommend any particular food or supplementation in the maternal diet	Avoidance of potent food allergens during pregnancy or lactation should NOT be made for the purpose of allergy prevention
Breastfeeding	There is no recommendation for or against using breastfeeding to prevent food allergy in infants and young children, but breastfeeding has many benefits for infants and mothers and should be encouraged wherever possible	Exclusive breastfeeding is universally recommended for all mothers, but there is no specific association between exclusive breastfeeding and the primary prevention of any specific food allergy	Exclusive breastfeeding should be recommended for the first 4–6 months of life if possible For mothers wishing to breastfeed, additional feeding of cow's milk-based formula during the first days of life should be avoided

(continued)

Table 29.1 (continued)

	EAACI Guidelines [7]	AAAAI/ACAAI/CSACI Consensus Statement [8]	S3 German Guidelines [9]
Human milk substitutes	The EAACI Task Force suggests avoiding supplementing with cow's milk formula in breastfed infants in the first week of life to prevent cow's milk allergy in infants and young children The EAACI Task Force suggests against introducing soy protein-based formula in the first 6 months of life to prevent cow's milk allergy in infants and young children For infants who need a breastmilk substitute, there is no recommendation for or against the use of regular cow's milk-based infant formula after the first week of life to prevent food allergy. There is no recommendation for or against using partially or extensively hydrolyzed formula to prevent food allergy in infants and young children	Do not routinely prescribe or recommend the use of any HFs for the specific prevention of food allergy or development of food sensitization	Soy-based baby foods should NOT be given for the purpose of allergy prevention Other animal milk including goat milk (not even as a basis for baby food), sheep, or horse milk should NOT be given for the purpose of allergy prevention Cereal drinks should NOT be given for the purpose of allergy prevention
Complementary feeding	Introduce well-cooked hen's egg, but not raw egg or uncooked pasteurized egg, into the infant diet as part of complementary feeding to prevent egg allergy in infants In populations where there is a high prevalence of peanut allergy, introduce peanuts into the infant diet in an age-appropriate form as part of complementary feeding to prevent peanut allergy in infants and young children. Peanut should not be the first solid to be introduced into the infant diet	Introduce egg or egg-containing products to all infants, irrespective of their relative risk of developing peanut allergy, starting around 6 months of life, though not before 4 months of life Introduce peanut-containing products to all infant, irrespective of their relative risk of developing peanut allergy, starting around 6 months of life, though not before 4 months of life Do not deliberately delay the introduction of other potentially allergenic complementary foods, once the introduction of complementary foods has commenced	The introduction of complementary food should start from the beginning of the 5th (at the earliest) to the beginning of the seventh month of life (at the latest) according to the willingness of the infants Dietary restriction should NOT be made because there is NO proof of preventive effect of dietary restriction by avoiding potent food allergens in the first year of life Heated-through but not raw chicken eggs or scrambled eggs should be added to complementary food and given regularly to prevent chicken egg allergy Introduction and regular consumption of peanut products can be considered in an age-appropriate format (i.e., peanut butter) when complementary feeding is started for preventing peanut allergy in infants with atopic dermatitis in families with regular peanut consumption

(continued)

Table 29.1 (continued)

	EAACI Guidelines [7]	AAAAI/ACAAI/CSACI Consensus Statement [8]	S3 German Guidelines [9]
Probiotics	There is no evidence to recommend that breastfeeding women should modify their diet or take any supplements such as probiotics to prevent food allergy in their children Probiotic supplements have been tested during infancy, but there is little evidence to support their effectiveness. Different microorganisms have been used in different studies, and it appears that different microbial strains may have different effects, which may explain the inconsistent results as regards a possible preventive effect of specific strains of probiotics	There is no conclusive evidence that the specific exclusion of particular foods, inclusion/dietary enrichment of certain foods, or the specific use of supplements or probiotics in the diets of breastfeeding mothers is associated with the development or prevention of food allergy in either at-risk or not at-risk children	Prebiotics and/or probiotics should not be given to pregnant women or infants for allergy prevention, not even as part of infant formula

allergic rhinitis, AD, asthma, and wheezing; however, there was no significant association between the mother's diet and food allergies in the offspring. On the other hand, a greater consumption of red meat, fried potatoes, rice/grains, cold cereals, and 100% fruit juice was linked to an increased risk of allergic diseases [11].

29.4 Breastfeeding

The practice of breastfeeding, while lacking any conclusive evidence as a preventive strategy for allergic diseases, has many benefits for mother and child, even for partially breastfed infants, and should be encouraged whenever possible [12–14]. Human milk meets all of the nutritional requirements needs of infants up to 6 months of age and is recommended by WHO [15].

Properties of substances found in human breast milk include immunological, anti-inflammatory, and tolerance-promoting activities and roles as agonists and antagonists of the innate immune responses. For these reasons, breast milk should be ideal for reducing the risk of allergic diseases. However, existing data on this issue are inconsistent [16], possibly due to several factors, which include the ethical inability to randomize subjects to breastfeeding or formula feeding [3]; the poor comparability between existing studies due to different designs, definitions of breastfeeding, and endpoint parameters; and potential confounding factors, such as parental smoking habits, age, level of education, socio-economic status, and introduction of complementary food, which may unrelatedly vary between exclusive breastfeeding and formula feeding [17, 18].

Most current studies show no indication of protective effects of breast milk against allergy development [19–24].

The association between breastfeeding and AD has been widely investigated; however, there is limited evidence to support the idea that exclusive breastfeeding for at least 3–4 months reduces the incidence of AD in both low- and high-risk infants.

Breastfeeding has been found to be associated with a reduced occurrence of recurrent wheezing in the first 2 years of life, potentially by decreasing the occurrence of symptomatic upper respiratory infections (URIs) [25–27]. URIs are a major cause of wheezing in infants and young children. However, the relationship between breastfeeding and the development of allergy-related wheezing or asthma in later childhood is not yet clear. Nevertheless, the advantages of breastfeeding for the overall health of the child outweigh any potential disadvantages, regardless of whether the mother or child has atopic conditions.

The effect of breastfeeding on the development of allergic rhinitis is still a topic of debate among researchers, as there is no evidence of a protective effect in AR prevention.

Likewise, investigations on the impact of breastfeeding on food allergy prevention have failed to produce conclusive evidence so far.

Despite these data, breastfeeding should be widely advocated for all infants due to its acknowledged advantages in terms of nutrition, gastrointestinal functionality, immediate defense against infectious diseases, as well as psychological well-being [5, 12–14]. Infants should be breastfed exclusively for the first 4–6 months, if possible, and breastfeeding should also be continued when complementary foods are introduced (Table 29.1).

29.5 Infant Milk Formulas

When breastfeeding is either not possible or insufficient to cover all the nutritional needs, infant milk formula should be administered at least until weaning is started and well tolerated. Cow's milk-derived infant formulas are preferred to standard cow's milk during the first year of life, due to their nutritional value and ease of digestion [20]. The use of hypoallergenic cow's milk formulas, such as partial and extensive hydrolysate milk formulas, in infancy has been investigated for the primary prevention of AD, food allergy, and respiratory allergies with conflicting results.

The latest EAACI guidelines of food allergy prevention, updated in 2020, suggest avoiding supplementation with regular cow's milk formulas in breastfed infants in the first week of life, to prevent the onset of cow's milk allergy (CMPA) in infants and young children [27]. This recommendation, however, has low certainty of evidence, because it is based on a single study [28] which reported a reduced risk of CMPA in Japanese infants who did not receive supplementation with infant formula in the first 3 days of life.

For infants who need a breast milk substitute, there is no recommendation for or against the use of regular cow's milk formula after the first week of life to prevent food allergy. In addition, there is no consistent evidence that hydrolyzed formulas reduce the risk of food allergy [27] and consequently, there is no recommendation for or against using a partially or extensively hydrolyzed formula to prevent CMPA in infants.

In addition, a recent systematic review concluded that there was insufficient evidence to support an association between cow's milk formula supplementation and the development of asthma and allergic rhinitis [29].

With regard to soy protein formula, another breast milk substitute for infants, the EAACI guidelines suggest against its introduction in the first 6 months of life to prevent CMPA in infants and young children [27]. Similarly, the allergy prevention guidelines published in 2021 defined that the use of soy-based infant formula cannot be recommended for allergy prevention [30]. Moreover, there are health concerns related to soy-based infant formula (high content of phytochemicals with a weak estrogenic effect and phytates, with possible disadvantages for nutrient absorption) [31, 32] which, however, are controversially discussed [33, 34].

In 2021, a collaborative consensus report involving the American Academy of Allergy, Asthma, and Immunology (AAAAI), the American College of Allergy, Asthma, and Immunology (ACAAI), and the Canadian Society for Allergy and Clinical Immunology (CSACI) determined that the utilization of a hydrolyzed milk formula does not provide any protective advantage in preventing food allergies or food sensitization [8] (Table 29.1).

29.6 Complementary Feeding: Weaning

Up to early 2000, the most endorsed recommendation on food allergy prevention was to delay the introduction of some allergenic foods in infants, especially those with a family history of atopy, after the first year of life. Such indication was mainly based on the theory that structural and functional immaturity of the guts, and consequent increased permeability, could lead to an increased risk of allergic sensitization [35].

However, following studies on animal models, have suggested that early exposure to such food allergens might be critical to achieve food tolerance, which is an antigen-driven process [36]. These data and subsequent epidemiological and clinical studies have shown that delaying the introduction of allergenic foods after the first year of life is not an effective strategy to prevent food allergy but could eventually increase its risk [35].

Current evidence suggests that the critical window for food tolerance is between 4 and 6 months, although the best timing for weaning for the prevention of food allergy is still debated [37]. The American and European allergy guidelines recommend not delaying the start of complementary feeding after 4–6 months of age in all infants, including the most common food allergens in children, preferably whilst breastfeeding [5, 38–40] (Table 29.1). However, the optimal timing of introducing allergenic solids for food allergy prevention is still debated. At present, there is no convincing evidence that early introduction of potentially allergenic foods can prevent food allergy to the same food, besides the introduction of peanuts between 4 and 11 months in infants living in areas with a high prevalence of peanut allergy and at high risk for peanut allergy (i.e., moderate-severe eczema and/or egg allergy) and cooked egg between 6 and 8 months [41–45].

Regarding the prevention of food allergy, based on a systematic review of the literature [41], the latest EAACI guidelines suggest introducing hen's eggs in a sufficiently heated form (e.g., hard-boiled) into the infant diet as part of complementary feeding to prevent egg allergy in infants. Once successfully introduced, hen's eggs should be given regularly twice a week in a sufficiently well-cooked form. Since the introduction of unheated or insufficiently heated eggs was not associated with any benefit, instead increasing by any chance risks of severe allergic reactions, the administration of raw (not fully heated) hen's eggs is not recommended for the prevention of egg allergy [27].

Concerning peanut allergy, EAACI guidelines support the introduction of peanut into the infant diet in populations with a high prevalence of peanut allergy, in an age-appropriate form, to avoid any risk of choking or inhalation, as part of complementary feeding [29, 46]. It appears that the most effective age to introduce is from 4 to 6 months of life. The evidence of benefit relates mainly to those at very increased risk, but this could be encouraged in those at general risk in populations with a high prevalence of peanut allergy [29].

Previous observational studies have also investigated the effect of the timing of fish introduction on the risk of allergic diseases [47, 48]. A recent systematic review provided limited evidence to suggest that the introduction of fish between 3 and 8 months of life may lower the risk of AD [29].

However, there currently is not sufficient evidence of a link between fish consumption and food allergy, asthma, or allergic rhinitis [49].

29.7 Overweight and Obesity

Obesity and overweight have been associated with an increased risk of asthma in children as well as adults. Prospective cohort studies show that overweight and obesity or a BMI ≥ 30 kg/m^2 before or at the beginning of pregnancy are positively associated with wheezing and/or asthma in the child [50, 51].

Several possible mechanisms have been postulated to explain the obesity–asthma relationship. Mediators or influencing factors under discussion for these associations include genetic factors and inflammatory molecules, like leptin, TNFalfa, IL-6, and TGFbeta1, highly expressed in obese individuals.

These molecules contribute to systemic inflammation and have direct effects on the airway, potentially leading to inflammation and asthma. The pro-inflammatory state of obese adipose tissue could directly impact airway inflammation and asthma development.

The relationship between BMI and asthma may differ based on gender. A meta-analysis suggested that overweight boys had a higher risk of asthma overall [52].

Further research is needed to fully elucidate the mechanisms underlying the relationship between high BMI and lung health and to investigate the potential gender differences in the relationship between obesity and asthma.

Therefore, promoting normal weight development in children is not only crucial for allergy prevention but also for their overall health and well-being.

29.8 Environmental Exposures

Interaction between environmental exposures in early life may add complexity to the risk of asthma and allergic disease. There is evidence to suggest that gene-environment interactions play a significant role in the development of these conditions. Prevention efforts should focus on reducing or eliminating exposure to known environmental allergens and irritants [53]. This includes measures such as reducing exposure to indoor and outdoor air pollution, tobacco smoke, and allergens such as dust mites.

The immune deviation has an important genetic component, even if the recent increase in food allergy and AD suggests that is mainly due to changes in epigenome driven by environmental exposure.

The complex interplay of environmental and genetic factors in the development of asthma and allergic disease highlights the need for a multifaceted approach to prevention and treatment [54]. Studies on farming families and religious traditional communities (Amish, Hutterites) suggest that early microbial exposure is important as a modulator of the development of childhood asthma and allergies [55]. Microbial exposure and its diversity depend on the environment and living habits. Urban soil materials have poorer microbial communities compared to rural ones. In urban environments where microbial diversity is lower, individuals may experience a less diverse and less robust immune response. The exposure to a diverse range of microorganisms helps to train the immune system and promote immune tolerance. Children living on farms are exposed to a wider range of microbes as compared to their rural peers [54, 55].

Environmental microbiota can be transferred to the mucosa of the upper airways, where they may interact with the local mucosa-associated immune system. Exploration of the world of microbiomes has revitalized the debates around the "hygiene hypothesis" and early priming of immune regulation, not only for atopy and allergy [54].

So far, not one single component conferring protection has been identified, and it seems quite possible that several factors with a multitude of exposure routes might be relevant and that asthma preventive approaches will focus on more than one facet.

Modifiable risk factors urgently require interventions to prevent increasing allergy rates in countries undergoing rapid urbanization. Exposure to beneficial environmental microbiota can be improved by increasing vegetation and reducing pollution.

29.9 Smoking

There is plenty of evidence that smoking increases the infant's chances of developing respiratory illness. Secondhand smoke exposure has also been known to cause worsening of childhood asthma with an impact on hospital admissions. The correlation between maternal secondhand smoke exposure during pregnancy and the development of childhood asthma has also been investigated [56]. Since smoking during and after pregnancy has demonstrated effects on disease progression in infants, mothers must be counseled appropriately to prevent respiratory pathology in their offspring. Since secondhand smoke has a role to play in this disease process, efforts to counsel the whole family against smoking to prevent diseases like asthma must be undertaken. This can prevent the disease process from developing, as well as control progression if an initial insult has already occurred.

The diseases are likely to be related to changes in lifestyle, environment, or both, including reduced microbial diversity, increased use of xenobiotics in industrial and consumer products, exposure to tobacco or nicotinic products, and variations in diets and nutritional elements.

29.10 Microbiota

The significant increase in the prevalence of allergic diseases reported over the last few years has closely paralleled substantial environmental changes both on a macro and microscale, which have led to reduced microbial exposure in early life and perturbation of the human microbiome composition. Increasing evidence shows that early life interactions between the human microbiome and the immune cells play a pivotal role in the development of the immune system. Therefore, the process of early colonization by a "healthy" microbiome is emerging as a key determinant of life-long health. In stark contrast, the perturbation of such a process, which results in changes in the host-microbiome biodiversity and metabolic activities, has been associated with greater susceptibility to immune-mediated disorders later in life, including allergic diseases [57]. So far, however, most studies on microbiota and allergic diseases are mainly observational assessing associations rather than causality.

Perinatal events, including cesarean section, season of birth, use of antibiotics, and neonatal jaundice, have been associated with the risk of developing allergic diseases [57]. As antibiotics are frequently prescribed during the neonatal period among preterm infants, an antibiotic-induced delay in intestinal bacterial colonization may increase the risk of developing allergic disorders. A relationship between the autumn-winter season of birth and the early onset of food allergy has been reported by a multicenter cross-sectional study [57]. Regarding food allergy, gut microbiota composition and an elevated *Enterobacteriaceae/Bacteroidaceae* ratio in early infancy were associated with food sensitization at 1 year of age. Correspondingly, food-sensitized children exhibited lower diversity of both, total microbiota and bacterial phylum *Bacteroidetes*, with an increased number of *Firmicutes* compared with healthy children. Alterations in bacterial taxa seem to be associated with a particular type of food allergy. Infants with CMPA have higher anaerobic bacteria, *Ruminococcaceae*, and *Lachnospiraceae*, and those allergic to peanuts have higher Bacteroides [58]. Loss of microbial diversity, with the predominance of *Staphylococcus aureus* over *Staphylococcus epidermidis*, is a characteristic feature at both acute and chronic skin sites of AD [59].

Patients with AD have lower concentrations of *Bifidobacterium* in the gut microbiome than healthy controls, and these counts are inversely related to the severity of the disease [60].

The prevention of allergic diseases is exploring possible strategies for correcting dysbiosis and enhancing exposure to beneficial microbes. From this perspective, probiotics, acting as promoters of an adequate balance in the gut microbiota, have been suggested as an intervention to prevent allergic diseases [61].

Although some studies have reported benefits in the treatment and prevention of atopic eczema, none has had any clear effects on the development of Th2-mediated allergic responses.

Current guidelines from prominent medical societies including the American Academy of Pediatrics, the European Academy of Allergy and Clinical Immunology, the National Institute of Allergy and Infectious Disease, and the European Society for Pediatric Gastroenterology, Hepatology, and Nutrition do not recommend the use of probiotics for primary prevention of allergic disease (Table 29.1). The World Allergy Organization (WAO) does not support the use of probiotics for primary prevention of allergic disease but does favor probiotic supplementation in pregnant/lactating women and infants with a family history of allergic disease [62–64].

The EAACI Food Allergy and Anaphylaxis Guidelines state that there is no evidence to recommend that breastfeeding women should modify their diet or take any supplements such as probiotics to prevent food allergy in their children [65].

29.11 Vitamin D and Other Vitamins

Environmental factors, including early neonatal nutrition, may have an important influence on allergy development and, thus, present an opportunity to prevent or delay the onset of allergies. Vitamin D may be an important environmental factor [66].

Vitamin D is crucial for bone metabolism, but it also has extraskeletal functions. Vitamin D has immunomodulatory effects and its receptor is expressed in a variety of immune cells, including B cells, T cells, dendritic cells, and macrophages. Several studies have documented a correlation between deficiencies in circulating vitamin D (25OHD) levels in early life and respiratory infections and wheezing in early childhood [67, 68]. Respiratory infections in the first years of life have been associated with an increased risk of allergic asthma in young children. Other studies have also found that lower 25OHD levels are associated with poor asthma control, lower lung function, the presence of exercise-induced bronchoconstriction in asthmatic children, and the severity of atopic dermatitis [69, 70]. Vitamin D Deficiency has been also suggested to impair epithelial barrier integrity, which in turn might lead to increased and inappropriate mucosal exposure to food antigens and increase the risk of food allergy.

The role of vitamin D in the prevention of allergic diseases has been largely investigated. However, despite a correlation between vitamin D deficiency and the risk of allergy, the supplementation of vitamin D, both in pregnant women and in their offspring, hasn't shown a preventive effect on allergic diseases [70, 71].

Few studies examine the impact of vitamin supplementation (vitamins A, E, C, and folic acid) during pregnancy or in infancy on the risk of developing an atopic disease. The available study data do not provide sufficient proof that supplementation of these vitamins is associated with the development of atopic diseases [72]. These vitamins should not be supplemented with the aim of allergy prevention [9].

29.12 Skin Barrier Dysfunction

The first manifestation of atopy is often atopic dermatitis (AD) in early infancy. In those patients following the so-called "atopic march," AD is followed by food allergy in the first year of life and asthma and allergic rhinitis in childhood or school age [73]. Very recently the impairment of the skin barrier early in life has been recognized as a crucial factor in the development of AD and the risk for allergic sensitization, suggesting that primary allergy prevention should start early and target barrier enhancement and the alimentary tract [73].

There are several factors that contribute to the skin barrier dysfunction. These include alterations in the lipid composition of the skin, changes in the expression of structural proteins such as filaggrin and involucrin, and disturbances in the microbial flora of the skin. Loss-of-function filaggrin (*FLG*) gene mutations are the strongest known genetic risk factor for AD [74]. In addition, there is evidence to suggest that defects in the immune system may also contribute to skin barrier dysfunction in AD. Specifically, there is an imbalance between Th2 and Th1 immune responses, with a predominance of Th2 cytokines such as IL-4 and IL-13 in AD skin lesions [75]. These cytokines inhibit the expression of filaggrin and other key structural proteins, compromising the skin barrier function. During the effector phase, activated mast cells and basophils release histamine, leukotrienes, and prostaglandins, which mediate the classic immediate-type allergic responses, including itching, sneezing, rhinorrhea, wheezing, dyspnea, and urticaria. The effector phase also involves the activation of Th2 cells, which secrete interleukin (IL)-4, IL-5, and IL-13, which promote B cell activation, IgE production, eosinophilic inflammation, and airway hyperresponsiveness.

Overall, the interplay between skin barrier dysfunction and immune dysregulation in AD leads to increased susceptibility to allergen penetration and subsequent sensitization, which may contribute to the development of allergic diseases such as food allergy and asthma.

Understanding these underlying mechanisms is important for the development of effective therapies to prevent or treat allergic diseases. The finding that cutaneous barrier dysfunction occurs in the nonlesional skin of children with AD, food allergy, and possibly childhood asthma, has important clinical implications. It suggests the need to institute early skincare even before the onset of clinical eczema and the potential importance of doing total body skin care beyond the inflammatory skin rash observed in AD [76]. These observations are further corroborated by a later study showing that increased forehead TEWL measurements at 1 week of age predict AD development and are associated with increased allergen sensitization [77]. All these results and the difficulties with systemic immune interventions put forward the potential for early interventional approaches targeting skin repair. Therefore, it has been proposed that intensive emollient use in early life, could prevent AD, especially in high-risk infants. Two prospective small studies have suggested that full-body application of moisturizers for 6–8 months, beginning within the first few weeks of life in high-risk infants, reduced the cumulative incidence of AD in a British/US cohort (relative risk, 50%) and a Japanese cohort (relative risk, 25%) [78, 79]. Another recently published cohort study showed a trend toward reduced incidence of AD and food sensitization at age 12 months, suggesting that the potential beneficial effects persisted for at least 6 months after stopping emollient treatment [80]. However, subsequent big clinical trials on skin care interventions have shown that emollients during the first year of life in healthy infants are probably not effective for preventing AD [81, 82]. There are trials underway on early skin care using emollients and prevention of food allergy [83].

Take-Home Messages

- Allergic diseases have been a public health issue in recent decades. Such diseases are highly prevalent among children and adults, especially in urbanized societies, and pose a significant socioeconomic burden for healthcare systems. The development of allergic diseases is a complex and dynamic process involving the interaction between genes, environment, allergen exposures, microbial imbalance, and immune dysregulation. Therefore, the prevention of allergic diseases is still challenging. Current preventive strategies for atopic diseases in children mainly focus on nutritional interventions, both in pregnant women and in children during early infancy, but the evidence is often limited. Targeting the exposome and the microbiome could be a future game changer in identifying infants at risk for developing atopic diseases and the critical window of opportunity for early preventive intervention.

References

1. Pawankar R, Canonica GW, Holgate ST, Lockey RF, Blaiss M. The WAO white book on allergy update. WAO; 2013.
2. Eichenfield LF, Hanifin JM, Beck LA, Lemanske RF Jr, Sampson HA, Weiss ST, et al. Atopic dermatitis and asthma: parallels in the evolution of treatment. Pediatrics. 2003;111:608.
3. Zeiger RS. Food allergen avoidance in the prevention of food allergy in infants and children. Pediatrics. 2003;111:1662.
4. Agostoni C, Decsi T, Fewtrell M, Goulet O, Kolacek S, Koletzko B, et al. Complementary feeding: a commentary by the ESPGHAN Committee on Nutrition. J Pediatr Gastroenterol Nutr. 2008;46:99.

5. Greer FR, Sicherer SH, Burks AW, COMMITTEE ON NUTRITION; SECTION ON ALLERGY AND IMMUNOLOGY. The effects of early nutritional interventions on the development of atopic disease in infants and children: the role of maternal dietary restriction, breastfeeding, hydrolyzed formulas, and timing of introduction of allergenic complementary foods. Pediatrics. 2019;143:e20190281.
6. Sicherer SH, Burks AW. Maternal and infant diets for prevention of allergic diseases: understanding menu changes in 2008. J Allergy Clin Immunol. 2008;122(1):29.
7. Halken S, Muraro A, de Silva D, Khaleva E, Angier E, Arasi S, et al., European Academy of Allergy and Clinical Immunology Food Allergy and Anaphylaxis Guidelines Group. EAACI guideline: preventing the development of food allergy in infants and young children (2020 update). Pediatr Allergy Immunol. 2021;32:843–58.
8. Fleischer DM, Chan ES, Venter C, Spergel JM, Abrams EM, Stukus D, et al. A consensus approach to the primary prevention of food allergy through nutrition: guidance from the American Academy of Allergy, Asthma, and Immunology; American College of Allergy, Asthma, and Immunology; and the Canadian Society for Allergy and Clinical Immunology. J Allergy Clin Immunol Pract. 2021;9(1):22–43.e4.
9. Kopp MV, Muche-Borowski C, Abou-Dakn M, Ahrens B, Beyer K, Blümchen K, et al. S3 guideline allergy prevention. Allergol Select. 2022;6:61–97.
10. Muraro A, Halken S, Arshad SH, Beyer K, Dubois AE, Du Toit G, et al. EAACI food allergy and anaphylaxis guidelines. Primary prevention of food allergy. Allergy. 2014;69:590.
11. Venter C, Palumbo MP, Glueck DH, Sauder KA, O'Mahony L, Fleischer DM, et al. The maternal diet index in pregnancy is associated with offspring allergic diseases: the Healthy Start study. Allergy. 2022;77:162.
12. Section on Breastfeeding. Breastfeeding and the use of human milk. Pediatrics. 2012;129:e827.
13. Department of Health and Human Services, Office on Women's Health. Breastfeeding: HHS blueprint for action on breastfeeding. Washington, DC: US Department of Health and Human Services; 2000.
14. American College of Obstetricians and Gynecologists. Breastfeeding: maternal and infant aspects. ACOG Educational Bulletin 258. Washington, DC: American College of Obstetricians and Gynecologists; 2000.
15. WHO. Maternal, infant and young child nutrition. 2016;EB138/8.
16. Minniti F, Comberiati P, Munblit D, Piacentini GL, Antoniazzi E, Zanoni L, et al. Breast-milk characteristics protecting against allergy. Endocr Metab Immune Disord Drug Targets. 2014;14(1):9–15.
17. Schoetzau A, Filipiak-Pittroff B, Franke K, Koletzko S, Von Berg A, Gruebl A, et al. Effect of exclusive breast-feeding and early solid food avoidance on the incidence of atopic dermatitis in high-risk infants at 1 year of age. Pediatr Allergy Immunol. 2002;13:234–42.
18. Berg A, Krämer U, Link E, Bollrath C, Heinrich J, Brockow I, et al. Impact of early feeding on childhood eczema: development after nutritional intervention compared with the natural course—the GINIplus study up to the age of 6 years. Clin Exp Allergy. 2010;40:627–36.
19. van Meel ER, de Jong M, Elbert NJ, den Dekker HT, Reiss IK, de Jongste JC,et al. Duration and exclusiveness of breastfeeding and schoolage lung function and asthma. Ann Allergy Asthma Immunol. 2017;119:21–26.e2.
20. Verduci E, D'Elios S, Cerrato L, Comberiati P, Calvani M, Palazzo S, et al. Cow's milk substitutes for children: nutritional aspects of milk from different mammalian species, special formula and plant-based beverages. Nutrients. 2019;11(8):1739.
21. Ajetunmobi OM, Whyte B, Chalmers J, Tappin DM, Wolfson L, Fleming M, et al. Breastfeeding is associated with reduced childhood hospitalization: evidence from a Scottish Birth Cohort (1997–2009). J Pediatr. 2015;166:620–625.e4.
22. Jelding-Dannemand E, Malby Schoos AM, Bisgaard H. Breast-feeding does not protect against allergic sensitization in early childhood and allergy-associated disease at age 7 years. J Allergy Clin Immunol. 2015;136:1302–1308.e1–13.
23. Leung JY, Kwok MK, Leung GM, Schooling CM. Breastfeeding and childhood hospitalizations for asthma and other wheezing disorders. Ann Epidemiol. 2016;26:21–27.e1–3.
24. Filipiak-Pittroff B, Koletzko S, Krämer U, Standl M, Bauer CP, Berdel D, et al. Full breastfeeding and allergies from infancy until adolescence in the GINIplus cohort. Pediatr Allergy Immunol. 2018;29:96–101.
25. Elliott L, Henderson J, Northstone K, Chiu GY, Dunson D, London SJ. Prospective study of breastfeeding in relation to wheeze, atopy, and bronchial hyperresponsiveness in the Avon Longitudinal Study of Parents and Children (ALSPAC). J Allergy Clin Immunol. 2008;122:49.
26. Wright AL, Holberg CJ, Martinez FD, Morgan WJ, Taussig LM. Breast feeding and lower respiratory tract illness in the first year of life. Group Health Medical Associates. BMJ. 1989;299:946.
27. Halken S, Muraro A, de Silva D, Khaleva E, Angier E, Arasi S, et al. EAACI guideline: preventing the development of food allergy in infants and young children (2020 update). Pediatr Allergy Immunol. 2021;32:843–58.
28. Urashima M, Mezawa H, Okuyama M, Urashima T, Hirano D, Gocho N, et al. Primary prevention of cow's milk sensitization and food allergy by avoiding supplementation with cow's milk formula at birth. JAMA Pediatr. 2019;173:1137.
29. Obbagy JE, English LK, Wong YP, Butte NF, Dewey KG, Fleischer DM, et al. Complementary feeding and food allergy, atopic dermatitis/eczema, asthma, and

allergic rhinitis: a systematic review. Am J Clin Nutr. 2019;109:890S–934S.
30. Osborn DA, Sinn J. Soy formula for prevention of allergy and food intolerance in infants. Cochrane Database Syst Rev. 2006;2006:CD003741.
31. Agostoni C, Axelsson I, Goulet O, Koletzko B, Michaelsen KF, Puntis J, et al. Soy protein infant formulae and follow-on formulae: a commentary by the ESPGHAN Committee on Nutrition. J Pediatr Gastroenterol Nutr. 2006;42:352–61.
32. Westmark CJ. Soy infant formula may be associated with autistic behaviors. Autism Open Access. 2013;3:20727.
33. Vandenplas Y, Castrellon PG, Rivas R, Gutiérrez CJ, Garcia LD, Jimenez JE, et al. Safety of soya-based infant formulas in children. Br J Nutr. 2014;111:1340–60.
34. Bhatia J, Greer F, American Academy of Pediatrics Committee on Nutrition. Use of soy protein-based formulas in infant feeding. Pediatrics. 2008;121:1062–8.
35. Comberiati P, Costagliola G, D'Elios S, Peroni D. Prevention of food allergy: the significance of early introduction. Medicina (Kaunas). 2019;55:323.
36. Fewtrell M, Bronsky J, Campoy C, Domellöf M, Embleton N, Fidler Mis N, et al. Complementary feeding: a position paper by the European Society for Paediatric Gastroenterology, Hepatology, and Nutrition (ESPGHAN) Committee on nutrition. J Pediatr Gastroenterol Nutr. 2017;64:119–32.
37. Prescott SL, Smith P, Tang M, Palmer DJ, Sinn J, Huntley SJ, et al. The importance of early complementary feeding in the development of oral tolerance: concerns and controversies. Pediatr Allergy Immunol. 2008;19:375–80.
38. Muraro A, Dreborg S, Halken S, Høst A, Niggemann B, Aalberse R, et al. Dietary prevention of allergic diseases in infants and small children. Part III: Critical review of published peer-reviewed observational and interventional studies and final recommendations. Pediatr Allergy Immunol. 2004;15(4):291.
39. Grimshaw KE, Allen K, Edwards CA, Beyer K, Boulay A, van der Aa LB, et al. Infant feeding and allergy prevention: a review of current knowledge and recommendations. A EuroPrevall state of the art paper. Allergy. 2009;64:1407.
40. Fleischer DM, Spergel JM, Assa'ad AH, Pongracic JA. Primary prevention of allergic disease through nutritional interventions. J Allergy Clin Immunol Pract. 2013;1:29.
41. de Silva D, Halken S, Singh C, Muraro A, Angier E, Arasi S, et al. Preventing food allergy in infancy and childhood: systematic review of randomised controlled trials. Pediatr Allergy Immunol. 2020;31:813–26.
42. Perkin MR, Logan K, Tseng A, Raji B, Ayis S, Peacock J, et al. Randomized trial of introduction of allergenic foods in breast-fed infants. N Engl J Med. 2016;374:1733–43.
43. Bellach J, Schwarz V, Ahrens B, Trendelenburg V, Aksünger Ö, Kalb B, et al. Randomized placebo-controlled trial of hen's egg consumption for primary prevention in infants. J Allergy Clin Immunol. 2017;139:1591–9.
44. Palmer DJ, Sullivan TR, Gold MS, Prescott SL, Makrides M. Randomized controlled trial of early regular egg intake to prevent egg allergy. J Allergy Clin Immunol. 2017;139:1600–7.
45. Palmer DJ, Metcalfe J, Makrides M, Gold MS, Quinn P, West CE, et al. Early regular egg exposure in infants with eczema: a randomized controlled trial. J Allergy Clin Immunol. 2013;132:387–92.
46. Du Toit G, Roberts G, Sayre PH, Bahnson HT, Radulovic S, Santos AF, et al. Randomized trial of peanut consumption in infants at risk for peanut allergy. N Engl J Med. 2015;372:803–13.
47. Nwaru BI, Takkinen HM, Niemela O, Kaila M, Erkkola M, Ahonen S, et al. Timing of infant feeding in relation to childhood asthma and allergic diseases. J Allergy Clin Immunol. 2013;131:78–86.
48. Hesselmar B, Saalman R, Rudin A, Adlerberth I, Wold A. Early fish introduction is associated with less eczema, but not sensitization, in infants. Acta Paediatr. 2010;99:1861–7.
49. Papamichael MM, Shrestha SK, Itsiopoulos C, Erbas B. The role of fish intake on asthma in children: a meta-analysis of observational studies. Pediatr Allergy Immunol. 2018;29:350–60.
50. Lang JE, Bunnell HT, Hossain MJ, Wysocki T, Lima JJ, Finkel TH, et al. Being overweight or obese and the development of asthma. Pediatrics. 2018;142:e20182119.
51. Nahhas M, Bhopal R, Anandan C, Elton R, Sheikh A. Investigating the association between obesity and asthma in 6- to 8-year-old Saudi children: a matched case-control study. NPJ Prim Care Respir Med. 2014;24:14004.
52. Chen YC, Dong GH, Lin KC, Lee YL. Gender difference of childhood overweight and obesity in predicting the risk of incident asthma: a systematic review and meta-analysis. Obes Rev. 2013;14:222–31.
53. Haahtela T, Alenius H, Lehtimäki J, Sinkkonen A, Fyhrquist N, Hyöty H, et al. Immunological resilience and biodiversity for prevention of allergic diseases and asthma. Allergy. 2021;76:3613–26.
54. Wahn U, Lau S, Eigenmann P, Melen E, Krauss-Etschmann S, Lex C, et al. Early priming of asthma and respiratory allergies: future aspects of prevention: a statement by the European Forum for Education and Research in Allergy and Airway Disease (EUFOREA) and the EAACI-Clemens von Pirquet Foundation. Pediatr Allergy Immunol. 2022;33:e13773.
55. Stein MM, Hrusch CL, Gozdz J, Igartua C, Pivniouk V, Murray SE, et al. Innate immunity and asthma risk in Amish and Hutterite farm children. N Engl J Med. 2016;375:411–21.
56. Eguiluz-Gracia I, Mathioudakis AG, Bartel S, Vijverberg SJH, Fuertes E, Comberiati P, et al. The need for clean air: the way air pollution and climate change affect allergic rhinitis and asthma. Allergy. 2020;75:2170–84.

57. Peroni DG, Nuzzi G, Trambusti I, Di Cicco ME, Comberiati P. Microbiome composition and its impact on the development of allergic diseases. Front Immunol. 2020;11:700.
58. Azad MB, Konya T, Guttman DS, Field CJ, Sears MR, HayGlass KT, et al. Infant gut microbiota and food sensitization: associations in the first year of life. Clin Exp Allergy. 2015;45:632–43.
59. Baurecht H, Rühlemann MC, Rodríguez E, Thielking F, Harder I, Erkens AS, et al. Epidermal lipid composition, barrier integrity, and eczematous inflammation are associated with skin microbiome configuration. J Allergy Clin Immunol. 2018;141:1668–76.
60. Watanabe S, Narisawa Y, Arase S, Okamatsu H, Ikenaga T, Tajiri Y, et al. Differences in fecal microflora between patients with atopic dermatitis and healthy control subjects. J Allergy Clin Immunol. 2003;111:587–91.
61. Lopez-Santamarina A, Gonzalez EG, Lamas A, Mondragon ADC, Regal P, Miranda JM. Probiotics as a possible strategy for the prevention and treatment of allergies. A narrative review. Foods. 2021;10:701.
62. Braegger C, Chmielewska A, Decsi T, Kolacek S, Mihatsch W, Moreno L, et al. Supplementation of infant formula with probiotics and/or prebiotics: a systematic review and comment by the ESPGHAN committee on nutrition. J Pediatr Gastroenterol Nutr. 2011;52:238–50.
63. West CE, Dzidic M, Prescott SL, Jenmalm MC. Bugging allergy; role of pre-, pro- and synbiotics in allergy prevention. Allergol Int. 2017;66:529–38.
64. Fiocchi A, Pawankar R, Cuello-Garcia CA, Ahn K, Al-Hammadi S, Agarwal A, et al. World Allergy Organization-McMaster University guidelines for allergic disease prevention (GLAD-P): probiotics. World Allergy Organ J. 2015;8:1–13.
65. Muraro A, Halken S, Arshad SH, Beyer K, Dubois AE, Du Toit G, et al. EAACI food allergy and anaphylaxis guidelines. Primary prevention of food allergy. Allergy. 2014;69:590–601.
66. Giannetti A, Bernardini L, Cangemi J, Gallucci M, Masetti R, Ricci G. Role of vitamin D in prevention of food allergy in infants. Front Pediatr. 2020;8:447.
67. Comberiati P, Tsabouri S, Piacentini GL, Moser S, Minniti F, Peroni DG. Is vitamin D deficiency correlated with childhood wheezing and asthma? Front Biosci (Elite Ed). 2014;6(1):31–9.
68. Bergman P, Lindh AU, Bjorkhem-Bergman L, Lindh JD. Vitamin D and respiratory tract infections: a systematic review and meta-analysis of randomized controlled trials. PLoS One. 2013;8:e65835.
69. Nuzzi G, Di Cicco M, Trambusti I, Agosti M, Peroni DG, Comberiati P. Primary prevention of pediatric asthma through nutritional interventions. Nutrients. 2022;14:754.
70. Comberiati P, Peroni DG. Vitamin D supplementation in pregnancy does not prevent school-age asthma. Allergy. 2020;75:2143–4.
71. Yepes-Nuñez JJ, Brożek JL, Fiocchi A, Pawankar R, Cuello-García C, Zhang Y, et al. Vitamin D supplementation in primary allergy prevention: systematic review of randomized and non-randomized studies. Allergy. 2018;73:37–49.
72. Peroni DG, Hufnagl K, Comberiati P, Roth-Walter F. Lack of iron, zinc, and vitamins as a contributor to the etiology of atopic diseases. Front Nutr. 2023;9:1032481.
73. Maiello N, Comberiati P, Giannetti A, Ricci G, Carello R, Galli E. New directions in understanding atopic march starting from atopic dermatitis. Children (Basel). 2022;9:450.
74. Irvine AD, McLean WH, Leung DY. Filaggrin mutations associated with skin and allergic diseases. N Engl J Med. 2011;365:1315–27.
75. Yang G, Seok JK, Kang HC, Cho YY, Lee HS, Lee JY. Skin barrier abnormalities and immune dysfunction in atopic dermatitis. Int J Mol Sci. 2020;21:2867.
76. Leung DYM, Berdyshev E, Goleva E. Cutaneous barrier dysfunction in allergic diseases. J Allergy Clin Immunol. 2020;145:1485–97.
77. Horimukai K, Morita K, Narita M, Kondo M, Kabashima S, Inoue E, et al. Transepidermal water loss measurement during infancy can predict the subsequent development of atopic dermatitis regardless of filaggrin mutations. Allergol Int. 2016;65:103–8.
78. Simpson EL, Chalmers JR, Hanifin JM, Thomas KS, Cork MJ, McLean WH, et al. Emollient enhancement of the skin barrier from birth offers effective atopic dermatitis prevention. J Allergy Clin Immunol. 2014;134:818.
79. Horimukai K, Morita K, Narita M, Kondo M, Kitazawa H, Nozaki M, et al. Application of moisturizer to neonates prevents development of atopic dermatitis. J Allergy Clin Immunol. 2014;134:824.
80. Lowe AJ, Su JC, Allen KJ, Abramson MJ, Cranswick N, Robertson CF, et al. A randomised trial of a barrier lipid replacement strategy for the prevention of atopic dermatitis and allergic sensitisation: the PEBBLES Pilot Study. Br J Dermatol. 2018;178:19–21.
81. Bradshaw LE, Wyatt LA, Brown SJ, Haines RH, Montgomery AA, Perkin MR, et al. Emollients for prevention of atopic dermatitis: 5-year findings from the BEEP randomized trial. Allergy. 2023;78:995–1006.
82. Kelleher MM, Phillips R, Brown SJ, Cro S, Cornelius V, Carlsen KCL, et al. Skin care interventions in infants for preventing eczema and food allergy. Cochrane Database Syst Rev. 2022;11:CD013534.
83. Lowe A, Su J, Tang M, Lodge CJ, Matheson M, Allen KJ, et al. PEBBLES study protocol: a randomised controlled trial to prevent atopic dermatitis, food allergy and sensitisation in infants with a family history of allergic disease using a skin barrier improvement strategy. BMJ Open. 2019;9:e024594.

Flashcards Questions (Right Answer in Bold)

Chapter 1

1. Please put the protagonists of the atopic march in the right order from the first to last:
   (a) Atopic dermatitis—asthma—food allergy—allergic rhinitis
   (b) Asthma—food allergy—allergic rhinitis—atopic dermatitis
   (c) **Atopic dermatitis—food allergy—asthma—allergic rhinitis**
   (d) Food allergy—asthma—allergic rhinitis—atopic dermatitis
2. Which of these can influence the development of childhood asthma?
   (a) Climate change
   (b) Air pollution
   (c) Allergens, biocontaminants, and their interplays
   (d) **All of them**
3. Which is the only treatment with long-lasting effects that prevents the allergic disease progression?
   (a) Oral corticosteroids
   (b) Antihistamines
   (c) **Allergen immunotherapy**
   (d) Biologics
4. In which area of allergy can CRD be most useful?
   (a) Hymenoptera venom allergy
   (b) Food allergy
   (c) Respiratory allergy
   (d) **All of them**
5. Biologic therapies represent a major advance in the treatment of difficult-to-treat diseases. For example:
   (a) **Severe asthma, atopic dermatitis, chronic spontaneous urticaria and most recently chronic rhinosinusitis with nasal polyps (CRSwNP) and eosinophil-driven diseases**
   (b) Allergic Rhinitis
   (c) Hereditary Angioedema
   (d) Systemic Mastocytosis

Chapter 2

1. Which type of immune response is primarily involved in allergy development?
   (a) Innate immunity
   (b) **Adaptive immunity**
   (c) Both innate and adaptive immunity
   (d) None of the above
2. Which immunoglobulin is specifically associated with allergic responses?
   (a) IgA
   (b) IgD
   (c) **IgE**
   (d) IgG
3. What is the role of CD4+ T cells in the immune response to allergens?
   (a) **They activate other immune cells**
   (b) They eliminate infected cells
   (c) They produce immunoglobulins
   (d) They inhibit immune responses

C. Caffarelli, G. L. Marseglia (eds.), *Textbook of Pediatric Allergy*,
https://doi.org/10.1007/978-3-031-71283-8

4. Which cytokine is responsible for inducing the isotypic class switch of IgM to IgE?
   (a) **IL-4**
   (b) IL-5
   (c) IL-9
   (d) IL-13
5. Which immune cells express receptors for IL-33?
   (a) Mast cells
   (b) Eosinophils
   (c) Basophils
   (d) **All of the above**
6. Which cytokine is primarily responsible for promoting Th2 immune deviation in allergic responses?
   (a) **IL-4**
   (b) IL-5
   (c) IL-10
   (d) IL-13
7. Which of the following is NOT a characteristic of the late-phase response in allergic inflammation?
   (a) Cellular infiltration
   (b) **Mast cell degranulation**
   (c) Eosinophil attraction
   (d) Edema and redness
8. Which of the following genetic regions is NOT associated with atopy?
   (a) 5q23–35 region
   (b) Chromosome 16
   (c) **Chromosome 6**
   (d) Chromosome 11q13 region
9. Which cytokine is primarily involved in the differentiation, survival, and activation of eosinophils?
   (a) IL-4
   (b) **IL-5**
   (c) IL-9
   (d) IL-13

Chapter 3

1. What is the recommended location for performing skin prick tests (SPT) in children?
   (a) Back
   (b) **Volar surface of the forearms**
   (c) Active lesions on the skin
   (d) Legs
2. What is the minimum distance that should be maintained between pricks during a skin prick test (SPT)?
   (a) 1 cm
   (b) **2 cm**
   (c) 5 cm
   (d) 10 cm
3. Which of the following statements is true about the measurement of specific IgE using microarrays?
   (a) Microarrays provide quantitative measurements of specific IgE
   (b) Microarrays are the first-line investigation in allergic diagnostics
   (c) **Microarrays can produce false-negative results in patients with low IgE concentrations**
   (d) Microarrays are not effective in diagnosing polysensitized patients
4. What is the advantage of using protein microarrays for determining specific IgE?
   (a) **They allow the investigation of a large number of allergens in parallel**
   (b) They provide quantitative measurements of specific IgE
   (c) They are more accurate in diagnosing single sensitizations
   (d) They can be compared with IgE measurements obtained with other analysis systems
5. What is the recommended time frame for testing antigens in the Basophil Activation Test (BAT) after the most recent exposure to an allergen?
   (a) Within 1 month
   (b) Within 3 months
   (c) **Within 6 months to 1 year**
   (d) Within 2 years
6. How is the measurement of the reaction during SPT calculated?
   (a) By adding the major and minor diameters of the wheal
   (b) By subtracting the major diameter from the minor diameter of the wheal
   (c) By multiplying the major and minor diameters of the wheal
   (d) **By dividing the sum of the major and minor diameters by two**

7. Why is Intradermal Test (IDT) not commonly performed for food allergies?
   (a) It is less accurate in detecting food sensitivities
   (b) It requires a larger volume of antigen injection
   (c) **It is more invasive and carries a higher risk of adverse reactions**
   (d) It does not elicit a wheal and flare response

Chapter 4

1. Pulmonary function tests are typically feasible:
   (a) Over 3 years of age
   (b) **Over 5 years of age**
   (c) Over 9 years of age
   (d) Over 12 years of age
2. Bronchodilator responsiveness test (albuterol) is positive when
   (a) FEV1 > 2% from baseline
   (b) FEV1 > 5% from baseline
   (c) FEV1 > 8% from baseline
   (d) **FEV1 > 12% from baseline**
3. The regular use of short-acting beta 2-agonists
   (a) Reduce severe exacerbations
   (b) Reduce airway inflammation
   (c) Reduce risk of asthma-related death
   (d) **Reduce the bronchodilator response**
4. When should the Asthma Treatment Step Down?
   (a) Asthma symptoms are well controlled for a week
   (b) Asthma symptoms are well controlled for at least 3 weeks
   (c) Asthma symptoms are well controlled for at least 6 weeks
   (d) **Asthma symptoms are well controlled for at least 3 months**

Chapter 5

1. How many children and adolescents suffer from asthma worldwide?
   (a) **2–5%**
   (b) 5–10%
   (c) 5%
   (d) 10%
2. The currently most used subclassification of pediatric severe-therapy-resistant asthma according to BAL characteristics is:
   (a) Allergic eosinophilic, nonallergic neutrophilic, paucigranulocytic
   (b) **Allergic eosinophilic, nonallergic eosinophilic, neutrophilic, paucigranulocytic, mixed**
   (c) Eosinophilic, neutrophilic, mixed
   (d) Allergic eosinophilic, nonallergic eosinophilic, mixed
3. What is the most common comorbidity in pediatric severe asthma?
   (a) **Allergic rhinitis**
   (b) Obesity
   (c) OSAS
   (d) Breathing pattern disorders
4. What are the most common HRCT findings of pediatric severe asthma?
   (a) Mucus plugging
   (b) Bronchiectasis
   (c) Airway thickening
   (d) **All of the above**
5. Which of the following biologic treatments is addressed against TSLP?
   (a) Omalizumab
   (b) Mepolizumab
   (c) **Tezepelumab**
   (d) Benralizumab

Chapter 6

1. Most wheezing episodes are triggered by viral infections of the airways, and they involve
   (a) **30–50% of preschool children**
   (b) 30–50% of school-aged children
   (c) 20% of school-aged children
   (d) 80% of preschool children
2. Recurrent wheezing is defined as
   (a) Two or more episodes in the previous month
   (b) Two or more episodes in the previous year
   (c) **Four or more episodes in the previous year**
   (d) Four or more episodes in the previous month

3. Which of the following is included in the spectrum of disorders underlying wheezing?
   (a) Congenital airway abnormalities
   (b) Chronic lung disease of prematurity
   (c) Airway tumours
   (d) **All the answers are correct**
4. "Episodic viral wheezing" (EVW) indicates:
   (a) Wheezing that occurs in every period of the year, with symptoms that are induced by heterogeneous output triggers
   (b) **Wheezing that occurs especially during autumn-winter seasons and presents with symptoms associated with viral respiratory tract infections**
   (c) All the answers are correct
   (d) Neither answer is correct
5. Which group of children with wheezing seem to respond better to ICS?
   (a) Children with primarily viral-associated wheezing
   (b) **Children sensitized to aeroallergens and with high peripheral eosinophilia**
   (c) Children with primarily exercise-induced wheezing
   (d) All the answers are correct

Chapter 7

1. Which are the most common infections in a patient with atopic dermatitis?
   (a) ***S. aureus* infections**
   (b) *S. pyogenes* infections
   (c) *S. pneumoniae* infections
   (d) Herpes simplex virus infections
2. Which are the most important cytokines in the pathogenesis of AD?
   (a) **IL-4, IL-13**
   (b) IL-2, IL-15
   (c) IL-17, IL 23
   (d) IL-1b, IL-10
3. For which areas of body topical calcineurine inhibitors (TCI) represent the most suitable treatment option?
   (a) **Eyelids and anogenital area**
   (b) Antecubital folds
   (c) Hands and feet
   (d) Trunk
4. What is the mechanism of action of dupilumab?
   (a) **It is a fully human IgG4κ monoclonal antibody that targets IL-4Rα, blocking both IL-4 and IL-13 signaling pathways through type 2 receptors, and also blocking IL-4 signaling through type 1 receptors**
   (b) It is an IgG4λ monoclonal antibody that inhibits IL-13 binding to IL-13Rα1 and α2 receptors, blocking type 2 signaling and interfering with IL-13 regulation mediated by IL-13Rα2 receptors
   (c) It is a humanized IgG4κ monoclonal antibody that binds IL-13, inhibiting the formation of the IL-13R1α/IL-4Rα heterodimer but not preventing IL-13 binding to the IL-13Rα2 receptor
   (d) It is a humanized monoclonal antibody against interleukin-5 (IL-5)
5. Infants (≤2 years) with AD, typically develop _______ lesions characterized by itchy papules and vesicles with poorly defined erythema, initially involving the______. These lesions often evolve with serous exudate, crusts, and forming large plaques.

   In children (>2 years), AD is characterized by ________ of the exudative component.

   Adolescents typically present with symmetrical papules and plaques, often associated with ________ and excoriations, affecting flexural regions, face, neck, and distal extremities.
   (a) **Acute**/chronic/moderate
   (b) **Cheeks**/feet/arms folds
   (c) **Reduction**/augmentation/maintenance
   (d) **Lichenification**/exudation/erythema

Chapter 8

1. Which of the following forms of allergic conjunctivitis is characterized by seasonal symptoms related to airborne allergens?
   (a) **Seasonal allergic conjunctivitis (SAC)**
   (b) Perennial allergic conjunctivitis (PAC)
   (c) Giant papillary conjunctivitis (GPC)
   (d) Atopic keratoconjunctivitis (AKC)

2. What are the typical symptoms of allergic conjunctivitis?
   (a) **Intense itching, redness, tearing, and photophobia**
   (b) Dryness, blurred vision, burning sensation and foreign body sensation
   (c) Eye pain, light sensitivity, mucus discharge and eyelid swelling
   (d) Blurred vision, increased heat sensitivity, thickened eyelids and skin irritation
3. What is a characteristic feature associated with the tarsal form of Vernal Keratoconjunctivitis (VKC)?
   (a) **Papillary hypertrophy "cobblestone-like" on the upper tarsal conjunctiva**
   (b) Absence of the lateral end of the eyebrows (Hertoghe's sign)
   (c) Presence of Horner-Trantas dots and limbal involvement
   (d) Dennie-Morgan lines on the lower eyelids
4. Which of the following is not a characteristic sign of Atopic keratoconjunctivitis (AKC)?
   (a) Eyelid eczema
   (b) Absence of the lateral end of the eyebrows (Hertoghe's sign)
   (c) **Multiple limbal or conjunctival gelatinous yellow-grey infiltrates**
   (d) Horizontal creases of the eyelids (Dennie-Morgan lines)
5. What are the main pharmacological treatments for allergic conjunctivitis in children?
   (a) Topical antibiotics
   (b) Eye drops containing vitamin C
   (c) Immunosuppressive drugs
   (d) **Topical antihistamines**

Chapter 9

1. Mild allergic rhinitis is defined by
   (a) Normal sleep, normal work and school, normal daily activity, disturbing symptoms
   (b) Normal sleep, normal work, normal daily activity, disturbing symptoms
   (c) **Normal sleep, normal work and school, normal daily activity, no disturbing symptoms**
   (d) Normal sleep, no disturbing symptoms
2. The diagnosis of allergic rhinitis is made by
   (a) History and physical examination
   (b) **History, physical examination, specific laboratory and functional tests**
   (c) Active anterior rhinomanometry and measuring nitric oxide nose (nFeNO)
   (d) Skin prick test only
3. According to ARIA document, initial treatment of allergic rhinitis consists of:
   (a) **Allergen avoidance measures, antihistamines and intranasal corticosteroids**
   (b) Omalizumab
   (c) Oral corticosteroids
   (d) Nasal decongestants
4. Main comorbidities of allergic rhinitis are:
   (a) Secondary immunodeficiencies
   (b) History of severe adverse reactions to AIT
   (c) **Asthma, allergic conjunctivitis, sinusitis, atopic eczema, adenoid hypertrophy**
   (d) Severe psychiatric disorders

Chapter 10

1. Systemic anaphylactic reactions associated with Hymenoptera venom represents
   (a) 5% of the general anaphylaxis among children
   (b) 15% of the general anaphylaxis among children
   (c) **20% of the general anaphylaxis among children**
   (d) 50% of the general anaphylaxis among children
2. Hymenoptera venom hypersensitivity can be associated with
   (a) Both nonimmunological and immunological (IgE- or non-IgE-mediated) mechanisms
   (b) Only IgE-mediated mechanisms
   (c) **Immunological (IgE- or non-IgE-mediated) mechanisms**
   (d) Only nonimmunological mechanisms

3. In case of anaphylaxis during the acute phase of an allergic reaction to Hymenoptera stings, first line treatment consists in
   (a) Corticosteroids and antihistamines
   (b) Intravenous corticosteroids
   (c) **Intramuscular adrenaline**
   (d) Intravenous adrenaline
4. Venom immunotherapy (VIT) to Hymenoptera venom lasts
   (a) 1 year
   (b) 5–10 years
   (c) 3 years
   (d) **3–5 years**

Chapter 11

1. What is the most frequent cause of anaphylaxis in children?
   (a) Drugs
   (b) **Food**
   (c) Insect bites
   (d) Physical exertion
2. The most effective drug in the treatment of anaphylaxis is
   (a) Cortisone
   (b) Beta2 agonists
   (c) Antihistamines
   (d) **Adrenaline**
3. The main risk factor for the severity of anaphylaxis is
   (a) Atopic dermatitis
   (b) **Bronchial asthma**
   (c) Cow's milk protein allergy
   (d) Urticaria
4. The most correct route of administration of adrenaline in anaphylaxis is
   (a) Aerosol
   (b) **Deep intramuscular on the lateral rectus muscle of the thigh**
   (c) Subcutaneous
   (d) Oral
5. The diagnosis of idiopathic anaphylaxis is
   (a) **A diagnosis of exclusion, after ruling out all causes of anaphylaxis**
   (b) A laboratory diagnosis
   (c) A diagnosis made by assaying tryptase
   (d) A clinical diagnosis

Chapter 12

1. Drug hypersensitivity reactions (DHR) represent
   (a) <10% of all Adverse Drug Reactions
   (b) **>20% of all Adverse Drug Reactions**
   (c) <5% of all Adverse Drug Reactions
   (d) <1% of all Adverse Drug Reactions
2. Patient related risk factors associated with DHRs include
   (a) Genetic factors and previous drug reaction
   (b) **Age, sex, genetic factors, concurrent medical illnesses, and previous drug reaction**
   (c) Age and sex
   (d) Concurrent medical illnesses
3. Severe Cutaneous Delayed Allergic Reactions (SCAR) include
   (a) Acute Generalized Exanthematous Pustulosis (AGEP)
   (b) Maculo-Papular Exanthema (MPE) and Erythema Multiforme (EM)
   (c) Serum Sickness-Like Reaction (SSLR)
   (d) **Steven-Johnson Syndrome/Toxic Epidermal Necrolysis (SJS/TEN), Acute Generalized Exanthematous Pustulosis (AGEP) and DRESS**
4. In children, the most confirmed drugs responsible for triggering a pediatric DHR are
   (a) Monoclonal Antibodies
   (b) NSAIDs
   (c) Anticonvulsivants
   (d) **BL-Antibiotics**

Chapter 13

1. Which one of the following tests is not useful for the diagnosis of food allergy?
   (a) Skin prick tests
   (b) Specific IgE dosing
   (c) **Specific IgG dosing**
   (d) Basophil activation test
   (e) Oral food challenge

2. An 8-year-old girl is allergic to cow's milk but doesn't present symptoms if she eats baked milk. Which one of the following allergens might be negative, when we dose specific IgE?
   (a) Whole milk
   (b) Alpha-lactalbumin
   (c) Beta-lactoglobulin
   (d) **Caseins**
   (e) Lactoferrin
3. A 3-year-old girl has negative specific IgE toward ovomucoid; what will she most likely tolerate?
   (a) Raw egg
   (b) Mayonnaise
   (c) Chocolate mousse
   (d) **Baked egg**
   (e) White egg, in any form
4. A 5-year-old boy is mono-sensitized to Ara h 2. Which one of the following sentences is correct?
   (a) He will surely present clinical symptoms if exposed to peanuts
   (b) The allergist should tell him that he can eat peanuts if he wishes
   (c) **He could present severe reactions if exposed to peanuts**
   (d) He could present an oral syndrome if exposed to peanuts, but no severe reactions
   (e) He should avoid all tree nuts and legumes
5. A 16-year-old boy presented an anaphylactic reaction after eating a peach. He used to eat peaches without presenting any clinical symptoms. He says that, in the previous year, he started consuming cannabinoids. Which one of the following proteins may be most likely involved in determining his present symptoms?
   (a) Pru p 1 (PR-10)
   (b) **Pru p 3 (nsLTP)**
   (c) Pru p 4 (Profilin)
   (d) Pru p 7 (GRP)
   (e) MUXF3 (CCD)

Chapter 14

1. The age of onset of food protein-induced allergic proctocolitis (FPIAP) is generally
   (a) Within the first year of life
   (b) Within the first 5 years of life
   (c) Within the first 3 years of life
   (d) **Within the first 6 months of life**
2. The most common foods triggering non-IgE-mediated gastrointestinal food allergies are
   (a) **Cow's milk, soy, and wheat**
   (b) Kiwi and cow's milk
   (c) Soy
   (d) Wheat and rice
3. Chronic FPIES clinical presentation include
   (a) Atopic eczema
   (b) Intense pallor and floppiness
   (c) **Failure to thrive or progressive weight loss**
   (d) Hypothermia and lethargy
4. The majority of infants with Food Protein-Induced Allergic Proctocolitis (FPIAP) develop tolerance
   (a) **By the first year of life**
   (b) By the second year of life
   (c) By the fifth year of life
   (d) By the fourth year of life

Chapter 15

1. Eosinophilic Esophagitis mainly affects
   (a) Adolescents younger than 16 years
   (b) Adults between 20 and 40 years
   (c) **Children between 5 and 10 years**
   (d) Children less than 5 years old
2. Typical toddler and young children symptoms include
   (a) Dysphagia
   (b) Food impaction
   (c) Recurrent vomiting and failure to thrive
   (d) **GERD-like symptoms**

3. Histologically, Eosinophilic Esophagitis is defined by the presence of
   (a) **≥15 eosinophils in one HPF**
   (b) ≥5 eosinophils in one HPF
   (c) ≥10 eosinophils in one HPF
   (d) ≥20 eosinophils in one HPF
4. The therapeutic options for Eosinophilic Esophagitis include
   (a) Medical therapy
   (b) Diet
   (c) Medical and mechanical therapy
   (d) **Drugs, diet, and mechanical therapy**

Chapter 16

1. Chronic urticaria is defined as a form of urticaria which lasts
   (a) >10 weeks
   (b) **>6 weeks**
   (c) >4 weeks
   (d) >12 weeks
2. Wheals, which are typical urticaria skin lesions, usually
   (a) **Resolves within 24 h**
   (b) Lasts over 48 h
   (c) Resolves within 12 h
   (d) Lasts over 36 h
3. First line therapy of acute urticaria is represented by
   (a) First-generation antihistamines
   (b) **Second-generation antihistamines**
   (c) Systemic corticosteroids
   (d) Omalizumb
4. Omalizumab recommended dose for urticaria is
   (a) 600 mg every 4 weeks
   (b) **300 mg every 4 weeks**
   (c) 150 mg every 2 weeks
   (d) 300 mg every 3 weeks

Chapter 17

1. Which is the main mediator of angioedema after histamine?
   (a) Platelet activating factor
   (b) Endothelial-derived growth factor
   (c) LTC4
   (d) **Bradykinin**
2. Which should be the next therapeutic step in pediatric patients with recurrent angioedema unresponsive to antihistamine prophylaxis?
   (a) Cyclosporine
   (b) Long term steroids
   (c) **Omalizumab**
   (d) Lanadelumab
3. How to assess hereditary angioedema?
   (a) **By C4 and C1 inhibitor assessment**
   (b) By chromosome 13 gene analysis
   (c) By dosing bradykinin urinary levels
   (d) By checking autoimmunity (ANA, ENA, anti-DNA)
4. Should you still suspect hereditary angioedema in children with recurrent swelling refractory to antihistamine prophylaxis and no family history?
   (a) **Yes, when also omalizumab fails to prevent angioedema recurrency**
   (b) No
   (c) Yes, but only in the female gender
   (d) Yes, but only in males
5. Which is the typical phenotype of hereditary angioedema due to factor XII mutation?
   (a) Male with early onset of symptoms, usually less than 5 years old
   (b) Children with very low C4 plasma levels
   (c) Children with Serping1 mutations
   (d) **Female with onset after puberty on introduction of contraceptive pill**

Chapter 18

1. Eosinophils
   (a) Eosinophils are normal constituents of the esophagus
   (b) **In physiological conditions, eosinophils are present in the small intestine**
   (c) In physiological conditions, eosinophils are not present in the small intestine
   (d) Eosinophil counts greater than 20,000 cells/μL are highly suggestive of allergic disorders
2. Select the Possible Cause of Eosinophilia
   (a) Allergic diseases
   (b) Lymphoid malignancies
   (c) Parasitic infections
   (d) **All the above are correct**

3. FeNO MEASUREMENT
   (a) Is an invasive method for evaluating airway inflammation in asthma
   (b) Is mandatory for the diagnosis of asthma
   (c) Is considered pathological when >50 ppb in children
   (d) **Is a non-invasive test for evaluating airway inflammation in asthma**
4. In Allergic Diseases, Peripheral Blood EOSINOPHILIA Is Usually
   (a) Absent
   (b) **Mild**
   (c) Moderate
   (d) Severe
5. In Patients with EOSINOPHILIC Esophagitis
   (a) Eosinophils can be absent in the esophagus
   (b) **Blood eosinophils can be normal**
   (c) The diagnostic threshold is >25 eosinophils/high power field
   (d) Endoscopy without biopsy is the gold standard for the diagnosis

Chapter 19

1. Which of the following symptoms may be indicative of mastocytosis in a pediatric patient?
   (a) Joint pain
   (b) **Skin lesions**
   (c) Vision changes
   (d) Increased appetite
2. What is a diagnostic test used for assessing mastocytosis in pediatric patients?
   (a) Magnetic resonance
   (b) **Skin biopsy**
   (c) Urine analysis
   (d) Echocardiogram
3. Which of the following is a potential complication of mastocytosis in pediatric patients?
   (a) Increased bone density
   (b) Decreased risk of infections
   (c) **Allergic reactions**
   (d) Improved cognitive function
4. What is the gene mutation associated with mastocytosis in both pediatric and adult cases?
   (a) **D816V**
   (b) BRCA1
   (c) TP53
   (d) EGFR
5. How can the quality of life be improved for pediatric patients with mastocytosis?
   (a) **Avoiding triggers and managing symptoms**
   (b) Increasing exposure to allergens
   (c) Decreasing physical activity
   (d) Avoiding routine medical check-ups

Chapter 20

1. Allergy contact dermatitis represents
   (a) 15% of all childhood dermatitis
   (b) 5% of all childhood dermatitis
   (c) 59% of all childhood dermatitis
   (d) **20% of all childhood dermatitis**
2. The triggering agent is identified by
   (a) Skin prick test
   (b) **Patch test**
   (c) Physical exam and medical history
   (d) Serum IgE
3. Patch testing is usually performed
   (a) In the lower back
   (b) In the upper arm
   (c) **In the upper back**
   (d) In the abdomen
4. During patch testing
   (a) Corticosteroids and other immunosuppressive drugs can be continued
   (b) It is allowed to practice martial art
   (c) Exposure to sunlight does not influence the results
   (d) **No bath or wash of the back is allowed during the period**

Chapter 21

1. What are the main red flags that should arise the suspicion of PADs/IEI and consequently lead to basic laboratory investigations?
   (a) **Atopy, infections, autoimmunity and malignancy**
   (b) Infections
   (c) Atopy and autoimmunity
   (d) Malignancy

2. In a patient with the suspicion of PADs/IEI the standard assessments and investigations should include:
   (a) Family and patient history
   (b) Laboratory findings
   (c) Clinical features
   (d) **All previous answers**
3. Atopic phenotypes are associated with all of the following IEI with the exception of:
   (a) Omenn Syndrome
   (b) Wiskott-Aldrich Syndrome
   (c) Hyper-IgE Syndrome
   (d) **Chronic granulomatous disease**
4. The most well-recognized IEIs associated with urticaria are:
   (a) Antibody defects
   (b) Innate immunity defects
   (c) **Autoinflammatory disorders**
   (d) Combined immunodeficiencies
5. Monogenic IEI associated to asthma are caused by mutations of the following genes except for:
   (a) SPINK5
   (b) CARMIL2
   (c) **BTK**
   (d) JAK1

Chapter 22

1. Increased circulating eosinophils:
   (a) Are always caused by hypereosinophilic syndromes
   (b) **Are a non-specific marker of type 2 inflammation**
   (c) Above 5000/μL are generally caused by atopic diseases
   (d) Are a specific marker of type 1 inflammation
2. Eosinophil cationic protein:
   (a) Is a protein released by inactive eosinophils
   (b) Can be measured only in serum
   (c) **Is a marker of eosinophil activity**
   (d) Is reduced in atopic conditions
3. Total serum IgE:
   (a) Are always increased in atopic subjects
   (b) Are not influenced by environmental factors
   (c) Are a marker of eosinophil activity
   (d) **Increase during childhood**
4. Specific IgE:
   (a) **Reveal the sensitization to the allergen**
   (b) Are influenced by antihistamine therapy
   (c) Reveal a condition of allergy even if the allergen does not cause clinical manifestations
   (d) Are a cheaper test than skin prick test
5. Basophil activation test:
   (a) Is not affected by any therapy
   (b) **Should be performed within 6–12 months of the reaction**
   (c) Is a functional test of IgG-mediated responses
   (d) Is positive when >1% of basophils are activated
6. Nasal cytology:
   (a) Is an expensive test
   (b) Can be performed only in adolescents and adults
   (c) **Allows to identify the "overlapped" rhinitis**
   (d) Is not useful in non-allergic rhinitis

Chapter 23

1. Growth charts of total IgE levels in childhood
   (a) **Show an increasing trend in the first decade of life, a plateau at adolescence followed by a slight decline**
   (b) Show an increasing trend until the puberty
   (c) Remain stable during the whole childhood
   (d) Show a slight decline from the birth to the adulthood
2. IgE sensitization to grass pollen starts with
   (a) **Phl p 2 and Phl p 11**
   (b) Phl p 6
   (c) Phl p 11
   (d) Phl p 1, alone or in combination with other molecules
3. Which are not primary food allergens?
   (a) Cor a 14
   (b) **Bet v 2**
   (c) Ara h 1
   (d) Pru p 3

4. Which are not panallergens with diagnostic relevance in childhood respiratory allergies?
   (a) **Cyclophilins**
   (b) Seed storage proteins
   (c) Profilins
   (d) Polcalcins

Chapter 24

1. Are corticosteroids the first-line treatment of anaphylaxis?
   (a) Yes
   (b) **No**
   (c) It depends on the severity of the reaction
   (d) Only after adrenaline administration
2. Which are the mechanisms of corticosteroids' action?
   (a) **Transrepression and transactivation**
   (b) Transrepression
   (c) Cis-repression
   (d) Cis-repression and cis-activation
3. Should corticosteroids be used in chronic urticaria?
   (a) Oral corticosteroids are recommended for chronic treatment of urticaria
   (b) **A short cycle of oral corticosteroids is used in severe exacerbations of chronic urticaria**
   (c) No
   (d) Yes, in mild exacerbations of chronic urticaria
4. Which is the less powerful topical corticosteroid useful in treating atopic dermatitis?
   (a) **Hydrocortisone acetate**
   (b) Betamethasone benzoate
   (c) Fluticasone propionate
   (d) Clobetasol propionate
5. Which is not a common adverse effect of oral corticosteroids?
   (a) Hypertrichosis
   (b) Osteoporosis
   (c) Glaucoma
   (d) **Sepsis**

Chapter 25

1. Which score is the most commonly used for evaluating chronic urticaria disease activity
   (a) **Urticaria Activity Score (UAS7)**
   (b) Urticaria score over a month
   (c) Urticaria-angioedema score
   (d) Oomalizumab score
2. What is the name of a fully human monoclonal antibody which acts by blocking receptors for IL-4 and IL-1?
   (a) Omalizumab
   (b) **Dupilumab**
   (c) Benralizumab
   (d) Infliximab
3. What are the most commonly observed adverse events in safety studies of mepolizumab? Would you classify it as having very severe side effects?
   (a) Pneumonia and meningitis
   (b) **Headache, injection site reactions, and back pain**
   (c) Atopic eczema, injection site reactions and psoriasis
   (d) injection site reactions, meningitis
4. What is the monoclonal antibody used for treating moderate to severe atopic dermatitis?
   (a) Benralizumab
   (b) Omalizumab
   (c) Infliximab
   (d) **Dupilumab**
5. Describe the action for omalizumab in food allergy?
   (a) **Prevent anaphylaxis**
   (b) Increase tolerance threshold of allergenic food
   (c) Reduce respiratory symptoms
   (d) Improve growth

Chapter 26

1. Allergen immunotherapy is recommended for treating
   (a) Allergic rhinitis only
   (b) Hymenoptera venom allergy only
   (c) **Allergic rhinitis, allergic asthma due to inhalant allergens, hymenoptera venom allergy, and food allergy**
   (d) Food allergy only

2. Considering the different types of Allergen immunotherapy to airborne allergens
   (a) SLIT is more efficacy than SCIT
   (b) **There is no evidence that there are differences in efficacy between SLIT and SCIT**
   (c) SCIT is more efficacy than SLIT
   (d) Only SCIT for seasonal allergic rhinitis prevent the development of asthma in children
3. To maintain benefits over time, both SCIT and SLIT therapy should be taken
   (a) **For at least 3 years to 5 years**
   (b) For at least 2 years
   (c) For at least 1 year
   (d) For at least 5 years
4. Which one of this is not a contraindication to AIT?
   (a) Primary immunodeficiencies
   (b) Severe chronic diseases
   (c) Uncontrolled asthma
   (d) **Beta-blocker treatment**

Chapter 27

1. Why are children more susceptible to climate change and air pollution?
   (a) Immature detoxifying systems
   (b) Higher respiratory rate
   (c) Narrower airways
   (d) **All the answers are correct**
2. Which of these diseases can be affected by air pollutants?
   (a) Atopic dermatitis
   (b) Allergic conjunctivitis
   (c) Only rhinitis and asthma
   (d) **Asthma, atopic dermatitis, and allergic rhinoconjunctivitis**
3. Which of these promote/favor asthmatic thunderstorms?
   (a) Pollens breakdown
   (b) Wind gusts
   (c) Alternaria sensitization
   (d) **All the answers are correct**
4. Which particulate matter (PM) type reaches the deeper part of the respiratory airways?
   (a) PM 25
   (b) PM 10
   (c) **PM 0.1**
   (d) No PM can reach the respiratory airways
5. Which of these conditions can favor asthma development?
   (a) Maternal smoking exposure
   (b) Traffic-related air pollution exposure
   (c) Breastfeeding
   (d) **Maternal smoking exposure, vaping, traffic-related air pollution exposure**

Chapter 28

1. What is the symptom in a child with severe atopic dermatitis that prevents him and his parents from sleeping:
   (a) The extension of eczema
   (b) The side effects of corticosteroid creams
   (c) **The itch**
   (d) Dry skin
2. What should the parent of a child with severe food allergy to cow's milk do immediately if he/she inadvertently has eaten a food containing cow's milk proteins and begins to have symptoms?
   (a) Make the child vomit
   (b) Call the pediatrician
   (c) Administer an antihistamine orally
   (d) **Inject epinephrine into the muscle**
3. With which element should contact be always avoided in a child suffering from bronchial asthma?
   (a) With dogs and cats
   (b) **With second-hand smoke**
   (c) With house dust mites
   (d) With molds

4. A child suffering from bronchial asthma but normally compensated by pharmacological therapy. What should be done immediately if he/she has an acute bronchospasm during a run?
   (a) Administer a cortisone tablet orally
   (b) **Multiple inhalations of pre-measured spray salbutamol applied to age-appropriate spacer**
   (c) Administer an intravenous vial of antihistamine
   (d) Call the emergency service
5. Who is responsible for the health of the child with severe food allergy or bronchial asthma at school?
   (a) **The head teacher**
   (b) The janitor
   (c) Classmates' parents
   (d) The teacher in the class

Chapter 29

1. Introduction of complementary food for food allergy prevention:
   (a) From the third month of life in "high-risk" infants
   (b) **In populations where there is a high prevalence of peanut allergy, introduce peanuts into the infant diet in an age-appropriate form as part of complementary feeding and not as the first solid food**
   (c) Eggs should be introduced after 12 months in all infants at risk
   (d) Peanuts should be introduced between 4 and 6 months in all infants irrespective of the prevalence of peanut allergy
2. During pregnancy and breastfeeding:
   (a) Women should avoid potentially allergenic foods
   (b) Atopic women should take probiotics with the intention of preventing atopy in their offspring
   (c) **Women should follow a balanced and healthy diet irrespective of their personal history of atopy**
   (d) The maternal diet should include the intake of multivitamins to prevent allergic diseases in their offspring
3. Human milk substitutes
   (a) Should be preferred to breastmilk
   (b) Are recommended in all infants with a family history of atopy
   (c) Partially hydrolyzed have less allergenic potential than extensively hydrolyzed milk formulas
   (d) **Cow's Milk-derived formulas for infants should not be routinely used for the prevention of food allergy**
4. The development of allergic diseases is caused by:
   (a) **Interaction between genetic predisposition, environmental and allergen exposure, immune dysfunction, and microbial imbalance**
   (b) Gain of function mutations in the filaggrin gene
   (c) The introduction of potentially allergenic complementary foods in the first year of life
   (d) Exposure to low-polluted environments
5. One of the following statements is correct:
   (a) The utilization of a hydrolyzed formula in high-risk infants provides a protective advantage in preventing food allergies
   (b) In high-risk infants in areas with a high prevalence of peanut allergy, peanuts should be avoided in the first year of life, to prevent peanut allergy
   (c) **Healthy microbiota can decrease the risk of allergy development**
   (d) Environmental factors do not influence the development of allergic diseases

Index

C. Caffarelli, G. L. Marseglia (eds.), *Textbook of Pediatric Allergy*,
https://doi.org/10.1007/978-3-031-71283-8

MIX
Papier aus verantwortungsvollen Quellen
Paper from responsible sources
FSC® C105338

If you have any concerns about our products,
you can contact us on
ProductSafety@springernature.com

In case Publisher is established outside the EU,
the EU authorized representative is:
Springer Nature Customer Service Center GmbH
Europaplatz 3, 69115 Heidelberg, Germany

Printed by Libri Plureos GmbH
in Hamburg, Germany